Tarascon Pocket Pharmacopoeia®

2013 Deluxe Lab-Coat Edition

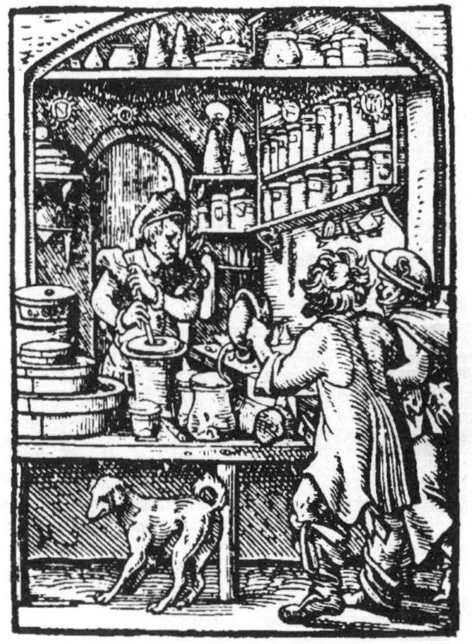

14TH EDITION

"Desire to take medicines ... distinguishes man from animals."
—Sir William Osler

Editor-in-Chief
Richard J. Hamilton, MD, FAAEM, FACMT, FACEP
Professor and Chair, Department of Emergency Medicine
Drexel University College of Medicine
Philadelphia, PA

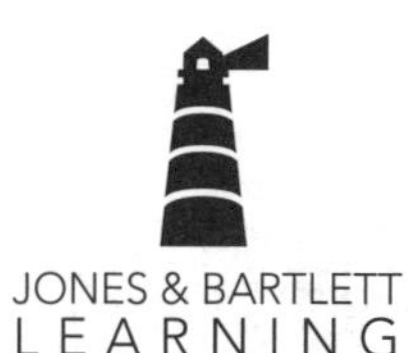

JONES & BARTLETT
LEARNING

World Headquarters
Jones & Bartlett Learning
5 Wall Street
Burlington, MA 01803
978-443-5000
info@jblearning.com
www.jblearning.com

Jones & Bartlett Learning books and products are available through most bookstores and online booksellers. To contact Jones & Bartlett Learning directly, call 800-832-0034, fax 978-443-8000, or visit our website www.jblearning.com.

Substantial discounts on bulk quantities of Jones & Bartlett Learning publications are available to corporations, professional associations, and other qualified organizations. For details and specific discount information, contact the special sales department at Jones & Bartlett Learning via the above contact information or send an email to specialsales@jblearning.com.

The information in the *Pocket Pharmacopoeia* is compiled from sources believed to be reliable, and exhaustive efforts have been put forth to make the book as accurate as possible. The *Pocket Pharmacopoeia* is edited by a panel of drug information experts with extensive peer review and input from more than 50 practicing clinicians of multiple specialties. Our goal is to provide health professionals focused, core prescribing information in a convenient, organized, and concise fashion. We include FDA-approved dosing indications and those off-label uses that have a reasonable basis to support their use. However, the accuracy and completeness of this work cannot be guaranteed. Despite our best efforts this book may contain typographical errors and omissions. The *Pocket Pharmacopoeia* is intended as a quick and convenient reminder of information you have already learned elsewhere. The contents are to be used as a guide only, and healthcare professionals should use sound clinical judgment and individualize therapy to each specific patient care situation. This book is not meant to be a replacement for training, experience, continuing medical education, or studying the latest drug prescribing literature. This book is sold without warranties of any kind, expressed or implied, and the publisher and editors disclaim any liability, loss, or damage caused by the contents. Although drug companies purchase and distribute our books as promotional items, the Tarascon editorial staff alone determines all book content.

Production Credits

Chief Executive Officer: Ty Field
President: James Homer
SVP, Chief Marketing Officer: Alison M. Pendergast
V.P., Design and Production: Anne Spencer
V.P., Manufacturing and Inventory Control: Therese Connell
Manufacturing and Inventory Control Supervisor: Amy Bacus
Executive Publisher: Christopher Davis
Senior Acquisitions Editor: Nancy Anastasi Duffy
Editorial Assistant: Marisa LaFleur
Production Editor: Daniel Stone
Digital Marketing Manager: Rebecca Leitch
Composition: Newgen
Text and Cover Design: Anne Spencer
Printing and Binding: Edward Brothers Malloy
Cover Printing: Edward Brothers Malloy

The cover woodcut is *The Apothecary* by Jost Amman, Frankfurt, 1574.

ISSN: 1945-9084
ISBN: 978-1-4496-7361-1

6048
Printed in the United States of America
16 15 14 13 12 10 9 8 7 6 5 4 3 2 1

For those of you still trying to solve last year's puzzle, here is the answer:

Do you recall the rather interesting dilemma of the prisoner's pants? A prisoner arrives in the emergency department with his ankles chained together. In his haste to escape from the police he put his pants on inside out, with the pocket flaps showing and the zipper in front. You've taken care of his injuries but before he can be discharged, he needs his pants reversed so they are back to the normal way to wear them. The police refuse to unshackle him and someone tells you that it is impossible to do this without unshackling the patient. Are they correct?

The answer is that you can reverse his pants pretty easily. First, pull the pants down over his legs so that they are on the chains, and push one of the legs through the other on the chains reversing the legs in the process. Then pull the trousers over the shackles by the waist to get them rightside out and put them back on the patient! Houdini meets topology in patient care. Note this only works if the ankles are not chained to anything else. Try it first at a friend's party before you attempt it with some in shackles.

We will send a free copy of next year's edition to the first 25 people who can solve the following interpersonal dilemma puzzle:

Here's one that is too easy – you should be able to do it in your head. A mother arrived at the Doctor's office with her two children. They cry inconsolably whenever she puts them down. To save everyone's ears when the nurse weighs them, she gets on the scale and says, "I forget how much they weigh, but I know that I weigh 40 pounds more than the combined weight of both children, and one of my children weighs half of the other." The scale says 160, what's everyone's weight?

TARASCON POCKET PHARMACOPOEIA EDITORIAL STAFF*

EDITOR IN CHIEF

Richard J. Hamilton, MD, FAAEM, FACMT, FACEP, Professor and Chair, Department of Emergency Medicine, Drexel University College of Medicine, Philadelphia, PA

ASSOCIATE EDITORS

Jill E. Allen, PharmD, BCPS, Pin Oak Associates, Drug Information Consultant, Salt Lake City, UT

Kim K. Birtcher, MS, PharmD, BCPS, Clinical Professor, University of Houston College of Pharmacy, Houston, TX

Jill S. Borchert, PharmD, BCPS, Professor, Pharmacy Practice, Director, PGY1 Residency Program, Midwestern University Chicago College of Pharmacy, Downers Grove, IL

Marie Cottman, PharmD, Owner, Pacific Compounding Pharmacy and Consultations, Inc., Lecturer, Department of Pharmaceutics and Medicinal Chemistry at Thomas J. Long School of Pharmacy and Health Sciences, University of the Pacific, Stockton, CA

David S. Craig, PharmD, H. Lee Moffitt Cancer Center and Research Institute, Tampa, FL

Deborah Hass, PharmD, BCOP, BCPS, Assistant Professor, Midwestern University Chicago College of Pharmacy, Downers Grove, IL

William A. Kehoe, PharmD, MA, BCPS, Professor of Pharmacy Practice and Psychology, University of the Pacific, Stockton, CA

Neeta Bahal O'Mara, PharmD, BCPS, Coldstream Consulting LLC, Skillman, NJ

Jeffrey T. Sherer, MPH, PharmD, BCPS, Clinical Associate Professor, University of Houston College of Pharmacy, Houston, TX

EDITORIAL BOARD

Steven R. Abel, PharmD, FASHP, Associate Dean for Clinical Programs, Bucke Professor and Head, Department of Pharmacy Practice , Purdue University College of Pharmacy, West Lafayette, IN

David R. Adams, MD, PharmD, Department of Dermatology, Penn State College of Medicine, Penn State Milton S. Hershey Medical Center, Hershey, PA

Heath P. Adams, PharmD, Department of Pharmacy, Trover Health Systems Regional Medical Center, Madisonville, KY

Giovannina M. Anthony, MD, Obstetrics and Gynecology, Women's Health Center of Jackson, Jackson, WY

Ouida Antle, PharmD, Carewest, Calgary, Alberta, Canada

*Affiliations are given for information purposes only, and no affiliation sponsorship is claimed.

CONTENTS

PAGE INDEX FOR TABLES

PREFACE TO THE TARASCON POCKET PHARMACOPOEIA®

The *Tarascon Pocket Pharmacopoeia®* arranges drugs by clinical class with a comprehensive index in the back. Trade names are italicized and capitalized. Drug doses shown in mg/kg are generally intended for children, while fixed doses represent typical adult recommendations. Brackets indicate currently available formulations, although not all pharmacies stock all formulations. The availability of generic, over-the-counter, and scored formulations is mentioned. We have set the disease or indication in red for the pharmaceutical agent. It is meant to function as an aid to find information quickly. Codes are as follows:

▸ **METABOLISM & EXCRETION: L** = primarily liver, **K** = primarily kidney, **LK** = both, but liver > kidney, **KL** = both, but kidney > liver.

♀ **SAFETY IN PREGNANCY: A** = Safety established using human studies, **B** = Presumed safety based on animal studies, **C** = Uncertain safety; no human studies and animal studies show an adverse effect, **D** = Unsafe - evidence of risk that may in certain clinical circumstances be justifiable, **X** = Highly unsafe - risk of use outweighs any possible benefit. For drugs that have not been assigned a category: **+** Generally accepted as safe, **?** Safety unknown or controversial, – Generally regarded as unsafe.

◗ **SAFETY IN LACTATION: +** Generally accepted as safe, **?** Safety unknown or controversial, – Generally regarded as unsafe. Many of our "+" listings are from the AAP policy "The Transfer of Drugs and Other Chemicals Into Human Milk" (see www.aap.org) and may differ from those recommended by the manufacturer.

© **DEA CONTROLLED SUBSTANCES: I** = High abuse potential, no accepted use (eg, heroin, marijuana), **II** = High abuse potential and severe dependence liability (eg, morphine, codeine, hydromorphone, cocaine, amphetamines, methylphenidate, secobarbital). Some states require triplicates. **III** = Moderate dependence liability (eg, *Tylenol #3, Vicodin*), **IV** = Limited dependence liability (benzodiazepines, propoxyphene, phentermine), **V** = Limited abuse potential (eg, *Lomotil*).

$ **RELATIVE COST:** Cost codes used are "per month" of maintenance therapy (eg, antihypertensives) or "per course" of short-term therapy (eg, antibiotics). Codes are calculated using average wholesale prices (at press time in US dollars) for the most common indication and route of each drug at a typical adult dosage. For maintenance therapy, costs are calculated based upon a 30-day supply or the quantity that might typically be used in a given month. For short-term therapy (ie, 10 days or less), costs are calculated on a single treatment course. When multiple forms are available (eg, generics), these codes reflect the least expensive generally available product. When drugs don't neatly fit into the classification scheme above, we have assigned codes based upon the relative cost of other similar drugs. *These codes should be used as a rough guide only*, as (1) they reflect cost, not charges, (2) pricing often varies substantially from location to location and time to time, and (3) HMOs, Medicaid, and buying groups often negotiate quite different pricing. Check with your local pharmacy if you have any questions.

Code	Cost
$	< $25
$$	$25 to $49
$$$	$50 to $99
$$$$	$100 to $199
$$$$$	≥ $200

🍁 CANADIAN TRADE NAMES: Unique common Canadian trade names not used in the US are listed after a maple leaf symbol. Trade names used in both nations or only in the US are displayed without such notation.

ABBREVIATIONS IN TEXT

AAP – American Academy of Pediatrics
ac – before meals
ACCP – American College of Chest Physicians
ADHD – attention deficit hyperactivity disorder
AHA – American Heart Association
Al – aluminum
ANC – absolute neutrophil count
ASA – aspirin
BP – blood pressure
BPH – benign prostatic hyperplasia
Ca – calcium
CAD – coronary artery disease
cap – capsule
cm – centimeter
CMV – cytomegalovirus
CNS – central nervous system
COPD – chronic obstructive pulmonary disease
CrCl – creatinine clearance
CVA – stroke
CYP – cytochrome P450
D5W – 5% dextrose
dL – deciliter
DM – diabetes mellitus
DPI – dry powder inhaler
ECG – electrocardiogram
EPS – extrapyramidal symptoms
ET – endotracheal
g – gram
GERD – gastroesophageal reflux disease
gtts – drops
GU – genitourinary
h – hour
HAART – highly active antiretroviral therapy
Hb – hemoglobin
HCTZ – hydrochlorothiazide
HIT – heparin-induced thrombocytopenia
hs – bedtime
HSV – herpes simplex virus
HTN – hypertension
IM – intramuscular
INR – international normalized ratio
IU – international units
IV – intravenous
JRA – juvenile rheumatoid arthritis
K+ – potassium
kg – kilogram
lbs – pounds
LFT – liver function test
LV – left ventricular
LVEF – left ventricular ejection fraction
m^2 – sqaure meters
MAOI – monoamine oxidase inhibitor
mcg – microgram
MDI – metered dose inhaler
mEq – milliequivalent
mg – milligram
Mg++ – magnesium
MI – myocardial infarction
min – minute
mIU – million International Units
mL – milliliter
mm – millimeter
mo – months old
MRSA – methicillin-resistant *Staphylococcus aureus*
ng – nanogram
NHLBI – National Heart, Lung, and Blood Institute
NS – normal saline
N/V – nausea/vomiting
NYHA – New York Heart Association
OA – osteoarthritis
oz – ounces
pc – after meals
PO – by mouth
PR – by rectum
prn – as needed
q – every
qam – every morning
qpm – every evening
RA – rheumatoid arthritis
RSV – respiratory synctial virus
SC – subcutaneous
sec – second
soln – solution
supp – suppository
susp – suspension
tab – tablet
TB – tuberculosis
TCA – tricyclic antidepressant
TNF – tumor necrosis factor
TPN – total parenteral nutrition
UTI – urinary tract infection
wt – weight
y – year
yo – years old

THERAPEUTIC DRUG LEVELS

Drug	Level	Optimal Timing
amikacin peak	20–35 mcg/mL	30 minutes after infusion
amikacin trough	<5 mcg/mL	Just prior to next dose
carbamazepine trough	4–12 mcg/mL	Just prior to next dose
cyclosporine trough	50–300 ng/mL	Just prior to next dose
digoxin	0.8–2.0 ng/mL	Just prior to next dose
ethosuximide trough	40–100 mcg/mL	Just prior to next dose
gentamicin peak	5–10 mcg/mL	30 minutes after infusion
gentamicin trough	<2 mcg/mL	Just prior to next dose
lidocaine	1.5–5 mcg/mL	12–24 hours after start of infusion
lithium trough	0.6–1.2 meq/L	Just prior to first morning dose
NAPA	10–30 mcg/mL	Just prior to next procainamide dose
phenobarbital trough	15–40 mcg/mL	Just prior to next dose
phenytoin trough	10–20 mcg/mL	Just prior to next dose
primidone trough	5–12 mcg/mL	Just prior to next dose
procainamide	4–10 mcg/mL	Just prior to next dose
quinidine	2–5 mcg/mL	Just prior to next dose
theophylline	5–15 mcg/mL	8–12 hours after once daily dose
tobramycin peak	5–10 mcg/mL	30 minutes after infusion
tobramycin trough	<2 mcg/mL	Just prior to next dose
valproate trough (epilepsy)	50–100 mcg/mL	Just prior to next dose
valproate trough (mania)	45–125 mcg/mL	Just prior to next dose
vancomycin trough[1]	10–20 mg/L	Just prior to next dose
zonisamide[2]	10–40 mcg/mL	Just prior to dose

[1] Maintain trough >10 mg/L to avoid resistance; optimal trough for complicated infections is 15–20 mg/L
[2] Ranges not firmly established but supported by clinical trial results

PEDIATRIC DRUGS		Age	2mo	4mo	6mo	9mo	12mo	15mo	2yo	3yo	5yo
		kg	5	6½	8	9	10	11	13	15	19
		lbs	11	15	17	20	22	24	28	33	42
med	**strength**	**freq**	**teaspoons of liquid per dose** (1 tsp= 5 mL)								
Tylenol (mg)		q4h	80	80	120	120	160	160	200	240	280
Tylenol (tsp)	160/t	q4h	½	½	¾	¾	1	1	1¼	1½	1¾
ibuprofen (mg)		q6h	-	-	75†	75†	100	100	125	150	175
ibuprofen (tsp)	100/t	q6h	-	-	¾†	¾†	1	1	1¼	1½	1¾
amoxicillin or	125/t	bid	1	1¼	1½	1¾	1¾	2	2¼	2¾	3½
Augmentin	200/t	bid	½	¾	1	1	1¼	1¼	1½	1¾	2¼
(not otitis media)	250/t	bid	½	½	¾	¾	1	1	1¼	1¼	1¾
	400/t	bid	¼	½	½	½	¾	¾	¾	1	1
amoxicillin,	200/t	bid	1	1¼	1¾	2	2	2¼	2¾	3	4
(otitis media)‡	250/t	bid	¾	1¼	1½	1½	1¾	1¾	2¼	2½	3¼
	400/t	bid	½	¾	¾	1	1	1¼	1½	1½	2
Augmentin ES‡	600/t	bid	?	½	½	¾	¾	¾	1	1¼	1½
azithromycin·§	100/t	qd	¼†	½†	½	½	½	½	¾	¾	1
(5-day Rx)	200/t	qd	--	¼†	¼	¼	¼	¼	½	½	½
Bactrim/Septra	---	bid	½	¾	1	1	1	1¼	1½	1½	2
cefaclor·	125/t	bid	1	1	1¼	1½	1½	1¾	2	2½	3
"	250/t	bid	½	½	¾	¾	¾	1	1	1¼	1½
cefadroxil	125/t	bid	½	¾	1	1	1¼	1¼	1½	1¾	2¼
"	250/t	bid	¼	½	½	½	¾	¾	¾	1	1
cefdinir	125/t	qd	--	¾†	1	1	1	1¼	1½	1¾	2
cefixime	100/t	qd	½	½	¾	¾	¾	1	1	1¼	1½
cefprozil*	125/t	bid	--	¾†	1	1	1¼	1½	1½	2	2¼
"	250/t	bid	--	½†	½	½	¾	¾	¾	1	1¼
cefuroxime	125/t	bid	-	¾	¾	1	1	1	1½	1¾	2¼
cephalexin	125/t	qid	--	½	¾	¾	1	1	1¼	1½	1¾
"	250/t	qid	-	¼	¼	½	½	½	¾	¾	1
clarithromycin	125/t	bid	½†	½†	½	½	¾	¾	¾	1	1¼
"	250/t	bid	--	--	--	¼	½	½	½	½	¾
dicloxacillin	62½/t	qid	½	¾	1	1	1¼	1¼	1½	1¾	2
nitrofurantoin	25/t	qid	¼	½	½	½	½	¾	¾	¾	1
Pediazole	---	tid	½	½	¾	¾	1	1	1	1¼	1½
penicillin V**	250/t	bid-tid	--	1	1	1	1	1	1	1	1
cetirizine	5/t	qd	-	-	½	½	½	½	½	½	½
Benadryl	12.5/t	q6h	½	½	¾	¾	1	1	1¼	1½	2
prednisolone	15/t	qd	¼	½	½	¾	¾	¾	1	1	1¼
prednisone	5/t	qd	1	1¼	1½	1¾	2	2¼	2½	3	3¾
Robitussin	---	q4h	-	-	¼†	¼†	½	½	¾	¾	1
Tylenol w/ codeine		q4h	-	-	-	-	-	-		1	1

*Dose shown is for otitis media only; see dosing in text for alternative indications.
†Dosing at this age/weight not recommended by manufacturer.
‡AAP now recommends high dose (80-90 mg/kg/d) for all otitis media in children; with Augmentin used as ES only.
§Give a double dose of azithromycin the first day.
**AHA dosing for streptococcal pharyngitis. Treat for 10 days.
tsp=teaspoon; t=teaspoon; q=every; h=hour; kg=kilogram; Lbs=pounds; mL=mililiter; bid=two times per day; tid=three times per day; qid=four times per day; qd=every day.

PEDIATRIC VITAL SIGNS AND INTRAVENOUS DRUGS												
Age		*Pre-matr*	*New-born*	*2m*	*4m*	*6m*	*9m*	*12m*	*15m*	*2y*	*3y*	*5y*
Weight	*(Kg)*	2	3½	5	6½	8	9	10	11	13	15	19
	(Lbs)	4½	7½	11	15	17	20	22	24	28	33	42
Maint fluids	*(mL/h)*	8	14	20	26	32	36	40	42	46	50	58
ET tube	*(mm)*	2½	3/3½	3½	3½	3½	4	4	4½	4½	4½	5
Defib	*(Joules)*	4	7	10	13	16	18	20	22	26	30	38
Systolic BP	*(high)*	70	80	85	90	95	100	103	104	106	109	114
	(low)	40	60	70	70	70	70	70	70	75	75	80
Pulse rate	*(high)*	145	145	180	180	180	160	160	160	150	150	135
	(low)	100	100	110	110	110	100	100	100	90	90	65
Resp rate	*(high)*	60	60	50	50	50	46	46	30	30	25	25
	(low)	35	30	30	30	24	24	20	20	20	20	20
adenosine	*(mg)*	0.2	0.3	0.5	0.6	0.8	0.9	1	1.1	1.3	1.5	1.9
atropine	*(mg)*	0.1	0.1	0.1	0.13	0.16	0.18	0.2	0.22	0.26	0.30	0.38
Benadryl	*(mg)*	-	-	-5	6½	8	9	10	11	13	15	19
Bicarbonate	(meq)	2	3½	5	6½	8	9	10	11	13	15	19
dextrose	*(g)*	1	2	5	6½	8	9	10	11	13	15	19
epinephrine	*(mg)*	.02	.04	.05	.07	.08	.09	0.1	0.11	0.13	0.15	0.19
lidocaine	*(mg)*	2	3½	5	6½	8	9	10	11	13	15	19
morphine	*(mg)*	0.2	0.3	0.5	0.6	0.8	0.9	1	1.1	1.3	1.5	1.9
mannitol	*(g)*	2	3½	5	6½	8	9	10	11	13	15	19
naloxone	*(mg)*	.02	.04	.05	.07	.08	.09	0.1	0.11	0.13	0.15	0.19
diazepam	*(mg)*	0.6	1	1.5	2	2.5	2.7	3	3.3	3.9	4.5	5
fosphenytoin*	*(PE)*	40	70	100	130	160	180	200	220	260	300	380
lorazepam	*(mg)*	0.1	0.2	0.3	0.35	0.4	0.5	0.5	0.6	0.7	0.8	1.0
phenobarb	*(mg)*	30	60	75	100	125	125	150	175	200	225	275
phenytoin*	*(mg)*	40	70	100	130	160	180	200	220	260	300	380
ampicillin	*(mg)*	100	175	250	325	400	450	500	550	650	750	1000
ceftriaxone	*(mg)*	-	-	250	325	400	450	500	550	650	750	1000
cefotaxime	*(mg)*	100	175	250	325	400	450	500	550	650	750	1000
gentamicin	*(mg)*	5	8	12	16	20	22	25	27	32	37	47

*Loading doses; fosphenytoin dosed in "phenytoin equivalents."

CONVERSIONS	*Liquid:*	*Weight:*
Temperature:	1 fluid ounce = 30 mL	1 kilogram = 2.2 lbs
F = (1.8) C + 32	1 teaspoon = 5 mL	1 ounce = 30 g
C = (F – 32)/1.8	1 tablespoon = 15 mL	1 grain = 65 mg

INHIBITORS, INDUCERS, AND SUBSTRATES OF CYTOCHROME P450 ISOZYMES

The cytochrome P450 (CYP) inhibitors and inducers below do not necessarily cause clinically important interactions with substrates listed. We exclude in vitro data which can be inaccurate. Refer to the *Tarascon Pocket Pharmacopoeia* drug interactions database (PDA edition) or other resources for more information if an interaction is suspected based on this chart. A drug that inhibits CYP subfamily activity can block the metabolism of substrates of that enzyme and substrate accumulation and toxicity may result. CYP inhibitors are classified by how much they increase the area-under-the-curve (AUC) of a substrate: weak (1.25-2 fold), moderate (2–5 fold), or strong (≥5 fold). A drug that induces CYP subfamily activity increases substrate metabolism and reduced substrate efficacy may result. CYP inducers are classified by how much they decrease the AUC of a substrate: weak (20-50%), moderate (50-80%), or strong (≥80%). A drug is considered a sensitive substrate if a CYP inhibitor increases the AUC of that drug by ≥5-fold. While AUC increases of >50% often do not affect patient response, smaller increases can be important if the therapeutic range is narrow (eg, theophylline, warfarin, cyclosporine). This table may be incomplete since new evidence about drug interactions is continually being identified.

CYP1A2

Inhibitors. ***Strong***: ciprofloxacin, fluvoxamine. ***Moderate***: methoxalan, mexiletine, oral contraceptives, phenylpropanolamine, vemurafenib, zileuton. ***Weak***: acyclovir, allopurinol, caffeine, cimetidine, disulfiram, echinacea, famotidine, norfloxacin, propafenone, propranolol, terbinafine, ticlopidine, verapamil.
Unclassified: amiodarone, atazanavir, citalopram, clarithromycin, deferasirox, erythromycin, estradiol, isoniazid, peginterferon alfa-2a.
Inducers: ***Moderate***: montelukast, phenytoin, smoking. ***Weak***: omeprazole, phenobarbital.
Unclassified: carbamazepine, charcoal-broiled foods, rifampin, ritonavir, tipranavir/ritonavir.
Substrates. ***Sensitive***: caffeine, duloxetine, melatonin, rameltion, tacrine, tizanidine.
Unclassified: acetaminophen, amitriptyline, asenapine, bendamustine, cinacalcet, clomipramine, clozapine, cyclobenzaprine, estradiol, fluvoxamine, haloperidol, imipramine, mexiletine, mirtazapine, naproxen, olanzapine, ondansetron, propranolol, rasagiline, riluzole, roflumilast, ropinirole, ropivacaine, R-warfarin, theophylline, zileuton, zolmitriptan.

CYP2B6

Inhibitors: ***Weak***: clopidogrel, prasugrel, ticlopidine.
Inducers. ***Moderate***: efavirenz, rifampin. ***Weak***: nevirapine. ***Unclassified***: baicalin (ingredient of Limbrel).
Substrates: ***Sensitive***: bupropion, efavirenz. ***Unclassified***: cyclophosphamide, methadone, nevirapine, prasugrel.

CYP 2C8

Inhibitors. ***Strong***: gemfibrozil. ***Moderate***: deferasirox. ***Weak***: fluvoxamine, ketoconazole, trimethoprim.
Inducers: ***Moderate***: rifampin. ***Unclassified***: barbiturates, carbamazepine, rifabutin.
Substrates. ***Sensitive***: repaglinide. ***Unclassified***: amiodarone, carbamazepine, ibuprofen, isotretinoin, loperamide, montelukast, paclitaxel, pioglitazone, treprostanil.

CYP 2C9

Inhibitors. ***Moderate***: amiodarone, fluconazole, miconazole, oxandrolone. ***Weak***: capecitabine, cotrimoxazole, etravirine, fluvastatin, fluvoxamine, metronidazole, sulfinpyrazone, tigecycline, voriconazole, zafirlukast. ***Unclassified***: cimetidine, fenofibrate, fenofibric acid, fluorouracil, imatinib, isoniazid, leflunomide,
Inducers: ***Moderate***: carbamazepine, rifampin. ***Weak***: aprepitant, bosentan, phenobarbital, St. John's wort. ***Unclassified***: rifapentine.
Substrates. ***Sensitive***: celecoxib. ***Unclassified***: azilsartan, bosentan, chlorpropamide, diclofenac, etravirine, fluoxetine, flurbiprofen, fluvastatin, formoterol, glimepiride, glipizide, glyburide, ibuprofen, irbesartan, losartan, mefenamic acid, meloxicam, montelukast, naproxen, nateglinide, phenytoin, piroxicam, ramelteon, sildenafil, tolbutamide, torsemide, vardenafil, voriconazole, S-warfarin, zafirlukast, zileuton.

CYP 2C19

Inhibitors. ***Strong***: fluconazole, fluvoxamine, ticlopidine. ***Moderate***: esomeprazole, fluoxetine, moclobemide, omeprazole, voriconazole. ***Weak***: armodafinil, carbamazepine, cimetidine, etravirine, felbamate, human growth hormone, ketoconazole, oral contraceptives. ***Unclassified***: chloramphenicol, isoniazid, modafinil, oxcarbazepine.
Inducers. ***Moderate***: rifampin. ***Unclassified***: St. John's wort.

Substrates. ***Sensitive***: lansoprazole, omeprazole. ***Unclassified***: amitriptyline, bortezomib, carisoprodol, cilostazol, citalopram, clobazam, clomipramine, clopidogrel, clozapine, cyclophosphamide, desipramine, dexlansoprazole, diazepam, escitalopram, esomeprazole, etravirine, formoterol, imipramine, lacosamide, methadone, moclobamide, nelfinavir, pantoprazole, phenytoin, progesterone, proguanil, propranolol, rabeprazole, sertraline, voriconazole, R-warfarin.

CYP 2D6

Inhibitors. ***Strong***: bupropion, fluoxetine, paroxetine, quinidine. ***Moderate***: cinacalcet, dronedarone, duloxetine, mirabegron, terbinafine. ***Weak***: amiodarone, asenapine, celecoxib, cimetidine, desvenlafaxine, diltiazem, diphenhydramine, echinacea, escitalopram, febuxostat, gefitinib, hydralazine, hydroxychloroquine, imitinib, methadone, oral contraceptives, propafenone, ranitidine, ritonavir, sertraline, telithromycin, venlafaxine, vemurafenib, verapamil. ***Unclassified***: abiraterone, chloroquine, clomipramine, fluphenazine, haloperidol, lorcaserin, lumefantrine, metoclopramide, moclobamide, perphenazine, quinine, ranolazine, thioridazine.

Inducers: None known.

Substrates. ***Sensitive***: atomoxetine, desipramine, dextromethorphan, metoprolol, nebivolol, perphenazine, tolterodine, venlafaxine. ***Unclassified***: amitriptyline, aripiprazole, carvedilol, cevimeline, chlorpheniramine, chlorpromazine, cinacalcet, clomipramine, codeine*, darifenacin, dihydrocodeine, dolasetron, donepezil, doxepin, duloxetine, fesoterodine, flecainide, fluoxetine, formoterol, galantamine, haloperidol, hydrocodone, iloperidone, imipramine, loratadine, maprotiline, methadone, methamphetamine, metoclopramide, mexiletine, mirtazapine, morphine, nortriptyline, ondansetron, paroxetine, promethazine, propafenone, propranolol, quetiapine, risperidone, ritonavir, tamoxifen, tetrabenazine, thioridazine, timolol, tramadol*, trazodone.

* Metabolism by CYP2D6 required to convert to active analgesic metabolite; analgesia may be impaired by CYP2D6 inhibitors.

CYP 3A4

Inhibitors. ***Strong***: boceprevir, clarithromycin, conivaptan, indinavir, itraconazole, ketoconazole, lopinavir-ritonavir, nefazodone, nelfinavir, posaconazole, ritonavir, saquinavir, telaprevir, telithromycin, voriconazole.

Moderate: aprepitant, atazanavir, crizotinib, darunavir-ritonavir, diltiazem, dronedarone, erythromycin, fluconazole, fosamprenavir, grapefruit juice (variable), imatinib, verapamil. ***Weak***: alprazolam, amiodarone, amlodipine, atorvastatin, bicalutamide, cilostazol, cimetidine, cyclosporine, fluoxetine, fluvoxamine, ginko, goldenseal, isoniazid, ivacaftor, nilotinib, oral contraceptives, ranitidine, ranolazine, ticagrelor, tipranavir-ritonavir, zileuton.

Unclassified: danazol, miconazole, quinine, quinupristin-dalfopristin, sertraline.

Inducers. ***Strong:*** carbamazepine, phenytoin, rifampin, St. Johns wort. ***Moderate***: bosentan, efavirenz, etravirine, modafinil, nafcillin. ***Weak:*** aprepitant, armodafinil, clobazam, echinacea, fosamprenavir, pioglitazone, rufinamide. ***Unclassified:*** artemether, barbiturates, dexamethasone, ethosuximide, oxcarbazepine, primidone, rifabutin, rifapentine, ritonavir vemurafenib.

Substrates. ***Sensitive***: alfentanil, aprepitant, budesonide, buspirone, conivaptan, darifenacin, darunavir, dasatinib, dronedarone, eletriptan, eplerenone, everolimus, felodipine, fluticasone, indinavir, ivacaftor, lopinavir, lovastatin, lurasidone, maraviroc, midazolam, nisoldipine, quetiapine, saquinavir, sildenafil, simvastatin, sirolimus, tipranavir, tolvaptan, triazolam, vardenafil. ***Unclassified***: alfuzosin, aliskiren, almotriptan, alprazolam, amiodarone, amlodipine, aripiprazole, armodafinil, artemether-lumefantrine, atazanavir, atorvastatin, avanafil, axitinib, boceprevir, bortezomib, bosentan, brentuximab, bromocriptine, buprenorphine, carbamazepine, cevimeline, cilostazol, cinacalcet, cisapride, citalopram, clarithromycin, clomipramine, clonazepam, clopidogrel, colchicine, clobazam, clozapine, corticosteroids, crizotinib, cyclophosphamide, cyclosporine, dapsone, desogestrel, desvenlafaxine, dexamethasone, dexlansoprazole, diazepam, dihydroergotamine, diltiazem, disopyramide, docetaxel, dofetilide, dolasetron, domperidone, donepezil, doxorubicin, dutasteride, efavirenz, ergotamine, erlotinib, erythromycin, escitalopram, esomeprazole, eszopiclone, ethinyl estradiol, etoposide, etravirine, fentanyl, fesoterodine, finasteride, fosamprenavir, fosaprepitant, galantamine, gefitinib, guanfacine, haloperidol, hydrocodone, ifosfamide, iloperidone, imatinib, imipramine, irinotecan, isradipine, itraconazole, ixabepilone, ketoconazole, lansoprazole, lapatinib, letrozole, lidocaine, loratadine, methylergonovine, mifepristone, mirtazapine, modafinil, mometasone, montelukast, nateglinide, nefazodone, nelfinavir, nevirapine, nicardipine, nifedipine, nilotinib, nimodipine, ondansetron, oxybutynin, oxycodone, paclitaxel, pantoprazole, pazopanib, pimozide, pioglitazone, prasugrel, praziquantel, quinidine, quinine, rabeprazole, ramelteon, ranolazine, repaglinide, rifabutin, rifampin, ritonavir, rivaroxaban, roflumilast, romidepsin, ruxolitinib, saxagliptin, sertraline, silodosin, solifenacin, sorafenib, sufentanil, sunitinib, tacrolimus, tadalafil, tamoxifen, telaprevir, telithromycin, temsirolimus, testosterone, tiagabine, ticagrelor, tinidazole, tolterodine, tramadol, trazodone, verapamil, vilazodone, vinblastine, vincristine, vinorelbine, voriconazole, R-warfarin, zaleplon, ziprasidone, zolpidem, zonisamide.

CORONARY ARTERY DISEASE 10-YEAR RISK

Framingham model for calculating 10–year risk for coronary artery disease (CAD) in patients without diabetes or clinically evident CAD. Diabetes is considered a CAD risk "equivalent", i.e., the prospective risk of CAD in diabetics is similar to those with established CAD. Automated calculator available at: http://hin.nhlbi.nih.gov/atpiii/calculator.asp?usertype=prof (NCEP, JAMA 2001; 285:2497)

MEN

Age	*Points*	*Age*	*Points*
20–34	-9	55–59	8
35–39	-4	60–64	10
40–44	0	65–69	11
45–49	3	70–74	12
50–54	6	75–79	13

Choles-terol*	Age (years)				
	20–39	*40–49*	*50–59*	*60–69*	*70–79*
<160	0	0	0	0	0
160–199	4	3	2	1	0
200–239	7	5	3	1	0
240–279	9	6	4	2	1
280+	11	8	5	3	1

Age (years)	*20–39*	*40–49*	*50–59*	*60–69*	*70–79*
Nonsmoker	0	0	0	0	0
Smoker	8	5	3	1	1

HDLmg/dL	*Points*	*HDLmg/dL*	*Points*
60+	-1	40–49	1
50–59	0	<40	2

Systolic BP	*If Untreated*	*If Treated*
<120mmHg	0	0
120–129 mmHg	0	1
130–139 mmHg	1	2
140–159 mmHg	1	2
160+ mmHg	2	3

Point Total	*10–Year Risk*	*Point Total*	*10–Year Risk*
0	1%	9	5%
1	1%	10	6%
2	1%	11	8%
3	1%	12	10%
4	1%	13	12%
5	2%	14	16%
6	2%	15	20%
7	3%	16	25%
8	4%	17+	30+%

WOMEN

Age	*Points*	*Age*	*Points*
20–34	-7	55–59	8
35–39	-3	60–64	10
40–44	0	65–69	12
45–49	3	70–74	14
50–54	6	75–79	16

Choles-terol*	Age (years)				
	20–39	*40–49*	*50–59*	*60–69*	*70–79*
<160	0	0	0	0	0
160–199	4	3	2	1	1
200–239	8	6	4	2	1
240–279	11	8	5	3	2
280+	13	10	7	4	2

Total in mg/dL

Age (years)	*20–39*	*40–49*	*50–59*	*60–69*	*70–79*
Nonsmoker	0	0	0	0	0
Smoker	9	7	4	2	1

HDLmg/dL	*Points*	*HDLmg/dL*	*Points*
60+	-1	40–49	1
50–59	0	<40	2

Systolic BP	*If Untreated*	*If Treated*
<120 mmHg	0	0
120–129 mmHg	1	3
130–139 mmHg	2	4
140–159 mmHg	3	5
160+ mmHg	4	6

Point Total	*10–Year Risk*	*Point Total*	*10–Year Risk*
<9	<1%	17	5%
9	1%	18	6%
10	1%	19	8%
11	1%	20	11%
12	1%	21	14%
13	2%	22	17%
14	2%	23	22%
15	3%	24	27%
16	4%	25+	30+%

DRUG THERAPY REFERENCE WEBSITES FORMULAS (selected)

Professional societies or governmental agencies with drug therapy guidelines		
AAP	American Academy of Pediatrics	www.aap.org
ACC	American College of Cardiology	www.acc.org
ACCP	American College of Chest Physicians	www.chestnet.org
ACCP	American College of Clinical Pharmacy	www.accp.com
ADA	American Diabetes Association	www.diabetes.org
AHA	American Heart Association	www.heart.org
AHRQ	Agency for Healthcare Research and Quality	www.ahcpr.gov
AIDSinfo	HIV Treatment, Prevention, and Research	www.aidsinfo.nih.gov
AMA	American Medical Association	www.ama-assn.org
APA	American Psychiatric Association	www.psych.org
APA	American Psychological Association	www.apa.org
ASHP	Amer. Society Health-Systems Pharmacists	www.ashp.org
ATS	American Thoracic Society	www.thoracic.org
CDC	Centers for Disease Control and Prevention	www.cdc.gov
CDC	CDC bioterrorism and radiation exposures	www.bt.cdc.gov
IDSA	Infectious Diseases Society of America	www.idsociety.org
MHA	Malignant Hyperthermia Association	www.mhaus.org
NHLBI	National Heart, Lung, and Blood Institute	www.nhlbi.nih.gov

Other therapy reference sites	
Cochrane library	www.cochrane.org
Emergency Contraception Website	www.not-2-late.com
Immunization Action Coalition	www.immunize.org
Int'l Registry for Drug-Induced Arrhythmias	www.qtdrugs.org
Managing Contraception	www.managingcontraception.com

ANALGESICS: Antirheumatic Agents—Biologic Response Modifiers

NOTE: Death, sepsis, and serious infections (eg, TB and invasive fungal infections) have been reported. Do not start if current serious infection, discontinue if serious infection develops, and closely monitor for any new infection. Screening for latent TB infection is recommended. Use caution if history of recurring infections or with underlying conditions (eg, DM) that predispose to infections. Combination use of these drugs increases the risk of serious infection and is contraindicated.

ABATACEPT (***Orencia***) ▶Serum ♀C ▶? $$$$$

WARNING – Do not use with TNF-blocking drugs such as adalimumab, etanercept, or infliximab or the IL-1 receptor antagonist anakinra.

ADULT – RA: Specialized dosing.

PEDS – Juvenile idiopathic arthritis age 6 yo or older: Specialized dosing.

NOTES – Monitor patients with COPD for exacerbation and pulmonary infections. Avoid live vaccines.

ADALIMUMAB (***Humira***) ▶Serum ♀B ▶– $$$$$

WARNING – Hypersensitivity. Combination use with other immunomodulators increases the risk of serious infections. Aplastic anemia, thrombocytopenia, and leukopenia. Rare CNS disorders (eg, multiple sclerosis, myelitis, optic neuritis) have been reported. May worsen heart failure; monitor signs/symptoms of heart failure.

ADULT – RA, psoriatic arthritis, ankylosing spondylitis: 40 mg SC q 2 weeks, alone or in combination with methotrexate or other disease-modifying antirheumatic drugs (DMARDs). May increase frequency to q week if not on methotrexate. Crohn's disease: 160 mg SC at week 0, 80 mg at week 2, then 40 mg q other week starting with week 4.

PEDS – Not approved in children.

FORMS – Trade only: 40 mg prefilled glass syringes or vials with needles, 2 per pack.

NOTES – Monitor CBC. Refrigerate and protect from light. Avoid live vaccines. Do not use in combination with anakinra.

ANAKINRA (***Kineret***) ▶K ♀B ▶? $$$$$

WARNING – Increased incidence of serious infections. Do not use in active infection or with other immunomodulators.

ADULT – RA: 100 mg SC daily, alone or in combination with other disease-modifying antirheumatic drugs (DMARDs) except TNF inhibitors.

PEDS – Not approved in children.

FORMS – Trade only: 100 mg prefilled glass syringes with needles, 7 or 28 per box.

NOTES – Monitor for neutropenia. Refrigerate and protect from light. Avoid live vaccines.

ETANERCEPT (***Enbrel***) ▶Serum ♀B ▶– $$$$$

WARNING – Combination use with other immunomodulators increases the risk of serious infections. Rare nervous system disorders (eg, multiple sclerosis, myelitis, optic neuritis) have been reported. May worsen heart failure; monitor closely.

ADULT – RA, psoriatic arthritis, ankylosing spondylitis: 50 mg SC q week, alone or in combination with methotrexate. Plaque psoriasis: 50 mg SC twice per week for 3 months, then 50 mg SC q week.

PEDS – JRA age 4 to 17 yo: 0.8 mg/kg SC q week, to max single dose of 50 mg.

UNAPPROVED PEDS – Plaque psoriasis age 4 to 17 yo: 0.8 mg/kg SC q week, to max single dose of 50 mg.

FORMS – Supplied in a carton containing four dose trays (four 25-mg vials with syringes) or single-use 50 mg prefilled syringes.

NOTES – Appropriate SC injection sites are thigh, abdomen, and upper arm. Rotate injection sites. Refrigerate. Avoid live vaccines. The needle cover contains latex; caution if allergy.

INFLIXIMAB (***Remicade***) ▶Serum ♀B ▶? $$$$$

WARNING – May worsen heart failure; monitor signs/symptoms of heart failure. May increase risk of lymphoma and other malignancies; caution if history of malignancy or if malignancy develops during treatment. Hypersensitivity reactions may occur. Combination use with other immunomodulators increases the risk of serious infections. Rare CNS disorders (eg, multiple sclerosis, myelitis, optic neuritis) have been reported.

ADULT – RA: 3 mg/kg IV in combination with methotrexate at 0, 2, and 6 weeks. Give q 8 weeks thereafter. May increase up to 10 mg/kg or q 4 weeks if incomplete response. Ankylosing spondylitis: 5 mg/kg IV at 0, 2, and 6 weeks. Give q 6 weeks thereafter. Plaque psoriasis, psoriatic arthritis, moderately to severely active Crohn's disease, ulcerative colitis, or fistulizing disease: 5 mg/kg IV at 0, 2, and 6 weeks, then q 8 weeks.

(cont.)

INFLIXIMAB (*cont.*)

PEDS – Moderately to severely active Crohn's disease or fistulizing disease: 5 mg/kg IV at 0, 2, and 6 weeks then q 8 weeks.

UNAPPROVED ADULT – Moderate to severe ulcerative colitis: Same dose as for Crohn's disease.

NOTES – Headache, dyspnea, urticaria, nausea, infections, abdominal pain, and fever. Avoid live vaccines. Three cases of toxic optic neuropathy reported. Refrigerate.

ANALGESICS: Antirheumatic Agents—Disease-Modifying Antirheumatic Drugs (DMARDs)

AURANOFIN (*Ridaura*) ▸K ♀C ▸+ $$$$$

WARNING – Gold toxicity may manifest as marrow suppression, proteinuria, hematuria, pruritus, rash, stomatitis, or persistent diarrhea. Monitor CBC and urinary protein q 4 to 12 weeks (oral) or q 1 to 2 weeks (injectable) due to the risk of myelosuppression and proteinuria.

ADULT – RA: Initial 3 mg PO two times per day or 6 mg PO daily. May increase to 3 mg PO three times per day after 6 months.

PEDS – RA: 0.1 to 0.15 mg/kg/day PO. Max dose 0.2 mg/kg/day. May be given daily or divided two times per day.

UNAPPROVED ADULT – Psoriatic arthritis: 3 mg PO two times per day or 6 mg PO daily.

FORMS – Trade only: Caps 3 mg.

NOTES – Contraindicated in patients with a history of any of the following gold-induced disorders: Anaphylactic reactions, necrotizing enterocolitis, pulmonary fibrosis, exfoliative dermatitis, bone marrow suppression. Not recommended in pregnancy. Proteinuria has developed in 3 to 9% of patients. Diarrhea, rash, stomatitis, chrysiasis (gray-to-blue pigmentation of skin) may occur. Minimize exposure to sunlight or artificial UV light. Auranofin may increase phenytoin levels.

AZATHIOPRINE (*Azasan, Imuran*) ▸LK ♀D ▸– $$$

WARNING – Chronic immunosuppression with azathioprine increases the risk of neoplasia. May cause marrow suppression or GI hypersensitivity reaction characterized by severe N/V.

ADULT – Severe RA: Initial dose 1 mg/kg (50 to 100 mg) PO daily or divided two times per day. Increase by 0.5 mg/kg/day at 6 to 8 weeks; if no serious toxicity and if initial response is unsatisfactory can then increase thereafter at 4-week intervals. Max dose 2.5 mg/kg/day. In patients with clinical response, use the lowest effective dose for maintenance therapy.

PEDS – Not approved in children.

UNAPPROVED ADULT – Crohn's disease: 75 to 100 mg PO daily. Myasthenia gravis, multiple sclerosis: 2 to 3 mg/kg/day PO. Behcet's syndrome, SLE: 2.5 mg/kg/day PO. Vasculitis: 2 mg/kg/day PO. Ulcerative colitis: 1.5 to 2.5 mg/kg/day PO. Inflammatory neuropathies: 1.5 to 3 mg/kg/day PO.

UNAPPROVED PEDS – JRA: Initial: 1 mg/kg/day PO. Increase by 0.5 mg/kg/day q 4 weeks until response or max dose of 2.5 to 3 mg/kg/day.

FORMS – Generic/Trade: Tabs 50 mg, scored. Trade only (Azasan): 75, 100 mg, scored.

NOTES – Monitor CBC q 1 to 2 weeks with dose changes, then q 1 to 3 months. ACE inhibitors, allopurinol, and methotrexate may increase activity and toxicity. Azathioprine may decrease the activity of anticoagulants, cyclosporine, and neuromuscular blockers.

GOLD SODIUM THIOMALATE (*Myochrysine*) ▸K ♀C ▸+ $$$$$

WARNING – Gold toxicity may manifest as marrow suppression, proteinuria, hematuria, pruritus, rash, stomatitis, or persistent diarrhea. Monitor CBC and urinary protein q 4 to 12 weeks (oral) or q 1 to 2 weeks (injectable) due to the risk of myelosuppression and proteinuria.

ADULT – RA: Weekly IM injections: First dose, 10 mg. Second dose, 25 mg. Third and subsequent doses, 25 to 50 mg. Continue the 25 to 50 mg dose weekly to a cumulative dose of 0.8 to 1 g. If improvement seen without toxicity, 25 to 50 mg q other week for 2 to 20 weeks. If stable, lengthen dosing intervals to q 3 to 4 weeks.

PEDS – JRA: Test dose 10 mg IM, then 1 mg/kg, not to exceed 50 mg for a single injection. Continue this dose weekly to a cumulative dose of 0.8 to 1 g. If improvement seen without toxicity, dose every other week for 2 to 20 weeks. If stable, lengthen dosing intervals to q 3 to 4 weeks.

UNAPPROVED ADULT – Load as per approved, but then continue weekly up to 1 year.

NOTES – Administer only IM, preferably intragluteally. Have patient remain recumbent for approximately 10 min after injection.

(cont.)

GOLD SODIUM THIOMALATE *(cont.)*

Contraindicated in pregnancy and in patients who have uncontrolled DM, severe debilitation, renal disease, hepatic dysfunction or hepatitis, marked HTN, uncontrolled heart failure, SLE, blood dyscrasias, patients recently irradiated and those with severe toxicity from previous exposure to gold or other heavy metals, urticaria, eczema, and colitis. Arthralgia and dermatitis may occur.

HYDROXYCHLOROQUINE (***Plaquenil***) ▶K ♀C ▶+ $

ADULT – RA: 400 to 600 mg PO daily to start, taken with food or milk. After clinical response, decrease to 200 to 400 mg PO daily. Discontinue if no objective improvement within 6 months. SLE: 400 mg PO one to two times per day to start. Decrease to 200 to 400 PO daily for prolonged maintenance.

PEDS – Not approved in children.

UNAPPROVED PEDS – JRA or SLE: 3 to 5 mg/kg/day, up to a max of 400 mg/day PO daily or divided two times per day. Max dose 7 mg/kg/day. Take with food or milk.

FORMS – Generic/Trade: Tabs 200 mg, scored.

NOTES – May exacerbate psoriasis or porphyria. Irreversible retinal damage possible with long-term or high dosage (greater than 6.5 mg/kg/day). Baseline and periodic eye exams recommended. Anorexia, nausea, and vomiting may occur. May increase digoxin and metoprolol levels.

LEFLUNOMIDE (***Arava***) ▶LK ♀X ▶– $$$$$

WARNING – Hepatotoxicity, interstitial lung disease. Rare reports of lymphoma, pancytopenia, agranulocytosis, thrombocytopenia, Stevens-Johnson syndrome, cutaneous necrotizing vasculitis, and severe HTN. Exclude pregnancy before starting. Women of childbearing potential must use reliable contraception.

ADULT – RA: Loading dose: 100 mg PO daily for 3 days. Maintenance dose: 10 to 20 mg PO daily.

PEDS – Not approved in children.

UNAPPROVED ADULT – Psoriatic arthritis: Initial: 100 mg PO daily for 3 days. Maintenance: 10 to 20 mg PO daily.

FORMS – Generic/Trade: Tabs 10, 20 mg. Trade only: Tabs 100 mg.

NOTES – Elimination of loading dose may reduce risk of hematologic and hepatic toxicity. Avoid in hepatic or renal insufficiency, severe immunodeficiency, bone marrow dysplasia, or severe infections. Consider interruption of therapy if serious infection occurs and administer cholestyramine (see below). Monitor LFTs, CBC, and creatinine monthly until stable, then q 1 to 2 months. Avoid in men wishing to father children or with concurrent live vaccines. May increase INR if on warfarin; check INR within 1 to 2 days of initiation, then weekly for 2 to 3 weeks and adjust the dose accordingly. Rifampin increases and cholestyramine decreases leflunomide levels. Give charcoal or cholestyramine in cases of overdose or drug toxicity. Cholestyramine: 8 g PO three times per day for up to 11 days. Activated charcoal: 50 g PO or NG q 6 h for 24 h. Administration on consecutive days is not necessary unless rapid elimination desired.

METHOTREXATE—RHEUMATOLOGY (***Rheumatrex, Trexall***) ▶LK ♀X ▶– $$

WARNING – Deaths have occurred from hepatotoxicity, pulmonary disease, intestinal perforation, and marrow suppression. According to the manufacturer, use is restricted to patients with severe, recalcitrant, disabling rheumatic disease unresponsive to other therapy. Use with extreme caution in renal insufficiency. May see diarrhea. Folate deficiency states may increase toxicity. The American College of Rheumatology recommends supplementation with 1 mg/day of folic acid.

ADULT – Severe RA, psoriasis: 7.5 mg/week PO single dose or 2.5 mg PO q 12 h for 3 doses given as a course once weekly. May be increased gradually to a max weekly dose of 20 mg. After clinical response, reduce to lowest effective dose. Psoriasis: 10 to 25 mg weekly IV/IM until response, then decrease to lowest effective dose. Supplement with 1 mg/day of folic acid. Chemotherapy doses vary by indication.

PEDS – Severe JRA: 10 mg/meters 2 PO q week. Chemotherapy doses vary by indication.

UNAPPROVED ADULT – Severe RA, psoriasis: 25 mg PO q week. After clinical response, reduce to lowest effective dose. Supplement with 1 mg/day of folic acid. Early ectopic pregnancy: 50 mg/m^2 IM single dose.

FORMS – Trade only (Trexall): Tabs 5, 7.5, 10, 15 mg. Dose Pak (Rheumatrex) 2.5 mg (# 8, 12, 16, 20, 24). Generic/Trade: Tabs 2.5 mg, scored.

NOTES – Contraindicated in pregnant and lactating women, alcoholism, liver disease, immunodeficiency, blood dyscrasias. Avoid ethanol. Monitor CBC q month, liver and renal function q 1 to 3 months.

ANALGESICS: Muscle Relaxants

NOTE: May cause drowsiness and/or sedation, which may be enhanced by alcohol and other CNS depressants.

BACLOFEN (*Lioresal, Kemstro*) ▶K ♀C ▶+ $$

WARNING – Abrupt discontinuation of intrathecal baclofen has been associated with life-threatening sequelae and/or death.

ADULT – Spasticity related to MS or spinal cord disease/injury: 5 mg PO three times per day for 3 days, 10 mg PO three times per day for 3 days, 15 mg PO three times per day for 3 days, then 20 mg PO three times per day for 3 days. Max dose: 20 mg PO four times per day. Spasticity related to spinal cord disease/injury, unresponsive to oral therapy: Specialized dosing via implantable intrathecal pump.

PEDS – Spasticity related to spinal cord disease/injury: Specialized dosing via implantable intrathecal pump.

UNAPPROVED ADULT – Trigeminal neuralgia: 30 to 80 mg/day PO divided three to four times per day. Tardive dyskinesia: 40 to 60 mg/day PO divided three to four times per day. Intractable hiccups: 15 to 45 mg PO divided three times per day.

UNAPPROVED PEDS – Spasticity age 2 yo or older: 10 to 15 mg/day PO divided q 8 h. Max doses 40 mg/day for age 2 to 7 yo, 60 mg/day for age 8 yo or older.

FORMS – Generic only: Tabs 10, 20 mg. Trade only (Kemstro): Tabs, orally disintegrating 10, 20 mg.

NOTES – Hallucinations and seizures with abrupt withdrawal. Administer with caution if impaired renal function. Efficacy not established for rheumatic disorders, CVA, cerebral palsy, or Parkinson's disease.

CARISOPRODOL (*Soma*) ▶LK ♀? ▶– $

ADULT – Acute musculoskeletal pain: 350 mg PO three to four times per day with meals and at bedtime.

PEDS – Not approved in children.

FORMS – Generic/Trade: Tabs 350 mg. Trade only: Tabs 250 mg.

NOTES – Contraindicated in porphyria, caution in renal or hepatic insufficiency. Abuse potential. Use with caution if addiction prone. Withdrawal and possible seizures with abrupt discontinuation. Sedative effects can result in impaired driving.

CHLORZOXAZONE (*Parafon Forte DSC*) ▶LK ♀C ▶? $

WARNING – If signs/symptoms of liver dysfunction are observed, discontinue use.

ADULT – Musculoskeletal pain: Start 500 mg PO three to four times per day, increase prn to 750 mg three to four times per day. After clinical improvement, decrease to 250 mg PO three to four times per day.

PEDS – Not approved in children.

UNAPPROVED PEDS – Musculoskeletal pain: 125 to 500 mg PO three to four times per day or 20 mg/kg/day divided three to four times per day depending on age and wt.

FORMS – Generic/Trade: Tabs 250, 500 mg (Parafon Forte DSC 500 mg tabs, scored).

NOTES – Use with caution in patients with history of drug allergies. Discontinue if allergic drug reactions occur or for signs/symptoms of liver dysfunction. May turn urine orange or purple-red.

CYCLOBENZAPRINE (*Amrix, Flexeril, Fexmid*) ▶LK ♀B ▶? $

ADULT – Musculoskeletal pain: 5 to 10 mg PO three times per day up to max dose of 30 mg/day or 15 to 30 mg (extended release) PO daily. Not recommended in elderly or for use longer than 2 to 3 weeks.

PEDS – Not approved in children.

FORMS – Generic/Trade: Tab 5, 10 mg. Generic only: Tabs 7.5 mg. Trade only: (Amrix $$$$$): Extended-release caps 15, 30 mg.

NOTES – Contraindicated with recent or concomitant MAOI use, immediately post MI, in patients with arrhythmias, conduction disturbances, heart failure, and hyperthyroidism. Not effective for cerebral or spinal cord disease or in children with cerebral palsy. May have similar adverse effects and drug interactions as TCAs. Caution with urinary retention, angle-closure glaucoma, increased intraocular pressure.

DANTROLENE (*Dantrium*) ▶LK ♀C ▶– $$$$

WARNING – Hepatotoxicity, monitor LFTs. Use the lowest possible effective dose.

ADULT – Chronic spasticity related to spinal cord injury, CVA, cerebral palsy, MS: 25 mg PO daily to start, increase to 25 mg two to four times per day, then by 25 mg up to max of 100 mg two to four times per day if necessary. Maintain each dosage level for 4 to 7 days to determine response. Use the lowest possible effective dose. Malignant hyperthermia: 2.5 mg/kg rapid IV push q 5 to 10 min continuing until symptoms subside or to a max 10 mg/kg. Doses of up to 40 mg/kg have been used.

(cont.)

DANTROLENE (*cont.*)

Follow with 4 to 8 mg/kg/day PO divided three to four times per day for 1 to 3 days to prevent recurrence.

PEDS – Chronic spasticity: 0.5 mg/kg PO two times per day to start; increase to 0.5 mg/kg three to four times per day, then by increments of 0.5 mg/kg up to 3 mg/kg two to four times per day. Max dose 100 mg PO four times per day. Malignant hyperthermia: Use adult dose.

UNAPPROVED ADULT – Neuroleptic malignant syndrome, heat stroke: 1 to 3 mg/kg/day PO/IV divided four times per day.

FORMS – Generic/Trade: Caps 25, 50, 100 mg.

NOTES – Photosensitization may occur. Warfarin may decrease protein binding of dantrolene and increase dantrolene's effect. Hyperkalemia and cardiovascular collapse have been reported with concomitant calcium channel blockers such as verapamil. The following website may be useful for malignant hyperthermia: www.mhaus.org.

METAXALONE (***Skelaxin***) ▸LK ♀? ▸? $$$$

ADULT – Musculoskeletal pain: 800 mg PO three to four times per day.

PEDS – Use adult dose for age older than 12 yo.

FORMS – Generic/Trade: Tabs 800 mg, scored.

NOTES – Contraindicated in serious renal or hepatic insufficiency or history of drug-induced hemolytic or other anemia. Beware of hypersensitivity reactions, leukopenia, hemolytic anemia, and jaundice. Monitor LFTs. Coadministration with food, especially a high-fat meal, enhances absorption significantly and may increase CNS depression.

METHOCARBAMOL (***Robaxin, Robaxin-750***) ▸LK ♀C ▸? $$

ADULT – Musculoskeletal pain, acute relief: 1500 mg PO four times per day or 1000 mg IM/IV three times per day for 48 to 72 h. Maintenance: 1000 mg PO four times per day, 750 mg PO q 4 h, or 1500 mg PO three times per day. Tetanus: Specialized dosing.

PEDS – Tetanus: Specialized dosing.

FORMS – Generic/Trade: Tabs 500 and 750 mg. OTC in Canada.

NOTES – Max IV rate of undiluted drug 3 mL/min to avoid syncope, hypotension, and bradycardia. Total parenteral dosage should not exceed 3 g/day for more than 3 consecutive days, except in the treatment of tetanus. Urine may turn brown, black, or green.

ORPHENADRINE (***Norflex***) ▸LK ♀C ▸? $$

ADULT – Musculoskeletal pain: 100 mg PO two times per day. 60 mg IV/IM two times per day.

PEDS – Not approved in children.

UNAPPROVED ADULT – Leg cramps: 100 mg PO at bedtime.

FORMS – Generic only: 100 mg extended-release. OTC in Canada.

NOTES – Contraindicated in glaucoma, pyloric or duodenal obstruction, BPH, and myasthenia gravis. Some products contain sulfites, which may cause allergic reactions. May increase anticholinergic effects of amantadine and decrease therapeutic effects of phenothiazines. Side effects include dry mouth, urinary retention and hesitancy, constipation, headache, and GI upset.

TIZANIDINE (***Zanaflex***) ▸LK ♀C ▸? $$$$

ADULT – Muscle spasticity due to MS or spinal cord injury: 4 to 8 mg PO q 6 to 8 h prn, max dose 36 mg/day.

PEDS – Not approved in children.

FORMS – Generic/Trade: Tabs 4 mg, scored. Trade only: Caps 2, 4, 6 mg. Generic only: Tabs 2 mg.

NOTES – Monitor LFTs. Avoid in hepatic or renal insufficiency. Alcohol, oral contraceptives, fluvoxamine, and ciprofloxacin increase tizanidine levels; may cause significant decreases in BP and increased drowsiness and psychomotor impairment. Concurrent antihypertensives may exacerbate hypotension. Dry mouth, somnolence, sedation, asthenia, and dizziness most common side effects.

ANALGESICS: Non-Opioid Analgesic Combinations

NOTE: Refer to individual components for further information. Carisoprodol and butalbital may be habit forming; butalbital contraindicated with porphyria. May cause drowsiness and/or sedation, which may be enhanced by alcohol and other CNS depressants. Avoid exceeding 4 g/day of acetaminophen in combination products. Caution people who drink 3 or more alcoholic drinks/day to limit acetaminophen use to 2.5 g/day due to additive liver toxicity.

ASCRIPTIN **(acetylsalicylic acid + aluminum hydroxide + magnesium hydroxide + calcium carbonate, *Aspir-Mox*)** ▸K ♀D ▸? $

WARNING – Multiple strengths; see FORMS.

ADULT – Pain: 1 to 2 tabs PO q 4 h.

PEDS – Not approved in children.

FORMS – OTC Trade only: Tabs 325 mg aspirin/50 mg Mg hydroxide/50 mg Al hydroxide/50

(cont.)

ASCRIPTIN *(cont.)*

mg Ca carbonate (Ascriptin and Aspir-Mox). 500 mg aspirin/33 mg Mg hydroxide/33 mg Al hydroxide/ 237 mg Ca carbonate (Ascriptin Maximum Strength).

NOTES – See NSAIDs—Salicylic Acid subclass warning.

BUFFERIN **(acetylsalicylic acid + calcium carbonate + magnesium oxide + magnesium carbonate)** ▶K ♀D ▶? $

ADULT – Pain: 1 to 2 tabs/caps PO q 4 h while symptoms persist. Max 12 in 24 h.

PEDS – Not approved in children.

FORMS – OTC Trade only: Tabs/caps 325 mg aspirin/158 mg Ca carbonate/63 mg of Mg oxide/34 mg of Mg carbonate. Bufferin ES: 500 mg aspirin/222.3 mg Ca carbonate/88.9 mg of Mg oxide/55.6 mg of Mg carbonate.

NOTES – See NSAIDs—Salicylic Acid subclass warning.

ESGIC **(acetaminophen + butalbital + caffeine)** ▶LK ♀C ▶? $

WARNING – Multiple strengths; see FORMS and write specific product on Rx.

ADULT – Tension or muscle contraction headache: 1 to 2 tabs or caps PO q 4 h. Max 6 in 24 h.

PEDS – Not approved in children.

FORMS – Generic only: Tabs/caps, 325 mg acetaminophen/50 mg butalbital/40 mg caffeine. Oral soln 325/50/40 mg per 15 mL. Generic/Trade: Tabs, Esgic Plus is 500/50/40 mg.

EXCEDRIN MIGRAINE **(acetaminophen + acetylsalicylic acid + caffeine)** ▶LK ♀D ▶? $

ADULT – Migraine headache: 2 tabs/caps/geltabs PO q 6 h while symptoms persist. Max 8 in 24 h.

PEDS – Use adult dose for age 12 yo or older.

FORMS – OTC Generic/Trade: Tabs/caps/geltabs 250 mg acetaminophen/250 mg aspirin/65 mg caffeine.

NOTES – See NSAIDs—Salicylic Acid subclass warning. Avoid concomitant use of other acetaminophen-containing products.

FIORICET **(acetaminophen + butalbital + caffeine)** ▶LK ♀C ▶? $

ADULT – Tension or muscle contraction headache: 1 to 2 tabs PO q 4 h. Max 6 in 24 h.

PEDS – Not approved in children.

FORMS – Generic/Trade: Tabs 325 mg acetaminophen/50 mg butalbital/40 mg caffeine.

FIORINAL **(acetylsalicylic acid + butalbital + caffeine,** ✤ ***Trianal*****)** ▶KL ♀D ▶–©III $

ADULT – Tension or muscle contraction headache: 1 to 2 tabs PO q 4 h. Max 6 tabs in 24 h.

PEDS – Not approved in children.

FORMS – Generic/Trade: Caps 325 mg aspirin/50 mg butalbital/40 mg caffeine.

NOTES – See NSAIDs—Salicylic Acid subclass warning.

GOODY'S EXTRA STRENGTH HEADACHE POWDER **(acetaminophen + acetylsalicylic acid + caffeine)** ▶LK ♀D ▶? $

ADULT – Headache: Place 1 powder on tongue and follow with liquid, or stir powder into a glass of water or other liquid. Repeat in 4 to 6 h prn. Max 4 powders in 24 h.

PEDS – Use adult dose for age 12 yo or older.

FORMS – OTC trade only: 260 mg acetaminophen/520 mg aspirin/32.5 mg caffeine per powder paper.

NOTES – See NSAIDs—Salicylic Acid subclass warning.

NORGESIC **(orphenadrine + acetylsalicylic acid + caffeine)** ▶KL ♀D ▶? $$

WARNING – Multiple strengths; see FORMS and write specific product on Rx.

ADULT – Musculoskeletal pain: Norgesic: 1 to 2 tabs PO three to four times per day. Norgesic Forte: 1 tab PO three to four times per day.

PEDS – Not approved in children.

FORMS – Generic/Trade: Tabs Norgesic 25 mg orphenadrine/385 mg aspirin/30 mg caffeine. Norgesic Forte 50/770/60 mg.

NOTES – See NSAIDs—Salicylic Acid subclass warning.

PHRENILIN **(acetaminophen + butalbital)** ▶LK ♀C ▶? $

WARNING – Multiple strengths; see FORMS and write specific product on Rx.

ADULT – Tension or muscle contraction headache: Phrenilin: 1 to 2 tabs PO q 4 h. Phrenilin Forte: 1 cap PO q 4 h. Max 6 in 24 h.

PEDS – Not approved in children.

FORMS – Generic/Trade: Tabs, Phrenilin 325 mg acetaminophen/50 mg butalbital. Caps, Phrenilin Forte 650/50 mg.

SEDAPAP **(acetaminophen + butalbital)** ▶LK ♀C ▶? $

ADULT – Tension or muscle contraction headache: 1 to 2 tabs PO q 4 h. Max 6 tabs in 24 h.

PEDS – Not approved in children.

FORMS – Generic only: Tabs 650 mg acetaminophen/50 mg butalbital.

SOMA COMPOUND **(carisoprodol + acetylsalicylic acid)** ▶LK ♀D ▶– $$$

ADULT – Musculoskeletal pain: 1 to 2 tabs PO four times per day.

PEDS – Not approved in children.

FORMS – Generic/Trade: Tabs 200 mg carisoprodol/325 mg aspirin.

(cont.)

SOMA COMPOUND *(cont.)*

NOTES – See NSAIDs—Salicylic Acid subclass warning. Carisoprodol may be habit forming. Withdrawal with abrupt discontinuation.

ULTRACET **(tramadol + acetaminophen, ✤ *Tramacet*)** ▶KL ♀C ▶– $$

ADULT – Acute pain: 2 tabs PO q 4 to 6 h prn, (up to 8 tabs/day for no more than 5 days). If CrCl is less than 30 mL/min, increase the dosing interval to 12 h. Consider a similar adjustment in elderly patients and in cirrhosis.

PEDS – Not approved in children.

FORMS – Generic/Trade: Tabs 37.5 mg tramadol/ 325 mg acetaminophen.

NOTES – Do not use with other acetaminophen-containing drugs due to potential for hepatotoxicity. Contraindicated in acute intoxication with alcohol, hypnotics, centrally acting analgesics, opioids, or psychotropic drugs. Seizures may occur with concurrent antidepressants or with seizure disorder. Use with great caution with MAOIs or in combination with SSRIs due to potential for serotonin syndrome; dose adjustment may be needed. Withdrawal symptoms may occur in patients dependent on opioids or with abrupt discontinuation. Overdose treated with naloxone may increase seizure risk. The most frequent side effects are somnolence and constipation.

ANALGESICS: Non-Steroidal Anti-Inflammatories—COX-2 Inhibitors

NOTE: The risk of serious cardiovascular events and GI bleeding may be increased in patients taking long-term, high-dose NSAIDs, both COX-2 inhibitors as well as non selective agents. All NSAIDs and COX-2 inhibitors are contraindicated immediately post-CABG surgery. The FDA advises evaluating alternative therapy or using the lowest effective dose of these drugs. Fewer GI side effects than 1st-generation NSAIDs and no effect on platelets, but other NSAID-related side effects (renal dysfunction, fluid retention, CNS) are possible. May cause fluid retention or exacerbate heart failure. May elevate BP or blunt effects of antihypertensives and loop diuretics. Not substitutes for aspirin for cardiovascular prophylaxis due to lack of antiplatelet effects. Monitor INR with warfarin. May increase lithium levels. Caution in aspirin-sensitive asthma. Use around the time of conception appears to increase the risk of miscarriage (use acetaminophen instead).

CELECOXIB (***Celebrex***) ▶L ♀C (D in 3rd trimester) ▶? $$$$$

WARNING – Increases the risk of serious cardiovascular events and GI bleeding. Contraindicated immediately post-CABG surgery.

ADULT – OA, ankylosing spondylitis: 200 mg PO daily or 100 mg PO two times per day. RA: 100 to 200 mg PO two times per day. Familial adenomatous polyposis (FAP), as an adjunct to usual care: 400 mg PO two times per day with food. Acute pain, dysmenorrhea: 400 mg once, then 200 mg PO two times per day. May take an additional 200 mg on day 1.

PEDS – JRA: Give 50 mg PO two times per day for age 2 to 17 yo and wt 10 to 25 kg, give 100 mg PO two times per day for wt greater than 25 kg.

FORMS – Trade only: Caps 50, 100, 200, 400 mg.

NOTES – Contraindicated in sulfonamide allergy. Decrease dose by 50% in hepatic dysfunction. Caps may be opened and sprinkled into 1 teaspoon of apple sauce and taken immediately with water. Drugs that inhibit CYP2C9, such as fluconazole, increase concentrations. Lithium concentrations increased.

ANALGESICS: Non-Steroidal Anti-Inflammatories—Salicylic Acid Derivatives

NOTE: The risk of serious cardiovascular events and GI bleeding may be increased in patients taking long-term, high-dose NSAIDs, COX-2 inhibitors, and nonselective agents (excluding aspirin). All NSAIDs and COX-2 inhibitors are contraindicated immediately post-CABG surgery. The FDA advises evaluating alternative therapy or using the lowest effective dose of these drugs. Avoid in aspirin allergy and in children younger than 17 yo with chickenpox or flu due to association with Reye's syndrome. May potentiate warfarin, heparin, valproic acid, methotrexate. Unlike aspirin, derivatives may have less GI toxicity and negligible effects on platelet aggregation and renal prostaglandins. Caution in aspirin-sensitive asthma. Ibuprofen and possibly other NSAIDs may antagonize antiplatelet effects of aspirin if given simultaneously. Use around the time of conception appears to increase the risk of miscarriage (use acetaminophen instead).

ACETYLSALICYLIC ACID (*Ecotrin, Empirin, Halfprin, Bayer, Anacin, ZORprin, Aspirin,* ✤ *Asaphen, Entrophen, Novasen*) ▶K ♀D ▶? $

ADULT – Mild to moderate pain, fever: 325 to 650 mg PO/PR q 4 h prn. Acute rheumatic fever: 5 to 8 g/day, initially. RA/OA: 3.2 to 6 g/day in divided doses. Platelet aggregation inhibition: 81 to 325 mg PO daily.

PEDS – Mild to moderate pain, fever: 10 to 15 mg/kg/dose PO q 4 to 6 h not to exceed 60 to 80 mg/kg/day. JRA: 60 to 100 mg/kg/day PO divided q 6 to 8 h. Acute rheumatic fever: 100 mg/kg/day PO/PR for 2 weeks, then 75 mg/kg/day for 4 to 6 weeks. Kawasaki disease: 80 to 100 mg/kg/day divided four times per day PO/PR until fever resolves, then 3 to 5 mg/kg/day PO q am for 7 weeks or longer if there is ECG evidence of coronary artery abnormalities.

UNAPPROVED ADULT – Primary prevention of cardiovascular events (10-year CHD risk more than 6 to 10% based on Framingham risk scoring): 75 to 325 mg PO daily. Post ST-elevation MI: 162 to 325 mg PO on day 1, continue indefinitely at 75 to 162 mg/day. Post non-ST-elevation MI: 162 to 325 mg PO on day 1, continue indefinitely at 75 to 162 mg/day. Long-term antithrombotic therapy for chronic atrial fib/flutter in patients with low to moderate risk of CVA (age younger than 75 yo without risk factors): 325 mg PO daily. Percutaneous coronary intervention pretreatment: Already taking daily aspirin therapy: 75 to 325 mg PO before procedure. Not already taking daily aspirin therapy: 300 to 325 mg PO at least 2 to 24 h before procedure. Post-percutaneous coronary intervention: 325 mg daily in combination with clopidogrel for at least 1 month after bare metal stent placement, at least 3 to 6 months after drug-eluting stent placement; then 75 to 162 mg PO daily indefinitely. Post-percutaneous coronary brachytherapy: 75 to 325 mg daily in combination with clopidogrel indefinitely.

FORMS – Generic/Trade (OTC): Tabs, 325, 500 mg; chewable 81 mg; enteric-coated 81, 162 mg (Halfprin), 81, 325, 500 mg (Ecotrin), 650, 975 mg. Trade only: Tabs, controlled-release 650, 800 mg (ZORprin, Rx). Generic only (OTC): Supps 60, 120, 200, 300, 600 mg.

NOTES – Consider discontinuation 1 week prior to surgery (except coronary bypass or in 1st year post-coronary stent implantation) because of the possibility of postop bleeding. Aspirin intolerance occurs in 4 to 19% of asthmatics. Use caution in liver damage, renal insufficiency, peptic ulcer, or bleeding tendencies. Crush or chew tabs (including enteric-coated products) in 1st dose with acute MI. Higher doses of aspirin (1.3 g/day) have not been shown to be superior to low doses in preventing TIAs and CVAs.

CHOLINE MAGNESIUM TRISALICYLATE (*Trilisate*) ▶K ♀C (D in 3rd trimester) ▶? $$

ADULT – RA/OA: 1500 mg PO two times per day. Mild to moderate pain, fever: 1000 to 1500 mg PO two times per day.

PEDS – RA, mild to moderate pain: 50 mg/kg/day (up to 37 kg) PO divided two times per day.

FORMS – Generic only: Tabs 500, 750, 1000 mg. Soln 500 mg/5 mL.

DIFLUNISAL (*Dolobid*) ▶K ♀C (D in 3rd trimester) ▶– $$$

ADULT – Mild to moderate pain: Initially: 500 mg to 1 g PO, then 250 to 500 mg PO q 8 to 12 h. RA/OA: 500 mg to 1 g PO divided two times per day. Max dose 1.5 g/day.

PEDS – Not approved in children.

FORMS – Generic/Trade: Tabs 250, 500 mg.

NOTES – Do not crush or chew tabs. Increases acetaminophen levels.

SALSALATE (*Salflex, Disalcid, Amigesic*) ▶K ♀C (D in 3rd trimester) ▶? $$

ADULT – RA/OA: 3000 mg/day PO divided q 8 to 12 h.

PEDS – Not approved in children.

FORMS – Generic only: Tabs 500, 750 mg, scored.

ANALGESICS: Non-Steroidal Anti-Inflammatories—Other

NOTE: The risk of serious cardiovascular events and GI bleeding may be increased in patients taking long-term, high-dose NSAIDs, both COX-2 inhibitors as well as non selective agents. All NSAIDs and COX-2 inhibitors are contraindicated immediately post-CABG surgery. The FDA advises evaluating alternative therapy or using the lowest effective dose of these drugs. Chronic use associated with renal insufficiency, gastritis, peptic ulcer disease, GI bleeds. Caution in liver disease. May cause fluid retention or exacerbate heart failure. May elevate BP or blunt effects of antihypertensives and loop diuretics. May increase levels of methotrexate, lithium, phenytoin, digoxin, and cyclosporine. May potentiate warfarin. Caution in aspirin-sensitive asthma. Ibuprofen or other NSAIDs may antagonize antiplatelet effects of aspirin if given simultaneously. Use around the time of conception appears to increase the risk of miscarriage (use acetaminophen instead).

ARTHROTEC **(diclofenac + misoprostol)** ▶LK ♀X ▶– $$$$$

WARNING – Because of the abortifacient property of the misoprostol component, it is contraindicated in women who are pregnant. Caution in women with childbearing potential; effective contraception is essential.

ADULT – OA: One 50/200 tab PO three times per day. RA: One 50/200 tab PO three to four times per day. If intolerant, may use 50/200 or 75/200 tabs PO two times per day.

PEDS – Not approved in children.

FORMS – Trade only: Tabs 50 mg/200 mcg, 75 mg/200 mcg, diclofenac/misoprostol.

NOTES – Refer to individual components. Abdominal pain and diarrhea may occur. Check LFTs at baseline, within 4 to 8 weeks of initiation, then periodically. Do not crush or chew tabs.

DICLOFENAC (***Voltaren, Voltaren XR, Cataflam, Flector, Zipsor, Cambia,*** ✤ ***Voltaren Rapide***) ▶L ♀B (D in 3rd trimester) ▶– $$$

WARNING – Multiple strengths; see FORMS and write specific product on Rx.

ADULT – OA: Immediate- or delayed-release 50 mg PO two to three times per day or 75 mg two times per day. Extended-release 100 mg PO daily. Gel: Apply 4 g to knees or 2 g to hands four times per day using enclosed dosing card. RA: Immediate- or delayed-release 50 mg PO three to four times per day or 75 mg two times per day. Extended-release 100 mg PO one to two times per day. Ankylosing spondylitis: Immediate- or delayed-release 25 mg PO four times per day and at bedtime. Analgesia and primary dysmenorrhea: Immediate- or delayed-release 50 mg PO three times per day. Acute pain of strains, sprains, or contusions: Apply 1 patch to painful area two times per day. Acute migraine with or without aura: 50 mg single dose (Cambia), mix packet with 30 to 60 mL water.

PEDS – Not approved in children.

UNAPPROVED PEDS – JRA: 2 to 3 mg/kg/day PO.

FORMS – Generic/Trade: Tabs, immediate-release (Cataflam) 50 mg, extended-release (Voltaren XR) 100 mg. Generic only: Tabs, delayed-release 25, 50, 75 mg. Trade only: Patch (Flector) 1.3% diclofenac epolamine. Topical gel (Voltaren) 1% 100 g tube. Trade only: Caps, liquid-filled (Zipsor) 25 mg. Trade only: Powder for oral soln (Cambia) 50 mg.

NOTES – Check LFTs at baseline, within 4 to 8 weeks of initiation, then periodically. Do not apply patch to damaged or non-intact skin. Wash hands and avoid eye contact when handling the patch. Do not wear patch while bathing or showering.

ETODOLAC ▶L ♀C (D in 3rd trimester) ▶– $$$

WARNING – Multiple strengths; write specific product on Rx.

ADULT – OA: 400 mg PO two to three times per day. 300 mg PO two to three times per day. 200 mg three to four times per day. Extended release 400 to 1200 mg PO daily. Mild to moderate pain: 200 to 400 mg q 6 to 8 h. (Up to 1200 mg/day or if wt 60 kg or less, 20 mg/kg/day).

PEDS – Not approved in children.

UNAPPROVED ADULT – RA, ankylosing spondylitis: 300 to 400 mg PO two times per day. Tendinitis, bursitis, and acute gout: 300 to 400 mg PO two to four times per day then taper.

FORMS – Generic only: Caps immediate-release 200, 300 mg, Tabs immediate-release 400, 500 mg, Tabs extended-release 400, 500, 600 mg.

NOTES – Brand name Lodine no longer marketed.

FENOPROFEN (***Nalfon***) ▶L ♀C (D in 3rd trimester) ▶- $

WARNING – Appears to represent a greater nephrotoxicity risk than other NSAIDs.

ADULT – RA/OA: 300 to 600 mg PO three to four times per day. Max dose: 3200 mg/day. Mild to moderate pain: 200 mg PO q 4 to 6 h prn.

PEDS – Not approved in children.

FORMS – Generic/Trade: Caps 200 and 300 mg. Generic only: Tab 600 mg.

FLURBIPROFEN (***Ansaid***) ▶L ♀B (D in 3rd trimester) ▶+ $$$

ADULT – RA/OA: 200 to 300 mg/day PO divided two to four times per day. Max single dose 100 mg.

PEDS – Not approved in children.

UNAPPROVED ADULT – Ankylosing spondylitis: 150 to 300 mg/day PO divided two to four times per day. Mild to moderate pain: 50 mg PO q 6 h. Primary dysmenorrhea: 50 mg PO daily at onset, discontinue when pain subsides. Tendinitis, bursitis, acute gout, acute migraine: 100 mg PO at onset, then 50 mg PO four times per day, then taper.

UNAPPROVED PEDS – JRA: 4 mg/kg/day PO.

FORMS – Generic/Trade: Tabs immediate-release 50, 100 mg.

IBUPROFEN (***Motrin, Advil, Nuprin, Rufen, NeoProfen, Caldolor***) ▶L ♀B (D in 3rd trimester) ▶+ $

ADULT – RA/OA, gout: 200 to 800 mg PO three to four times per day. Mild to moderate pain: 400 mg PO q 4 to 6 h. 400 to 800 mg IV

(cont.)

IBUPROFEN (*cont.*)

(Caldolor) q 6 h prn. 400 mg IV (Caldolor) q 4 to 6 h or 100 to 200 mg q 4 h prn. Primary dysmenorrhea: 400 mg PO q 4 h prn. Fever: 200 mg PO q 4 to 6 h prn. Migraine pain: 200 to 400 mg PO not to exceed 400 mg in 24 h unless directed by a physician (OTC dosing). Max dose 3.2 g/day.

PEDS – JRA: 30 to 50 mg/kg/day PO divided q 6 h. Max dose 2400 mg/24 h. 20 mg/kg/day may be adequate for milder disease. Analgesic/antipyretic age older than 6 mo: 5 to 10 mg/kg PO q 6 to 8 h, prn. Max dose 40 mg/kg/day. Patent ductus arteriosus in neonates age 32 weeks gestational age or younger weighing 500 to 1500 g (NeoProfen): Specialized dosing.

FORMS – OTC: Caps/Liqui-Gel Caps 200 mg. Tabs 100, 200 mg. Chewable tabs 50, 100 mg. Susp (infant gtts) 50 mg/1.25 mL (with calibrated dropper), 100 mg/5 mL. Rx Generic/Trade: Tabs 300, 400, 600, 800 mg. Vials: 400 mg/4 mL or 800 mg/8 mL.

NOTES – May antagonize antiplatelet effects of aspirin if given simultaneously. Take aspirin 2 h prior to ibuprofen. Administer IV (Caldolor) over at least 30 min; hydration important.

INDOMETHACIN (***Indocin, Indocin SR, Indocin IV,*** ✤ ***Indocid-P.D.A.***) ▶L ♀B (D in 3rd trimester) ◗+ $

WARNING – Multiple strengths; see FORMS and write specific product on Rx. Use during labor increases risk of fetal and maternal complications: premature closure of the ductus arteriosus, fetal pulmonary HTN, oligohydramnios, higher rate of postpartum hemorrhage.

ADULT – RA/OA, ankylosing spondylitis: 25 mg PO two to three times per day to start. Increase incrementally to a total daily dose of 150 to 200 mg. Bursitis/tendinitis: 75 to 150 mg/day PO divided three to four times per day. Acute gout: 50 mg PO three times per day until pain tolerable, rapidly taper dose to discontinue. Sustained-release: 75 mg PO one to two times per day.

PEDS – Closure of patent ductus arteriosus in neonates: Initial dose 0.2 mg/kg IV, if additional doses necessary, dose and frequency (q 12 h or q 24 h) based on neonate's age and urine output.

UNAPPROVED ADULT – Primary dysmenorrhea: 25 mg PO three to four times per day. Cluster headache: 75 to 150 mg SR PO daily. Polyhydramnios: 2.2 to 3 mg/kg/day PO based on maternal wt; premature closure of the ductus arteriosus has been reported. Preterm labor: Initial 50 to 100 mg PO followed by 25 mg PO q 6 to 12 h up to 48 h.

UNAPPROVED PEDS – JRA: 1 to 3 mg/kg/day three to four times per day to start. Increase prn to max dose of 4 mg/kg/day or 200 mg/day, whichever is less.

FORMS – Generic/Trade: Caps, sustained-release 75 mg. Generic only: Caps, immediate-release 25, 50 mg. Suppository 50 mg. Trade only: Oral susp 25 mg/5 mL (237 mL)

NOTES – May aggravate depression or other psychiatric disturbances. Do not crush sustained-release cap.

KETOPROFEN (***Orudis, Orudis KT, Actron, Oruvail,*** ✤ ***Orudis SR***) ▶L ♀B (D in 3rd trimester) ◗– $$$

ADULT – RA/OA: 75 mg PO three times per day or 50 mg PO four times per day. Extended-release 200 mg PO daily. Mild to moderate pain, primary dysmenorrhea: 25 to 50 mg PO q 6 to 8 h prn.

PEDS – Not approved in children.

UNAPPROVED PEDS – JRA: 100 to 200 mg/m²/day PO. Max dose 320 mg/day.

FORMS – OTC: Tabs, immediate-release 12.5 mg. Rx Generic only: Caps, extended-release 100, 150, 200 mg. Caps, immediate-release 25, 50, 75 mg.

KETOROLAC (***Toradol***) ▶L ♀C (D in 3rd trimester) ◗+ $

WARNING – Indicated for short-term (up to 5 days) therapy only. Ketorolac is a potent NSAID and can cause serious GI and renal adverse effects. It may also increase the risk of bleeding by inhibiting platelet function. Contraindicated in patients with active peptic ulcer disease, recent GI bleeding or perforation, a history of peptic ulcer disease or GI bleeding, or advanced renal impairment.

ADULT – Moderately severe, acute pain, single-dose treatment: 30 to 60 mg IM or 15 to 30 mg IV. Multiple-dose treatment: 15 to 30 mg IV/IM q 6 h. IV/IM doses are not to exceed 60 mg/day for age 65 yo or older, wt less than 50 kg, and patients with moderately elevated serum creatinine. Oral continuation therapy: 10 mg PO q 4 to 6 h prn, max dose 40 mg/day. Combined duration IV/IM and PO is not to exceed 5 days.

PEDS – Not approved in children.

UNAPPROVED PEDS – Pain: 0.5 mg/kg/dose IM/IV q 6 h (up to 30 mg q 6 h or 120 mg/day), give 10 mg PO q 6 h prn (up to 40 mg/day) for wt greater than 50 kg.

FORMS – Generic only: Tabs 10 mg.

MECLOFENAMATE ▶L ♀B (D in 3rd trimester) ▶– $$$

ADULT – Mild to moderate pain: 50 mg PO q 4 to 6 h prn. Max dose 400 mg/day. Menorrhagia and primary dysmenorrhea: 100 mg PO three times per day for up to 6 days. RA/OA: 200 to 400 mg/day PO divided three to four times per day.

PEDS – Not approved in children.

UNAPPROVED PEDS – JRA: 3 to 7.5 mg/kg/day PO. Max dose 300 mg/day.

FORMS – Generic only: Caps 50, 100 mg.

NOTES – Reversible autoimmune hemolytic anemia with use for longer than 12 months.

MEFENAMIC ACID (***Ponstel, ✤Ponstan***) ▶L ♀D ▶– $$$$$

ADULT – Mild to moderate pain, primary dysmenorrhea: 500 mg PO initially, then 250 mg PO q 6 h prn for up to 1 week.

PEDS – Use adult dose for age older than 14 yo.

FORMS – Trade only: Caps 250 mg.

MELOXICAM (***Mobic, ✤Mobicox***) ▶L ♀C (D in 3rd trimester) ▶? $

ADULT – RA/OA: 7.5 mg PO daily. Max dose 15 mg/day.

PEDS – JRA age 2 yo or older: 0.125 mg/kg PO daily to max of 7.5 mg.

FORMS – Generic/Trade: Tabs 7.5, 15 mg. Susp 7.5 mg/5 mL (1.5 mg/mL).

NOTES – Shake susp gently before using. This is not a selective COX-2 inhibitor.

NABUMETONE (***Relafen***) ▶L ♀C (D in 3rd trimester) ▶– $$$

ADULT – RA/OA: Initial: Two 500 mg tabs (1000 mg) PO daily. May increase to 1500 to 2000 mg PO daily or divided two times per day. Dosages greater than 2000 mg/day have not been studied.

PEDS – Not approved in children.

FORMS – Generic only: Tabs 500, 750 mg.

NAPROXEN (***Naprosyn, Aleve, Anaprox, EC-Naprosyn, Naprelan, Prevacid, NapraPac***) ▶L ♀B (D in 3rd trimester) ▶+ $$$

WARNING – Multiple strengths; see FORMS and write specific product on Rx.

ADULT – RA/OA, ankylosing spondylitis, pain, dysmenorrhea, acute tendinitis and bursitis, fever: 250 to 500 mg PO two times per day. Delayed-release: 375 to 500 mg PO two times per day (do not crush or chew). Controlled-release: 750 to 1000 mg PO daily. Acute gout: 750 mg PO once, then 250 mg PO q 8 h until the attack subsides. Controlled-release: 1000 to 1500 mg PO once, then 1000 mg PO daily until the attack subsides.

PEDS – JRA: 10 to 20 mg/kg/day PO divided two times per day (up to 1250 mg/24 h). Pain for age older than 2 yo: 5 to 7 mg/kg/dose PO q 8 to 12 h.

UNAPPROVED ADULT – Acute migraine: 750 mg PO once, then 250 to 500 mg PO prn. Migraine prophylaxis, menstrual migraine: 500 mg PO two times per day beginning 1 day prior to onset of menses and ending on last day of period.

FORMS – OTC Generic/Trade (Aleve): Tabs immediate-release 200 mg. OTC Trade only (Aleve): Caps, Gelcaps immediate-release 200 mg. Rx Generic/Trade: Tabs immediate-release (Naprosyn) 250, 375, 500 mg, (Anaprox) 275, 550 mg. Tabs delayed-release enteric-coated (EC-Naprosyn) 375, 500 mg. Tabs, controlled-release (Naprelan) 375, 500, 750 mg. Susp (Naprosyn) 125 mg/5 mL. Prevacid NapraPac: 7 lansoprazole 15 mg caps packaged with 14 naproxen tabs 375 mg or 500 mg.

NOTES – All dosing is based on naproxen content; 500 mg naproxen is equivalent to 550 mg naproxen sodium.

OXAPROZIN (***Daypro***) ▶L ♀C (D in 3rd trimester) ▶– $$$

ADULT – RA/OA: 1200 mg PO daily. Max dose 1800 mg/day or 26 mg/kg/day, whichever is lower.

PEDS – Not approved in children.

FORMS – Generic/Trade: Tabs 600 mg, trade scored.

PIROXICAM (***Feldene, Fexicam***) ▶L ♀B (D in 3rd trimester) ▶+ $$$

ADULT – RA/OA: 20 mg PO daily or divided two times per day.

PEDS – Not approved in children.

UNAPPROVED ADULT – Primary dysmenorrhea: 20 to 40 mg PO daily for 3 days.

FORMS – Generic/Trade: Caps 10, 20 mg.

SULINDAC (***Clinoril***) ▶L ♀B (D in 3rd trimester) ▶– $$$

ADULT – RA/OA, ankylosing spondylitis: 150 mg PO two times per day. Bursitis, tendinitis, acute gout: 200 mg PO two times per day, decrease after response. Max dose: 400 mg/day.

PEDS – Not approved in children.

UNAPPROVED PEDS – JRA: 4 mg/kg/day PO divided two times per day.

FORMS – Generic/Trade: Tabs 200 mg. Generic only: Tabs 150 mg.

NOTES – Sulindac-associated pancreatitis and a potentially fatal hypersensitivity syndrome have occurred.

TIAPROFENIC ACID (***✤Surgam, Surgam SR***) ▶K ♀C (D in 3rd trimester) ▶– $$

ADULT – No longer manufactured in United States. Canada only. RA or OA: 600 mg PO daily of sustained release, or 300 mg PO two

(cont.)

TIAPROFENIC ACID (*cont.*)

times per day of regular release. Some OA patients may be maintained on 300 mg/day.

PEDS – Not approved in children.

FORMS – Generic/Trade: Tabs 300 mg. Trade only: Caps, sustained-release 300 mg. Generic only: Tabs 200 mg.

NOTES – No longer manufactured in United States. Caution in renal insufficiency. Cystitis has been reported more frequently than with other NSAIDs.

TOLMETIN (***Tolectin***) ▶L ♀C (D in 3rd trimester) ▶+ $$$$

ADULT – RA/OA: 400 mg PO three times per day to start. Range 600 to 1800 mg/day PO divided three times per day.

PEDS – JRA age 2 yo or older: 20 mg/kg/day PO divided three to four times per day to start. Range 15 to 30 mg/kg/day divided three to four times per day. Max dose 2 g/24 h.

UNAPPROVED PEDS – Pain age 2 yo or older: 5 to 7 mg/kg/dose PO q 6 to 8 h. Max dose 2 g/24 h.

FORMS – Generic/Trade: Tabs 200 (trade scored), 600 mg. Caps 400 mg.

NOTES – Rare anaphylaxis.

ANALGESICS: Opioid Agonist-Antagonists

NOTE: May cause drowsiness and/or sedation, which may be enhanced by alcohol and other CNS depressants. Opioid agonist-antagonists may result in inadequate pain control and/or withdrawal effects in the opioid-dependent. Reserve IM for when alternative routes are not feasible.

BUPRENORPHINE (***Buprenex, Butrans, Subutex***) ▶L ♀C ▶– ©III $ IV, $$$$$ SL

ADULT – Moderate to severe pain: 0.3 to 0.6 mg IM or slow IV, q 6 h prn. Max single dose 0.6 mg. Treatment of opioid dependence: Induction 8 mg SL on day 1, 16 mg SL on day 2. Maintenance: 16 mg SL daily. Can individualize to range of 4 to 24 mg SL daily. Moderate to severe chronic pain: 5 to 20 mcg/h patch changed q 7 days.

PEDS – Moderate to severe pain: 2 to 12 yo: 2 to 6 mcg/kg/dose IM or slow IV q 4 to 6 h. Max single dose 6 mcg/kg. Patch not approved for use in children.

FORMS – Generic/Trade (Subutex): SL Tabs 2, 8 mg. Trade only (Butrans): transdermal patches 5, 10, 20 mcg/h.

NOTES – May cause bradycardia, hypotension, and respiratory depression. Concurrent use with diazepam has resulted in respiratory and cardiovascular collapse. For opioid dependence Subutex is preferred over Suboxone for induction. Suboxone preferred for maintenance. Prescribers must complete training and apply for special DEA number. See www.suboxone.com.

BUTORPHANOL (***Stadol, Stadol NS***) ▶LK ♀C ▶+ ©IV $$$

WARNING – Approved as a nasal spray in 1991 and has been promoted as a safe treatment for migraine headaches. There have been numerous reports of dependence addiction and major psychological disturbances. These problems have been documented by the FDA. Stadol NS should be used for patients with infrequent but severe migraine attacks for whom all other common abortive treatments have failed. Experts recommend restriction to no more than 2 bottles (30 sprays) per month in patients who are appropriate candidates for this medication.

ADULT – Pain, including postop pain: 0.5 to 2 mg IV q 3 to 4 h prn. 1 to 4 mg IM q 3 to 4 h prn. Obstetric pain during labor: 1 to 2 mg IV/IM at full term in early labor, repeat after 4 h. Last resort for migraine pain: 1 mg nasal spray (1 spray in 1 nostril). If no pain relief in 60 to 90 min, may give a 2nd spray in the other nostril. Additional doses q 3 to 4 h prn.

PEDS – Not approved in children.

FORMS – Generic only: Nasal spray 1 mg/spray, 2.5 mL bottle (14 to 15 doses/bottle).

NOTES – May increase cardiac workload.

NALBUPHINE (***Nubain***) ▶LK ♀? ▶? $

ADULT – Moderate to severe pain: 10 to 20 mg SC/IM/IV q 3 to 6 h prn. Max dose 160 mg/day.

PEDS – Not approved in children.

PENTAZOCINE (***Talwin NX***) ▶LK ♀C ▶? ©IV $$$

WARNING – The oral form (Talwin NX) may cause fatal reactions if injected.

ADULT – Moderate to severe pain: Talwin: 30 mg IM/IV q 3 to 4 h prn, max dose 360 mg/day. Talwin NX: 1 tab PO q 3 to 4 h, max 12 tabs/day.

PEDS – Not approved in children.

FORMS – Generic/Trade: Tabs 50 mg with 0.5 mg naloxone, trade scored.

NOTES – Rotate injection sites. Can cause hallucinations, disorientation, and seizures. Concomitant sibutramine may precipitate serotonin syndrome.

ANALGESICS: Opioid Agonists

NOTE: May cause life-threatening respiratory depression. May cause drowsiness and/or sedation, which may be enhanced by alcohol and other CNS depressants. Patients with chronic pain may require more frequent and higher dosing. Opioids commonly cause constipation. All opioids are pregnancy class D if used for prolonged periods or in high doses at term.

CODEINE (♣ *Onsolis, Abstra*) ▶LK ♀C ▶–©II $$

WARNING – Do not use IV in children due to large histamine-release and cardiovascular effects. Use in nursing mothers has led to infant death.

ADULT – Mild to moderate pain: 15 to 60 mg PO/IM/IV/SC q 4 to 6 h. Max dose 360 mg in 24 h. Antitussive: 10 to 20 mg PO q 4 to 6 h prn. Max dose 120 mg in 24 h.

PEDS – Mild to moderate pain in age 1 yo or older: 0.5 to 1 mg/kg PO/SC/IM q 4 to 6 h, max dose 60 mg/dose. Antitussive: Give 2.5 to 5 mg PO q 4 to 6 h prn (up to 30 mg/day) for age 2 to 5 yo, give 5 to 10 mg PO q 4 to 6 h prn (up to 60 mg/day) for age 6 to 12 yo.

FORMS – Generic only: Tabs 15, 30, 60 mg. Oral soln: 15 mg/5 mL.

FENTANYL (*Duragesic, Actiq, Fentora, Sublimaze, IONSYS, Abstral, Subsys, Lazanda*) ▶L ♀C ▶+©II $$$$$

WARNING – Duragesic patches, Actiq, Fentora, Abstral, Subsys, and Lazanda are contraindicated in the management of acute or postop pain due to potentially life-threatening respiratory depression in opioid non-tolerant patients. Instruct patients and their caregivers that even used patches/lozenges on a stick can be fatal to a child or pet. Dispose via toilet. Actiq and Fentora are not interchangeable. IONSYS: For hospital use only; remove prior to discharge. Can cause life-threatening respiratory depression.

ADULT – Duragesic patches: Chronic pain: 12 to 100 mcg/h patch q 72 h. Titrate dose to the needs of the patient. Some patients require q 48 h dosing. May wear more than 1 patch to achieve the correct analgesic effect. Actiq: Breakthrough cancer pain: 200 to 1600 mcg sucked over 15 min, if 200 mcg ineffective for 6 units use higher strength. Goal is 4 lozenges on a stick/day in conjunction with long-acting opioid. Buccal tab (Fentora) for breakthrough cancer pain: 100 to 800 mcg, titrated to pain relief; may repeat once after 30 min during single episode of breakthrough pain. See prescribing information for dose conversion from transmucosal lozenges. Buccal soluble film (Onsolis) for breakthrough cancer pain: 200 to 1200 mcg, titrated to pain relief; no more than 4 doses/day separated by at least 2 h. Postop analgesia: 50 to 100 mcg IM; repeat in 1 to 2 h prn. Sublingual tab (Abstral) for breakthrough cancer pain: 100 mcg, may repeat once after 30 minutes. Specialized titration. Sublingual spray (Subsys) for breakthrough cancer pain: 100 mcg, may repeat once after 30 minutes. Specialized titration. Nasal spray (Lazanda) for breakthrough cancer pain: 100 mcg. Specialized titration. IONSYS: Acute postop pain: Specialized dosing.

PEDS – Transdermal (Duragesic): Not approved in children younger than 2 yo or in opioid-naive. Use adult dosing for age older than 2 yo. Children converting to a 25 mcg patch should be receiving 45 mg or more oral morphine equivalents/day. Actiq: Not approved for age younger than 16 yo. IONSYS not approved in children. Abstral, Subsys, and Lazanda: Not approved for age younger than 18.

UNAPPROVED ADULT – Analgesia/procedural sedation: 50 to 100 mcg slow IV over 1 to 2 min; carefully titrate to effect. Analgesia: 50 to 100 mcg IM q 1 to 2 h prn.

UNAPPROVED PEDS – Analgesia: 1 to 2 mcg/kg/dose IV/IM q 30 to 60 min prn or continuous IV infusion 1 to 3 mcg/kg/h (not to exceed adult dosing). Procedural sedation: 2 to 3 mcg/kg/dose for age 1 to 3 yo; 1 to 2 mcg/kg/dose for age 3 to 12 yo, 0.5 to 1 mcg/kg/dose (not to exceed adult dosing) for age older than 12 yo, procedural sedation doses may be repeated q 30 to 60 min prn.

FORMS – Generic/Trade: Transdermal patches 12, 25, 50, 75, 100 mcg/h. Actiq lozenges on a stick, berry flavored 200, 400, 600, 800, 1200, 1600 mcg. Trade only: IONSYS: Iontophoretic transdermal system: 40 mcg fentanyl per activation; max 6 doses/h. Max per system is eighty 40 mcg doses over 24 h. Trade only: (Fentora) buccal tab 100, 200, 300, 400, 600, 800 mcg. Trade only: (Onsolis) buccal soluble film 200, 400, 600, 800, 1200 mcg in child-resistant, protective foil. Trade only: (Abstral) sublingual tab: 100, 200, 300, 400, 600, 800 mcg, packs of 12 or 32 (32 only for 600 and 800 mcg) . Trade only: (Subsys) sublingual spray: 100, 200, 400, 600, 800 mcg blister packs in cartons of 6, 14, and 28. Trade only: (Lazanda) nasal spray: 100, 400 mcg/spray, 8 sprays/bottle, cartons of 1 or 4.

(cont.)

FENTANYL (*cont.*)

NOTES – Do not use patches for acute pain or in opioid-naive patients. Oral transmucosal fentanyl doses of 5 mcg/kg provide effects similar to 0.75 to 1.25 mcg/kg of fentanyl IM. Lozenges on a stick should be sucked, not chewed. Flush lozenge remnants (without stick) down the toilet. For transdermal systems: Apply patch to non-hairy skin. Clip (not shave) hair if you have to apply to hairy area. Fever or external heat sources may increase fentanyl released from patch. Patch should be removed prior to MRI and reapplied after the test. Dispose of a used patch by folding with the adhesive side of the patch adhering to itself, then flush it down the toilet immediately. Do not cut the patch in half. For Duragesic patches and Actiq lozenges on a stick: Titrate dose as high as necessary to relieve cancer or nonmalignant pain where chronic opioids are necessary. Do not suck, chew, or swallow buccal tab. IONSYS: Apply to intact skin on the chest or upper arm. Each dose, activated by the patient, is delivered over a 10-min period. Remove prior to hospital discharge. Do not allow gel to touch mucous membranes. Dispose using gloves. Keep all forms of fentanyl out of the reach of children or pets. Concomitant use with potent CYP3A4 inhibitors such as ritonavir, ketoconazole, itraconazole, troleandomycin, clarithromycin, nelfinavir, and nefazodone may result in an increase in fentanyl plasma concentrations, which could increase or prolong adverse drug effects and may cause potentially fatal respiratory depression. Onsolis is available only through the FOCUS Program and requires prescriber, pharmacy, and patient enrollment. Used films should be discarded into toilet. Abstral, Subsys, and Lazanda: outpatients, prescribers, pharmacies, and distributors must be enrolled in TIRF REMS Access program before patient may receive medication.

HYDROMORPHONE (***Dilaudid, Dilaudid-5, Exalgo*** ♣ ***Hydromorph Contin***) ▶L ♀C ▶?©II $$

ADULT – Moderate to severe pain: 2 to 4 mg PO q 4 to 6 h. Initial dose (opioid-naive) 0.5 to 2 mg SC/IM or slow IV q 4 to 6 h prn. 3 mg PR q 6 to 8 h. Controlled-release tabs: 8 to 64 mg daily.

PEDS – Not approved in children.

UNAPPROVED PEDS – Pain age 12 yo or younger: 0.03 to 0.08 mg/kg PO q 4 to 6 h prn. 0.015 mg/kg/dose IV q 4 to 6 h prn, use adult dose for older than 12 yo.

FORMS – Generic/Trade: Tabs 2, 4, 8 mg (8 mg trade scored). Oral soln 5 mg/5 mL. Suppository 3 mg. Controlled-release tabs (Exalgo): 8, 12, 16 mg.

NOTES – In opioid-naive patients, consider an initial dose of 0.5 mg or less IM/SC/IV. SC/IM/IV doses after initial dose should be individualized. May be given by slow IV injection over 2 to 5 min. Titrate dose as high as necessary to relieve cancer or nonmalignant pain where chronic opioids are necessary. 1.5 mg IV = 7.5 mg PO. Exalgo intended for opioid-tolerant patients only.

OPIOID EQUIVALENCY*

Opioid	PO	IV/SC/IM	Opioid	PO	IV/SC/IM
buprenorphine	n/a	0.3–0.4 mg	meperidine	300 mg	75 mg
butorphanol	n/a	2 mg	methadone	5–15 mg	2.5–10 mg
codeine	130 mg	75 mg	morphine	30 mg	10 mg
fentanyl	?	0.1 mg	nalbuphine	n/a	10 mg
hydrocodone	20 mg	n/a	oxycodone	20 mg	n/a
hydromorphone	7.5 mg	1.5 mg	oxymorphone	10 mg	1 mg
levorphanol	4 mg	2 mg	pentazocine	50 mg	30 mg

*Approximate equianalgesic doses as adapted from the 2003 American Pain Society (www.ampainsoc.org) guidelines and the 1992 AHCPR guidelines. Not available = "n/a." See drug entries themselves for starting doses. Many recommend initially using lower than equivalent doses when switching between different opioids. IV doses should be titrated slowly with appropriate monitoring. All PO dosing is with immediate-release preparations. Individualize all dosing, especially in the elderly, children, and in those with chronic pain, opioid naïve, or hepatic/renal insufficiency.

FENTANYL TRANSDERMALDOSE (Dosing based on ongoing morphine requirement.)

Morphine (IV/IM)	Morphine (PO)	Transdermal fentanyl
10–22 mg/day	60–134 mg/day	25 mcg/h
23–37 mg/day	135–224 mg/day	50 mcg/h
38–52 mg/day	225–314 mg/day	75 mcg/h
53–67 mg/day	315–404 mg/day	100 mcg/h

For higher morphine doses, see product insert for transdermal fentanyl equivalencies.

LEVORPHANOL (*Levo-Dromoran*) ▶L ♀C ▶?©II $$$$

ADULT – Moderate to severe pain: 2 mg PO q 6 to 8 h prn. Increase to 4 mg if necessary.

PEDS – Not approved in children.

FORMS – Generic only: Tabs 2 mg, scored.

MEPERIDINE (***Demerol*, pethidine**) ▶LK ♀C but + ▶+©II $$$

ADULT – Moderate to severe pain: 50 to 150 mg IM/SC/PO q 3 to 4 h prn. OB analgesia: When pains become regular, 50 to 100 mg IM/SC q 1 to 3 h. May also be given slow IV diluted to 10 mg/mL, or by continuous IV infusion diluted to 1 mg/mL.

PEDS – Moderate to severe pain: 1 to 1.8 mg/kg IM/SC/PO or slow IV (see adult dosing) up to adult dose, q 3 to 4 h prn.

FORMS – Generic/Trade: Tabs 50 (trade scored), 100 mg. Syrup 50 mg/5 mL (trade banana flavored).

NOTES – Avoid in renal insufficiency and in elderly due to risk of metabolite accumulation and increased risk of CNS disturbance and seizures. Multiple drug interactions including MAOIs and SSRIs. Poor oral absorption/efficacy. 75 mg meperidine IV/IM/SC = 300 mg meperidine PO. Take syrup with ½ glass (4 oz) water. Due to the risk of seizures at high doses, meperidine is not a good choice for treatment of chronic pain. Not recommended in children.

METHADONE (***Diskets, Dolophine, Methadose,* ✤ *Metadol***) ▶L ♀C ▶?©II $

WARNING – High doses (mean approximately 200 mg/day) have been inconclusively associated with arrhythmia (torsades de pointes), particularly in those with preexisting risk factors. Caution in opioid-naive patients. Elimination half-life (8 to 59 h) far longer than its duration of analgesic action (4 to 8 h); monitor for respiratory depression and titrate accordingly. Use caution with escalating doses.

ADULT – Severe pain in opioid-tolerant patients: Initial dose is 2.5 mg IM/SC/PO q 8 to 12 h prn. Titrate up by 2.5 mg per dose every 5 to 7 days as necessary to relieve cancer or nonmalignant pain where chronic opioids are necessary. May start as high as 10 mg per dose if opioid dependent patient and dosing is managed by experienced practitioner using an opioid converson formula. Opioid dependence: Typical dose to prevent withdrawal is 20 mg PO daily but must be managed by an experienced practitioner. Treatment longer than 3 weeks is maintenance and only permitted in approved treatment programs. Opioid-naive patients: Not recommended in opioid naive patients, as first line treatment of acute pain, mild chronic pain, postoperative pain, or as a PRN medication.

UNAPPROVED PEDS – Pain age 12 yo or younger: 0.7 mg/kg/24 h divided q 4 to 6 h PO/SC/IM/IV prn. Max 10 mg/dose.

FORMS – Generic/Trade: Tabs 5, 10 mg. Dispersible tabs 40 mg (for opioid dependence only). Oral concentrate (Intensol): 10 mg/mL. Generic only: Oral soln 5, 10 mg/5 mL.

NOTES – Titrate dose as high as necessary to relieve cancer or nonmalignant pain where chronic opioids are necessary. Every 8 to 12 h dosing may decrease the risk of drug accumulation and overdose. Treatment for opioid dependence longer than 3 weeks is maintenance and only permitted in approved treatment programs. Drug interactions leading to decreased methadone levels with enzyme-inducing HIV drugs (eg, efavirenz, nevirapine) and other potent inducers such as rifampin. Monitor for opiate withdrawal symptoms and increase methadone if necessary. Rapid metabolizers may require more frequent daily dosing.

MORPHINE (***MS Contin, Kadian, Avinza, Roxanol, Oramorph SR, MSIR, DepoDur* ✤ *Statex, M.O.S., Doloral, M-Eslon***) ▶LK ♀C ▶+©II $$$$

WARNING – Multiple strengths; see FORMS and write specific product on Rx. Drinking alcohol while taking Avinza may result in a rapid release of a potentially fatal dose of morphine.

ADULT – Moderate to severe pain: 10 to 30 mg PO q 4 h (immediate-release tabs, or oral soln). Controlled-release (MS Contin, Oramorph SR): 30 mg PO q 8 to 12 h. (Kadian): 20 mg PO q 12 to 24 h. Extended-release caps (Avinza): 30 mg PO daily. 10 mg q 4 h IM/SC. 2.5 to 15 mg/70 kg IV over 4 to 5 min. 10 to 20 mg PR q 4 h. Pain with major surgery (DepoDur): 10 to 15 mg once epidurally at the lumbar level prior to surgery (max dose 20 mg), or 10 mg epidurally after clamping of the umbilical cord with cesarean section.

PEDS – Moderate to severe pain: 0.1 to 0.2 mg/kg up to 15 mg IM/SC/IV q 2 to 4 h.

UNAPPROVED PEDS – Moderate to severe pain: 0.2 to 0.5 mg/kg/dose PO (immediate-release) q 4 to 6 h. 0.3 to 0.6 mg/kg/dose PO (controlled-release) q 12 h.

FORMS – Generic/Trade: Tabs, immediate-release 15, 30 mg. Oral soln: 10 mg/5 mL, 20 mg/5 mL, 20 mg/mL (concentrate). Rectal supps 5, 10, 20, 30 mg. Controlled-release tabs (MS Contin) 15, 30, 60, 100, 200 mg. Trade only: Controlled-release caps (Kadian) 10, 20, 30, 50, 60, 80, 100, 200 mg. Controlled-release tabs (Oramorph SR) 15, 30, 60, 100 mg. Extended-release caps (Avinza) 30, 45, 60, 75, 90, 120 mg.

(cont.)

MORPHINE (*cont.*)

NOTES – Titrate dose as high as necessary to relieve cancer or nonmalignant pain where chronic opioids are necessary. The active metabolites may accumulate in hepatic/renal insufficiency and the elderly leading to increased analgesic and sedative effects. Do not break, chew, or crush MS Contin or Oramorph SR. Kadian and Avinza caps may be opened and sprinkled in applesauce for easier administration; however, the pellets should not be crushed or chewed. Doses more than 1600 mg/day of Avinza contain a potentially nephrotoxic quantity of fumaric acid. Do not mix DepoDur with other medications; do not administer any other medications into epidural space for for at least 48 h. Severe opiate overdose with respiratory depression has occurred with intrathecal leakage of DepoDur.

OXYCODONE (***Roxicodone, OxyContin, Percolone, OxyIR, OxyFAST, Oxecta, ✤Endocodone, Supeudol, OxyNEO***) ▶L ♀B ▶– ©II $$$$$

WARNING – Do not prescribe OxyContin tabs on a prn basis. 80 mg tabs for use in opioid-tolerant patients only. Multiple strengths; see FORMS and write specific product on Rx. Do not break, chew, or crush controlled-release preparations.

ADULT – Moderate to severe pain: 5 mg PO q 4 to 6 h prn. Controlled-release tabs: 10 to 40 mg PO q 12 h (no supporting data for shorter dosing intervals for controlled-release tabs).

PEDS – Not approved in children.

UNAPPROVED PEDS – Pain age 12 yo or younger: 0.05 to 0.3 mg/kg/dose q 4 to 6 h PO prn to max of 10 mg/dose.

FORMS – Generic/Trade: Immediate-release: Tabs 5 mg, scored. Caps 5 mg. Tabs 15, 30 mg. Oral soln 5 mg/5 mL. Oral concentrate 20 mg/mL. Generic only: Immediate-release tabs 10, 20 mg. Trade only: Immediate-release tabs: 7.5 mg. Controlled-release tabs: 10, 15, 20, 30, 40, 60, 80 mg.

NOTES – Titrate dose as high as necessary to relieve cancer or nonmalignant pain where chronic opioids are necessary.

OXYMORPHONE (***Opana***) ▶L ♀C ▶? ©II $$$$

WARNING – Do not break, chew, dissolve, or crush extended-release tabs due to a rapid release and absorption of a potentially fatal dose of oxymorphone.

ADULT – Moderate to severe pain: 10 to 20 mg PO q 4 to 6 h (immediate-release) or 5 mg q 12 h (extended-release) 1 h before or 2 h after meals. Titrate q 3 to 7 days until adequate pain relief. 1 to 1.5 mg IM/SC q 4 to 6 h prn. 0.5 mg IV initial dose in healthy patients then q 4 to 6 h prn, increase dose until pain adequately controlled.

PEDS – Not approved in children.

FORMS – Trade only: Extended-release tabs (Opana ER) 5, 7.5, 10, 15, 20, 30, 40 mg. Immediate-release tabs (Opana IR) 5, 10 mg.

NOTES – Contraindicated in moderate to severe hepatic dysfunction. Decrease dose in elderly and with CrCl less than 50 mL/min. Avoid alcohol.

ANALGESICS: Opioid Analgesic Combinations

NOTE: Refer to individual components for further information. May cause drowsiness and/or sedation, which may be enhanced by alcohol and other CNS depressants. Opioids, carisoprodol, and butalbital may be habit forming. Avoid exceeding 4 g/day of acetaminophen in combination products. Caution people who drink 3 or more alcoholic drinks/day to limit acetaminophen use to 2.5 g/day due to additive liver toxicity. Opioids commonly cause constipation; concurrent laxatives are recommended. All opioids are pregnancy class D if used for prolonged periods or in high doses at term.

ANEXSIA **(hydrocodone + acetaminophen)** ▶LK ♀C ▶– ©III $$

WARNING – Multiple strengths; see FORMS and write specific product on Rx.

ADULT – Moderate pain: 1 tab PO q 4 to 6 h prn.

PEDS – Not approved in children.

FORMS – Generic/Trade: Tabs 5/325, 5/500, 7.5/325, 7.5/650, 10/750 mg hydrocodone/mg acetaminophen, scored.

CAPITAL WITH CODEINE SUSPENSION **(acetaminophen + codeine)** ▶LK ♀C ▶? ©V $

ADULT – Moderate pain: 15 mL PO q 4 h prn.

PEDS – Moderate pain: Give 5 mL PO q 4 to 6 h prn for age 3 to 6 yo, give 10 mL PO q 4 to 6 h prn for age 7 to 12 yo, use adult dose for age older than 12 yo.

FORMS – Generic equivalent to oral soln. Trade equivalent to susp. Both codeine 12 mg and acetaminophen 120 mg per 5 mL (trade, fruit punch flavor).

COMBUNOX **(oxycodone + ibuprofen)** ▶L ♀C (D in 3rd trimester) ▶?©II $$$

ADULT – Moderate to severe pain: 1 tab PO q 6 h prn for no more than 7 days. Max dose 4 tabs/24 h.

PEDS – Moderate to severe pain for age 14 yo or older: Use adult dose.

FORMS – Generic/Trade: Tabs 5 mg oxycodone/400 mg ibuprofen.

NOTES – For short-term (no more than 7 days) management of pain. See NSAIDs—Other subclass warning and individual components.

EMPIRIN WITH CODEINE **(acetylsalicylic acid + codeine,** ✤ ***292 tab*****)** ▶LK ♀D ▶–©III $

WARNING – Multiple strengths; see FORMS and write specific product on Rx.

ADULT – Moderate pain: 1 to 2 tabs PO q 4 h prn.

PEDS – Not approved in children.

FORMS – Generic only: Tabs 325/30, 325/60 mg aspirin/mg codeine. Empirin brand no longer made.

FIORICET WITH CODEINE **(acetaminophen + butalbital + caffeine + codeine)** ▶LK ♀C ▶–©III $$$

ADULT – Moderate pain: 1 to 2 caps PO q 4 h prn, max dose 6 caps/day.

PEDS – Not approved in children.

FORMS – Generic/Trade: Caps 325 mg acetaminophen/50 mg butalbital/40 mg caffeine/30 mg codeine.

FIORINAL WITH CODEINE **(acetylsalicylic acid + butalbital + caffeine + codeine,** ✤ ***Fiorinal C-1/4, Fiorinal C-1/2, Trianal C-1/4, Trianal C-1/2*****)** ▶LK ♀D ▶–©III $$$

ADULT – Moderate pain: 1 to 2 caps PO q 4 h prn, max dose 6 caps/day.

PEDS – Not approved in children.

FORMS – Generic/Trade: Caps 325 mg aspirin/50 mg butalbital/40 mg caffeine/30 mg codeine.

IBUDONE **(hydrocodone + ibuprofen)** ▶LK ♀– ▶?©III $$$

ADULT – Moderate pain: 1 tab PO q 4 to 6 h prn, max dose 5 tabs/day.

PEDS – Not approved in children.

FORMS – Generic/Trade: Tabs 5/200 mg and 10/200 mg hydrocodone/ibuprofen.

NOTES – See NSAIDs—Other subclass warning.

LORCET **(hydrocodone + acetaminophen)** ▶LK ♀C ▶–©III $

WARNING – Multiple strengths; see FORMS and write specific product on Rx.

ADULT – Moderate pain: 1 to 2 caps (5/500) PO q 4 to 6 h prn, max dose 8 caps/day. 1 tab PO q 4 to 6 h prn (7.5/650 and 10/650), max dose 6 tabs/day.

PEDS – Not approved in children.

FORMS – Generic/Trade: Caps 5/500 mg, Tabs 7.5/ 650, 10/650 mg hydrocodone/acetaminophen.

LORTAB **(hydrocodone + acetaminophen)** ▶LK ♀C ▶–©III $$

WARNING – Multiple strengths; see FORMS and write specific product on Rx.

ADULT – Moderate pain: 1 to 2 tabs 2.5/500 and 5/500 PO q 4 to 6 h prn, max dose 8 tabs/day. 1 tab 7.5/500 and 10/500 PO q 4 to 6 h prn, max dose 5 tabs/day. Elixir 15 mL PO q 4 to 6 h prn, max 6 doses/day.

PEDS – Not approved in children.

FORMS – Generic/Trade: Lortab 5/500 (scored), Lortab 7.5/500 (trade scored), Lortab 10/500 mg hydrocodone/mg acetaminophen. Elixir: 7.5/500 mg hydrocodone/mg acetaminophen/15 mL. Trade only: Tabs 2.5/500 mg.

MAGNACET **(oxycodone + acetaminophen)** ▶L ♀C ▶–©II $$$$

WARNING – Multiple strengths; see FORMS and write specific product on Rx.

ADULT – Moderate to severe pain: 1 to 2 tabs PO q 6 h prn (2.5/400). 1 tab PO q 6 h prn (5/400, 7.5/400, 10/400).

PEDS – Not approved in children.

FORMS – Trade only: Tabs 2.5/400, 5/400, 7.5/400, 10/400 mg oxycodone/acetaminophen.

MAXIDONE **(hydrocodone + acetaminophen)** ▶LK ♀C ▶–©III $$$

ADULT – Moderate pain: 1 tab PO q 4 to 6 h prn, max dose 5 tabs/day.

PEDS – Not approved in children.

FORMS – Trade only: Tabs 10/750 mg hydrocodone/mg acetaminophen.

MERSYNDOL WITH CODEINE **(acetaminophen + codeine + doxylamine,** ✤**)** ▶LK ♀C ▶? $

ADULT – Canada only. Headaches, cold symptoms, muscle aches, neuralgia: 1 to 2 tabs PO q 4 to 6 h prn. Maximum 12 tabs/24 h.

PEDS – Not approved in children.

FORMS – Canada trade only: OTC tab 325 mg acetaminophen/8 mg codeine phosphate/5 mg doxylamine.

NOTES – May be habit forming. Hepatotoxicity may be increased with acetaminophen overdose and may be enhanced with concomitant chronic alcohol ingestion.

NORCO **(hydrocodone + acetaminophen)** ▶L ♀C ▶?©III $$$

WARNING – Multiple strengths; see FORMS and write specific product on Rx.

(cont.)

NORCO *(cont.)*

ADULT – Moderate to severe pain: 1 to 2 tabs PO q 4 to 6 h prn (5/325), max dose 12 tabs/day. 1 tab (7.5/325 and 10/325) PO q 4 to 6 h prn, max dose 8 and 6 tabs/day, respectively.

PEDS – Not approved in children.

FORMS – Trade only: Tabs 5/325, 7.5/325, 10/325 mg hydrocodone/acetaminophen, scored.

PERCOCET **(oxycodone + acetaminophen, ✤ *Percocet-demi, Oxycocet, Endocet*)** ▶L ♀C ▶–©II $

WARNING – Multiple strengths; see FORMS and write specific product on Rx.

ADULT – Moderate to severe pain: 1 to 2 tabs PO q 4 to 6 h prn (2.5/325 and 5/325). 1 tab PO q 4 to 6 h prn (7.5/325, 7.5/500, 10/325 and 10/650).

PEDS – Not approved in children.

FORMS – Trade only: Tabs 2.5/325 oxycodone/acetaminophen. Generic/Trade: Tabs 5/325, 7.5/325, 7.5/500, 10/325, 10/650 mg. Generic only: 2.5/300, 5/300, 7.5/300, 10/300, 2.5/400, 5/400, 7.5/400, 10/400, 10/500 mg.

PERCODAN **(oxycodone + acetylsalicylic acid, ✤ *Oxycodan*)** ▶LK ♀D ▶–©II $$

ADULT – Moderate to severe pain: 1 tab PO q 6 h prn.

PEDS – Not approved in children.

FORMS – Generic/Trade: Tabs 4.88/325 mg oxycodone/aspirin (trade scored).

ROXICET **(oxycodone + acetaminophen)** ▶L ♀C ▶–©II $

WARNING – Multiple strengths; see FORMS and write specific product on Rx.

ADULT – Moderate to severe pain: 1 tab PO q 6 h prn. Oral soln: 5 mL PO q 6 h prn.

PEDS – Not approved in children.

FORMS – Generic/Trade: Tabs 5/325 mg. Caps/Caplets 5/500 mg. Soln 5/325 per 5 mL, mg oxycodone/acetaminophen.

SOMA COMPOUND WITH CODEINE **(carisoprodol + acetylsalicylic acid + codeine)** ▶L ♀D ▶–©III $$$

ADULT – Moderate to severe musculoskeletal pain: 1 to 2 tabs PO four times per day prn.

PEDS – Not approved in children.

FORMS – Generic/Trade: Tabs 200 mg carisoprodol/ 325 mg aspirin/16 mg codeine.

NOTES – Refer to individual components. Withdrawal with abrupt discontinuation.

SYNALGOS-DC **(dihydrocodeine + acetylsalicylic acid + caffeine)** ▶L ♀C ▶–©III $

WARNING – Case reports of prolonged erections when taken concomitantly with sildenafil.

ADULT – Moderate to severe pain: 2 caps PO q 4 h prn.

PEDS – Not approved in children.

FORMS – Trade only: Caps 16 mg dihydrocodeine/ 356.4 mg aspirin/30 mg caffeine. "Painpack" = 12 caps.

NOTES – Most common use is dental pain. Refer to individual components.

TALACEN **(pentazocine + acetaminophen)** ▶L ♀C ▶?©IV $$$

ADULT – Moderate pain: 1 tab PO q 4 h prn.

PEDS – Not approved in children.

FORMS – Generic/Trade: Tabs 25 mg pentazocine/ 650 mg acetaminophen, trade scored.

NOTES – Serious skin reactions, including erythema multiforme and Stevens-Johnson syndrome, have been reported.

TYLENOL WITH CODEINE **(codeine + acetaminophen, ✤ *Tylenol #1, Tylenol #2, Tylenol #3, Tylenol #4, Atasol 8, Atasol 15, Atasol 30*)** ▶LK ♀C ▶?©III $

WARNING – Multiple strengths; see FORMS and write specific product on Rx.

ADULT – Moderate pain: 1 to 2 tabs PO q 4 h prn.

PEDS – Moderate pain: Elixir: Give 5 mL q 4 to 6 h prn for age 3 to 6 yo, give 10 mL q 4 to 6 h prn for age 7 to 12 yo, use adult dose for age older than 12 yo.

(cont.)

Analgesics—NSAIDs

Salicylic acid derivatives	ASA, diflunisal, salsalate, Trilisate
Propionic acids	flurbiprofen, ibuprofen, ketoprofen, naproxen, oxaprozin
Acetic acids	diclofenac, etodolac, indomethacin, ketorolac, nabumetone, sulindac, tolmetin
Fenamates	meclofenamate
Oxicams	meloxicam, piroxicam
COX-2 inhibitors	celecoxib

Note: If one class fails, consider another.

TYLENOL WITH CODEINE *(cont.)*

FORMS – Generic only: Tabs Tylenol #2 (15/300). Tylenol with Codeine Elixir 12/120 per 5 mL, mg codeine/mg acetaminophen. Generic/Trade: Tabs Tylenol #3 (30/300), Tylenol #4 (60/300). Canadian forms come with (Lenoltec, Tylenol) or without (Empracet, Emtec) caffeine.

TYLOX **(oxycodone + acetaminophen)** ▶L ♀C ▶–©II $

ADULT – Moderate to severe pain: 1 cap PO q 6 h prn.

PEDS – Not approved in children.

FORMS – Generic/Trade: Caps 5 mg oxycodone/500 mg acetaminophen.

VICODIN **(hydrocodone + acetaminophen)** ▶LK ♀C ▶?©III $

WARNING – Multiple strengths; see FORMS and write specific product on Rx.

ADULT – Moderate pain: 5/500 (max dose 8 tabs/day) and 7.5/750 (max dose of 5 tabs/day): 1 to 2 tabs PO q 4 to 6 h prn. 10/660: 1 tab PO q 4 to 6 h prn (max of 6 tabs/day).

PEDS – Not approved in children.

FORMS – Generic/Trade: Tabs Vicodin (5/500), Vicodin ES (7.5/750), Vicodin HP (10/660), scored, mg hydrocodone/mg acetaminophen.

VICOPROFEN **(hydrocodone + ibuprofen)** ▶LK ♀– ▶?©III $$$

ADULT – Moderate pain: 1 tab PO q 4 to 6 h prn, max dose 5 tabs/day.

PEDS – Not approved in children.

FORMS – Generic/Trade: Tabs 7.5/200 mg hydrocodone/ibuprofen. Generic only: Tabs 2.5/200, 5/200, 10/200 mg.

NOTES – See NSAIDs—Other subclass warning.

XODOL **(hydrocodone + acetaminophen)** ▶LK ♀C ▶–©III $$

ADULT – Moderate pain: 1 tab PO q 4 to 6 h prn, max 6 doses/day.

PEDS – Not approved in children.

FORMS – Trade only: Tabs 5/300, 7.5/300, 10/300 mg hydrocodone/acetaminophen.

ZYDONE **(hydrocodone + acetaminophen)** ▶LK ♀C ▶?©III $$

WARNING – Multiple strengths; see FORMS and write specific product on Rx.

ADULT – Moderate pain: 1 to 2 tabs (5/400) PO q 4 to 6 h prn, max dose 8 tabs/day. 1 tab (7.5/400, 10/400) q 4 to 6 h prn, max dose 6 tabs/day.

PEDS – Not approved in children.

FORMS – Trade only: Tabs 5/400, 7.5/400, 10/400 mg hydrocodone/mg acetaminophen.

ANALGESICS: Opioid Antagonists

NOTE: May result in withdrawal in the opioid dependent, including life-threatening withdrawal if administered to neonates born to opioid-dependent mothers. Rarely pulmonary edema, cardiovascular instability, hypotension, HTN, ventricular tachycardia, and ventricular fibrillation have been reported in connection with opioid reversal.

NALOXONE (***Narcan***) ▶LK ♀B ▶? $

ADULT – Management of opioid overdose: 0.4 to 2 mg IV. May repeat IV at 2 to 3 min intervals up to 10 mg. Use IM/SC/ET if IV not available. IV infusion: 2 mg in 500 mL D5W or NS (0.004 mg/mL); titrate according to response. Partial postop opioid reversal: 0.1 to 0.2 mg IV at 2 to 3 min intervals; repeat IM doses may be required at 1 to 2 h intervals.

PEDS – Management of opioid overdose: 0.01 mg/kg IV. Give a subsequent dose of 0.1 mg/kg if inadequate response. Use IM/SC/ET if IV not available. Partial postop opioid reversal: 0.005 to 0.01 mg IV at 2- to 3-min intervals.

NOTES – Watch patients for reemergence of opioid effects.

ANALGESICS: Other Analgesics

ACETAMINOPHEN (***Tylenol, Panadol, Tempra, Ofirmev,*** **paracetamol,** ♣***Abenol, Atasol, Pediatrix***) ▶LK ♀B ▶+ $

ADULT – Analgesic/antipyretic: 325 to 1000 mg PO q 4 to 6 h prn. 650 mg PR q 4 to 6 h prn. Max dose 4 g/day. OA: Extended-release: 2 caps PO q 8 h around the clock. Max dose 6 caps/day.

PEDS – Analgesic/antipyretic: 10 to 15 mg/kg q 4 to 6 h PO/PR prn. Max 5 doses/day.

UNAPPROVED ADULT – OA: 1000 mg PO four times per day.

FORMS – OTC: Tabs 325, 500, 650 mg. Chewable Tabs 80 mg. Oral disintegrating Tabs 80, 160 mg. Caps/Gelcaps/Caps 500 mg. Extended-release caplets 650 mg. Liquid

(cont.)

ACETAMINOPHEN (*cont.*)

160 mg/5 mL, 500 mg/15 mL. Supps 80, 120, 325, 650 mg.

NOTES – Risk of hepatotoxicity with chronic use, especially in alcoholics. Caution in those who drink 3 or more drinks/day. Rectal administration may produce lower/less reliable plasma levels.

CANNIBIS SATIVA L. EXTRACT (✤ ***Sativex***) ▶LK ♀X ▶– $$$$

ADULT – Canada only. Adjunctive treatment for the symptomatic relief of neuropathic pain in multiple sclerosis: Start: 1 spray q 4 h (max 4 times per day), and titrate upward as tolerated. Limited experience with more than 12 sprays/day.

PEDS – Not approved in children.

FORMS – Canada Trade only: Buccal spray, 27 mg/mL delta-9-tetrahydrocannabinol and 25 mg/mL cannabidiol, delivers 100 mcL per actuation, 5.5 mL vials containing up to 51 actuations per vial.

NOTES – Contraindicated in pregnancy, childbearing potential without birth control, history of psychosis, serious heart disease. Contains ethanol. Use cautiously if history of substance abuse.

CLONIDINE—EPIDURAL (***Duraclon***) ▶LK ♀C ▶– $$$$$

WARNING – Not recommended for obstetrical, postpartum, or perioperative pain management due to hypotension and bradycardia. Abrupt discontinuation may result in a rapid BP rise.

ADULT – Severe cancer pain in combination with opioids: Specialized epidural dosing.

PEDS – Severe cancer pain in combination with opioids: Specialized epidural dosing.

NOTES – Bradycardia and hypotension common. May be exacerbated by beta-blockers, certain calcium channel blockers, and digoxin.

HYALURONATE (***Hyalgan, Supartz,*** ✤ ***Neovisc, Orthovisc***) ▶KL ♀? ▶? $$$$$

WARNING – Do not inject extra-articularly; avoid the synovial tissues and cap. Do not use disinfectants containing benzalkonium chloride for skin preparation.

ADULT – OA (knee): Hyalgan: 2 mL intra-articular injection q week for 3 to 5 weeks. Supartz: 2.5 mL intra-articular injection q week for 5 weeks. Orthovisc and Neovisc (Canada): 2 mL intra-articular injection q week for 3 weeks. Inject a local anesthetic SC prior to injections.

PEDS – Not approved in children.

FORMS – Trade only: Hyalgan, Neovisc, Orthovisc: 2 mL vials, prefilled syringes. Supartz: 2.5 mL prefilled syringes.

NOTES – For those who have failed conservative therapy. Caution in allergy to eggs, avian proteins, or feathers (except Neovisc—synthetic). Remove synovial fluid or effusion before each injection. Knee pain and swelling most common side effects.

HYLAN GF-20 (***Synvisc***) ▶KL ♀? ▶? $$$$$

WARNING – Do not inject extra-articularly; avoid the synovial tissues and cap. Do not use disinfectants containing benzalkonium chloride for skin preparation.

ADULT – OA (knee): 2 mL intra-articular injection q week for 3 weeks.

PEDS – Not approved in children.

FORMS – Trade only: 2.25 mL glass syringe with 2 mL drug; 3/pack.

NOTES – For those who have failed conservative therapy. Caution in allergy to eggs, avian proteins, or feathers. Remove synovial fluid or effusion before each injection. Knee pain and swelling most common side effects.

TAPENTADOL (***Nucynta, Nucynta ER***) ▶LK ♀C ▶–©II $$$$

WARNING – Abuse potential.

ADULT – Moderate to severe acute pain: Immediate rellease: 50 to 100 mg PO q 4 to 6 h prn. Max dose 600 mg/day. If moderate hepatic impairment, decrease dose to 50 mg PO q 8 h. Moderate to severe chronic pain: Extended release: 50 to 250 mg PO twice daily. Start at 50 mg PO twice daily if patient not currently taking opioids. Do not use in severe renal or hepatic impairment.

PEDS – Not approved in children younger than 18 yo.

FORMS – Trade only: Immediate release: Tabs 50, 75, 100 mg. Extended release: Tabs 50, 100, 150, 200, 250 mg.

NOTES – When switching from immediate-release to extended-release form, use same total daily dose. Contraindicated in acute intoxication with alcohol, hypnotics, centrally acting analgesics, opioids, or psychotropic drugs and with respiratory depression. Use with caution in patients with known seizure disorders. Seizures and/or serotonin syndrome may occur with concurrent antidepressants, triptans, linezolid, lithium, St. John's wort.

TRAMADOL (***Ultram, Ultram ER, Ryzolt,*** ✤ ***Zytram XL, Tridural, Ralivia***) ▶KL ♀C ▶– $$$

ADULT – Moderate to moderately severe pain: 50 to 100 mg PO q 4 to 6 h prn. Max dose 400 mg/day. If older than 75 yo, use less than 300 mg/day PO in divided doses. If CrCl less than 30 mL/min, increase the dosing interval to 12 h. If cirrhosis, decrease dose to 50 mg PO q 12 h. Chronic pain, extended-release:

(cont.)

TRAMADOL (*cont.*)

100 to 300 mg PO daily. Do not use if CrCl is less than 30 mL/min or with severe hepatic dysfunction.

PEDS – Not approved in children younger than 16 yo.

FORMS – Generic/Trade: Tabs, immediate-release 50 mg. Trade only (Ultram ER, Ryzolt): Extended-release tabs 100, 200, 300 mg.

NOTES – Contraindicated in acute intoxication with alcohol, hypnotics, centrally acting analgesics, opioids, or psychotropic drugs. Seizures and/or serotonin syndrome may occur with concurrent antidepressants, triptans, linezolid, lithium, St. John's wort, or enzyme-inducing drugs such as ketoconazole and erythromycin; use with caution and adjust dose. Withdrawal symptoms may occur in patients dependent on opioids or with abrupt discontinuation. Overdose treated with naloxone may increase seizures. Carbamazepine decreases tramadol levels. The most frequent side effects are nausea and constipation. ER tabs cannot be crushed, chewed, or split.

WOMEN'S TYLENOL MENSTRUAL RELIEF **(acetaminophen + pamabrom)** ▸LK ♀B ▸+ $

ADULT – Menstrual cramps: 2 caps PO q 4 to 6 h.

PEDS – Use adult dose for age older than 12 yo.

FORMS – OTC: Caps 500 mg acetaminophen/ 25 mg pamabrom (diuretic).

NOTES – Hepatotoxicity with chronic use, especially in alcoholics.

ZICONOTIDE (***Prialt***) ▸Plasma ♀C ▸? $$$$$

WARNING – Severe psychiatric and neurologic impairment may occur. Monitor for mood changes, hallucinations, or cognitive changes. Contraindicated if history of psychosis.

ADULT – Severe intractable chronic pain: Specialized intrathecal dosing.

PEDS – Not approved in children younger than 16 yo.

NOTES – Contraindicated in patients with history of psychosis, uncontrolled bleeding, spinal canal obstruction, or infection at the infusion site. Does not prevent opioid withdrawal; gradually taper while instituting ziconotide therapy. Monitor CK periodically.

ANESTHESIA: Anesthetics and Sedatives

ALFENTANIL (***Alfenta***) ▸L ♀C ▸?©II $

ADULT – IV general anesthesia adjunct; specialized dosing.

PEDS – Not approved in children.

DESFLURANE (***Suprane***) ▸Respiratory ♀B ▸+ Varies

ADULT – General anesthetic gas: specialized dosing.

PEDS – Not recommended for induction due to high rate of laryngospasm.

NOTES – Minimum alveolar concentration (MAC) 6.0%. Known trigger of malignant hyperthermia; see mhaus.org.

DEXMEDETOMIDINE (***Precedex***) ▸LK ♀C ▸? $$$$

ADULT – ICU sedation less than 24 h: Load 1 mcg/kg over 10 min followed by infusion 0.2 to 0.7 mcg/kg/h titrated to desired sedation endpoint.

PEDS – Not recommended for age younger than 18 yo.

NOTES – Alpha-2-adrenergic agonist with sedative properties. Beware of bradycardia and hypotension. Avoid in advanced heart block.

ENFLURANE (***Ethrane***) ▸Respiratory/L ♀B ▸? Varies

ADULT – Rarely used general anesthetic gas: specialized dosing.

PEDS – Age younger than 5 yo: Rarely used general anesthetic gas: specialized dosing.

NOTES – Minimum alveolar concentration (MAC) 1.68%. Known trigger of malignant hyperthermia; see mhaus.org.

ETOMIDATE (***Amidate***) ▸L ♀C ▸? $

ADULT – Anesthesia induction/rapid sequence intubation: 0.3 mg/kg IV.

PEDS – Age younger than 10 yo: Not approved. Age 10 yo or older: Use adult dosing.

UNAPPROVED PEDS – Anesthesia induction/ rapid sequence intubation: 0.3 mg/kg IV.

NOTES – Adrenocortical suppression, but rarely of clinical significance.

FOSPROPOFOL (***Lusedra***) ▸L ♀– ▸? $$$$

WARNING – Beware of respiratory depression/apnea. Administer with appropriate monitoring.

ADULT – Deep sedation (age younger than 65 yo): 6.5 mg/kg IV (not to exceed 16.5 mL), 1.6 mg/kg supplemental dose q 4 min (not to exceed 4 mL). Age older than 65 yo or severe systemic disease (aspirin P3 or P4) use 75% of initial and supplemental doses. Wt greater than 90 kg, dose at 90 kg; wt less than 60 kg, dose at 60 kg.

PEDS – Not recommended.

NOTES – Prodrug which is compatible with standard IV fluids.

HALOTHANE (*Fluothane*) ▶Respiratory/L ♀C ▶? Varies
ADULT – Rarely used general anesthetic gas: specialized dosing.
PEDS – Rarely used general anesthetic gas: specialized dosing.
NOTES – Minimum alveolar concentration (MAC) 0.77%. Known trigger of malignant hyperthermia; see mhaus.org.

ISOFLURANE (*Forane*) ▶Respiratory ♀C ▶? Varies
ADULT – General anesthetic gas: specialized dosing.
PEDS – General anesthetic gas: specialized dosing.
NOTES – Minimum alveolar concentration (MAC) 1.15%. Known trigger of malignant hyperthermia; see mhaus.org.

KETAMINE (*Ketalar*) ▶L ♀? ▶?©III $
WARNING – Emergence delirium limits value of ketamine in adults; such reactions are rare in children.
ADULT – Dissociative sedation: 1 to 2 mg/kg IV over 1 to 2 min or 4 to 5 mg/kg IM.
PEDS – Dissociative sedation: 1 to 2 mg/kg IV over 1 to 2 min or 4 to 5 mg/kg IM.
NOTES – Raises BP and intracranial pressure; avoid if CAD, HTN, head, or eye injury. Concurrent atropine minimizes hypersalivation; can be combined in same syringe with ketamine for IM use.

METHOHEXITAL (*Brevital*) ▶L ♀B ▶?©IV $
ADULT – Anesthesia induction: 1 to 1.5 mg/kg IV.
PEDS – Anesthesia induction: 6.6 to 10 mg/kg IM or 25 mg/kg PR.
UNAPPROVED PEDS – Sedation for diagnostic imaging: 25 mg/kg PR.

MIDAZOLAM (*Versed*) ▶LK ♀D ▶–©IV $
WARNING – Beware of respiratory depression/apnea. Administer with appropriate monitoring.
ADULT – Sedation/anxiolysis: 0.07 to 0.08 mg/kg IM (5 mg in average adult); or 1 mg IV slowly q 2 to 3 min up to 5 mg. Anesthesia induction: 0.3 to 0.35 mg/kg IV over 20 to 30 sec.
PEDS – Sedation/anxiolysis: Oral route 0.25 to 1 mg/kg (0.5 mg/kg most effective) to maximum of 20 mg PO, IM route 0.1 to 0.15 mg/kg IM. IV route initial dose 0.05 to 0.1 mg/kg IV, then titrated to max 0.6 mg/kg for age 6 mo to 5 yo, initial dose 0.025 to 0.05 mg/kg IV, then titrated to max 0.4 mg/kg for age 6 to 12 yo.
UNAPPROVED PEDS – Sedation/anxiolysis: Intranasal 0.2 to 0.4 mg/kg. Rectal: 0.25 to 0.5 mg/kg PR. Status epilepticus: Load 0.15 mg/kg IV followed by infusion 1 mcg/kg/min and titrate dose upward q 5 min prn.
FORMS – Generic only: Oral liquid 2 mg/mL.
NOTES – Use lower doses in the elderly, chronically ill, and those receiving concurrent CNS depressants.

NITROUS OXIDE (*Entonox*) ▶Respiratory ♀– ▶? Varies
ADULT – General anesthetic gas: specialized dosing.
PEDS – General anesthetic gas: specialized dosing.
NOTES – Always maintain at least 20% oxygen administration.

PENTOBARBITAL (*Nembutal*) ▶LK ♀D ▶?©II $$
ADULT – Rarely used; other drugs preferred. Hypnotic: 150 to 200 mg IM or 100 mg IV at a rate of 50 mg/min, maximum dose is 500 mg.
PEDS – FDA approved for active seizing, but other agents preferred.
UNAPPROVED PEDS – Procedural sedation: 1 to 6 mg/kg IV, adjusted in increments of 1 to 2 mg/kg to desired effect, or 2 to 6 mg/kg IM, max 100 mg. Do not exceed 50 mg/min.

PROPOFOL (*Diprivan*) ▶L ♀B ▶– $$$
WARNING – Beware of respiratory depression/apnea. Administer with appropriate monitoring.
ADULT – Anesthesia (age younger than 55 yo): 40 mg IV q 10 sec until induction onset (typical 2 to 2.5 mg/kg). Follow with maintenance infusion generally 100 to 200 mcg/kg/min. Lower doses in elderly or for sedation. ICU ventilator sedation: Infusion 5 to 50 mcg/kg/min.
PEDS – Anesthesia age 3 yo or older: 2.5 to 3.5 mg/kg IV over 20 to 30 sec, followed with infusion 125 to 300 mcg/kg/min. Not recommended if age younger than 3 yo or for prolonged ICU use.
UNAPPROVED ADULT – Deep sedation: 1 mg/kg IV over 20 to 30 sec. Repeat 0.5 mg/kg IV prn. Intubation adjunct: 2.0 to 2.5 mg/kg IV.
UNAPPROVED PEDS – Deep sedation: 1 mg/kg IV (max 40 mg) over 20 to 30 sec. Repeat 0.5 mg/kg (max 20 mg) IV prn.
NOTES – Avoid with egg or soy allergies. Prolonged infusions may lead to hypertriglyceridemia. Injection pain can be treated or pretreated with lidocaine 40 to 50 mg IV.

REMIFENTANIL (*Ultiva*) ▶L ♀C ▶?©II $$
ADULT – IV general anesthesia adjunct; specialized dosing.
PEDS – IV general anesthesia adjunct; specialized dosing.

SEVOFLURANE (*Ultane*, ✤*Sevorane*) ▶Respiratory/L ♀B ▶? Varies
ADULT – General anesthetic gas; specialized dosing.
PEDS – General anesthetic gas; specialized dosing.
NOTES – Minimum Alveolar Concentration (MAC) 2.05%. Known trigger of malignant hyperthermia; see mhaus.org.

SUFENTANIL (*Sufenta*) ▶L ♀C ▶?©II $$
ADULT – IV anesthesia adjunct: Specialized dosing.
PEDS – IV anesthesia adjunct: Specialized dosing.

ANESTHESIA: Local Anesthetics

ARTICAINE (*Septocaine, Zorcaine*) ▶LK ♀C ▶? $
ADULT – Dental local anesthesia: 4% injection.
PEDS – Dental local anesthesia age 4 yo or older: 4% injection.
FORMS – 4% (includes epinephrine 1:100,000).
NOTES – Do not exceed 7 mg/kg total dose.

BUPIVACAINE (*Marcaine, Sensorcaine*) ▶LK ♀C ▶? $
ADULT – Local anesthesia, nerve block: 0.25% injection.
PEDS – Not recommended in children age younger than 12 yo.
FORMS – 0.25%, 0.5%, 0.75%, all with or without epinephrine.
NOTES – Onset 5 min, duration 2 to 4 h (longer with epi). Amide group. Max dose 2.5 mg/kg alone, or 3.0 mg/kg with epinephrine.

CHLOROPROCAINE (*Nesacaine*) ▶LK ♀C ▶? $
ADULT – Local and regional anesthesia: 1 to 3% injection.
PEDS – Local and regional anesthesia if 3 yo or older: 1 to 3% injection.
FORMS – 1%, 2%, 3%.
NOTES – Maximum local dose: 11 mg/kg.

DUOCAINE **(bupivacaine + lidocaine—local anesthetic)** ▶LK ♀C ▶? $
ADULT – Local anesthesia, nerve block for eye surgery.
PEDS – Not recommended in children younger than 12 yo.
FORMS – Vials contain bupivacaine 0.375% + lidocaine 1%.
NOTES – Use standard precautions including maximum dosing without epi for both bupivacaine and lidocaine.

LIDOCAINE—LOCAL ANESTHETIC (*Xylocaine*) ▶LK ♀B ▶? $
ADULT – Local anesthesia: 0.5 to 1% injection.
PEDS – Local anesthesia: 0.5 to 1% injection.
FORMS – 0.5, 1, 1.5, 2%. With epi: 0.5, 1, 1.5, 2%.
NOTES – Onset within 2 min, duration 30 to 60 min (longer with epi). Amide group. Potentially toxic dose 3 to 5 mg/kg without epinephrine, and 5 to 7 mg/kg with epinephrine. Use "cardiac lidocaine" (ie, IV formulation) for Bier blocks at maximum dose of 3 mg/kg so that neither epinephrine nor methylparaben are injected IV.

MEPIVACAINE (*Carbocaine, Polocaine*) ▶LK ♀C ▶? $
ADULT – Nerve block: 1% to 2% injection.
PEDS – Nerve block: 1% to 2% injection. Use less than 2% concentration if age younger than 3 yo or wt less than 30 pounds.
FORMS – 1%, 1.5%, 2%, 3%.
NOTES – Onset 3 to 5 min, duration 45 to 90 min. Amide group. Max local dose 5 to 6 mg/kg.

ORAQIX **(prilocaine + lidocaine—local anesthetic)** ▶LK ♀B ▶? $$
ADULT – Local anesthetic gel applied to periodontal pockets using blunt-tipped applicator: 4% injection.
PEDS – Not approved in children.
FORMS – Gel 2.5% + 2.5% with applicator.
NOTES – Do not exceed maximum dose for lidocaine or prilocaine.

PRILOCAINE (*Citanest*) ▶LK ♀B ▶? $
ADULT – Nerve block and dental procedures: 4% injection.
PEDS – Nerve block and dental procedures, age older than 9 mo: 4% injection.
FORMS – 4%, 4% with epinephrine.
NOTES – Contraindicated if younger than 6 to 9 mo. If younger than 5 yo, maximum local dose is 3 to 4 mg/kg (with or without epinephrine). If 5 yo or older, maximum local dose is 5 mg/kg without epinephrine and 7 mg/kg with epinephrine.

PROCAINE (*Novocain*) ▶Plasma ♀C ▶? $
ADULT – Local and regional anesthesia: 1% to 2% injection. Spinal anesthesia: 10%.
PEDS – Local and regional anesthesia: 1% to 2% injection. Spinal anesthesia: 10%.
FORMS – 1%, 2%, 10%.

ROPIVACAINE (*Naropin*) ▶LK ♀B ▶? $
WARNING – Inadvertent intravascular injection may result in arrhythmia or cardiac arrest.
ADULT – Local and regional anesthesia: 0.2% to 1% injection.
PEDS – Not approved in children.
FORMS – 0.2%, 0.5%, 0.75%, 1%.

TETRACAINE (*Pontocaine*, ✤amethocaine) ▶Plasma ♀C ▶? $
ADULT – Spinal anesthesia.
PEDS – Not approved in children.
FORMS – 0.2%, 0.3%, 1%.

ANESTHESIA: Neuromuscular Blockers

NOTE: Should be administered only by those skilled in airway management and respiratory support.

ATRACURIUM (*Tracrium*) ▶Plasma ♀C ▶? $
ADULT – Paralysis: 0.4 to 0.5 mg/kg IV.
PEDS – Paralysis age 2 yo or older: 0.4 to 0.5 mg/kg IV.
NOTES – Duration 15 to 30 min. Hoffman degradation.

CISATRACURIUM (*Nimbex*) ▶Plasma ♀B ▶? $$
ADULT – Paralysis: 0.15 to 0.2 mg/kg IV.
PEDS – Paralysis: 0.1 mg/kg IV over 5 to 10 sec.
NOTES – Duration 30 to 60 min. Hoffman degradation.

PANCURONIUM (*Pavulon*) ▶LK ♀C ▶? $
ADULT – Paralysis: 0.04 to 0.1 mg/kg IV.
PEDS – Paralysis (beyond neonatal age): 0.04 to 0.1 mg/kg IV.
NOTES – Duration 45 min. Decrease dose if renal disease.

ROCURONIUM (*Zemuron*) ▶L ♀B ▶? $$
ADULT – Paralysis: 0.6 mg/kg IV. Rapid sequence intubation: 0.6 to 1.2 mg/kg IV. Continuous infusion: 10 to 12 mcg/kg/min; first verify spontaneous recovery from bolus dose.
PEDS – Paralysis (age older than 3 mo): 0.6 mg/kg IV. Continuous infusion: 12 mcg/kg/min; first verify spontaneous recovery from bolus dose.
NOTES – Duration 30 min. Decrease dose if severe liver disease.

SUCCINYLCHOLINE (*Anectine, Quelicin*) ▶Plasma ♀C ▶? $
ADULT – Paralysis: 0.6 to 1.1 mg/kg IV.
PEDS – Paralysis age younger than 5 yo: 2 mg/kg IV. Paralysis age 5 yo or older: 1 mg/kg IV.
NOTES – Avoid in hyperkalemia, myopathies, eye injuries, rhabdomyolysis, subacute burn, and syndromes of denervated or disused musculature (eg, paralysis from spinal cord injury or major CVA). If immediate cardiac arrest and ET tube is in correct place and no tension pneumothorax evident, strongly consider empiric treatment for hyperkalemia. Succinylcholine can trigger malignant hyperthermia; see www.mhaus.org.

VECURONIUM (*Norcuron*) ▶LK ♀C ▶? $
ADULT – Paralysis: 0.08 to 0.1 mg/kg IV bolus. Continuous infusion: 0.8 to 1.2 mcg/kg/min; first verify spontaneous recovery from bolus dose.
PEDS – Age younger than 7 weeks: Safety has not been established. Age 7 weeks to 1 yo: Moderately more sensitive on a mg/kg dose compared to adults and take 1.5 for longer to recover. Age 1 to 10 yo: May require a slightly higher initial dose and may also require supplementation slightly more often than older patients. Paralysis age 10 yo or older: 0.08 to 0.1 mg/kg IV bolus. Continuous infusion: 0.8 to 1.2 mcg/kg/min; first verify spontaneous recovery from bolus dose.
NOTES – Duration 15 to 30 min. Decrease dose in severe liver disease.

ANTIMICROBIALS: Aminoglycosides

NOTE: See also Dermatology and Ophthalmology.

AMIKACIN ▶K ♀D ▶? $$$
WARNING – Nephrotoxicity, ototoxicity.
ADULT – Gram-negative infections: 15 mg/kg/day (up to 1500 mg/day) IM/IV divided q 8 to 12 h.
PEDS – Gram-negative infections: 15 mg/kg/day (up to 1500 mg/day) IM/IV divided q 8 to 12 h. Neonates: 10 mg/kg load, then 7.5 mg/kg IM/IV q 12 h.
UNAPPROVED ADULT – Once-daily dosing: 15 mg/kg IV q 24 h. TB (2nd-line treatment): 15 mg/kg (up to 1 g) IM/IV daily; 10 mg/kg (up to 750 mg) IM/IV daily for age older than 59 yo.
UNAPPROVED PEDS – Severe infections: 15 to 22.5 mg/kg/day IV divided q 8 h. Some experts recommend 30 mg/kg/day. Once-daily dosing: 15 mg/kg IV q 24 h. Some experts consider once-daily dosing of aminoglycosides investigational in children. TB (2nd-line treatment): 15 to 30 mg/kg (up to 1 g) IM/IV daily.
NOTES – May enhance effects of neuromuscular blockers. Avoid other ototoxic/nephrotoxic

(cont.)

AMIKACIN (*cont.*)

drugs. Individualize dose in renal dysfunction, burn patients. Base dose on average of actual and ideal body wt in obesity. Peak 20 to 35 mcg/mL, trough is less than 5 mcg/mL.

GENTAMICIN ▶K ♀D ▶+ $

WARNING – Nephrotoxicity, ototoxicity.

ADULT – Gram-negative infections: 3 to 5 mg/kg/day IM/IV divided q 8 h. See table for prophylaxis of bacterial endocarditis.

PEDS – Gram-negative infections: 2.5 mg/kg IM/IV q 12 h for age younger than 1 week old and wt greater than 2 kg; 2 to 2.5 mg/kg IM/IV q 8 h for age 1 week old or older and wt greater than 2 kg. Cystic fibrosis: 9 mg/kg/day IV in divided doses with target peak of 8 to 12 mcg/mL.

UNAPPROVED ADULT – Once-daily dosing for gram-negative infections: 5 to 7 mg/kg IV q 24 h. Endocarditis: 3 mg/kg/day for synergy with another agent. Give once daily for viridans streptococci, 2 to 3 divided doses for staphylococci, 3 divided doses for enterococci.

UNAPPROVED PEDS – Once-daily dosing: 5 to 7 mg/kg IV q 24 h. Give 4 mg/kg IV q 24 h for age younger than 1 week old and full term. Some experts consider once-daily dosing of aminoglycosides investigational in children.

NOTES – May enhance effects of neuromuscular blockers. Avoid other ototoxic/nephrotoxic drugs. Individualize dose in renal dysfunction, burn patients. Base dose on average of actual and ideal body wt in obesity. Peak 5 to 10 mcg/mL, trough is less than 2 mcg/mL.

STREPTOMYCIN ▶K ♀D ▶+ $$$$$

WARNING – Nephrotoxicity, ototoxicity. Monitor audiometry, renal function, and electrolytes.

ADULT – Combined therapy for TB: 15 mg/kg (up to 1 g) IM/IV daily. 10 mg/kg (up to 750 mg) IM/IV daily if age 60 yo or older.

PEDS – Combined therapy for TB: 20 to 40 mg/kg (up to 1 g) IM daily.

UNAPPROVED ADULT – Same IM dosing can be given IV. Streptococcal endocarditis: 7.5 mg/kg IV/IM two times per day. Go to www.americanheart.org for further info.

NOTES – Contraindicated in pregnancy. Obtain baseline audiogram, vestibular, and Romberg testing, and renal function. Monitor renal function and vestibular and auditory symptoms monthly. May enhance effects of neuromuscular blockers. Avoid other ototoxic/nephrotoxic drugs. Individualize dose in renal dysfunction.

TOBRAMYCIN (*TOBI*) ▶K ♀D ▶? $$

WARNING – Nephrotoxicity, ototoxicity.

ADULT – Gram-negative infections: 3 to 5 mg/kg/day IM/IV divided q 8 h. Parenteral for cystic fibrosis: 10 mg/kg/day IV divided q 6 h with target peak of 8 to 12 mcg/mL. Nebulized for cystic fibrosis (TOBI): 300 mg nebulized two times per day 28 days on, then 28 days off.

PEDS – Gram-negative infections: 2 to 2.5 mg/kg IV q 8 h or 1.5 to 1.9 mg/kg IV q 6 h. Give 4 mg/kg/day divided q 12 h for premature/full-term neonates age 1 week old or younger. Parenteral for cystic fibrosis: 10 mg/kg/day IV divided q 6 h with target peak of 8 to 12 mcg/mL. Nebulized for cystic fibrosis (TOBI) age 6 yo or older: 300 mg nebulized two times per day, 28 days on, then 28 days off.

UNAPPROVED ADULT – Once-daily dosing: 5 to 7 mg/kg IV q 24 h.

UNAPPROVED PEDS – Once-daily dosing: 5 to 7 mg/kg IV q 24 h. Some experts consider once-daily dosing of aminoglycosides investigational in children.

FORMS – Trade only: TOBI 300 mg ampules for nebulizer.

NOTES – May enhance effects of neuromuscular blockers. Avoid other ototoxic/nephrotoxic drugs. Individualize dose in renal dysfunction, burn patients. Base dose on average of actual and ideal body wt in obesity. Routine monitoring of tobramycin levels not required with nebulized TOBI. Peak 5 to 10 mcg/mL, trough is less than 2 mcg/mL.

ANTIMICROBIALS: Antifungal Agents—Azoles

NOTE: See www.idsociety.org for guidelines on the management of fungal infections. See www.aidsinfo.nih.gov for management of fungal infections in HIV-infected patients.

CLOTRIMAZOLE (*Mycelex*) ▶L ♀C ▶? $$$$

ADULT – Oropharyngeal candidiasis: 1 troche dissolved slowly in mouth 5 times per day for 14 days. Prevention of oropharyngeal candidiasis in immunocompromised patients: 1 troche dissolved slowly in mouth three times per day until end of chemotherapy or high-dose corticosteroids.

PEDS – Oropharyngeal candidiasis age 3 yo or older: Use adult dose.

FORMS – Generic/Trade: Oral troches 10 mg.

FLUCONAZOLE (*Diflucan,* ✤ *CanesOral*) ▶K ♀C for single-dose treatment of vaginal candidiasis, D for all other indications ▶+ $$$$

ADULT – Vaginal candidiasis: 150 mg PO single dose ($). All other dosing regimens IV/PO. Oropharyngeal candidiasis: 200 mg first day, then 100 mg daily for at least 2 weeks. Esophageal candidiasis: 200 mg first day, then 100 mg daily (up to 400 mg/day) for at least 3 weeks and continuing for 2 weeks past symptom resolution. Systemic candidiasis: Up to 400 mg daily. Candidal UTI, peritonitis: 50 to 200 mg daily. See UNAPPROVED ADULT for IDSA regimens for Candida infections. Cryptococcal meningitis: 400 mg daily until 10 to 12 weeks after cerebrospinal fluid is culture negative (see UNAPPROVED ADULT for first-line regimen). Suppression of cryptococcal meningitis relapse in AIDS: 200 mg daily until immune system reconstitution. Prevention of candidiasis after bone marrow transplant: 400 mg daily starting several days before neutropenia and continuing until ANC is greater than 1000 cells/mm^3 for 7 days.

PEDS – All dosing regimens IV/PO. Oropharyngeal candidiasis: 6 mg/kg first day, then 3 mg/kg daily for at least 2 weeks. Esophageal candidiasis: 6 mg/kg first day, then 3 mg/kg daily (up to 12 mg/kg daily) for at least 3 weeks and continuing for 2 weeks past symptom resolution. Systemic candidiasis: 6 to 12 mg/kg daily. See UNAPPROVED PEDS for alternative regimens for Candida infections. Cryptococcal meningitis: 12 mg/kg on first day, then 6 to 12 mg/kg daily until 10 to 12 weeks after cerebrospinal fluid is culture negative. Suppression of cryptococcal meningitis relapse in AIDS: 6 mg/kg daily. Peds/adult dose equivalents: 3 mg/kg peds equivalent to 100 mg adult; 6 mg/kg peds equivalent to 200 mg adult; 12 mg/kg peds equivalent to 400 mg adult; max peds dose is 600 mg/day.

UNAPPROVED ADULT – Onychomycosis, fingernail: 150 to 300 mg PO q week for 3 to 6 months. Onychomycosis, toenail: 150 to 300 mg PO q week for 6 to 12 months. Recurrent vaginal candidiasis: 100 to 200 mg PO q 3rd day for 3 doses, then 100 to 200 mg PO q week for 6 months. Oropharyngeal candidiasis: 100 to 200 mg daily for 7 to 14 days. Esophageal candidiasis: 200 to 400 mg daily for 14 to 21 days. Candidemia: 800 mg first day, then 400 mg once a day. Treat for 14 days after first negative blood culture and resolution of signs/symptoms. Candida pyelonephritis: 200 to 400 mg (3 to 6 mg/kg) daily for 14 days. Prevention of candidal infections in high-risk neutropenic patients: 400 mg/day during period of risk for neutropenia. Cryptococcal meningitis (per IDSA guideline): Amphotericin B preferably in combo with flucytosine for at least 2 weeks (induction), followed by fluconazole 400 mg PO once daily for 8 weeks (consolidation), then chronic suppression with fluconazole 200 mg PO once daily until immune system reconstitution. Treatment/suppression of coccidioidomycosis in HIV infection: 400 mg PO once daily.

UNAPPROVED PEDS – Oropharyngeal candidiasis: 6 mg/kg first day, then 3 mg/kg once daily for 7 to 14 days. Esophageal candidiasis: 12 mg/kg first day, then 6 mg/kg once daily for 14 to 21 days. Systemic Candida infection: 12 mg/kg on first day, then 6 to 12 mg/kg once daily. Cryptococcal meningitis: Amphotericin B preferably in combo with flucytosine for 2 weeks (induction), followed by fluconazole 12 mg/kg on first day, then 6 to 12 mg/kg (max 800 mg) IV/PO once a day for at least 8 weeks (consolidation), then chronic suppression with lower dose of fluconazole.

FORMS – Generic/Trade: Tabs 50, 100, 150, 200 mg. 150 mg tab in single-dose blister pack. Susp 10, 40 mg/mL (35 mL).

NOTES – Many drug interactions, including increased levels of cyclosporine, phenytoin, theophylline, and increased INR with warfarin. May inhibit metabolism of fluvastatin (limit fluvastatin to 20 mg/day), and possibly simvastatin/lovastatin at higher doses. Dosing in renal dysfunction: Reduce maintenance dose by 50% for CrCl 11 to 50 mL/min. Hemodialysis: Give recommended dose after each dialysis. Single dose during first trimester of pregnancy does not appear to increase risk of congenital birth defects.

ITRACONAZOLE (*Onmel, Sporanox*) ▶L ♀C ▶– $$$$$

WARNING – Inhibition of CYP3A4 metabolism by itraconazole can lead to dangerously high levels of some drugs. High levels of some can prolong QT interval (see QT drugs table). Contraindicated with felodipine, dofetilide, ergot alkaloids, lovastatin, PO midazolam, methadone, nisoldipine, pimozide, quinidine, simvastatin, triazolam. Negative inotrope (may be additive with calcium channel blockers); reassess treatment if signs/symptoms of heart failure develop. Not for use in ventricular dysfunction (CHF or history of CHF) unless for life-threatening or serious infection. Do not use caps for onychomycosis in patients with left ventricular dysfunction.

(cont.)

ITRACONAZOLE (*cont.*)

ADULT – Caps: Take caps or tabs with full meal. Onychomycosis, toenails: 200 mg PO daily for 12 weeks. Onychomycosis "pulse dosing" for fingernails: 200 mg PO two times per day for 1st week of month for 2 months. Test nail specimen to confirm diagnosis before prescribing. Aspergillosis in patients intolerant/refractory to amphotericin, blastomycosis, histoplasmosis: 200 mg PO one to two times per day. Treat for at least 3 months. For life-threatening infections, load with 200 mg PO three times per day for 3 days. Oral soln: Swish and swallow in 10-mL increments on empty stomach. Oropharyngeal candidiasis: 200 mg PO daily for 1 to 2 weeks. Oropharyngeal candidiasis unresponsive to fluconazole: 100 mg PO two times per day. Esophageal candidiasis: 100 to 200 mg PO daily for at least 3 weeks and continuing for 2 weeks past symptom resolution.

PEDS – Not approved in children.

UNAPPROVED ADULT – Caps: Onychomycosis "pulse dosing" for toenails: 200 mg PO two times per day for 1st week of month for 3 to 4 months. Confirm diagnosis with nail specimen lab testing before prescribing. Prevention of histoplasmosis in HIV infection: 200 mg PO once daily. Treatment/suppression of coccidioidomycosis in HIV infection: 200 mg PO two times per day. Fluconazole-refractory oropharyngeal or esophageal candidiasis: 200 mg PO of oral soln daily for 14 to 21 days.

UNAPPROVED PEDS – Oropharyngeal candidiasis, age 5 yo or older: Oral soln 2.5 mg/kg PO two times per day (max 200 to 400 mg/day) for 7 to 14 days. Esophageal candidiasis, age 5 yo or older: Oral soln 2.5 mg/kg PO two times per day or 5 mg/kg PO once daily for minimum of 14 to 21 days. Caps usually ineffective for esophageal candidiasis.

FORMS – Trade: Tabs 200 mg. Oral soln 10 mg/mL (150 mL). Generic/Trade: Caps 100 mg.

NOTES – Hepatotoxicity, even during 1st weeks of therapy. Monitor LFTs if baseline abnormal LFTs or history of drug-induced hepatotoxicity; consider monitoring in all patients. Decreased absorption of itraconazole with antacids, buffered didanosine, H2 blockers, proton pump inhibitors, or achlorhydria. Itraconazole levels reduced by carbamazepine, isoniazid, nevirapine, phenobarbital, phenytoin, rifabutin and rifampin, and potentially efavirenz. Itraconazole inhibits CYP3A4 metabolism of many drugs. Not more than 200 mg two times per day of itraconazole with unboosted indinavir. May increase adverse effects of trazodone; consider reducing trazodone dose. May increase QT interval with disopyramide. Caps and oral soln not interchangeable. Oral soln may be preferred in serious infections due to greater absorption. Oral soln may not achieve adequate levels in cystic fibrosis patients; consider alternative if no response. Start therapy for onychomycosis on days 1 to 2 of menses in women of childbearing potential and advise against pregnancy until 2 months after therapy ends.

KETOCONAZOLE (***Nizoral***) ▶L ♀C ▶?+ $$$

WARNING – Hepatotoxicity: Inform patients of risk and monitor. Do not use with midazolam, pimozide, triazolam.

ADULT – Systemic fungal infections: 200 to 400 mg PO daily.

PEDS – Systemic fungal infections, age 2 yo or older: 3.3 to 6.6 mg/kg PO daily.

UNAPPROVED ADULT – Tinea versicolor: 400 mg PO single dose or 200 mg PO daily for 7 days.

FORMS – Generic/Trade: Tabs 200 mg.

NOTES – Decreased absorption of ketoconazole by antacids, H2 blockers, proton pump inhibitors, buffered didanosine, and achlorhydria. Ketoconazole levels reduced by isoniazid, rifampin, and potentially efavirenz. Do not exceed 200 mg/day of ketoconazole with ritonavir or Kaletra. Ketoconazole inhibits CYP3A4 metabolism of many drugs. May increase adverse effects of trazodone; consider reducing trazodone dose.

MICONAZOLE—BUCCAL (***Oravig***) ▶L ♀C ▶? $$$$$

ADULT – Oropharyngeal candidiasis: Apply 50 mg buccal tab to gums once daily for 14 days. Apply rounded side of tab to upper gum above incisor in the morning after brushing teeth. Hold in place for 30 seconds. Tab can be used if it sticks to cheek, inside of lip, or gum. Apply to new site each day.

PEDS – Not approved in children. Not recommended for younger children due to potential risk of choking.

FORMS – Trade only: Buccal tabs, 50 mg.

NOTES – Contraindicated if hypersensitivity to milk protein concentrate. Increased INR with warfarin. Buccal tab is intended to remain in place until it dissolves. If it falls off within 6 hours of application, reposition tab. If it does not stay in place, apply a new tab. If tab is swallowed within first 6 hours, drink a glass of water and apply a new tab. No action is needed if tab falls off or is swallowed after it has been in place for at least 6 hours. Do not chew gum while tab is in place.

POSACONAZOLE (*Noxafil,* ♣ *Posanol*) ▶Glucuronidation ♀C ▶– $$$$$

ADULT – Prevention of invasive Aspergillus or Candida infection: 200 mg (5 mL) PO three times per day. Oropharyngeal candidiasis: 100 mg (2.5 mL) PO twice on day 1, then 100 mg PO once daily for 13 days. Oropharyngeal candidiasis resistant to itraconazole/fluconazole: 400 mg (10 mL) PO two times per day; duration of therapy based on severity of underlying disease and clinical response. Take during or within 20 min of full meal or liquid nutritional supplement.

PEDS – Prevention of invasive Aspergillus or Candida infection, age 13 yo or older: 200 mg (5 mL) PO three times per day. Oropharyngeal candidiasis, age 13 yo or older: 100 mg (2.5 mL) PO twice on day 1, then 100 mg PO once daily for 13 days. Oropharyngeal candidiasis resistant to itraconazole/fluconazole, age 13 yo or older: 400 mg (10 mL) PO two times per day; duration of therapy based on severity of underlying disease and clinical response. Take during or within 20 min of full meal or liquid nutritional supplement.

UNAPPROVED ADULT – Invasive pulmonary aspergillosis: 200 mg PO four times per day, then 400 mg PO two times per day when stable. Treat invasive pulmonary aspergillosis for at least 6 to 12 weeks; treat immunosuppressed patients throughout immunosuppression and until lesions resolved. Fluconazole-refractory oropharyngeal candidiasis: 400 mg PO two times per day for 3 days, then 400 mg PO once daily for up to 28 days. Fluconazole-refractory esophageal candidiasis: 400 mg PO two times per day for 14 to 21 days.

FORMS – Trade only: Oral susp 40 mg/mL (105 mL).

NOTES – Consider alternative or monitor for breakthrough fungal infection if patient cannot take during or within 20 min of a full meal or liquid nutritional supplement. If meal or liquid supplement not tolerated, consider giving with acidic carbonated drink (eg, ginger ale). Monitor for breakthrough fungal infection if severe vomiting/diarrhea, posaconazole is given by NG tube, or proton pump inhibitor or metoclopramide is coadministered. Posaconazole is a strong CYP3A4 inhibitor. Contraindicated with atorvastatin, ergot alkaloids, lovastatin, simvastatin, sirolimus, and CYP3A4 substrates that prolong the QT interval, including pimozide and quinidine. Monitor for adverse effects of atazanavir, ritonavir, alprazolam, midazolam, triazolam. Consider dosage reduction of vinca alkaloids, calcium channel blockers. Reduce cyclosporine dose by 25% and tacrolimus dose by 66% when posaconazole started; monitor levels of cyclosporine, tacrolimus. Posaconazole levels reduced by efavirenz, rifabutin, phenytoin, and cimetidine; phenytoin and rifabutin levels increased by posaconazole. Do not coadminister unless benefit exceeds risk. Monitor for rifabutin adverse effects. Posaconazole levels reduced by fosamprenavir; monitor for breakthrough fungal infection.

VORICONAZOLE (*Vfend*) ▶L ♀D ▶? $$$$$

ADULT – Invasive aspergillosis: 6 mg/kg IV q 12 h for 2 doses, then 4 mg/kg IV q 12 h. Systemic candidiasis: 6 mg/kg IV q 12 h for 2 doses, then 3 to 4 mg/kg IV q 12 h. Treat until at least 14 days past resolution of signs/symptoms or last positive blood culture. Maintenance therapy, aspergillosis or candidiasis: 200 mg PO two times per day. For wt less than 40 kg, reduce to 100 mg PO two times per day. See prescribing information for dosage adjustments for poor response/adverse effects. Esophageal candidiasis: 200 mg PO q 12 h for at least 14 days and 7 days past resolution of signs/symptoms. For wt less than 40 kg, reduce to 100 mg PO two times per day. Dosage adjustment for efavirenz: Voriconazole 400 mg PO two times per day with efavirenz 300 mg (use caps) PO once daily. Take tabs or susp 1 h before or after meals.

PEDS – Safety and efficacy not established in children younger than 12 yo. Use adult dose age 12 yo or older.

UNAPPROVED ADULT – Fluconazole-refractory oropharyngeal or esophageal candidiasis: 200 mg PO two times per day for 14 to 21 days. For wt less than 40 kg, reduce to 100 mg PO two times per day.

UNAPPROVED PEDS – In children younger than 12 yo, 7 mg/kg IV q 12 h is comparable to 4 mg/kg IV q 12 h in adults. Invasive aspergillosis: 7 mg/kg (max 400 mg) IV q 12 h for 2 doses, then 7 mg/kg (max 200 mg) IV/PO q 12 h. AAP oral regimen for fungal infections: 10 mg/kg PO q 12 h for 2 doses, then 7 mg/kg PO q 12 h.

FORMS – Trade only: Tabs 50, 200 mg (contains lactose). Susp 40 mg/mL (75 mL).

NOTES – Anaphylactoid reactions (IV only), QT interval prolongation, severe skin reactions and photosensitivity, hepatotoxicity rarely. Transient visual disturbances common; advise against hazardous tasks (if vision impaired), night driving, and strong, direct sunlight. Monitor visual (if treated for

(cont.)

VORICONAZOLE (*cont.*)

more than 28 days), liver, and renal function. Monitor pancreatic function if at risk for acute pancreatitis (recent chemotherapy/bone marrow transplant). Many drug interactions. Substrate and inhibitor of CYP2C9, 2C19, and 3A4. Do not use with carbamazepine, ergot alkaloids, fluconazole, lopinavir-ritonavir (Kaletra), phenobarbital, pimozide, quinidine, rifabutin, rifampin, ritonavir 400 mg two times per day, sirolimus, or St. John's wort. Ritonavir decreases voriconazole levels; avoid coadministration unless benefit exceeds risk. Dosage adjustments for drug interactions with cyclosporine, omeprazole, phenytoin, tacrolimus in prescribing information. Increased INR with warfarin. Could inhibit metabolism of benzodiazepines, calcium channel blockers, fentanyl, ibuprofen, methadone, oxycodone, and statins. When combining voriconazole with oral contraceptives, monitor for adverse effects from increased levels of voriconazole, estrogen, and progestin. Dilute IV to 5 mg/mL or less; max infusion rate is 3 mg/kg/h over 1 to 2 h. Do not infuse IV voriconazole at same time as a blood product/concentrated electrolytes even if given by separate IV lines. IV voriconazole can be infused at the same time as non concentrated electrolytes/total parenteral nutrition if given by separate lines; give TPN by different port if multi-lumen catheter is used. Vehicle in IV form may accumulate in renal impairment; oral preferred if CrCl is less than 50 mL/min. Mild/moderate cirrhosis (Child-Pugh class A/B): Same loading dose and reduce maintenance dose by 50%. Oral susp stable for 14 days at room temperature.

ANTIMICROBIALS: Antifungal Agents—Echinocandins

NOTE: See www.idsociety.org for guidelines on the management of fungal infections. See www.aidsinfo.nih.gov for management of fungal infections in HIV-infected patients.

ANIDULAFUNGIN (***Eraxis***) ▶Degraded chemically ♀C ▶? $$$$$

ADULT – Candidemia, other systemic candidal infections: 200 mg IV load on day 1, then 100 mg IV once daily until at least 14 days after last positive culture. Esophageal candidiasis: 100 mg IV load on day 1, then 50 mg IV once daily for at least 14 days, and continuing for at least 7 days after symptoms resolved.

PEDS – Not approved in children.

UNAPPROVED PEDS – 0.75 to 1.5 mg/kg IV once daily. Systemic Candida infections, age 2 yo or older: 1.5 mg/kg IV once daily.

NOTES – Max infusion rate of 1.1 mg/min to prevent histamine reactions. Diluent contains dehydrated alcohol.

CASPOFUNGIN (***Cancidas***) ▶KL ♀C ▶? $$$$$

ADULT – Infuse IV over 1 h. Aspergillosis, candidemia, empiric therapy in febrile neutropenia: 70 mg loading dose on day 1, then 50 mg once daily. Patients taking rifampin: 70 mg once daily. Consider this dose with other enzyme inducers (such as carbamazepine, dexamethasone, efavirenz, nevirapine, phenytoin) or if inadequate response to lower dose in febrile neutropenia or aspergillosis. Esophageal candidiasis: 50 mg daily. Duration of therapy in invasive aspergillosis is based on severity, treatment response, and resolution of immunosuppression. Treat candidal infections for at least 14 days after last positive culture. For empiric therapy of febrile neutropenia, treat until neutropenia resolved. If fungal infection confirmed, treat for at least 14 days and continue treatment for at least 7 days after symptoms and neutropenia resolved.

PEDS – Infuse IV over 1 h. Aspergillosis, candidemia, esophageal candidiasis, empiric therapy in febrile neutropenia, 3 mo to 17 yo: 70 mg/m^2 loading dose on day 1, then 50 mg/m^2 once daily. Consider increasing daily dose to 70 mg/m^2 up to max of 70 mg once daily if coadministered with enzyme inducers (eg, carbamazepine, dexamethasone, efavirenz, nevirapine, phenytoin, or rifampin) or if inadequate response to lower dose in febrile neutropenia or aspergillosis. Duration of therapy in invasive aspergillosis is based on severity, treatment response, and resolution of immunosuppression. Treat Candida infections for at least 14 days after last positive culture. For empiric therapy of febrile neutropenia, treat until neutropenia resolved. If fungal infection confirmed, treat for at least 14 days and continue treatment for at least 7 days after symptoms and neutropenia resolved. If vial strength is available, in order to improve dosing accuracy, use 50 mg vial (5 mg/mL) for pediatric dose less than 50 mg and 70 mg vial (7 mg/mL) for pediatric dose greater than 50 mg.

NOTES – Abnormal LFTs reported; possible risk of hepatitis. Monitor hepatic function if abnormal LFTs. Cyclosporine increases caspofungin levels and hepatic transaminases; risk of concomitant

(cont.)

CASPOFUNGIN (*cont.*)

use unclear. Caspofungin decreases tacrolimus levels. Dosage adjustment in adults with moderate liver dysfunction (Child-Pugh score 7 to 9): 35 mg IV daily (after 70 mg loading dose in patients with invasive aspergillosis).

MICAFUNGIN (*Mycamine*) ▶L, feces ♀C ▶? $$$$$

ADULT – Esophageal candidiasis: 150 mg IV once daily. Candidemia, acute disseminated candidiasis, Candida peritonitis/abscess: 100 mg IV once daily. Prevention of candidal infections in bone marrow transplant patients: 50 mg IV once daily. Infuse over 1 h. Histamine-mediated reactions possible with more rapid infusion. Flush existing IV lines with NS before micafungin infusion.

PEDS – Not approved in children.

UNAPPROVED ADULT – Prophylaxis of invasive aspergillosis: 50 mg IV once daily. Infuse IV over 1 h.

UNAPPROVED PEDS – Esophageal candidiasis: 3 mg/kg up to 150 mg IV once daily for wt less than 50 kg; 150 mg IV once daily for wt greater than 50 kg. Systemic candidiasis: 2 to 3 mg/kg up to 150 mg IV once daily for wt less than 40 kg; 100 to 150 mg IV once daily for wt 40 kg or greater. Higher doses may be needed in infants, but specific dose is not established.

NOTES – Increases levels of sirolimus and nifedipine. Not dialyzed. Protect diluted soln from light. Do not mix with other meds; it may precipitate.

ANTIMICROBIALS: Antifungal Agents—Polyenes

NOTE: See www.idsociety.org for guidelines on the management of fungal infections. See www.aidsinfo.nih.gov for management of fungal infections in HIV-infected patients.

AMPHOTERICIN B DEOXYCHOLATE (*Fungizone*) ▶Tissues ♀B ▶? $$$$

WARNING – Do not use IV route for noninvasive fungal infections (oral thrush, vaginal or esophageal candidiasis) in patients with normal neutrophil counts.

ADULT – Life-threatening systemic fungal infections: Test dose 1 mg slow IV. Wait 2 to 4 h, and if tolerated start 0.25 mg/kg IV daily. Advance to 0.5 to 1.5 mg/kg/day depending on fungal type. Maximum dose 1.5 mg/kg/day. Infuse over 2 to 6 h. Hydrate with 500 mL NS before and after infusion to decrease risk of nephrotoxicity.

PEDS – No remaining FDA-approved indications.

UNAPPROVED ADULT – Alternative regimen, life-threatening systemic fungal infections: 1 mg test dose as part of first infusion (no need for separate IV bag); if tolerated continue infusion, giving target dose of 0.5 to 1.5 mg/kg on first day. Candidemia: 0.5 to 1 mg/kg IV daily. Treat until 14 days after first negative blood culture and resolution of signs/symptoms. Symptomatic Candida cystitis: 0.3 to 0.6 mg/kg IV for 1 to 7 days. Candida pyelonephritis: 0.5 to 0.7 mg/kg IV daily (± flucytosine). Cryptococcal meningitis in HIV infection: 0.7 mg/kg/day IV preferably in combo with flucytosine 25 mg/kg PO q 6 h for 2 weeks. Follow with fluconazole consolidation, then fluconazole chronic suppression until immune reconstitution.

UNAPPROVED PEDS – Systemic life-threatening fungal infections: Test dose 0.1 mg/kg (max of 1 mg) slow IV. Wait 2 to 4 h, and if tolerated start 0.25 mg/kg IV once daily. Advance to 0.5 to 1.5 mg/kg/day depending on fungal type. Maximum dose 1.5 mg/kg/day. Infuse over 2 to 6 h. Hydrate with 10 to 15 mL/kg NS before infusion to decrease risk of nephrotoxicity. Alternative dosing regimen: Give test dose as part of first infusion (separate IV bag not needed); if tolerated continue infusion, giving target dose of 0.5 to 1.5 mg/kg on first day. Cryptococcal infection in HIV-infected patients: 0.7 to 1 mg/kg IV once daily; may add flucytosine depending on site and severity of infection.

NOTES – Acute infusion reactions, anaphylaxis, nephrotoxicity, hypokalemia, hypomagnesemia, acidosis, anemia. Monitor renal and hepatic function, CBC, serum electrolytes. Lipid formulations better tolerated, preferred in renal dysfunction.

AMPHOTERICIN B LIPID FORMULATIONS (*Amphotec, Abelcet, AmBisome*) ▶? ♀B ▶? $$$$$

ADULT – Lipid formulations used primarily in patients refractory/intolerant to amphotericin deoxycholate. Abelcet: Invasive fungal infections: 5 mg/kg/day IV at 2.5 mg/kg/h. Shake infusion bag q 2 h. AmBisome: Infuse IV over 2 h. Empiric therapy of fungal infections in febrile neutropenia: 3 mg/kg/day. Aspergillus, candidal, cryptococcal infections: 3 to 5 mg/kg/day. Cryptococcal meningitis in HIV infection: 6 mg/kg/day. Amphotec: Aspergillosis: Test dose of 10 mL over 15 to 30 min, observe for 30 min, then 3 to 4 mg/kg/day IV at 1 mg/kg/h.

(cont.)

AMPHOTERICIN B LIPID FORMULATIONS (*cont.*)

PEDS – Lipid formulations used primarily in patients refractory/intolerant to amphotericin deoxycholate. Abelcet: Invasive fungal infections: 5 mg/kg/day IV at 2.5 mg/kg/h. Shake infusion bag q 2 h. AmBisome: Infuse IV over 2 h. Empiric therapy of fungal infections in febrile neutropenia: 3 mg/kg/day. Aspergillus, candidal, cryptococcal infections: 3 to 5 mg/kg/day. Cryptococcal meningitis in HIV infection: 6 mg/kg/day. Amphotec: Aspergillosis: Test dose of 10 mL over 15 to 30 min, observe for 30 min, then 3 to 4 mg/kg/day IV at 1 mg/kg/h.

NOTES – Acute infusion reactions, anaphylaxis, nephrotoxicity, hypokalemia, hypomagnesemia, acidosis. Lipid formulations better tolerated than amphotericin deoxycholate, preferred in renal dysfunction. Monitor renal and hepatic function, CBC, electrolytes.

ANTIMICROBIALS: Antifungal Agents—Other

NOTE: See www.idsociety.org for guidelines on the management of fungal infections. See www.aidsinfo.nih.gov for management of fungal infections in HIV-infected patients.

FLUCYTOSINE (*Ancobon*) ▶K ♀C ▶– $$$$$

WARNING – Extreme caution in renal or bone marrow impairment. Monitor hematologic, hepatic, renal function in all patients.

ADULT – Candidal/cryptococcal infections: 50 to 150 mg/kg/day PO divided four times per day. Candida UTI: 100 mg/kg/day PO divided four times per day for 7 to 10 days for symptomatic cystitis, for 14 days (± amphotericin deoxycholate) for pyelonephritis. Initial therapy for cryptococcal meningitis: 100 mg/kg/day PO divided four times per day.

PEDS – Not approved in children.

UNAPPROVED PEDS – Candidal/cryptococcal infections: 50 to 150 mg/kg/day PO divided four times per day.

FORMS – Generic/Trade: Caps 250, 500 mg.

NOTES – Flucytosine is given with other antifungal agents. Myelosuppression. Reduce nausea by taking caps a few at a time over 15 min. Monitor flucytosine levels. Peak 70 to 80 mg/L, trough 30 to 40 mg/L. Reduce dose in renal dysfunction. Avoid in children with severe renal dysfunction.

GRISEOFULVIN (*Grifulvin V*) ▶Skin ♀C ▶? $$$$

ADULT – Tinea: 500 mg PO daily for 4 to 6 weeks for capitis, 2 to 4 weeks for corporis, 4 to 8 weeks for pedis, 4 months for fingernails, 6 months for toenails. Can use 1 g/day for pedis and unguium.

PEDS – Tinea: 11 mg/kg PO daily for 4 to 6 weeks for capitis, 2 to 4 weeks for corporis, 4 to 8 weeks for pedis, 4 months for fingernails, 6 months for toenails.

UNAPPROVED PEDS – Tinea capitis: AAP recommends 10 to 20 mg/kg (max 1 g) PO daily for 4 to 6 weeks, continuing for 2 weeks past symptom resolution. Some infections may require 20 to 25 mg/kg/day or ultramicrosize griseofulvin 5 to 10 mg/kg (max 750 mg) PO daily.

FORMS – Generic/Trade: Susp 125 mg/5 mL (120 mL). Trade only: Tabs 250, 500 mg.

NOTES – Do not use in liver failure, porphyria. May cause photosensitivity, lupus-like syndrome/exacerbation of lupus. Decreased INR with warfarin, decreased efficacy of oral contraceptives. Ultramicrosize formulations have greater GI absorption, and are available with different strengths and dosing.

GRISEOFULVIN ULTRAMICROSIZE (*Gris-PEG*) ▶Skin ♀C ▶? $$$$

ADULT – Tinea: 375 mg PO daily for 4 to 6 weeks for capitis, 2 to 4 weeks for corporis, 4 to 8 weeks for pedis, 4 months for fingernails, 6 months for toenails. Can use 750 mg/day for pedis and unguium. Best absorption when given after meal containing fat.

PEDS – Tinea, age 2 yo or older: 7.3 mg/kg PO daily for 4 to 6 weeks for capitis, 2 to 4 weeks for corporis, 4 to 8 weeks for pedis, 4 months for fingernails, 6 months for toenails. Give 82.5 to 165 mg PO daily for 13.6 to 22.6 kg. Give 165 to 330 mg for wt greater than 22.6 kg. Tinea capitis: AAP recommends 5 to 15 mg/kg (up to 750 mg) PO daily for 4 to 6 weeks, continuing for 2 weeks past symptom resolution. Best absorption when given after meal containing fat.

FORMS – Trade only: Tabs 125, 250 mg.

NOTES – Do not use in liver failure, porphyria. May cause photosensitivity, lupus-like syndrome/exacerbation of lupus. Decreased INR with warfarin, decreased efficacy of oral contraceptives. Microsize formulations, which have lower GI absorption, are available with different strengths and dosing.

NYSTATIN (♣ *Nilstat*) ▶Not absorbed ♀B ▶? $$

ADULT – Thrush: 4 to 6 mL PO swish and swallow four times per day or suck on 1 to 2 troches 4 to 5 times per day.

(cont.)

NYSTATIN (*cont.*)

PEDS – Thrush, infants: 2 mL/dose PO with 1 mL in each cheek four times per day. Premature and low-wt infants: 0.5 mL PO in each cheek four times per day. Thrush, older children: 4 to 6 mL PO swish and swallow four times per day or suck on 1 to 2 troches 4 to 5 times per day.

FORMS – Generic only: Susp 100,000 units/mL (60, 480 mL). Troches 500,000 units/tab.

TERBINAFINE (*Lamisil*) ▶LK ♀B ▶– $

ADULT – Onychomycosis: 250 mg PO daily for 6 weeks for fingernails, for 12 weeks for toenails.

PEDS – Tinea capitis, age 4 yo or older: Give granules once daily with food for 6 weeks: 125 mg for wt less than 25 kg, 187.5 mg for wt 25 to 35 kg, 250 mg for wt greater than 35 kg.

UNAPPROVED PEDS – Onychomycosis: 67.5 mg PO daily for wt less than 20 kg, 125 mg PO once daily for wt 20 to 40 kg, 250 mg PO once daily for wt greater than 40 kg. Treat for 6 weeks for fingernails, for 12 weeks for toenails.

FORMS – Generic/Trade: Tabs 250 mg. Trade only: Oral granules 125, 187.5 mg/packet.

NOTES – Hepatotoxicity; monitor AST and ALT at baseline. Neutropenia. May rarely cause or exacerbate lupus. Do not use in liver disease or CrCl less than 50 mL/min. Test nail specimen to confirm diagnosis before prescribing. Inhibitor of CYP2D6.

ANTIMICROBIALS: Antimalarials

NOTE: For help treating malaria or getting antimalarials, see www.cdc.gov/malaria or call the CDC "malaria hotline" 770-488–7788 Monday through Friday 9 am to 5 pm EST; after hours/weekend 770-488–7100. Pediatric doses of antimalarials should never exceed adult doses.

CHLOROQUINE (*Aralen*) ▶KL ♀C but + ▶+ $

WARNING – Review product labeling for precautions and adverse effects before prescribing.

ADULT – Doses as chloroquine phosphate. Malaria prophylaxis, chloroquine-sensitive areas: 500 mg PO q week from 1 to 2 weeks before exposure to 4 weeks after. Malaria treatment, chloroquine-sensitive areas: 1 g PO once, then 500 mg PO at 6, 24, and 48 h. Total dose is 2.5 g. Extraintestinal amebiasis: 1 g PO daily for 2 days, then 500 mg PO daily for 2 to 3 weeks.

PEDS – Doses as chloroquine phosphate. Malaria prophylaxis, chloroquine-sensitive areas: 8.3 mg/kg (up to 500 mg) PO q week from 1 to 2 weeks before exposure to 4 weeks after. Malaria treatment, chloroquine-sensitive areas: 16.7 mg/kg PO once, then 8.3 mg/kg at 6, 24, and 48 h. Do not exceed adult dose. Chloroquine phosphate 8.3 mg/kg is equivalent to chloroquine base 5 mg/kg.

FORMS – Generic only: Tabs 250 mg. Generic/Trade: Tabs 500 mg (500 mg phosphate equivalent to 300 mg base).

NOTES – Can prolong QT interval and cause torsades. Retinopathy with chronic/high doses; eye exams required. May cause seizures (caution advised if epilepsy); ototoxicity (caution advised if hearing loss); myopathy (discontinue if muscle weakness develops); bone marrow toxicity (monitor CBC if long-term use); exacerbation of psoriasis. Concentrates in liver; caution advised if hepatic disease, alcoholism, or hepatotoxic drugs. Antacids reduce absorption; give at least 4 h apart. Chloroquine reduces ampicillin absorption; give at least 2 h apart. May increase cyclosporine levels. As little as 1 g can cause fatal overdose in a child. Fatal malaria reported after chloroquine used as malaria prophylaxis in areas with chloroquine resistance; use only in areas without resistance. Other agents are superior for severe chloroquine-sensitive malaria. Maternal antimalarial prophylaxis does not harm breastfed infant or protect infant from malaria. Use with primaquine phosphate for treatment of *P. vivax* or *P. ovale*.

COARTEM **(artemether + lumefantrine, coartemether)** ▶L ♀C ▶? $$$

ADULT – Uncomplicated malaria, wt 35 kg or greater: 4 tabs PO two times per day for 3 days. On day 1, give 2nd dose 8 h after 1st dose. Take with food.

PEDS – Uncomplicated malaria, wt greater than 5 kg and age 2 mo or older: Take with food two times per day for 3 days. On day 1, give 2nd dose 8 h after 1st dose. Dose based on wt: 1 tab for 5 to 14 kg; 2 tabs for 15 to 24 kg; 3 tabs for 25 to 34 kg; 4 tab for 35 kg or greater.

FORMS – Trade only: Tabs, artemether 20 mg + lumefantrine 120 mg.

NOTES – Can prolong QT interval; avoid using in proarrhythmic conditions or with drugs

(cont.)

***COARTEM** (cont.)*

that prolong QT interval. May inhibit CYP2D6; avoid with drugs metabolized by CYP2D6 that have cardiac effects and caution with CYP3A4 inhibitors as both interactions may prolong QT interval. Do not use Coartem and halofantrine within 1 month of each other. Repeat the dose if vomiting occurs within 1 to 2 h; use another antimalarial if second dose is vomited. Can crush tabs and mix with 1 to 2 tsp water immediately before the dose.

MALARONE **(atovaquone + proguanil)** ▶Fecal excretion; LK ♀C ▶? $$$$$

ADULT – Malaria prophylaxis: 1 adult tab PO once daily from 1 to 2 days before exposure until 7 days after. Malaria treatment: 4 adult tabs PO once daily for 3 days. Take with food/milky drink at same time each day. Repeat dose if vomiting within 1 h after the dose. CDC recommends for presumptive self-treatment of malaria (same dose as for treatment, but not for patients currently taking it for prophylaxis).

PEDS – Safety and efficacy established in children with wt 11 kg or greater for prevention, and 5 kg or greater for treatment. Prevention of malaria: Give following dose based on wt PO once daily from 1 to 2 days before exposure until 7 days after: 1 ped tab for 11 to 20 kg; 2 ped tabs for 21 to 30 kg; 3 ped tabs for 31 to 40 kg; 1 adult tab for greater than 40 kg. Treatment of malaria: Give following dose based on wt PO once daily for 3 days: 2 ped tabs for 5 to 8 kg; 3 ped tabs for 9 to 10 kg; 1 adult tab for 11 to 20 kg; 2 adult tabs for 21 to 30 kg; 3 adult tabs for 31 to 40 kg; 4 adult tabs for greater than 40 kg. Take with food or milky drink at same time each day. Repeat dose if vomiting occurs within 1 h after dose.

UNAPPROVED PEDS – CDC doses for prevention of malaria: Give PO daily from 1 to 2 days before exposure until 7 days after: ½ ped tab for wt 5 to 8 kg; ¾ ped tab for wt 9 to 10 kg. Not advised for infants less than 5 kg.

FORMS – Generic/Trade: Adult tabs atovaquone 250 mg + proguanil 100 mg. Trade only: Pediatric tabs 62.5 mg + 25 mg.

NOTES – Vomiting common with malaria treatment doses (consider antiemetic). Monitor parasitemia. Atovaquone levels may be decreased by tetracycline, metoclopramide (use another antiemetic if possible), and rifampin (avoid). Atovaquone can reduce indinavir trough levels. Proguanil may increase the INR with warfarin. If CrCl is less than 30 mL/min avoid for malaria prophylaxis and use cautiously for treatment. CDC recommends against use by women breastfeeding infant weighing less than 5 kg.

MEFLOQUINE ▶L ♀B ▶? $$

ADULT – Malaria prophylaxis, chloroquine-resistant areas: 250 mg PO once weekly from 1 week before exposure until 4 weeks after. Malaria treatment: 1250 mg PO single dose. Take on full stomach with at least 8 oz water.

PEDS – Malaria treatment: 20 to 25 mg/kg PO; given in 1 to 2 divided doses 6 to 8 h apart to reduce risk of vomiting. Repeat full dose if vomiting within 30 min after dose; repeat ½ dose if vomiting within 30 to 60 min after dose. Experience limited in infants age younger than 3 mo or wt less than 5 kg. Malaria prophylaxis: Give the following dose based on wt PO once a week starting 1 week before exposure until 4 weeks after. For 9 kg or less give 5 mg/kg; for wt greater than 9 to 19 kg give ¼ tab; for wt greater than 19 to 30 kg give ½ tab; for wt greater than 31 to 45 kg give ¾ tab; for wt 45 kg or greater give 1 tab. Take on full stomach. Pharmacist needs to compound 5 mg/kg dose.

UNAPPROVED ADULT – CDC regimen for malaria: 750 mg PO followed by 500 mg PO 6 to 12 h later, for total of 1250 mg. Quinine plus doxycycline/tetracycline/clindamycin or atovaquone-proguanil preferred over mefloquine because of high rate of neuropsychiatric adverse effects with malaria treatment doses of mefloquine.

UNAPPROVED PEDS – Malaria prophylaxis, chloroquine-resistant areas: CDC recommends these PO doses once weekly starting 1 week before exposure until 4 weeks after: 5 mg/kg for wt 15 kg or less; ¼ tab for 15 to 19 kg; ½ tab for 20 to 30 kg; ¾ tab for 31 to 45 kg; 1 tab for 45 kg or greater. Malaria treatment for wt less than 45 kg: 15 mg/kg PO, then 10 mg/kg PO given 8 to 12 h after 1st dose. Take on full stomach with at least 8 oz water.

FORMS – Generic only: Tabs 250 mg.

NOTES – Cardiac conduction disturbances. Do not use with ziprasidone. Do not give until 12 h after the last dose of quinidine, quinine, or chloroquine; may cause ECG changes and seizures. Contraindicated for prophylaxis if depression (active/recent), generalized anxiety disorder, psychosis, schizophrenia, other major psychiatric disorder, or history of seizures. Tell patients to discontinue if psychiatric symptoms occur during prophylaxis.

(cont.)

MEFLOQUINE (*cont.*)

May cause drowsiness (warn about hazardous tasks). Can crush tabs and mix with a little water, milk, or other liquid. Pharmacists can put small doses into caps to mask bitter taste. Decreases valproate levels. Rifampin decreases mefloquine levels. Maternal use of antimalarial prophylaxis does not harm or protect breastfed infant from malaria.

PRIMAQUINE ▶L ♀– ▶– $$

WARNING – Review product labeling for precautions and adverse effects and document normal G6PD level before prescribing.

ADULT – Prevention of relapse, P. vivax/ovale malaria: 30 mg base PO daily for 14 days.

PEDS – Not approved in children.

UNAPPROVED ADULT – Pneumocystis in patients intolerant to trimethoprim-sulfamethoxazole: 15 to 30 mg primaquine base PO daily plus clindamycin 600 to 900 mg IV q 6 to 8 h or 300 to 450 mg PO q 6 to 8 h for 21 days. Primary prevention of malaria in special circumstances: 30 mg base PO once daily beginning 1 to 2 days before exposure until 7 days after (consult with malaria expert; contact CDC at 770–488–7788 for info).

UNAPPROVED PEDS – Prevention of relapse, *P. vivax/ovale* malaria: 0.5 mg/kg (up to 30 mg) base PO once daily for 14 days. Primary prevention of malaria in special circumstances: 0.5 mg/kg (up to 30 mg) base PO once daily beginning 1 to 2 days before exposure until 7 days after (consult with malaria expert; contact CDC at 770-488-7788 for info).

FORMS – Generic only: Tabs 26.3 mg (equiv alent to 15 mg base).

NOTES – Causes hemolytic anemia in G6PD deficiency, methemoglobinemia in NADH methemoglobin reductase deficiency. Contraindicated in pregnancy and G6PD deficiency; screen for deficiency before prescribing. Stop if dark urine or anemia. Avoid in patients with RA or SLE, recent quinacrine use, or use of other bone marrow suppressants.

QUININE (***Qualaquin***) ▶L ♀C ▶+? $$$$

WARNING – FDA has repeatedly warned that the risks of using quinine for management of nocturnal leg cramps (an unapproved indication) exceed any potential benefit. Risks include life-threatening hematological reactions, especially thrombocytopenia and hemolytic-uremic syndrome/thrombotic thrombocytopenic purpura (HUS/TTP). HUS/TTP can cause chronic renal impairment.

ADULT – Malaria: 648 mg PO three times per day for 3 days (Africa/South America) or 7 days (Southeast Asia). Also give 7-day course of doxycycline, tetracycline, or clindamycin.

PEDS – Not approved in children.

UNAPPROVED ADULT – Nocturnal leg cramps: 260 to 325 mg PO at bedtime. FDA warns that risks outweigh benefits for this indication.

UNAPPROVED PEDS – Malaria: 25 to 30 mg/kg/day (up to 2 g/day) PO divided q 8 h for 3 days (Africa/South America) or 7 days (Southeast Asia). Also give 7-day course of doxycycline, tetracycline, or clindamycin.

FORMS – Trade only: Caps 324 mg.

NOTES – Thrombocytopenia, hemolytic uremic syndrome/thrombotic thrombocytopenic purpura, cinchonism, hemolytic anemia with G6PD deficiency, cardiac conduction disturbances, hearing impairment. Contraindicated if prolonged QT interval, optic neuritis, myasthenia gravis, or hypersensitivity to quinine, quinidine, or mefloquine. Many drug interactions. Do not use with clarithromycin, erythromycin, rifampin, ritonavir, neuromuscular blockers. May increase digoxin levels. May decrease theophylline levels. Monitor INR with warfarin. Antacids decrease quinine absorption. Rule out G6PD deficiency in breastfed at-risk infant before giving quinine to mother.

ANTIMICROBIALS: Antimycobacterial Agents

NOTE: Treat active mycobacterial infection with at least 2 drugs. See guidelines at www.thoracic.org/statements/ and www.aidsinfo.nih.gov. Get baseline LFTs, creatinine, and platelet count before treating TB. Evaluate at least monthly for adverse drug reactions. Routine liver and renal function tests not needed unless baseline dysfunction or increased risk of hepatotoxicity.

CLOFAZIMINE ▶Fecal excretion ♀C ▶?–

ADULT – Approved for leprosy therapy.

PEDS – Not approved in children.

UNAPPROVED ADULT – *Mycobacterium avium* complex in immunocompetent patients: 100 to 200 mg PO daily until "tan," then 50 mg PO daily or 100 mg PO three times per week. Use in combination with other antimycobacterial agents. Not for general use in AIDS patients due to increased mortality.

FORMS – Caps 50 mg. Distributed only through investigational new drug application.

(cont.)

CLOFAZIMINE (*cont.*)

For leprosy, contact National Hansen's Disease Program (phone 800–642–2477). For non-leprosy indications, contact FDA Division of Special Pathogen and Transplant Products Program (phone 301–796–1600).

NOTES – Abdominal pain common; rare reports of splenic infarction, bowel obstruction, and GI bleeding. Pink to brownish-black skin pigmentation that may persist for months to years after drug is discontinued. Discoloration of urine, body secretions.

DAPSONE (*Aczone*) ▶LK ♀C ▶– $

ADULT – Leprosy: 100 mg PO daily with rifampin ± clofazimine or ethionamide. Acne (Aczone; $$$$): Apply two times per day.

PEDS – Leprosy: 1 mg/kg (up to 100 mg) PO daily with other antimycobacterial agents. Acne, 12 to 17 yo (Aczone; $$$$): Apply two times per day.

UNAPPROVED ADULT – Pneumocystis prophylaxis: 100 mg PO daily. Pneumocystis treatment: 100 mg PO daily with trimethoprim 5 mg/kg PO three times per day for 21 days.

UNAPPROVED PEDS – Pneumocystis prophylaxis, age 1 mo or older: 2 mg/kg (up to 100 mg/day) PO once daily or 4 mg/kg/week (up to 200 mg/week) PO once weekly.

FORMS – Generic only: Tabs 25, 100 mg. Trade only (Aczone): Topical gel 5% 30 or 60 g.

NOTES – Oral: Blood dyscrasias, severe allergic skin reactions, sulfone syndrome, hemolysis in G6PD deficiency, hepatotoxicity, neuropathy, photosensitivity, leprosy reactional states. Monitor CBC weekly for 4 weeks, then monthly for 6 months, then twice a year. Monitor LFTs.

ETHAMBUTOL (*Myambutol*, ✤*Etibi*) ▶LK ♀C but + ▶+ $$$$

ADULT – TB: ATS and CDC recommend 15 to 20 mg/kg PO daily. Dose with whole tabs: 800 mg PO daily for wt 40 to 55 kg, 1200 mg PO daily for wt 56 to 75 kg, 1600 mg PO daily for wt 76 to 90 kg. Base dose on estimated lean body wt. Max dose regardless of wt is 1600 mg/day.

PEDS – TB: ATS and CDC recommend 15 to 20 mg/kg (up to 1 g) PO daily. Use cautiously if visual acuity cannot be monitored. Manufacturer recommends against use in children younger than 13 yo.

UNAPPROVED ADULT – Treatment or prevention of recurrent *Mycobacterium avium* complex disease in HIV infection: 15 to 25 mg/kg (up to 1600 mg) PO daily with clarithromycin/azithromycin ± rifabutin.

UNAPPROVED PEDS – Treatment or prevention of recurrent *Mycobacterium avium* complex disease in HIV infection: 15 mg/kg (up to 900 mg) PO daily with clarithromycin/azithromycin ± rifabutin.

FORMS – Generic/Trade: Tabs 100, 400 mg.

NOTES – Can cause retrobulbar neuritis. Avoid, if possible, in patients with optic neuritis. Test visual acuity and color discrimination at baseline. Ask about visual disturbances monthly. Monitor visual acuity and color discrimination monthly if dose is greater than 15 to 20 mg/kg, duration is longer than 2 months, or renal dysfunction. Advise patients to report any change in vision immediately; do not use in those who cannot report visual symptoms (eg, children, unconscious). Do not give aluminum hydroxide antacid until at least 4 h after ethambutol dose. Reduce dose in renal impairment.

ISONIAZID (*INH*) ▶LK ♀C but + ▶+ $

WARNING – Hepatotoxicity. Obtain baseline LFTs. Monitor LFTs monthly in high-risk patients (HIV, signs/history of liver disease, abnormal LFTs at baseline, pregnancy/postpartum, alcoholism/regular alcohol use, some patients older than 35 yo). Tell all patients to stop isoniazid and call prescriber at once if hepatotoxicity symptoms develop. Discontinue if ALT at least 3 times the upper limit of normal with hepatotoxicity symptoms or ALT at least 5 times the upper limit of normal without hepatotoxicity symptoms.

ADULT – TB treatment: 5 mg/kg (up to 300 mg) PO daily or 15 mg/kg (up to 900 mg) twice a week. Latent TB: 300 mg PO daily.

PEDS – TB treatment: 10 to 15 mg/kg (up to 300 mg) PO daily. Latent TB: 10 mg/kg (up to 300 mg) PO daily.

UNAPPROVED ADULT – American Thoracic Society regimen, latent TB: 5 mg/kg (up to 300 mg) PO daily for 9 months (6 months adequate if HIV-negative, but less effective than 9 months). This is preferred regimen for age 2 to 11 yo. Weekly regimen for latent TB: Give once weekly for 12 weeks isoniazid 15 mg/kg PO rounded up to nearest 50 or 100 mg (max 900 mg) plus rifapentine 750 mg for wt 32.1 to 49.9 kg or rifapentine 900 mg for wt 50 kg or greater. Regimen intended for directly observed therapy; not recommended for HIV-infected patients treated with antiretrovirals, or for use during pregnancy.

UNAPPROVED PEDS – American Thoracic Society regimen for latent TB: 10 to 20 mg/kg

(cont.)

ISONIAZID (*cont.*)

(up to 300 mg) PO daily for 9 months. Weekly regimen for latent TB, age 12 yo or older: Give once weekly for 12 weeks isoniazid 15 mg/kg PO rounded up to nearest 50 or 100 mg (max 900 mg) + rifapentine dosed according to wt. Rifapentine dose is 300 mg for 10 to 14 kg; 450 mg for 14.1 to 25 kg; 600 mg for 25.1 to 32 kg; 750 mg for wt 32.1 to 49.9 kg; 900 mg for wt 50 kg or greater. Regimen intended for directly observed therapy; not recommended for HIV-infected patients treated with antiretrovirals, or use during pregnancy.

FORMS – Generic only: Tabs 100, 300 mg. Syrup 50 mg/5 mL.

NOTES – To reduce risk of peripheral neuropathy, give pyridoxine if alcoholism, diabetes, HIV, uremia, malnutrition, seizure disorder, pregnant/breastfeeding woman, breastfed infant of INH-treated mother. Many drug interactions.

PYRAZINAMIDE (***PZA***) ▶LK ♀C ▶? $$$$

WARNING – The ATS and CDC recommend against general use of 2-month regimen of rifampin plus pyrazinamide for latent TB due to reports of fatal hepatotoxicity.

ADULT – TB: ATS and CDC recommend 20 to 25 mg/kg PO daily. Dose with whole tabs: Give 1000 mg PO daily for wt 40 to 55 kg, 1500 mg daily for wt 56 to 75 kg, 2000 mg for wt 76 to 90 kg. Base dose on estimated lean body wt. Max dose regardless of wt is 2000 mg PO daily.

PEDS – TB: 15 to 30 mg/kg (up to 2000 mg) PO daily.

FORMS – Generic only: Tabs 500 mg.

NOTES – Hepatotoxicity, hyperuricemia (avoid in acute gout). Obtain LFTs at baseline. Monitor periodically in high-risk patients (HIV infection, alcoholism, pregnancy, signs/history of liver disease, abnormal LFTs at baseline). Discontinue if ALT is at least 3 times the upper limit of normal with hepatotoxicity symptoms or ALT is at least 5 times upper limit of normal without hepatotoxicity symptoms. Consider reduced dose in renal dysfunction.

RIFABUTIN (***Mycobutin***) ▶L ♀B ▶? $$$$$

ADULT – Prevention of disseminated *Mycobacterium avium* complex disease in AIDS: 300 mg PO daily; can give 150 mg PO two times per day if GI upset. Per HIV guidelines, reduce rifabutin dose for coadministration with unboosted atazanavir or fosamprenavir; or ritonavir-boosted atazanavir, darunavir, fosamprenavir, lopinavir (Kaletra), saquinavir, or tipranavir: 150 mg PO once daily or 300 mg PO three times per week. For ritonavir-boosted regimens, monitor antimycobacterial activity and consider therapeutic drug monitoring. Reduce dose for nelfinavir (use nelfinavir 1250 mg PO two times per day), unboosted indinavir (increase indinavir to 1000 mg PO q 8 h): 150 mg PO daily. Dosage increase for efavirenz: 450 to 600 mg PO daily or 600 mg PO three times per week. Use standard rifabutin dose with etravirine (without ritonavir-boosted protease inhibitor) or nevirapine. Avoid rifabutin in patients receiving etravirine with a ritonavir-boosted protease inhibitor or rilpivirine. Monitor CBC at least weekly. Consider dosage adjustment based on rifabutin levels for patients receiving antiretroviral drugs.

PEDS – Not approved in children.

UNAPPROVED ADULT – TB or *Mycobacterium avium* complex disease treatment in AIDS: 300 mg PO daily. Dosage reduction for ritonavir-boosted protease inhibitors: 150 mg once daily or three times weekly. For ritonavir-boosted regimens, monitor antimycobacterial activity and consider therapeutic drug monitoring.

UNAPPROVED PEDS – *Mycobacterium avium* complex disease. Prophylaxis: Give 5 mg/kg (up to 300 mg) PO daily for age younger than 6 yo; give 300 mg PO daily for age 6 yo or older. Treatment: 10 to 20 mg/kg (max 300 mg/day) PO once daily. TB: 10 to 20 mg/kg (up to 300 mg/day) PO once daily.

FORMS – Trade only: Caps 150 mg.

NOTES – Uveitis (with high doses or if metabolism inhibited by other drugs), hepatotoxicity, thrombocytopenia, neutropenia. Obtain CBC and LFTs at baseline. Monitor periodically in high-risk patients (HIV infection, alcoholism, pregnancy, signs/history of liver disease, abnormal LFTs at baseline). May induce liver metabolism of other drugs including oral contraceptives, protease inhibitors, and azole antifungals. Substrate of CYP3A4; azole antifungals, clarithromycin, and protease inhibitors increase rifabutin levels. Urine, body secretion, soft contact lenses may turn orange-brown. Consider dosage reduction for hepatic dysfunction.

RIFAMATE (**isoniazid + rifampin**) ▶LK ♀C but + ▶+ $$$$

WARNING – Hepatotoxicity.

ADULT – TB: 2 caps PO daily on empty stomach.

PEDS – Not approved in children.

FORMS – Generic/Trade: Caps isoniazid 150 mg plus rifampin 300 mg.

NOTES – See components. Monitor LFTs at baseline and periodically during therapy.

RIFAMPIN (*Rifadin*) ▶L ♀C but + ▶+ $$$

WARNING – The ATS and CDC recommend against general use of 2-month regimen of rifampin plus pyrazinamide for latent TB due to reports of fatal hepatotoxicity.

ADULT – TB: 10 mg/kg (up to 600 mg) PO/IV daily. Neisseria meningitidis carriers: 600 mg PO two times per day for 2 days. Take oral doses on empty stomach. IV and PO doses are the same.

PEDS – TB: 10 to 20 mg/kg (up to 600 mg) PO/IV daily. Neisseria meningitidis carriers: Age younger than 1 mo, 5 mg/kg PO two times per day for 2 days; age 1 mo or older, 10 mg/kg (up to 600 mg) PO two times per day for 2 days. Take oral doses on empty stomach. IV and PO doses are the same.

UNAPPROVED ADULT – Prophylaxis of H. *influenzae* type b infection: 20 mg/kg (up to 600 mg) PO daily for 4 days. Leprosy: 600 mg PO q month with dapsone. ATS regimen for latent TB: 10 mg/kg up to 600 mg PO daily for 4 months. Staphylococcal prosthetic valve endocarditis: 300 mg PO q 8 h in combination with gentamicin plus nafcillin, oxacillin, or vancomycin. Take on empty stomach.

UNAPPROVED PEDS – Prophylaxis of H. *influenzae* type b infection: Age younger than 1 mo, 10 mg/kg PO daily for 4 days; age 1 mo or older, 20 mg/kg up to 600 mg PO daily for 4 days. Prophylaxis of invasive meningococcal disease: Age younger than 1 mo, 5 mg/kg PO two times per day for 2 days; age 1 mo or older, 10 mg/kg (up to 600 mg) PO two times per day for 2 days. ATS regimen for latent tuberculosis: 10 to 20 mg/kg (up to 600 mg) PO daily for 4 months. Take on empty stomach.

FORMS – Generic/Trade: Caps 150, 300 mg. Pharmacists can make oral susp.

NOTES – Hepatotoxicity, thrombocytopenia. When treating TB, obtain baseline CBC, LFTs. Monitor periodically in high-risk patients (HIV infection, alcoholism, pregnancy, signs/history of liver disease, abnormal LFTs at baseline). Discontinue if ALT is at least 3 times the upper limit of normal with hepatotoxicity symptoms or ALT is at least 5 times the upper limit of normal without hepatotoxicity symptoms. Avoid interruptions in rifampin therapy; rare renal hypersensitivity reactions can occur after resumption. Induces hepatic metabolism of many drugs; check other sources for dosage adjustments before prescribing. If used with rifampin, consider increasing efavirenz to 800 mg once daily at bedtime if wt greater than 60 kg. Do not use rifampin with protease inhibitors. Decreased efficacy of oral contraceptives; use nonhormonal method. Decreased INR with warfarin; monitor daily or as needed. Adjust dose for hepatic impairment. Colors urine, body secretions, soft contact lenses red-orange. Give prophylactic vitamin K 10 mg IM single dose to newborns of women taking rifampin. IV rifampin is stable for 4 h after dilution in dextrose 5%.

RIFAPENTINE (*Priftin, RPT*) ▶Esterases, fecal ♀C ▶? $$$$

ADULT – TB: 600 mg PO twice a week for 2 months, then once a week for 4 months. Use only for continuation therapy in selected HIV-negative patients.

PEDS – Not approved in children younger than 12 yo.

UNAPPROVED ADULT – Weekly regimen for latent TB: Give once weekly for 12 weeks isoniazid 15 mg/kg PO rounded up to nearest 50 or 100 mg (max 900 mg) plus rifapentine 750 mg for wt 32.1 to 49.9 kg or 900 mg for wt 50 kg or greater. Regimen intended for directly observed therapy; not recommended for HIV-infected patients treated with antiretrovirals or for use during pregnancy.

UNAPPROVED PEDS – Weekly regimen for latent TB, age 12 yo or older: Give once weekly for 12 weeks isoniazid 15 mg/kg PO rounded up to nearest 50 or 100 mg (max 900 mg) plus rifapentine PO dosed according to wt. Rifapentine dose is 300 mg for 10 to 14 kg; 450 mg for 14.1 to 25 kg; 600 mg for 25.1 to 32 kg; 750 mg for wt 32.1 to 49.9 kg; 900 mg for wt 50 kg or greater. Regimen intended for directly observed therapy; not recommended for HIV-infected patients treated with antiretrovirals or for use during pregnancy.

FORMS – Trade only: Tabs 150 mg.

NOTES – Hepatotoxicity, thrombocytopenia, exacerbation of porphyria. Obtain CBC and LFTs at baseline. Monitor LFTs periodically in high-risk patients (alcoholism, pregnancy, signs/history of liver disease, abnormal LFTs at baseline). Do not use in porphyria. Urine, body secretions, contact lenses, and dentures may turn red-orange. May induce liver metabolism of other drugs including oral contraceptives. Advise women taking hormonal contractive to use barrier contraceptive during treatment. Avoid with protease inhibitors, NNRTIs, and maraviroc.

RIFATER **(isoniazid + rifampin + pyrazinamide)** ▶LK ♀C ▶? $$$$$
WARNING – Hepatotoxicity.
ADULT – TB, initial 2 months of treatment: 4 tabs daily for wt less than 45 kg, 5 tabs daily for 45 to 54 kg, 6 tabs daily for 55 kg or greater. Additional pyrazinamide tabs required to provide adequate dose for wt greater than 90 kg. Take on empty stomach. Can finish treatment with Rifamate.
PEDS – Ratio of formulation may not be appropriate for children younger than 15 yo.
FORMS – Trade only: Tabs isoniazid 50 mg plus rifampin 120 mg plus pyrazinamide 300 mg.
NOTES – See components. Monitor LFTs at baseline and during therapy. Do not use in patients with renal dysfunction.

ANTIMICROBIALS: Antiparasitics

ALBENDAZOLE (*Albenza*) ▶L ♀C ▶? $$$
ADULT – Hydatid disease, neurocysticercosis: 15 mg/kg/day (up to 800 mg/day) PO divided in two doses for wt less than 60 kg, 400 mg PO two times per day for wt 60 kg or greater. Treatment duration varies. Take with food.
PEDS – Hydatid disease, neurocysticercosis: 15 mg/kg/day (up to 800 mg/day) PO divided in two doses for wt less than 60 kg, 400 mg PO two times per day for wt 60 kg or greater. Treatment duration varies. Take with food.
UNAPPROVED ADULT – Hookworm, whipworm, pinworm, roundworm: 400 mg PO single dose. Repeat in 2 weeks for pinworm. Cutaneous larva migrans: 200 mg PO two times per day for 3 days. Giardia: 400 mg PO daily for 5 days. Intestinal/disseminated microsporidiosis in HIV infection (not for ocular or caused by *E. bienuesi/V. corneae*): 400 mg PO two times per day until CD4 count higher than 200 for more than 6 months after starting antiretrovirals.
UNAPPROVED PEDS – Roundworm, hookworm, pinworm, whipworm: 400 mg PO single dose. Repeat in 2 weeks for pinworm. Cutaneous larva migrans: 200 mg PO two times per day for 3 days. Giardia: 400 mg PO daily for 5 days.
FORMS – Trade only: Tabs 200 mg.
NOTES – Associated with bone marrow suppression (especially if liver disease), increased LFTs (common with long-term use), and hepatotoxicity (rare). Monitor CBC and LFTs before starting and then q 2 weeks; discontinue if significant changes. Consider corticosteroids and anticonvulsants in neurocysticercosis. Consider diagnosis of preexisting neurocysticercosis if patient develops neurologic symptoms soon after albendazole treatment for another indication. Get negative pregnancy test before treatment and warn against getting pregnant until 1 month after treatment. Treat close contacts for pinworms. Can crush/chew tabs and swallow with water.

ATOVAQUONE (*Mepron*) ▶Fecal ♀C ▶? $$$$$
ADULT – Pneumocystis pneumonia in patients intolerant to trimethoprim-sulfamethoxazole: Treatment 750 mg PO two times per day for 21 days. Prevention 1500 mg PO daily. Take with meals.
PEDS – Pneumocystis pneumonia in patients intolerant to trimethoprim-sulfamethoxazole, 13 to 16 yo: Treatment, 750 mg PO two times per day for 21 days. Prevention, 1500 mg PO daily. Take with meals.
UNAPPROVED PEDS – Prevention of recurrent Pneumocystis pneumonia in HIV infection: 30 mg/kg PO daily for age 1 to 3 mo; 45 mg/kg PO daily for age 4 to 24 mo; 30 mg/kg PO daily for age 25 mo or older. Take with meals.
FORMS – Trade only: Susp 750 mg/5 mL (210 mL), foil pouch 750 mg/5 mL (5, 10 mL).
NOTES – Efficacy of atovaquone may be decreased by rifampin (consider using alternative), rifabutin, or rifapentine.

IODOQUINOL (*Yodoxin*, diiodohydroxyquin ✦ *Diodoquin*) ▶Not absorbed ♀? ▶? $$$
ADULT – Intestinal amebiasis: 650 mg PO three times per day after meals for 20 days.
PEDS – Intestinal amebiasis: 40 mg/kg/day PO divided three times per day for 20 days. Do not exceed adult dose.
FORMS – Trade only (Yodoxin): Tabs 210, 650 mg.
NOTES – Optic neuritis/atrophy, peripheral neuropathy with prolonged high doses. Interference with some thyroid function tests for up to 6 months after treatment.

IVERMECTIN (*Stromectol*) ▶L ♀C ▶+ $$
ADULT – Strongyloidiasis: 200 mcg/kg PO single dose. Onchocerciasis: 150 mcg/kg PO single dose q 3 to 12 months. Take on empty stomach with water.
PEDS – Strongyloidiasis: 200 mcg/kg PO single dose. Onchocerciasis: 150 mcg/kg PO single dose q 3 to 12 months. Take on empty stomach with water. Safety and efficacy not established in children less than 15 kg.

(cont.)

IVERMECTIN (*cont.*)

UNAPPROVED ADULT – Scabies: 200 mcg/kg PO repeated in 2 weeks. Pubic lice: 250 mcg/kg PO repeated in 2 weeks. Cutaneous larva migrans: 150 to 200 mcg/kg PO single dose. Take on empty stomach with water.

UNAPPROVED PEDS – Scabies: 200 mcg/kg PO single dose (dose may need to be repeated in 10 to 14 days). Head lice: 200 to 400 mcg/kg PO single dose; repeat in 7 days. Cutaneous larva migrans: 150 to 200 mcg/kg PO single dose. Take on empty stomach with water. Not for wt less than 15 kg.

FORMS – Trade only: Tabs 3 mg.

NOTES – Mazzotti and ophthalmic reactions with treatment for onchocerciasis. May need repeat/monthly treatment for strongyloidiasis in immunocompromised/HIV-infected patients. Increased INRs with warfarin reported rarely.

NITAZOXANIDE (*Alinia*) ▶L ♀B ▶? $$$$

ADULT – Cryptosporidial or giardial diarrhea: 500 mg PO two times per day with food for 3 days.

PEDS – Cryptosporidial or giardial diarrhea: 100 mg two times per day for 1 to 3 yo; 200 mg two times per day for 4 to 11 yo; 500 mg two times per day for 12 yo or older. Give PO with food for 3 days. Use susp if younger than 12 yo.

UNAPPROVED ADULT – *C. difficile*-associated diarrhea: 500 mg PO two times per day for 10 days. Cryptosporidiosis in HIV infection (alternative therapy in addition to concurrent HAART): 500 to 1000 mg PO two times per day with food for 14 days.

FORMS – Trade only: Oral susp 100 mg/5 mL, 60 mL bottle. Tabs 500 mg.

NOTES – Turns urine bright yellow. Susp contains 1.5 g sucrose/5 mL. Store susp at room temperature for up to 7 days.

PAROMOMYCIN ▶Not absorbed ♀C ▶– $$$$

ADULT – Intestinal amebiasis: 25 to 35 mg/kg/day PO divided three times per day with or after meals for 5 to 10 days.

PEDS – Intestinal amebiasis: 25 to 35 mg/kg/day PO divided three times per day with or after meals for 5 to 10 days.

UNAPPROVED ADULT – Giardiasis: 500 mg PO three times per day for 7 days.

UNAPPROVED PEDS – Giardiasis: 25 to 35 mg/kg/day PO divided three times per day with or after meals for 7 days.

FORMS – Generic only: Caps 250 mg.

NOTES – Nephrotoxicity possible in inflammatory bowel disease due to increased systemic absorption. Not effective for extraintestinal amebiasis.

PENTAMIDINE (*Pentam, NebuPent*) ▶K ♀C ▶– $$$

ADULT – Pneumocystis pneumonia treatment: 4 mg/kg IM/IV daily for 21 days. Some experts reduce to 3 mg/kg IM/IV daily if toxicity. IV infused over 60 to 90 min. NebuPent for Pneumocystis pneumonia prevention: 300 mg nebulized q 4 weeks.

PEDS – Pneumocystis pneumonia treatment: 4 mg/kg IM/IV daily for 21 days. NebuPent not approved in children.

UNAPPROVED PEDS – Pneumocystis pneumonia prevention, age 5 yo or older: 300 mg NebuPent nebulized q 4 weeks.

FORMS – Trade only: Aerosol 300 mg.

NOTES – Contraindicated with ziprasidone. Fatalities due to severe hypotension, hypoglycemia, cardiac arrhythmias with IM/IV. Have patient lie down, check BP, and keep resuscitation equipment nearby during IM/IV injection. May cause torsades, hyperglycemia, neutropenia, nephrotoxicity, pancreatitis, and hypocalcemia. Monitor BUN, serum creatinine, blood glucose, CBC, LFTs, serum calcium, and ECG. Bronchospasm with inhalation (consider bronchodilator). Reduce IM/IV dose in renal dysfunction.

PRAZIQUANTEL (*Biltricide*) ▶LK ♀B ▶– $$$

ADULT – Schistosomiasis: 20 mg/kg PO q 4 to 6 h for 3 doses. Liver flukes: 25 mg/kg PO q 4 to 6 h for 3 doses.

PEDS – Schistosomiasis: 20 mg/kg PO q 4 to 6 h for 3 doses. Liver flukes: 25 mg/kg PO q 4 to 6 h for 3 doses.

UNAPPROVED ADULT – Fish, dog, beef, pork intestinal tapeworms: 10 mg/kg PO single dose.

UNAPPROVED PEDS – Fish, dog, beef, pork intestinal tapeworms: 10 mg/kg PO single dose.

FORMS – Trade only: Tabs 600 mg.

NOTES – Contraindicated in ocular cysticercosis. May cause drowsiness; do not drive or operate machinery for 48 h. Phenytoin, carbamazepine, rifampin (contraindicated), and dexamethasone may lower praziquantel levels enough to cause treatment failure. Albendazole is preferred for neurocysticercosis because it avoids these drug interactions. Take with liquids during a meal. Do not chew tabs. Manufacturer advises against breastfeeding until 72 h after treatment.

PYRANTEL (*Pin-X, Pinworm,* ✤ *Combantrin*) ▶Not absorbed ♀– ▶? $

ADULT – Pinworm, roundworm: 11 mg/kg (up to 1 g) PO single dose. Repeat in 2 weeks for pinworm.

PEDS – Pinworm, roundworm: 11 mg/kg (up to 1 g) PO single dose. Repeat in 2 weeks for pinworm.

UNAPPROVED ADULT – Hookworm: 11 mg/kg (up to 1 g) PO daily for 3 days.

UNAPPROVED PEDS – Hookworm: 11 mg/kg (up to 1 g) PO daily for 3 days.

FORMS – OTC Trade only (Pin-X): Susp 144 mg/mL (equivalent to 50 mg/mL of pyrantel base) 30, 60 mL. Tabs 720.5 mg (equivalent to 250 mg of pyrantel base). OTC Generic only: Caps 180 mg (equivalent to 62.5 mg of pyrantel base).

NOTES – Purging not necessary. Treat close contacts for pinworms.

PYRIMETHAMINE (*Daraprim*) ▶L ♀C ▶+ $$

ADULT – Toxoplasmosis, immunocompetent patients: 50 to 75 mg PO daily for 1 to 3 weeks, then reduce dose by 50% for 4 to 5 more weeks. Give with leucovorin (10 to 15 mg daily) and sulfadiazine. Reduce initial dose in seizure disorders.

PEDS – Toxoplasmosis: 1 mg/kg/day PO divided two times per day for 2 to 4 days, then reduce by 50% for 1 month. Give with sulfadiazine and leucovorin. Reduce initial dose in seizure disorders.

UNAPPROVED ADULT – CNS toxoplasmosis in AIDS. Acute therapy: See regimen for acute treatment of CNS toxoplasmosis in Sulfadiazine entry.

UNAPPROVED PEDS – Acquired toxoplasmosis: 2 mg/kg (up to 50 mg) PO once daily for 3 days, then 1 mg/kg (up to 25 mg) PO once daily plus sulfadiazine 25 to 50 mg/kg PO (up to 1 to 1.5 g/dose) PO four times per day. Give leucovorin 10 to 25 mg/day PO. Treat for at least 6 weeks followed by chronic suppressive therapy.

FORMS – Trade only: Tabs 25 mg.

NOTES – Hemolytic anemia in G6PD deficiency, dose-related folate deficiency, hypersensitivity. Monitor CBC.

TINIDAZOLE (*Tindamax*) ▶KL ♀C ▶?– $

WARNING – Metronidazole, a related drug, was carcinogenic in animal studies.

ADULT – Trichomoniasis or giardiasis: 2 g PO single dose. Amebiasis: 2 g PO once daily for 3 days. Bacterial vaginosis: 2 g PO once daily for 2 days or 1 g PO once daily for 5 days. Take with food.

PEDS – Giardiasis, age older than 3 yo: 50 mg/kg (up to 2 g) PO single dose. Amebiasis, age older than 3 yo: 50 mg/kg (up to 2 g) PO once daily for 3 days. Take with food.

UNAPPROVED ADULT – Recurrent/persistent urethritis: 2 g PO single dose.

FORMS – Generic/Trade: Tabs 250, 500 mg. Pharmacists can compound oral susp.

NOTES – Give iodoquinol/paromomycin after treatment for amebic dysentery or liver abscess. Disulfiram reaction; avoid alcohol for at least 3 days after treatment. Can minimize infant exposure by withholding breastfeeding for 3 days after maternal single dose. May increase levels of cyclosporine, fluorouracil, lithium, phenytoin, tacrolimus. May increase INR with warfarin. Do not give at same time as cholestyramine. For patients undergoing hemodialysis: Give supplemental dose after dialysis session.

ANTIMICROBIALS: Antiviral Agents—Anti-CMV

CIDOFOVIR (*Vistide*) ▶K ♀C ▶– $$$$$

WARNING – Severe nephrotoxicity. Granulocytopenia: Monitor neutrophil counts.

ADULT – CMV retinitis: 5 mg/kg IV weekly for 2 weeks, then 5 mg/kg every other week. Give probenecid 2 g PO 3 h before and 1 g PO 2 h and 8 h after infusion. Give NS with each infusion.

PEDS – Not approved in children.

NOTES – Fanconi-like syndrome. Stop nephrotoxic drugs at least 1 week before cidofovir. Get serum creatinine, urine protein before each dose. See prescribing information for dosage adjustments based on renal function. Do not use if creatinine is greater than 1.5 mg/dL, CrCl 55 mL/min or less, or urine protein 100 mg/dL (2+) or greater. Hold/decrease zidovudine dose by 50% on day cidofovir is given. Tell women not to get pregnant until 1 month after and men to use barrier contraceptive until 3 months after cidofovir. Ocular hypotony: Monitor intraocular pressure.

FOSCARNET ▶K ♀C ▶? $$$$$

WARNING – Nephrotoxicity; seizures due to mineral/electrolyte imbalance.

ADULT – Hydrate before infusion. CMV retinitis: 60 mg/kg IV (over 1 h) q 8 h or 90 mg/kg IV (over 1.5 to 2 h) q 12 h for 2 to 3 weeks, then 90 to 120 mg/kg IV daily over 2 h. Acyclovir-resistant HSV infection: 40 mg/kg IV (over 1 h) q 8 to 12 h for 2 to 3 weeks or until healed.

(cont.)

FOSCARNET (*cont.*)

PEDS – Not approved in children. Deposits into teeth and bone of young animals.

NOTES – Granulocytopenia, anemia, vein irritation, penile ulcers. Decreased ionized serum calcium, especially with IV pentamidine. Must use IV pump to avoid rapid administration. Monitor renal function, serum calcium, magnesium, phosphate, potassium. Reduce dose in renal impairment. Stop foscarnet if CrCl decreases to less than 0.4 mL/min/kg.

GANCICLOVIR (*Cytovene*) ▶K ♀C ▶– $$$$$

WARNING – Neutropenia, anemia, thrombocytopenia. Do not use if ANC is less than 500/mm^3 or platelets are less than 25,000/mm^3.

ADULT – CMV retinitis. Induction: 5 mg/kg IV q 12 h for 14 to 21 days. Maintenance: 6 mg/kg IV daily for 5 days/week or 5 mg/kg IV daily. Prevention of CMV disease after organ transplant: 5 mg/kg IV q 12 h for 7 to 14 days, then 6 mg/kg IV daily for 5 days/week. Give IV infusion over 1 h.

PEDS – Safety and efficacy not established in children; potential carcinogenic or reproductive adverse effects.

UNAPPROVED PEDS – CMV retinitis. Induction: 5 mg/kg IV q 12 h for 14 to 21 days. Maintenance: 5 mg/kg IV daily or 6 mg/kg IV daily for 5 days/weeks. Symptomatic congenital CMV infection: 6 mg/kg IV q 12 h for 6 weeks.

NOTES – Neutropenia (worsened by zidovudine), phlebitis/pain at infusion site, increased seizure risk with imipenem. Monitor CBC, renal function. Reduce dose if CrCl is less than 70 mL/min. Adequate hydration required. Potential teratogen. Tell women not to get pregnant during and men to use barrier contraceptive at least 3 months after treatment. Potential carcinogen. Follow guidelines for handling/disposal of cytotoxic agents.

VALGANCICLOVIR (*Valcyte*) ▶K ♀C ▶– $$$$$

WARNING – Myelosuppression may occur at any time. Monitor CBC and platelet count frequently. Do not use if ANC is less than 500/mm^3, platelets less than 25,000/mm^3, hemoglobin less than 8 g/dL.

ADULT – CMV retinitis: 900 mg PO two times per day for 21 days, then 900 mg PO daily. Prevention of CMV disease in high-risk transplant patients: 900 mg PO daily given within 10 days post-transplant until 100 days post-transplant for heart or kidney-pancreas or 200 days for kidney transplant. Give with food.

PEDS – Prevention of CMV disease in high-risk kidney/heart transplant patients 4 months of age and older: Daily dose in mg is 7 × body surface area × CrCl (calculated with modified Schwartz formula). Give PO once daily from within 10 days post transplant to 100 days post-transplant. Max dose of 900 mg/day. Give with food.

FORMS – Trade only: Tabs 450 mg. Oral soln 50 mg/mL.

NOTES – Contraindicated in ganciclovir allergy. Potential teratogen. Tell women not to get pregnant until 1 month after and men to use barrier contraceptive until at least 3 months after treatment. CNS toxicity; warn against hazardous tasks. May increase serum creatinine; monitor renal function. Reduce dose if CrCl is less than 60 mL/min. Use ganciclovir instead in hemodialysis patients. Potential drug interactions with didanosine, mycophenolate, zidovudine. Potential carcinogen. Avoid direct contact with broken/crushed tabs; do not intentionally break/crush tabs. Follow guidelines for handling/disposal of cytotoxic agents.

ANTIMICROBIALS: Antiviral Agents—Anti-Herpetic

ACYCLOVIR (*Zovirax*) ▶K ♀B ▶+ $

ADULT – Genital herpes: 200 mg PO q 4 h (five times per day) for 10 days for first episode, for 5 days for recurrent episodes. Chronic suppression: 400 mg PO two times per day. Zoster: 800 mg PO q 4 h (five times per day) for 7 to 10 days. Chickenpox: 800 mg PO four times per day for 5 days. IV: 5 to 10 mg/kg IV q 8 h, each dose over 1 h. Zoster in immunocompromised patients: 10 mg/kg IV q 8 h for 7 days. Herpes simplex encephalitis: 10 mg/kg IV q 8 h for 10 days. Mucosal/cutaneous herpes simplex in immunocompromised patients: 5 mg/kg IV q 8 h for 7 days.

PEDS – Safety and efficacy of PO acyclovir not established in children younger than 2 yo. Chickenpox: 20 mg/kg PO four times per day for 5 days. Use adult dose if wt greater than 40 kg. AAP does not recommend routine treatment of chickenpox with acyclovir, but it should be considered in patients older than 12 yo or with chronic cutaneous or pulmonary disease, chronic salicylate use, or short, intermittent, or inhaled courses of

(cont.)

ACYCLOVIR (*cont.*)

corticosteroid. Possibly also for secondary household cases. IV: 250 to 500 mg/m^2 q 8 h, each dose over 1 h. Zoster in immunocompromised patients younger than 12 yo: 20 mg/kg IV q 8 h for 7 days. Herpes simplex encephalitis: 20 mg/kg IV q 8 h for 10 days for age 3 mo to 12 yo; adult dose for age 13 yo or older. Neonatal herpes simplex (birth to 3 mo): 10 mg/kg IV q 8 h for 10 days; CDC regimen is 20 mg/kg IV q 8 h for 21 days for disseminated/CNS disease, for 14 days for skin/mucous membranes. Mucosal/cutaneous herpes simplex in immunocompromised patients: 10 mg/kg IV q 8 h for 7 days for age younger than 12 yo, adult dose for 13 yo or older. Treat ASAP after symptom onset.

UNAPPROVED ADULT – Genital herpes: 400 mg PO three times per day for 7 to 10 days for first episode, for 5 days for recurrent episodes, for 5 to 10 days for recurrent episodes in HIV+ patients. Alternative regimens for recurrent episodes in HIV-negative patients: 800 mg PO two times per day for 5 days or 800 mg PO three times per day for 2 days. Chronic suppression of genital herpes in HIV+ patients: 400 to 800 mg PO two to three times per day. Orolabial herpes: 400 mg PO 5 times a day.

UNAPPROVED PEDS – Primary herpes gingivostomatitis: 15 mg/kg PO 5 times a day for 7 days. First episode genital herpes: 80 mg/kg/day PO divided three times per day (max 1.2 g/day) for 7 to 10 days. Use dose in unapproved adult for adolescents.

FORMS – Generic/Trade: Caps 200 mg. Tabs 400, 800 mg. Susp 200 mg/5 mL.

NOTES – Maintain adequate hydration. Severe drowsiness with acyclovir plus zidovudine. Consider suppressive therapy for patients with at least 6 episodes of genital herpes per year. Reduce dose in renal dysfunction and in elderly. Base IV dose on ideal body wt in obese adults.

FAMCICLOVIR (*Famvir*) ▶K ♀B ▶? $$

ADULT – Recurrent genital herpes: 1000 mg PO two times per day for 2 days. Chronic suppression of genital herpes: 250 mg PO two times per day. Recurrent herpes labialis: 1500 mg PO single dose. Recurrent orolabial/genital herpes in HIV patients: 500 mg PO two times per day for 7 days. Zoster: 500 mg PO three times per day for 7 days. Treat ASAP after symptom onset.

PEDS – Not approved in children.

UNAPPROVED ADULT – First episode genital herpes: 250 mg PO three times per day for 7 to 10 days. Chronic suppression of genital herpes in HIV+ patients: 500 mg PO two times per day. Chickenpox in young adults: 500 mg PO three times per day for 5 days. Bell's palsy: 750 mg PO three times per day plus prednisone 1 mg/kg PO daily for 7 days. Treat ASAP after symptom onset.

UNAPPROVED PEDS – Chickenpox in adolescents: 500 mg PO three times per day for 5 days. First episode genital herpes in adolescents: Use dose in unapproved adult.

FORMS – Generic/Trade: Tabs 125, 250, 500 mg.

NOTES – Consider suppressive therapy for patients with at least 6 episodes of genital herpes per year. Reduce dose for CrCl less than 60 mL/min.

VALACYCLOVIR (*Valtrex*) ▶K ♀B ▶+ $$$$$

ADULT – First episode genital herpes: 1 g PO two times per day for 10 days. Recurrent genital herpes: 500 mg PO two times per day for 3 days. Chronic suppression of genital herpes in immunocompetent patients: 1 g PO daily. Can use 500 mg PO daily if 9 or fewer recurrences per year; transmission of genital herpes reduced with use of this regimen by source partner, in conjunction with safer sex practices. Chronic suppression of genital herpes in HIV-infected patients: 500 mg PO two times per day. Herpes labialis: 2 g PO q 12 h for 2 doses. Zoster: 1 g PO three times per day for 7 days. Treat ASAP after symptom onset.

PEDS – Herpes labialis, age 12 yo or older: 2 g PO q 12 h for 2 doses. Chickenpox, age 2 to 17 yo: 20 mg/kg (max of 1 g) PO three times per day for 5 days. Treat ASAP after symptom onset.

UNAPPROVED ADULT – Recurrent genital herpes: 1 g PO daily for 5 days. Recurrent genital herpes in HIV+ patients: 1 g PO two times per day for 5 to 10 days. Bell's palsy: 1 g PO two times per day plus prednisone 1 mg/kg PO daily for 7 days. Orolabial herpes in immunocompromised patients, including HIV infection: 1 g PO three times per day for 7 days. Chickenpox in young adults: 1 g PO three times per day for 5 days. Treat ASAP after symptom onset.

UNAPPROVED PEDS – First episode genital herpes in adolescents: Use adult dose. Treat ASAP after symptom onset.

FORMS – Generic/Trade: Tabs 500, 1000 mg.

NOTES – Consider suppressive therapy for patients with at least 6 episodes of genital herpes per year. Maintain adequate hydration. CNS and renal adverse effects more common

(cont.)

VALACYCLOVIR (*cont.*)
if elderly or renal impairment; avoid inappropriately high doses in these patients. Reduce dose for CrCl less than 50 mL/min. Thrombotic thrombocytopenic purpura/hemolytic uremic syndrome at dose of 8 g/day.

ANTIMICROBIALS: Antiviral Agents—Anti-HIV—CCR5 Antagonists

MARAVIROC (*Selzentry, MVC,* ♣ *Celsentri*) ▶LK ♀B ▶– $$$$$

WARNING – Hepatotoxicity with allergic features, including DRESS. May have prodrome of severe rash or systemic allergic reaction. Monitor LFTs at baseline and if rash, allergic reaction, or signs/symptoms of hepatitis. Consider discontinuation if signs/symptoms of hepatitis, or increased LFTs with rash or other systemic symptoms. Caution if baseline liver dysfunction or coinfection with hepatitis B/C.

ADULT – Combination therapy for HIV infection: 150 mg PO two times per day with strong CYP3A4 inhibitors (most protease inhibitors, ketoconazole, itraconazole, clarithromycin); 300 mg PO two times per day with drugs that are not strong CYP3A4 inducers/inhibitors (NRTIs, tipranavir-ritonavir, nevirapine, enfuvirtide, raltegravir; rifabutin without a strong CYP3A4 inhibitor or inducer); 600 mg PO two times per day with strong CYP3A4 inducers (efavirenz, etravirine, rifampin, carbamazepine, phenobarbital, phenytoin). Tropism test before treatment; not for dual/mixed or CXCR4-tropic HIV infection.

PEDS – Not recommended for age younger than 16 yo based on lack of data.

FORMS – Trade only: Tabs 150, 300 mg.

NOTES – May increase risk of myocardial ischemia or MI. Theoretical risk of infection/malignancy due to effects on immune system. Metabolized by CYP3A4; do not use with St. John's wort. Contraindicated in patients with CrCl less than 30 mL/min who are taking a strong CYP3A4 inhibitor or inducer. Consider dosage reduction to 150 mg two times per day if postural hypotension occurs in patients with CrCL less than 30 mL/min.

ANTIMICROBIALS: Antiviral Agents—Anti-HIV—Combinations

ATRIPLA **(efavirenz + emtricitabine + tenofovir)** ▶KL ♀D ▶– $$$$$

WARNING – Tenofovir: Potentially fatal lactic acidosis and hepatosteatosis. Emtricitabine and tenofovir: severe acute exacerbation of hepatitis B after discontinuation in patients coinfected with HIV and hepatitis B.

ADULT – Combination therapy for HIV infection: 1 tab PO once daily on empty stomach, preferably at bedtime. Atripla can be used alone or in combination with other antiretrovirals that are not already in the tab.

PEDS – Safety and efficacy not established.

UNAPPROVED PEDS – Combination therapy for HIV infection, adolescents 40 kg or greater: 1 tab PO once daily on empty stomach, preferably at bedtime. Atripla can be used alone or in combination with other antiretrovirals.

FORMS – Trade only: Tabs efavirenz 600 mg + emtricitabine 200 mg + tenofovir 300 mg.

NOTES – See components. Do not give Atripla with lamivudine. Not for CrCl less than 50 mL/min. Efavirenz induces CYP3A4, causing many drug interactions.

COMBIVIR **(lamivudine + zidovudine)** ▶LK ♀C ▶– $$$$$

WARNING – Zidovudine: Bone marrow suppression, myopathy. Lamivudine: Severe acute exacerbation of hepatitis B can occur after discontinuation of lamivudine in patients coinfected with HIV and hepatitis B. Monitor closely for at least 2 months after discontinuing lamivudine in such patients; consider treating hepatitis B. Zidovudine and lamivudine: Lactic acidosis and hepatic steatosis.

ADULT – Combination therapy for HIV infection: 1 tab PO twice daily.

PEDS – Combination therapy for HIV infection, wt 30 kg or greater: 1 tab PO twice daily.

FORMS – Generic/Trade: Tabs lamivudine 150 mg plus zidovudine 300 mg.

NOTES – See components. Monitor CBC. Not for wt less than 30 kg, CrCl < 50 mL/min, hepatic dysfunction, or if dosage adjustment required.

COMPLERA **(emtricitabine + rilpivirine + tenofovir)** ▶KL ♀B ▶– $$$$$

WARNING – Tenofovir: Potentially fatal lactic acidosis and hepatosteatosis. Emtricitabine and tenofovir: severe acute exacerbation of hepatitis B after discontinuation in patients coinfected with HIV and hepatitis B.

ADULT – Combination therapy of HIV: 1 tab PO once daily with a meal.

PEDS – Safety and efficacy not established in children.

(cont.)

COMPLERA (*cont.*)

FORMS – Trade only: Tabs emtricitabine 200 mg + rilpivirine 25 mg + tenofovir 300 mg.

NOTES – See components. Not for CrCl <50 mL/min. Monitor CrCl before treatment. Dosage adjustment not required for mild/moderate hepatic impairment (Child-Pugh Class A/B). Rilpivirine has higher virologic failure rate than efavirenz in patients with baseline HIV RNA greater than 100,000 copies/mL. Contraindicated with carbamazepine, dexamethasone (more than a single dose), oxcarbazepine, phenobarbital, phenytoin, proton pump inhibitors, rifabutin, rifampin, rifapentine, St. John's wort.

EPZICOM (**abacavir + lamivudine,** ✦ ***Kivexa***) ▶LK ♀C ▶– $$$$$

WARNING – Abacavir: Potentially fatal hypersensitivity reactions. HLA-B*5701 predisposes to hypersensitivity; screen before starting abacavir and avoid if positive test. Never rechallenge with abacavir after suspected reaction. Abacavir and lamivudine: Lactic acidosis and hepatosteatosis. Lamivudine: Exacerbation of hepatitis B after discontinuation in patients coinfected with HIV and hepatitis B.

ADULT – Combination therapy for HIV infection: 1 tab PO daily.

PEDS – Safety and efficacy not established in children.

FORMS – Trade only: Tabs abacavir 600 mg + lamivudine 300 mg.

NOTES – See components. Not for patients with CrCl less than 50 mL/min, hepatic dysfunction, or if dosage adjustment required.

STRIBILD (**elvitegravir + cobicistat + emtricitabine + tenofovir**) ▶KL ♀B ▶– $$$$$

WARNING – Tenofovir: Potentially fatal lactic acidosis and hepatosteatosis. Emtricitabine and tenofovir: Severe acute exacerbation of hepatitis B after discontinuation in patients coinfected with HIV and hepatitis B.

ADULT – Combination therapy for HIV infection: 1 tab PO once daily with food. Do not use Stribild with other antiretroviral drugs.

PEDS – Safety and efficacy not established in children.

FORMS – Trade only: Tabs elvitegravir 150 mg + cobicistat 150 mg + emtricitibine 200 mg + tenofovir 300 mg.

NOTES – See components. Monitor CrCl, urine glucose, urine protein. Do not start if CrCl < 70 mL/min; stop if CrCl declines to < 50 mL/min. Contraindicated with alfuzosin, ergot alkaloids, lovastatin, oral midazolam, pimozide, rifabutin, rifampin, rifapentine, high-dose sildenafil for pulmonary hypertension, simvastatin, St John's wort, triazolam.

TRIZIVIR (**abacavir + lamivudine + zidovudine**) ▶LK ♀C ▶– $$$$$

WARNING – Abacavir: Life-threatening hypersensitivity. HLA-B*5701 predisposes to hypersensitivity; screen before starting abacavir and avoid if positive test. Never rechallenge with abacavir after suspected reaction. Abacavir and lamivudine: Lactic acidosis and hepatosteatosis. Zidovudine: Bone marrow suppression, myopathy.

ADULT – HIV infection, alone (not a preferred regimen) or in combination with other agents: 1 tab PO two times per day.

PEDS – HIV infection in adolescents 40 kg or greater, alone (not a preferred regimen) or in combination with other agents: 1 tab PO two times per day.

FORMS – Trade only: Tabs abacavir 300 mg + lamivudine 150 mg + zidovudine 300 mg.

NOTES – See components. Monitor CBC. Not for wt less than 40 kg, CrCl less than 50 mL/min or if dosage adjustment required.

TRUVADA (**emtricitabine + tenofovir**) ▶K ♀B ▶– $$$$$

WARNING – Tenofovir: Potentially fatal lactic acidosis and hepatosteatosis. Emtricitabine and tenofovir: Severe acute exacerbation of hepatitis B after discontinuation in patients coinfected with HIV and hepatitis B.

ADULT – Pre-exposure prophylaxis of HIV in adults at high risk for sexual acquisition of HIV: 1 tab PO once daily. Confirm negative HIV status before use as prophylaxis. Combination therapy for HIV infection: 1 tab PO daily.

PEDS – Combination therapy for HIV infection (age 12 yo or older and wt 35 kg or greater): 1 tab PO daily.

UNAPPROVED ADULT – Antiviral-resistant chronic hepatitis B in HIV-coinfected patients: 1 tab PO daily.

FORMS – Trade only: Tabs emtricitabine 200 mg + tenofovir 300 mg.

NOTES – See components. Do not use in a triple nucleoside regimen. Not for patients with CrCl less than 30 mL/min or hemodialysis; hepatic dysfunction; or if dosage adjustment required. Increase dosing interval to q 48 h if CrCl is 30 to 49 mL/min. Use with didanosine cautiously; reduce didanosine dose to 250 mg for adults over 60 kg, monitor for adverse effects and discontinue didanosine if they occur. Dosage adjustment

(cont.)

***TRUVADA** (cont.)*

of didanosine unclear if wt less than 60 kg. Give Videx EC + Truvada on empty stomach or with light meal. Give buffered didanosine plus Truvada on empty stomach. Atazanavir and lopinavir-ritonavir increase tenofovir levels; monitor and discontinue Truvada if tenofovir adverse effects. Tenofovir decreases atazanavir levels. If atazanavir is used with Truvada, use 300 mg atazanavir plus 100 mg ritonavir. Do not use Truvada with lamivudine.

ANTIMICROBIALS: Antiviral Agents—Anti-HIV—Fusion Inhibitors

ENFUVIRTIDE (***Fuzeon, T-20***) ▸Serum ♀B ▸– $$$$$

ADULT – Combination therapy for HIV infection: 90 mg SC two times per day. Give each injection at new site in upper arm, anterior thigh, or abdomen, avoiding areas with current injection site reaction.

PEDS – Combination therapy for HIV infection, 6 to 16 yo: 2 mg/kg (up to 90 mg) SC two times per day. Give each injection at new site in upper arm, anterior thigh, or abdomen, avoiding areas with current injection site reaction.

FORMS – 30-day kit with vials, diluent, syringes, alcohol wipes. Single-dose vials contain 108 mg to provide delivery of 90 mg enfuvirtide.

NOTES – Increased risk of bacterial pneumonia; monitor for signs and symptoms of pneumonia. Biojector 2000 can cause persistent nerve pain if used near large nerves, bruising, hematomas. Anticoagulants, hemophilia, or other coagulation disorder may increase risk of postinjection bleeding. Reconstitute with 1.1 mL sterile water for injection. Allow vial to stand until powder dissolves completely (up to 45 min). Do not shake. Inject 1 mL (90 mg) and discard unused soln. Discard unused soln.

ANTIMICROBIALS: Antiviral Agents—Anti-HIV—Integrase Strand Transfer Inhibitor

RALTEGRAVIR (***Isentress, RAL***) ▸Glucuronidation ♀C ▸– $$$$$

ADULT – Combination therapy for HIV infection: 400 mg PO two times per day. Increase to 800 mg PO two times per day if given with rifampin.

PEDS – Combination therapy for HIV infection: Film-coated tabs, age 6 yo and older and wt 25 kg or greater: 400 mg PO two times per day. Chew tabs, 2 to 11 yo: Give PO two times per day at a dose of 75 mg for 10 kg to less than 14 kg; 100 mg for 14 kg to less than 20 kg; 150 mg for 20 kg to less than 28 kg; 200 mg for 28 kg to less than 40 kg; 300 mg for 40 kg or more. Do not substitute chew tabs for 400 mg film-coated tabs.

FORMS – Trade only: Film-coated tabs 400 mg. Chewable tabs (contain phenylalanine): 25 mg, 100 mg.

NOTES – Myopathy and rhabdomyolysis reported; caution advised for coadministration with drugs that cause myopathy. Can cause severe skin and hypersensitivity reactions including Stevens-Johnson syndrome; stop raltegravir if signs or symptoms occur. Do not cut or crush 400 mg film-coated tabs.

ANTIMICROBIALS: Antiviral Agents—Anti-HIV—Non-Nucleoside Reverse Transcriptase Inhibitors

NOTE: Many serious drug interactions—always check before prescribing!

EFAVIRENZ (***Sustiva, EFV***) ▸L ♀D ▸– $$$$$

ADULT – Combination therapy for HIV infection: 600 mg PO once daily on empty stomach, preferably at bedtime. Coadministration with voriconazole: Use voriconazole maintenance dose of 400 mg PO two times per day and reduce efavirenz to 300 mg (use caps) PO once daily. Avoid with high-fat meal.

PEDS – Consider antihistamine rash prophylaxis before starting. Combination therapy for HIV infection, age 3 yo or older: Give PO once daily on empty stomach, preferably at bedtime. Dose based on wt: 200 mg for 10 kg to less than 15 kg; 250 mg for 15 kg to less than 20 kg; 300 mg for 20 kg to less than 25 kg; 350 mg for 25 kg to less than 32.5 kg;

(cont.)

EFAVIRENZ (*cont.*)

400 mg for 32.5 kg to less than 40 kg; 600 mg for wt 40 kg or greater. Do not give with high-fat meal.

FORMS – Trade only: Caps 50, 100, 200 mg. Tabs 600 mg.

NOTES – Psychiatric/CNS reactions (warn about hazardous tasks), rash (stop treatment if severe), increased cholesterol (monitor). False-positive with Microgenics cannabinoid screening test. Monitor LFTs if given with ritonavir, hepatotoxic drugs, or to patients with hepatitis B/C. Induces CYP3A4. Many drug interactions, including decreased levels of anticonvulsants, atorvastatin, bupropion, diltiazem, itraconazole, methadone, posaconazole, pravastatin, simvastatin, and probably cyclosporine, ketoconazole, sirolimus, and tacrolimus. Do not give with pimozide, triazolam, ergot alkaloids, or St. John's wort. Do not give with atazanavir to treatment-experienced patients. Midazolam contraindicated in labeling, but can use single-dose IV cautiously with monitoring for procedural sedation. If used with rifampin, increase efavirenz to 800 mg once daily at bedtime if wt 50 kg or greater. High risk of rash when taken with clarithromycin; consider alternative antimicrobial. Potentially teratogenic; get negative pregnancy test before use by women of child-bearing potential and recommend barrier contraceptive until 12 weeks after efavirenz is stopped.

ETRAVIRINE (***Intelence, ETR***) ▶L ♀B ▶– $$$$$

ADULT – Combination therapy for treatment-resistant HIV infection: 200 mg PO two times per day after meals.

PEDS – Combination therapy for treatment-resistant HIV infection age 6 yo and older: Give PO two times per day after meals at 100 mg per dose for 16 kg to less than 20 kg; 125 mg per dose for 20 kg to less than 25 kg; 150 mg per dose for 25 kg to less than 30 kg; 200 mg per dose for 30 kg or greater.

FORMS – Trade only: Tabs 25, 100, 200 mg.

NOTES – Severe skin reactions, Stevens-Johnson syndrome, hypersensitivity. Induces CYP3A4 and inhibits CYP2C9 and 2C19; substrate of CYP2C9, 2C19, and 3A4. Do not give with efavirenz, nevirapine, ritonavir 600 mg two times per day; ritonavir-boosted tipranavir/fosamprenavir/atazanavir; St. John's wort, rifampin, rifapentine, carbamazepine, phenobarbital, phenytoin. Give rifabutin 300 mg once daily with etravirine (without ritonavir-boosted protease inhibitor). Avoid rifabutin in patients receiving etravirine with a protease inhibitor. Monitor INR with warfarin. May need dosage reduction of fluvastatin or diazepam. Consider alternative to clarithromycin for *Mycobacterium avium* complex treatment or prevention. Consider monitoring antiarrhythmic blood levels. Can disperse tabs in water and take immediately if swallowing difficulty. Do not disperse tabs in grapefruit juice or warm or carbonated drinks.

NEVIRAPINE (***Viramune, Viramune XR, NVP***) ▶LK ♀C ▶– $$$$$

WARNING – Life-threatening skin reactions, hypersensitivity, and hepatotoxicity. Monitor clinical and lab status intensively during first 18 weeks of therapy (risk of rash and/or hepatotoxicity greatest during first 6 weeks of therapy) and frequently thereafter. Consider LFTs at baseline, before and 2 weeks after dose increase, and at least once a month. Rapidly progressive liver failure can occur after only a few weeks of therapy. Stop nevirapine and never rechallenge if clinical hepatitis, severe rash, or rash with constitutional symptoms/increased LFTs. Obtain LFTs if rash occurs. Risk of hepatotoxicity with rash high in women or high CD4 count (women with CD4 count greater than 250 especially high risk, including pregnant women). Do not use if CD4 count greater than 250 in women or greater than 400 in men unless benefit clearly outweighs risk. Elevated LFTs or hepatitis B/C infection at baseline increases risk of hepatotoxicity. Hepatotoxicity not reported after single doses of nevirapine or in children.

ADULT – Combination therapy for HIV infection: 200 mg PO daily for 14 days, then 200 mg PO two times per day or Viramune XR 400 mg PO once daily. Patients maintained on immediate-release tabs can switch directly to Viramune XR. Dose titration reduces risk of rash. If rash develops, do not increase dose until it resolves. If stopped for more than 7 days, restart with initial dose.

PEDS – Combination therapy for HIV infection, age 15 days old or older: 150 mg/m^2 PO once daily for 14 days, then 150 mg/m^2 two times per day (max dose 200 mg two times per day). Dose titration reduces risk of rash. If rash develops, do not increase dose until it resolves. If stopped for more than 7 days, restart with initial dose. Per HIV guidelines, children 8 yo or younger may require up to 200 mg/m^2 PO two times per day (max dose 200 mg two times per day).

(cont.)

NEVIRAPINE (*cont.*)

UNAPPROVED ADULT – Combination therapy for HIV infection: 200 mg PO daily for 14 days, then 400 mg PO daily. Prevention of maternal–fetal HIV transmission, maternal dosing: 200 mg PO single dose at onset of labor. Do not add single-dose nevirapine to standard HIV regimens in pregnant women in the United States.

UNAPPROVED PEDS – Prevention of maternal–fetal HIV transmission, neonatal dose: 2 mg/kg PO single dose within 3 days of birth.

FORMS – Generic/Trade: Tabs 200 mg. Trade only: Susp 50 mg/5 mL (240 mL), extended-release tabs (Viramune XR) 400 mg.

NOTES – CYP3A4 inducer. May require increased methadone dose. Do not give with atazanavir, ketoconazole, hormonal contraceptives, St. John's wort. Granulocytopenia more common in children receiving zidovudine and nevirapine. Contraindicated if Child-Pugh Class B/C liver failure. Give supplemental dose of 200 mg after dialysis session. Do not use for postexposure prophylaxis in HIV-uninfected patients. Do not use in infants who have been exposed to nevirapine as part of maternal–infant prophylaxis. Do not chew, crush, or split Viramine XR tabs.

RILPIVIRINE (*Edurant, RPV*) ▶L ♀B ▶– $$$$$

ADULT – Combination therapy of treatment-naive HIV infection: 25 mg PO once daily with a meal.

PEDS – Safety and efficacy not established in children.

FORMS – Trade only: Tabs 25 mg.

NOTES – Higher virologic failure rate than efavirenz in patients with baseline HIV RNA greater than 100,000 copies/mL. NNRTI cross-resistance is likely in patients who develop virologic failure and resistance to rilpivirine. More lamivudine/emtricitabine resistance with rilpivirine than efavirenz. Metabolized by CYP3A4. Contraindicated with carbamazepine, dexamethasone (more than single dose), oxcarbazepine, phenobarbital, phenytoin, proton pump inhibitors, rifampin, rifabutin, rifapentine, St. John's wort. Use cautiously with drugs that cause torsades; supratherapeutic doses of rilpivirine prolonged QT interval. Give antacids at least 2 h before or 4 h after rilpivirine. Give H2 blockers at least 12 h before or 4 h after rilpivirine. Monitor for reduced response to methadone. Store in original bottle to protect from light.

ANTIMICROBIALS: Antiviral Agents—Anti-HIV—Nucleoside/Nucleotide Reverse Transcriptase Inhibitors

NOTE: Black Box Warning for all drugs in this class: Can cause lactic acidosis and hepatic steatosis.

ABACAVIR (*Ziagen, ABC*) ▶L ♀C ▶– $$$$$

WARNING – Potentially fatal hypersensitivity (look for fever, rash, GI symptoms, cough, dyspnea, pharyngitis, or other respiratory symptoms). Stop at once and never rechallenge after suspected reaction. Fatal reactions can recur within hours of rechallenge in patients with previously unrecognized reaction. HLA-B*5701 predisposes to hypersensitivity; screen before starting abacavir and avoid if positive test. Label HLA-B*5701-positive patients as abacavir-allergic in medical record.

ADULT – Combination therapy for HIV infection: 300 mg PO two times per day or 600 mg PO daily. Severe hypersensitivity may be more common with single daily dose.

PEDS – Combination therapy for HIV. Oral soln, age 3 mo or older: 8 mg/kg (up to 300 mg) PO two times per day. Tabs: 150 mg PO two times per day for wt 14 to 21 kg; 150 mg PO q am and 300 mg PO q pm for wt 22 kg to 29 kg; 300 mg PO two times per day for wt 30 kg or greater.

FORMS – Trade only: Tabs 300 mg scored. Oral soln 20 mg/mL (240 mL).

NOTES – Reduce dose for mild hepatic dysfunction (Child-Pugh score 5 to 6): 200 mg (10 mL of oral soln) PO two times per day. FDA safety review did not find increased risk of myocardial infarction with abacavir.

DIDANOSINE (*Videx, Videx EC, DDI*) ▶LK ♀B ▶– $$$$

WARNING – Potentially fatal pancreatitis; avoid other drugs that can cause pancreatitis. Avoid didanosine and stavudine in pregnancy due to reports of fatal lactic acidosis with pancreatitis or hepatic steatosis.

ADULT – Combination therapy for HIV infection: Buffered powder: 167 mg PO two times per day for wt less than 60 kg, 250 mg PO two times per day for wt 60 kg or greater. Videx EC: 250 mg PO daily for wt less than 60 kg. 400 mg PO daily for wt 60 kg or greater. All formulations usually taken on empty stomach. If taken with tenofovir, reduce dose to 200 mg for wt less than 60 kg and 250 mg for 60 kg or greater. Dosage reduction unclear with

(cont.)

DIDANOSINE (*cont.*)

tenofovir if CrCl is less than 60 mL/min. Give tenofovir and Videx EC on empty stomach or with light meal; give tenofovir and buffered didanosine on empty stomach.

PEDS – Combination therapy for HIV infection: 100 mg/m² PO two times per day for age 2 weeks to 8 mo. 120 mg/m² PO two times per day for age older than 8 mo. Videx EC: 200 mg PO once daily for wt 20 to 24 kg, 250 mg for wt 25 to 59 kg, 400 mg for wt 60 kg or greater.

FORMS – Generic/Trade: Pediatric powder for oral soln 10 mg/mL (buffered with antacid). Delayed-release caps (Videx EC): 125, 200, 250, 400 mg.

NOTES – Peripheral neuropathy (use cautiously with other neurotoxic drugs), retinal changes, optic neuritis, retinal depigmentation in children, hyperuricemia. Risk of lactic acidosis, pancreatitis, and peripheral neuropathy increased by concomitant stavudine. Diarrhea with buffered powder. See prescribing information for reduced dose if CrCl is less than 60 mL/min. Do not use with allopurinol. Give some medications at least 1 h (indinavir), 2 h (atazanavir, ciprofloxacin, levofloxacin, norfloxacin, ofloxacin, itraconazole, ketoconazole, ritonavir, dapsone, tetracyclines), or 4 h (moxifloxacin, gatifloxacin) before buffered didanosine. Contraindicated with ribavirin due to risk of didanosine toxicity. Methadone may reduce efficacy of didanosine, especially with buffered pediatric powder; use Videx EC instead of powder with methadone and monitor for reduced didanosine efficacy.

EMTRICITABINE (*Emtriva, FTC*) ▶K ♀B ◗– $$$$$

WARNING – Severe acute exacerbation of hepatitis B can occur after discontinuation in patients coinfected with HIV and hepatitis B. Monitor closely for at least 2 months; consider treating hepatitis B.

ADULT – Combination therapy for HIV infection: 200 mg cap PO daily. Oral soln: 240 mg (24 mL) PO daily.

PEDS – Combination therapy for HIV: Give 3 mg/kg oral soln PO once daily for age birth to 3 mo; 6 mg/kg PO once daily (up to 240 mg) for age older than 3 mo. Give 200 mg cap PO once daily for wt greater than 33 kg.

FORMS – Trade only: Caps 200 mg. Oral soln 10 mg/mL (170 mL).

NOTES – Reduce dose in adults with renal dysfunction. Caps: Give 200 mg PO q 96 h if CrCl less than 15 mL/min or hemodialysis; 200 mg PO q 72 h if CrCl 15 to 29 mL/min; 200 mg PO q 48 h if CrCl 30 to 49 mL/min. Oral soln: 60 mg q 24 h if CrCl less than 15 mL/min or hemodialysis; 80 mg q 24 h if CrCl is 15 to 29 mL/min; 120 mg q 24 h if CrCl is 30 to 49 mL/min; refrigerate oral soln if possible; stable for 3 months at room temp.

LAMIVUDINE (*Epivir, Epivir-HBV, 3TC,* ✤ *Heptovir*) ▶K ♀C ◗– $$$$$

WARNING – Lower dose of lamivudine in Epivir-HBV can cause HIV resistance; test for HIV before prescribing Epivir-HBV. Severe acute exacerbation of hepatitis B can occur after discontinuation of lamivudine in patients coinfected with HIV and hepatitis B. Monitor closely for at least 2 months after discontinuing lamivudine in such patients; consider treating hepatitis B.

ADULT – Epivir for combination therapy for HIV infection: 300 mg PO daily or 150 mg PO two times per day. Epivir-HBV for chronic hepatitis B: 100 mg PO daily. Coinfection with HIV and hepatitis B requires higher dose of lamivudine for HIV infection.

PEDS – Epivir for HIV infection: 3 mo to 16 yo, 4 mg/kg (up to 150 mg) PO two times per day. Epivir tabs: 75 mg two times per day for 14 to 21 kg, 75 mg q am and 150 mg q pm for 22 to 29 kg; 150 mg two times per day for 30 kg or greater; 300 mg PO once daily or 150 mg PO two times per day for age 16 yo or older. Epivir-HBV for chronic hepatitis B: 3 mg/kg (up to 100 mg) PO daily for age 2 yo or older. Coinfection with HIV and hepatitis B requires higher dose of lamivudine for HIV infection.

UNAPPROVED PEDS – Epivir for combination therapy for HIV infection. Infants, age younger than 30 days old: 2 mg/kg PO two times per day.

FORMS – Generic/Trade: Tabs 150 (scored), 300 mg. Trade only (Epivir): Oral soln 10 mg/mL. Trade only (Epivir-HBV, Heptovir): Tabs 100 mg, Oral soln 5 mg/mL.

NOTES – Lamivudine-resistant hepatitis B reported. Epivir: Pancreatitis in children. Monitor for hepatic decompensation (potentially fatal), neutropenia, and anemia if also receiving interferon for hepatitis C. If hepatic decompensation occurs, consider

(cont.)

LAMIVUDINE (*cont.*)

discontinuing lamivudine and reducing or discontinuing interferon and/or ribavirin. Dosage reduction for CrCl less than 50 mL/min in prescribing information.

TENOFOVIR (*Viread, TDF*) ▶K ♀B ▶– $$$$$

WARNING – Stop tenofovir if hepatomegaly or steatosis occur, even if LFTs normal. Severe acute exacerbation of hepatitis B can occur after discontinuation of tenofovir in patients coinfected with HIV and hepatitis B. Monitor closely for at least 2 months after discontinuing tenofovir in such patients; consider treating hepatitis B.

ADULT – Combination therapy for HIV, chronic hepatitis B: 300 mg PO daily without regard to food. For adults who cannot swallow tabs, use 7.5 scoops of oral powder once daily. High rate of virologic failure with tenofovir plus didanosine and lamivudine for HIV infection; avoid this regimen.

PEDS – Combination therapy for HIV: Oral powder, 2 yo and older: 8 mg/kg PO once daily (max 300 mg/day). Dosing scoop for oral powder delivers 40 mg tenofovir per scoop. Mix powder with 2 to 4 ounces of soft food that does not require chewing (applesauce, baby food, yogurt). Use immediately after mixing. Do not mix powder with liquid. Tabs, 2 yo and older and wt 17 kg or greater: Give PO once daily at dose of 150 mg for wt 17 kg to less than 22 kg; 200 mg for wt 22 kg to less than 28 kg; 250 mg for wt 28 kg to less than 35 kg; 300 mg for wt 35 kg or greater.

FORMS – Trade only: Tabs 150, 200, 250, 300 mg. Oral powder 40 mg tenofovir/g.

NOTES – Decreased bone mineral density; consider bone mineral density monitoring if history of pathologic fracture or high risk of osteopenia. Consider calcium and vitamin D supplement. Tenofovir increases didanosine levels and possibly serious didanosine adverse effects (eg, pancreatitis, lactic acidosis, hyperlactatemia, neuropathy). If atazanavir is used with tenofovir, use 300 mg atazanavir plus 100 mg ritonavir PO once daily. Atazanavir and lopinavir-ritonavir increase tenofovir levels; monitor and discontinue tenofovir if adverse effects. Tenofovir can cause renal impairment including acute renal failure and Fanconi syndrome. Monitor CrCl before starting tenofovir. Avoid tenofovir if current/recent nephrotoxic drug use. Drugs that reduce renal function or undergo renal elimination (eg, acyclovir, adefovir, ganciclovir) may increase tenofovir levels; do not use with adefovir. Monitor CrCl and phosphate if risk/history of renal insufficiency or nephrotoxic drug. Reduce dose for renal dysfunction: 300 mg once weekly (given after dialysis) for dialysis; 300 mg twice weekly if CrCl is 10 to 29 mL/min; 300 mg q 48 h if CrCl is 30 to 49 mL/min.

ZIDOVUDINE (*Retrovir, AZT, ZDV*) ▶LK ♀C ▶– $$$$$

WARNING – Bone marrow suppression, myopathy.

ADULT – Combination therapy for HIV infection: 600 mg/day PO divided two or three times per day. IV dosing: 1 mg/kg IV administered over 1 h five to six times per day. Prevention of maternal–fetal HIV transmission, maternal dosing (after 14 weeks of pregnancy): 600 mg/day PO divided two or three times per day until start of labor. During labor, 2 mg/kg (total body wt) IV over 1 h, then 1 mg/kg/h until delivery.

PEDS – Combination therapy for HIV infection, age 4 weeks or older: Give 24 mg/kg/day divided two or three times per day for wt 4 to 8 kg; give 18 mg/kg/day divided two or three times per day for wt 9 kg to 29 kg; give 600 mg/day divided two or three times per day for wt 30 kg or greater. Alternative dose: 480 mg/m^2/day PO divided two or three times per day. Prevention of maternal–fetal HIV transmission, infant dosing: 2 mg/kg PO q 6 h from within 12 h of birth until 6 weeks old. Can also give infants 1.5 mg/kg IV over 30 min q 6 h.

FORMS – Generic/Trade: Caps 100 mg. Tabs 300 mg. Syrup 50 mg/5 mL (240 mL).

NOTES – Hematologic toxicity; monitor CBC. Increased bone marrow suppression with ganciclovir or valganciclovir. Granulocytopenia more common in children receiving zidovudine and nevirapine. Monitor for hepatic decompensation, neutropenia, and anemia if also receiving interferon regimen for hepatitis C. If hepatic decompensation occurs, consider discontinuing zidovudine, interferon, and/or ribavirin. See prescribing information for dosage adjustments for renal dysfunction or hematologic toxicity.

ANTIMICROBIALS: Antiviral Agents—Anti-HIV—Protease Inhibitors

NOTE: Many serious drug interactions: Always check before prescribing. Protease inhibitors inhibit CYP3A4. Contraindicated with most antiarrhythmics, alfuzosin, ergot alkaloids, lovastatin, pimozide, rifampin, rifapentine, salmeterol, high-dose sildenafil for pulmonary hypertension, simvastatin, St. John's wort, triazolam. Midazolam contraindicated in labeling, but can use single-dose IV cautiously with monitoring for procedural sedation. Monitor INR with warfarin. Avoid inhaled/nasal fluticasone with ritonavir if possible; increased fluticasone levels can cause Cushing's syndrome/adrenal suppression. Other protease inhibitors may increase fluticasone levels; find alternatives for long-term use. Reduce colchicine dose; do not coadminister colchicine and protease inhibitors in patients with renal or hepatic dysfunction. Adjust dose of bosentan or tadalafil for pulmonary hypertension. Erectile dysfunction: Single dose of sildenafil 25 mg q 48 h, tadalafil 5 mg (not more than 10 mg) q 72 h, or vardenafil initially 2.5 mg q 72 h. Adverse effects include spontaneous bleeding in hemophiliacs, hyperglycemia, hyperlipidemia, immune reconstitution syndrome, and fat redistribution. Coinfection with hepatitis C or other liver disease increases the risk of hepatotoxicity with protease inhibitors; monitor LFTs at least twice in first month of therapy, then q 3 months.

ATAZANAVIR (*Reyataz, ATV*) ▶L ♀B ▶– $$$$$

ADULT – Combination therapy for HIV infection. Therapy-naive patients: Atazanavir 300 mg + ritonavir 100 mg PO once daily OR atazanavir 400 mg PO once daily if ritonavir-intolerant. With tenofovir, therapy-naive: 300 mg + ritonavir 100 mg PO once daily. With efavirenz, therapy-naive: 400 mg + ritonavir 100 mg once daily. Therapy-experienced: 300 mg + ritonavir 100 mg once daily. Do not give atazanavir with efavirenz in therapy-experienced patients. Pregnancy or postpartum: Usual dose is 300 mg + 100 mg ritonavir PO once daily; do not use unboosted atazanavir. If given with tenofovir or an H2 blocker in treatment-experienced patients in 2nd or 3rd trimester, give atazanavir 400 mg plus ritonavir 100 mg PO once daily. Atazanavir exposure can increase during the first 2 months post-partum; monitor for adverse effects. Give atazanavir with food; give 2 h before or 1 h after buffered didanosine.

PEDS – Combination therapy for HIV infection, age 6 yo and older: Give atazanavir/ritonavir PO once daily 150/100 mg for wt 15 to less than 20 kg; 200/100 mg for wt 20 kg to less than 40 kg; 300/100 mg for wt 40 kg or greater. Not for patients with wt less than 40 kg taking tenofovir, H2 blockers, or proton pump inhibitors. Therapy-naive, ritonavir-intolerant, age 13 yo or older and wt 40 kg or greater: 400 mg PO once daily with food. Do not give unboosted atazanavir to patients taking tenofovir, H2 blockers, or proton pump inhibitors. Give atazanavir with food. Max dose for atazanavir/ritonavir of 300/100 mg. Do not use in infants; may cause kernicterus.

FORMS – Trade only: Caps 100, 150, 200, 300 mg.

NOTES – Does not appear to increase cholesterol or triglycerides. Asymptomatic increases in indirect bilirubin due to inhibition of UDP-glucuronosyl transferase (UGT); may cause jaundice/scleral icterus. Do not use with indinavir; both may increase bilirubin. Do not use with nevirapine. May inhibit irinotecan metabolism. Can prolong PR interval and rare cases of 2nd degree AV block reported; caution advised for patients with AV block or on drugs that prolong PR interval, especially if metabolized by CYP3A4. Monitor ECG with calcium channel blockers; consider reducing diltiazem dose by 50%. Reduce clarithromycin dose by 50%; consider alternative therapy for indications other than *Mycobacterium avium* complex. Acid required for absorption; acid-suppressing drugs can cause treatment failure. Proton pump inhibitors: In treatment-naive patients do not exceed dose equivalent of omeprazole 20 mg; give PPI 12 h before atazanavir 300 mg + ritonavir 100 mg. Do not use PPIs with unboosted atazanavir or in treatment-experienced patients. H2 blockers: Give atazanavir 300 mg + ritonavir 100 mg simultaneously with H2 blocker and/or at least 10 h after H2 blocker, with max dose equivalent of famotidine 40 mg two times per day for treatment-naive patients and 20 mg two times per day for treatment-experienced patients. For treatment-experienced patients receiving tenofovir and H2 blocker, give atazanavir 400 mg + ritonavir 100 mg once daily with food. If treatment-naive and ritonavir-intolerant, give atazanavir 400 mg PO once daily with food given at least 2 h before and at least 10 h after H2 blocker (max dose equivalent to famotidine 20 mg two times per day). For treatment-experienced pregnant women in 2nd or 3rd trimester receiving tenofovir or H2 blocker, give atazanavir 400 mg + ritonavir 100 mg once daily. Give atazanavir 2 h before or 1 h after antacids

(cont.)

ATAZANAVIR (*cont.*)

or buffered didanosine. Give atazanavir and EC didanosine at different times. Inhibits CYP1A2, 2C9, and 3A4. Do not use unboosted atazanavir with buprenorphine; monitor for sedation if buprenorphine given with atazanavir/ritonavir. Use lowest possible dose of rosuvastatin (limit to 10 mg/day) or atorvastatin. Monitor levels of immunosuppressants, TCAs. Use oral contraceptive with at least 35 mcg ethinyl estradiol with ritonavir-boosted atazanavir. Use oral contraceptive with 25 to 30 mcg ethinyl estradiol if atazanavir is not boosted by ritonavir. In mild to moderate hepatic impairment (Child-Pugh class B), consider dosage reduction to 300 mg PO daily with food. Do not use in Child-Pugh Class C. Dosage adjustment for hemodialysis: Atazanavir 300 mg + ritonavir 100 mg if treatment-naive; do not use atazanavir during hemodialysis if treatment-experienced.

DARUNAVIR (***Prezista, DRV***) ▶L ♀B ▶– $$$$$

ADULT – Combination therapy for HIV infection. Therapy-naive or experienced with no darunavir resistance substitutions: 800 mg + ritonavir 100 mg PO once daily. Therapy-experienced with at least 1 darunavir resistance substitution: 600 mg + ritonavir 100 mg PO two times per day. Take with food.

PEDS – Combination therapy for HIV infection: age 3 yo or older: 375 mg + ritonavir 50 mg both two times per day for wt 15 to 29 kg; 450 mg + ritonavir 60 mg both two times per day for wt 30 to 39 kg; 600 mg + ritonavir 100 mg both two times per day for wt 40 kg or greater. Oral soln, 10 kg to less than 15 kg: darunavir 20 mg/kg with ritonavir 3 mg/kg both two times per day. Do not exceed adult dose. Take PO with food.

FORMS – Trade only: Tabs 75, 150, 400, 600 mg. 100 mg/mL (200 mL).

NOTES – Cross-sensitivity with sulfonamides possible; use caution in sulfonamide-allergic patients. Hepatotoxicity; monitor AST/ALT more frequently (especially during first few months of therapy) if patient already has liver dysfunction. Do not give with lopinavir-ritonavir or saquinavir. Reduce dose of clarithromycin if CrCl is less than 60 mL/min (see clarithromycin entry for details). Do not use with more than 200 mg/day of ketoconazole or itraconazole. Ritonavir decreases voriconazole levels; do not use voriconazole with darunavir-ritonavir unless benefit exceeds risk. May decrease oral contraceptive efficacy; consider additional or alternative method. Give didanosine 1 h before or 2 h after darunavir/ritonavir. Use lowest possible dose of atorvastatin (not more than 20 mg/day), pravastatin, or rosuvastatin.

FOSAMPRENAVIR (***Lexiva, FPV,*** ✤ ***Telzir***) ▶L ♀C ▶– $$$$$

ADULT – Combination therapy for HIV infection. Therapy-naive patients: Fosamprenavir 1400 mg PO two times per day (without ritonavir) OR fosamprenavir 1400 mg PO once daily + ritonavir 100 to 200 mg PO once daily OR fosamprenavir 700 mg PO + ritonavir 100 mg PO both two times per day. Protease inhibitor-experienced patients: 700 mg fosamprenavir + 100 mg ritonavir PO both two times per day. Do not use once-daily regimen. If once-daily ritonavir-boosted regimen given with efavirenz, increase ritonavir to 300 mg/day; no increase of ritonavir dose needed for two times per day regimen with efavirenz. Can give nevirapine with fosamprenavir only if two times per day ritonavir-boosted regimen used. No meal restrictions for tabs; take susp with food. Re-dose if vomiting occurs within 30 min of giving oral susp.

PEDS – Combination therapy for HIV infection. Fosamprenavir/ritonavir for protease inhibitor–naïve patients 4 wks or older, or protease inhibitor–experienced patients, 6 mo or older: Give PO two times per day according to wt: Fosamprenavir 45 mg/kg plus ritonavir 7 mg/kg for wt less than 11 kg; fosamprenavir 30 mg/kg plus ritonavir 3 mg/kg for wt 11 kg to less than 15 kg; fosamprenavir 23 mg/kg plus ritonavir 3 mg/kg for 15 kg to less than 20 kg; fosamprenavir 18 mg/kg plus ritonavir 3 mg/kg for 20 kg or greater. Do not exceed adult dose of fosamprenavir 700 mg plus ritonavir 100 mg, both PO two times per day. For fosamprenavir/ritonavir, can use fosamprenavir tabs if wt 39 kg or greater and ritonavir caps if wt 33 kg or greater. Fosamprenavir monotherapy for protease inhibitor–naïve patients, 2 yo and older: 30 mg/kg PO two times per day; can give 1400 mg as tabs PO two times per day if wt 47 kg or greater. Fosamprenavir is only for infants born at 38 wks gestation or more who have attained postnatal age of 28 days. Do not use once-daily dosing of fosamprenavir in children. Give susp with food. Take tabs without regard to meals. Re-dose if vomiting occurs within 30 min of giving oral susp.

FORMS – Trade only: Tabs 700 mg. Susp 50 mg/mL.

NOTES – Life-threatening skin reactions possible (reported with amprenavir). Cross-sensitivity with sulfonamides possible; use

(cont.)

FOSAMPRENAVIR (*cont.*)

caution in sulfonamide-allergic patients. Increased cholesterol and triglycerides; monitor lipids. Use lowest possible dose of atorvastatin (not more than 20 mg/day). Monitor CBC at least weekly if taking rifabutin. Monitor levels of immunosuppressants, TCAs. May need to increase dose of methadone. Do not use more than 200 mg/day ketoconazole/itraconazole with fosamprenavir + ritonavir; may need to reduce antifungal dose if patient is receiving more than 400 mg/day itraconazole or ketoconazole with unboosted fosamprenavir. Do not use more than 2.5 mg vardenafil q 24 h with unboosted fosamprenavir or q 72 h for fosamprenavir + ritonavir. Do not use hormonal contraceptives. More adverse reactions when fosamprenavir is given with Kaletra; appropriate dose for combination therapy unclear. Mild hepatic dysfunction (Child-Pugh score 5 to 6): 700 mg PO two times per day unboosted (for treatment-naive) or 700 mg PO two times per day plus ritonavir 100 mg PO once daily (for treatment-naive or -experienced). Moderate hepatic dysfunction (Child-Pugh score 7 to 9): 700 mg PO two times per day unboosted (for treatment-naive) or 450 mg PO two times per day plus ritonavir 100 mg PO once daily (for treatment-naive or -experienced). Severe hepatic dysfunction: fosamprenavir 350 mg PO two times per day unboosted (for treatment-naive) or 300 mg PO two times per day plus ritonavir 100 mg PO once daily (for treatment-naive or -experienced). No dosage adjustments available for peds patients with hepatic dysfunction. Refrigeration not required, but may improve taste of oral susp.

INDINAVIR (*Crixivan, IDV*) ▶LK ♀C ▶– $$$$$

ADULT – Combination therapy for HIV infection: 800 mg PO q 8 h between meals with water (at least 48 oz/day).

PEDS – Not approved in children. Do not use in infants; may cause kernicterus.

UNAPPROVED ADULT – Combination therapy for HIV infection: Indinavir 800 mg PO with ritonavir 100 to 200 mg PO both two times per day; or indinavir 400 mg with ritonavir 400 mg both two times per day; or indinavir 600 mg PO with Kaletra 400/100 mg PO both two times per day. Can be given without regard to meals when given with ritonavir.

UNAPPROVED PEDS – Combination therapy for HIV infection: 350 to 500 mg/m²/dose (max of 800 mg/dose) PO q 8 h for children; 800 mg PO q 8 h between meals with water (at least 48 oz/day) for adolescents.

FORMS – Trade only: Caps 100, 200, 400 mg.

NOTES – Nephrolithiasis (especially in children), hemolytic anemia, indirect hyperbilirubinemia, possible hepatitis, interstitial nephritis with asymptomatic pyuria. Do not use with atazanavir; both may increase bilirubin. Avoid using with carbamazepine if possible. Give indinavir and buffered didanosine 1 h apart on empty stomach. Reduce indinavir dose to 600 mg PO q 8 h when given with ketoconazole or itraconazole 200 mg two times per day. Increase indinavir dose to 1000 mg PO q 8 h when given with efavirenz or nevirapine. Use lowest possible dose of atorvastatin or rosuvastatin. For mild to moderate hepatic cirrhosis, give 600 mg PO q 8 h. Indinavir not recommended in pregnancy because of dramatic reduction in blood levels.

LOPINAVIR-RITONAVIR (*Kaletra, LPV/r*) ▶L ♀C ▶– $$$$$

ADULT – Combination therapy for HIV infection: 400/100 mg PO two times per day (tabs or oral soln). Can use 800/200 mg PO once daily in patients with less than 3 lopinavir resistance–associated substitutions. Dosage adjustment for coadministration with efavirenz, nevirapine, fosamprenavir, or nelfinavir: 500/125 mg tabs (use two 200/50 mg + one 100/25 mg tab) or 533/133 mg oral soln (6.5 mL) PO two times per day. No once-daily dosing for pregnant patients; coadministration with carbamazepine, phenobarbital, phenytoin, efavirenz, nevirapine, fosamprenavir, or nelfinavir; or in patients with 3 or more lopinavir resistance–associated substitutions (L10F/I/R/V, K20M/N/R, L24I, L33F, M36I, I47V, G48V, I54L/T/V, V82A/C/F/S/T, and I84V). Give tabs without regard to meals; give oral soln with food.

PEDS – Combination therapy for HIV infection, age 14 days to 6 mo: Lopinavir 300 mg/m² or 16 mg/kg PO two times per day. Propylene glycol in oral soln can cause life-threatening toxicity in infants (especially preterm); do not give oral soln to neonates before postmenstrual age of 42 weeks and postnatal age of at least 14 days. Age 6 mo to 12 yo: Lopinavir 230 mg/m² or 12 mg/kg PO two times per day if wt less than 15 kg; 10 mg/kg PO two times per day if wt 15 to 40 kg. Dosage adjustment for coadministration with efavirenz, nevirapine, fosamprenavir, or nelfinavir: Lopinavir 300 mg/m² PO two times per day or 13 mg/kg PO two times per day for wt less than 15 kg; 11 mg/kg PO two times per day for wt 15 to 45 kg. Do not exceed adult dose. Give tabs without regard

(cont.)

LOPINAVIR-RITONAVIR (*cont.*)

to meals; give oral soln with food. Beware of medication errors with oral soln; fatal overdose reported in infant given excessive volume of soln.

FORMS – Trade only: Tabs 200/50 mg, 100/25 mg. Oral soln 80/20 mg/mL (160 mL).

NOTES – Medication errors can occur if Keppra (levetiracetam) confused with Kaletra. May cause pancreatitis. Ritonavir included in formulation to inhibit metabolism and boost levels of lopinavir. Increases tenofovir levels; monitor for adverse reactions. Many other drug interactions including decreased efficacy of oral contraceptives. Limit rosuvastatin dose to 10 mg/day; use lowest possible dose of atorvastatin. Ritonavir decreases voriconazole levels; do not give with voriconazole unless benefit exceeds risk. Expected to increase fentanyl exposure. May require higher methadone dose. Reduce dose of clarithromycin if CrCl is less than 60 mL/min (see clarithromycin entry for details). Give buffered didanosine 1 h before or 2 h after Kaletra oral soln. Kaletra tabs can be given at same time as didanosine without food. Do not give Kaletra with tipranavir 500 mg + ritonavir 200 mg both two times per day. Do not give Kaletra once daily with phenytoin, phenobarbital, or carbamazepine; monitor for reduced phenytoin levels. Oral soln contains alcohol. Use oral soln within 2 months if stored at room temperature. Tabs do not require refrigeration. Do not crush, cut, or chew tabs.

NELFINAVIR (*Viracept, NFV*) ▶L ♀B ▶– $$$$$

ADULT – Combination therapy for HIV infection: 750 mg PO three times per day or 1250 mg PO two times per day with meals. Absorption improved when meal contains at least 500 calories with 11 to 28 g of fat.

PEDS – Combination therapy for HIV infection: 45 to 55 mg/kg PO two times per day or 25 to 35 mg/kg PO three times per day (up to 2500 mg/day) for age 2 yo or older. Take with meals. Absorption improved when meal contains at least 500 calories with 11 to 28 g of fat. Use powder or 250 mg tabs which can be crushed and mixed with water or other liquids. Do not mix with acidic foods/juice; will taste bitter.

FORMS – Trade only: Tabs 250, 625 mg. Oral powder 50 mg/g (114 g).

NOTES – Diarrhea common. Use lowest possible dose of atorvastatin (not more than 40 mg/day) or rosuvastatin or consider pravastatin/fluvastatin. Decreases efficacy of oral contraceptives. May require higher methadone dose. Do not use with proton pump inhibitors. Give nelfinavir 2 h before or 1 h after buffered didanosine. Oral powder stable for 6 h after mixing if refrigerated. No dosage adjustment for mild hepatic impairment (Child-Pugh Class A); not recommended for more severe hepatic failure (Child-Pugh B/C).

RITONAVIR (*Norvir, RTV*) ▶L ♀B ▶– $$$$$

WARNING – Contraindicated with many drugs due to risk of drug interactions.

ADULT – Adult doses of 100 mg PO daily to 400 mg PO two times per day used to boost levels of other protease inhibitors. Full-dose regimen (600 mg PO two times per day) poorly tolerated. Best tolerated regimen with saquinavir may be ritonavir 400 mg + saquinavir 400 mg, both two times per day. Saquinavir 1000 mg + ritonavir 100 mg, both two times per day also used. Take tabs with meals.

PEDS – Combination therapy for HIV infection: Start with 250 mg/m^2 and increase q 2 to 3 days by 50 mg/m^2 twice daily to achieve usual dose of 350 to 400 mg/m^2 (up to 600 mg/dose) PO two times per day for age older than 1 mo. If 400 mg/m^2 twice daily not tolerated, consider other alternatives. Give with meals.

UNAPPROVED ADULT – Combination therapy for HIV infection: Ritonavir 100 to 200 mg PO two times per day with indinavir 800 mg PO two times per day or ritonavir 400 mg plus indinavir 400 mg both two times per day.

UNAPPROVED PEDS – Used at lower than labeled doses to boost levels of other protease inhibitors.

FORMS – Trade only: Caps 100 mg, tabs 100 mg. Oral soln 80 mg/mL (240 mL).

NOTES – N/V, pancreatitis, alterations in AST, ALT, GGT, CPK, uric acid. Do not give with quinine. Ritonavir decreases voriconazole levels. Do not use ritonavir doses of 400 mg two times per day or greater with voriconazole; use ritonavir 100 mg two times per day with voriconazole only if benefit exceeds risk. Do not use more than 200 mg/day of ketoconazole with ritonavir. Decreases efficacy of combined oral or patch contraceptives; consider alternative. May increases fentanyl levels; monitor for increase in fentanyl effects. Increases methadone dosage requirements. May cause serotonin syndrome with fluoxetine. Can prolong PR interval and rare cases of 2nd or 3rd degree AV block reported; caution advised for patients at risk for conduction problems or taking drugs that prolong PR interval, especially if metabolized by CYP3A4. Reduce clarithromycin dose if CrCl is less than 60 mL/min (see clarithromycin entry for details).

(cont.)

RITONAVIR (*cont.*)

Give ritonavir 2.5 h before and after buffered didanosine. Monitor for increased digoxin levels. Caps and oral soln contain alcohol. Do not refrigerate oral soln. Try to refrigerate caps, but stable for 30 days at less than 77°F. Tabs do not require refrigeration, but must be taken with food.

SAQUINAVIR (***Invirase, SQV***) ▶L ♀B ▶? $$$$$

ADULT – Combination therapy for HIV infection. Regimen must contain ritonavir. Saquinavir 1000 mg + ritonavir 100 mg PO, both two times per day taken within 2 h after meals. Saquinavir 1000 mg plus lopinavir-ritonavir (Kaletra) 400/100 mg PO both two times per day. If serious toxicity occurs, do not reduce Invirase dose; efficacy unclear for lower doses.

PEDS – Combination therapy for HIV, for age 16 yo or older: Use adult dose.

FORMS – Trade only: Invirase (hard gel) Caps 200 mg. Tabs 500 mg.

NOTES – Can prolong QT (increase more than some other boosted protease inhibitors) and PR intervals; rare cases of torsades and 2nd/3rd degree AV block. Get ECG at baseline, after 3 to 4 days of therapy, and periodically in at-risk patients. Do not use if baseline QT interval is longer than 450 msec. Discontinue if on-treatment QT interval is longer than 480 msec or interval increases by more than 20 msec over baseline. Do not use if refractory hypokalemia/hypomagnesemia, congenital long QT syndrome, complete AV block without pacemaker or at high risk for complete AV block, or severe hepatic impairment. Do not use with Class IA or III antiarrhythmics, neuroleptics or antimicrobials that prolong QT interval, trazodone, drugs that increase saquinavir levels and prolong the QT interval, or if QT interval increases by more than 20 msec after starting a drug that might increase the QT interval. Monitor if used with other drugs that prolong the PR interval (beta blockers, calcium channel blockers, digoxin, atazanavir). Do not use saquinavir with garlic supplements or tipranavir-ritonavir. Use lowest possible dose of atorvastatin (not more than 20 mg/day) or rosuvastatin. Proton pump inhibitors may increase saquinavir levels. Do not exceed 200 mg/day ketoconazole. Monitor for increased digoxin levels. May reduce methadone levels. Reduce dose of clarithromycin if CrCl is less than 60 mL/min (see clarithromycin entry for details).

TIPRANAVIR (***Aptivus, TPV***) ▶Feces ♀C ▶– $$$$$

WARNING – Potentially fatal hepatotoxicity. Monitor clinical status and LFTs frequently. Risk increased by coinfection with hepatitis B/C. Contraindicated in moderate to severe (Child-Pugh B/C) hepatic failure. Intracranial hemorrhage can occur with tipranavir + ritonavir; caution if at risk of bleeding from trauma, surgery, other medical conditions, or receiving antiplatelet agents or anticoagulants.

ADULT – HIV infection, boosted by ritonavir in treatment-experienced patients with strains resistant to multiple protease inhibitors: 500 mg + ritonavir 200 mg PO both two times per day. Take tipranavir plus ritonavir capsules/soln without regard to meals; take tipranavir plus ritonavir tabs with meals.

PEDS – HIV infection, boosted by ritonavir in treatment-experienced patients age 2 yo or older with strains resistant to multiple protease inhibitors: 14 mg/kg with 6 mg/kg ritonavir (375 mg/m^2 with ritonavir 150 mg/m^2) PO two times per day to max of 500 mg with ritonavir 200 mg two times per day. Dosage reduction for toxicity in patients infected with virus that is not resistant to multiple protease inhibitors: 12 mg/kg with 5 mg/kg ritonavir (290 mg/m^2 with 115 mg/m^2 ritonavir) PO two times per day. Take tipranavir plus ritonavir caps/soln without regard to meals; take tipranavir plus ritonavir tabs with meals.

FORMS – Trade only: Caps 250 mg. Oral soln 100 mg/mL (95 mL in unit-of-use amber glass bottle).

NOTES – Contains sulfonamide moiety; potential for cross-sensitivity unknown. Al/Mg antacids may decrease absorption of tipranavir; separate doses. Contraindicated with CYP3A4 substrates that can cause life-threatening toxicity at high concentrations. Do not use atorvastatin. Monitor levels of immunosuppressants, TCAs. May need higher methadone dose. Ritonavir decreases voriconazole levels; do not give together unless benefit exceeds risk. Do not use tipranavir-ritonavir with Kaletra or saquinavir. Decreases ethinyl estradiol levels; consider nonhormonal contraception. Reduce clarithromycin dose if CrCl is less than 60 mL/min (see clarithromycin entry for details). Caps contain alcohol. Refrigerate bottle of caps before opening. Use caps and oral soln within 60 days of opening container. Oral soln contains 116 international units/mL of vitamin E; advise patients not to take supplemental vitamin E other than a multivitamin.

ANTIMICROBIALS: Antiviral Agents—Anti-Influenza

NOTE: Whenever possible, immunization is the preferred method of prophylaxis. Avoid anti-influenza antivirals from 48 h before until 2 weeks after a dose of live influenza vaccine (FluMist) unless medically necessary. Patients with suspected influenza may have primary/concomitant bacterial pneumonia; antibiotics may be indicated.

AMANTADINE (***Symmetrel***) ▶K ♀C ▶? $$

ADULT – Influenza A: 100 mg PO two times per day; reduce dose to 100 mg PO daily for age 65 yo or older. The CDC generally recommends against amantadine or rimantadine for treatment or prevention of influenza A in the United States due to high levels of resistance. Parkinsonism: 100 mg PO two times per day. Max 400 mg/day divided three to four times per day. Drug-induced extrapyramidal disorders: 100 mg PO two times per day. Max 300 mg/day divided three to four times per day.

PEDS – Safety and efficacy not established in infants age younger than 1 yo. Influenza A, treatment or prophylaxis: 5 mg/kg/day (up to 150 mg/day) PO divided two times per day for age 1 to 9 yo and any child wt less than 40 kg. 100 mg PO two times per day for age 10 yo or older. The CDC generally recommends against amantadine or rimantadine for treatment or prevention of influenza A in the United States due to high levels of resistance.

FORMS – Generic only: Caps 100 mg. Tabs 100 mg. Syrup 50 mg/5 mL (480 mL).

NOTES – CNS toxicity, suicide attempts, neuroleptic malignant syndrome with dosage reduction/withdrawal, anticholinergic effects, orthostatic hypotension. Do not stop abruptly in Parkinson's disease. Dosage reduction in adults with renal dysfunction: 200 mg PO once a week for CrCl less than 15 mL/min or hemodialysis. 200 mg PO 1st day, then 100 mg PO every other day for CrCl 15 to 29 mL/min. 200 mg PO 1st day, then 100 mg PO daily for CrCl 30 to 50 mL/min.

OSELTAMIVIR (***Tamiflu***) ▶LK ♀C, but + ▶? $$$

ADULT – Influenza A/B, treatment: 75 mg PO two times per day for 5 days starting within 2 days of symptom onset. Prophylaxis: 75 mg PO daily. Start within 2 days of exposure and continue for 10 days. Take with food to improve tolerability.

PEDS – Influenza A/B: Dose is 30 mg for age 1 yo or older and wt 15 kg or less, 45 mg for wt 16 to 23 kg, 60 mg for wt 24 to 40 kg, 75 mg for wt greater than 40 kg or age 13 yo and older. Treatment: Give dose twice daily for 5 days starting within 2 days of symptom onset. Prophylaxis: Give once daily for 10 days starting within 2 days of exposure.

UNAPPROVED PEDS – Influenza treatment in infants younger than 1 yo: 3 mg/kg/dose PO two times per day for 5 days starting within 2 days of symptom onset. Influenza treatment, premature infants: 2 mg/kg/day PO divided two times per day. Influenza prophylaxis in infants 3 to 11 mo: 3 mg/kg/dose PO once daily for 10 days starting within 2 days of exposure. Due to limited data, prophylaxis is not recommended for infants younger than 3 mo unless the situation is critical. Take with food to improve tolerability. The new 10 mL dosing syringe appears capable of measuring smaller doses.

FORMS – Trade only: Caps 30, 45, 75 mg. Susp 6 mg/mL (60 mL) with 10 mL dosing device. Pharmacist can also compound susp (6 mg/mL). Before July 2011, Tamiflu susp concentration was 12 mg/mL and pharmacists compounded 15 mg/mL susp. Instructions for compounding new 6 mg/mL susp are in Tamiflu prescribing information.

NOTES – Previously not used in children younger than 1 yo; immature blood-brain barrier could lead to high oseltamivir levels in CNS. Increased INR with warfarin. Postmarketing reports (mostly from Japan) of self-injury and delirium, primarily among children and adolescents; monitor for abnormal behavior. Dosage adjustment for adults with CrCl 10 to 30 mL/min: 75 mg PO daily for 5 days for treatment, 75 mg PO every other day or 30 mg PO once daily for prophylaxis. Susp stable for 10 days at room temperature, 17 days refrigerated.

RIMANTADINE (***Flumadine***) ▶LK ♀C ▶– $$

ADULT – Prophylaxis/treatment of influenza A: 100 mg PO two times per day. Start treatment within 2 days of symptom onset and continue for 7 days. Reduce dose to 100 mg PO once daily if severe hepatic dysfunction, CrCl less than 30 mL/min, or age older than 65 yo. The CDC generally recommends against amantadine/rimantadine for treatment/prevention of influenza A in the United States due to high levels of resistance.

PEDS – Influenza A prophylaxis: 5 mg/kg (up to 150 mg/day) PO once daily for age 1 to 9

(cont.)

RIMANTADINE (*cont.*)

yo; 100 mg PO two times per day for age 10 yo and older. The CDC generally recommends against amantadine/rimantadine for treatment/prevention of influenza A in the United States due to high levels of resistance.

UNAPPROVED PEDS – Influenza A treatment: 6.6 mg/kg (up to 150 mg/day) PO divided two times per day for age 1 to 9 yo; 100 mg PO two times per day for age 10 yo and older. Start treatment within 2 days of symptom onset and continue for 7 days.

FORMS – Generic/Trade: Tabs 100 mg. Pharmacist can compound suspension.

ZANAMIVIR (***Relenza***) ▸K ♀C ▸? $$$

ADULT – Influenza A/B treatment: 2 puffs two times per day for 5 days. Take 2 doses on day 1 at least 2 h apart. Start within 2 days of symptom onset. Influenza A/B prevention: 2 puffs once daily for 10 days, starting within 2 days of exposure.

PEDS – Influenza A/B treatment: 2 puffs two times per day for 5 days for age 7 yo or older. Take 2 doses on day 1 at least 2 h apart. Start within 2 days of symptom onset. Influenza A/B prevention: 2 puffs once daily for 10 days for age 5 yo or older, starting within 2 days of exposure.

FORMS – Trade only: Rotadisk inhaler 5 mg/puff (20 puffs).

NOTES – Contains lactose; contraindicated in patients with milk protein allergy. May cause bronchospasm and worsen pulmonary function in asthma or COPD; avoid if underlying airways disease. Stop if bronchospasm/decline in respiratory function. Show patient how to use inhaler.

ANTIMICROBIALS: Antiviral Agents—Other

See www.idsociety.org for guidelines on management of hepatitis B and C. See www.aidsinfo.nih.gov for guidelines on the management of hepatitis B and C in HIV-infected patients.

ADEFOVIR (***Hepsera***) ▸K ♀C ▸– $$$$$

WARNING – Nephrotoxic; monitor renal function. May result in HIV resistance in untreated HIV infection; test for HIV before prescribing. Lactic acidosis with hepatic steatosis. Severe acute exacerbation of hepatitis B can occur after discontinuation of adefovir in patients with HIV and hepatitis B coinfection. Monitor closely for at least 2 months after discontinuing adefovir in such patients; consider re-treating hepatitis B.

ADULT – Chronic hepatitis B: 10 mg PO daily.

PEDS – Chronic hepatitis B: 10 mg PO daily for age 12 yo or older.

FORMS – Trade only: Tabs 10 mg.

NOTES – Monitor renal function. See prescribing information for dosage reduction if CrCl < 50 mL/min. Other nephrotoxic drugs may increase risk of nephrotoxicity; do not use with tenofovir. Use adefovir plus lamivudine instead of adefovir alone in patients with lamivudine-resistant hepatitis B. Adefovir resistance can cause viral load rebound. Consider change in therapy if persistent serum hepatitis B DNA > 1000 copies/mL.

BOCEPREVIR (***Victrelis***) ▸L ♀B ▸– $$$$$

ADULT – Chronic hepatitis C (genotype 1): 800 mg PO three times per day (q 7 to 9 h) in combination with peginterferon and ribavirin. Take with food. Start boceprevir after 4 weeks of peginterferon plus ribavirin. Treatment duration is based on response at weeks 8, 12, and 24. Stop boceprevir if HCV-RNA is 100 International units/mL or greater at week 12 or confirmed detectable at week 24.

PEDS – Safety and efficacy not established in children.

FORMS – Trade only: Caps 200 mg.

NOTES – Not for monotherapy. Strong inhibitor of CYP3A4. Many drug interactions. Contraindicated with alfuzosin, atorvastatin doses greater than 20 mg/day, carbamazepine, colchicine in patients with renal or hepatic impairment, drosperinone, ergot alkaloids, high-dose itraconazole or ketoconazole (>200 mg/day), lovastatin, oral midazolam, phenobarbital, phenytoin, pimozide, rifampin, salmeterol, high-dose sildenafil or tadalafil for pulmonary hypertension, simvastatin, St. John's wort, triazolam. Do not use with efavirenz, ritonavir-boosted atazanavir, ritonavir-darunavir, or lopinavir-ritonavir. Reduce doses of phosphodiesterase inhibitors for erectile dysfunction to not more than sildenafil 25 mg q 48 h, tadalafil 10 mg q 72 h, or vardenafil 2.5 mg q 24 h. Avoid pregnancy in female patients or female partners of male patients because of ribavirin teratogenicity. May impair efficacy of hormonal contraceptives; use 2 nonhormonal contraceptives. Can cause anemia and neutropenia; monitor CBC at baseline, weeks 4, 8, 12, and prn. Patients with compensated cirrhosis: 800 mg PO three times per day for 44 weeks in combination with peginterferon and ribavirin. Start boceprevir after 4 weeks of peginterferon plus

(cont.)

BOCEPREVIR (*cont.*)

ribavirin. Store in refrigerator before dispensing; patients can store at room temperature for 3 months.

ENTECAVIR (*Baraclude*) ▶K ♀C ▶– $$$$$

WARNING – Nucleoside analogues can cause lactic acidosis with hepatic steatosis. Severe acute exacerbation of hepatitis B can occur after discontinuation. Monitor closely for at least 2 months after discontinuation. Patients coinfected with HIV and hepatitis B should not receive entecavir for hepatitis B unless they also receive HAART for HIV; failure to treat HIV in such patients could lead to HIV resistance to NRTIs.

ADULT – Chronic hepatitis B: 0.5 mg PO once daily if treatment-naive; 1 mg if lamivudine- or telbivudine-resistant, history of viremia despite lamivudine treatment, decompensated liver disease, or HIV coinfected. Give on empty stomach (2 h after last meal and 2 h before next meal).

PEDS – Chronic hepatitis B, age 16 yo or older: 0.5 mg PO once daily if treatment-naive; 1 mg if lamivudine-or telbivudine-resistant, history of viremia despite lamivudine treatment, decompensated liver disease, or HIV coinfected. Give on empty stomach (2 h after last meal and 2 h before next meal).

FORMS – Trade only: Tabs 0.5, 1 mg. Oral soln 0.05 mg/mL (210 mL).

NOTES – Entecavir treatment of coinfected patients not receiving HIV treatment may increase the risk of resistance to lamivudine or emtricitabine. Do not mix oral soln with water or other liquid. Reduce dose if CrCl is less than 50 mL/min or dialysis. Give dose after dialysis sessions.

INTERFERON ALFA-2B (*Intron A*) ▶K ♀C ▶?+ $$$$$

WARNING – May cause or worsen serious neuropsychiatric, autoimmune, ischemic, and infectious diseases. Frequent clinical and lab monitoring required. Stop interferon if signs/symptoms of these conditions are persistently severe or worsen.

ADULT – Chronic hepatitis B: 5 million units/day or 10 million units three times per week SC/IM for 16 weeks if HBeAg positive. Chronic hepatitis C: 3 million units SC/IM three times per week for 16 weeks. Continue for 18 to 24 months if ALT normalized. In combination with ribavirin for hepatitis C, peginterferon is preferred over interferon alfa-2b because of substantially higher response rate. Other indications: Condylomata acuminata, AIDS-related Kaposi's sarcoma, hairy-cell leukemia, melanoma, and follicular lymphoma—see prescribing information for specific dose.

PEDS – Chronic hepatitis B: 3 million units/m² three times per week for 1st week, then 6 million units/m² (max 10 million units/dose) SC three times per week for age 1 yo or older. Chronic hepatitis C: Interferon alfa-2b 3 million units/m² SC three times per week for age 3 yo or older with PO ribavirin according to wt. Ribavirin: 200 mg two times per day for wt 25 to 36 kg; 200 mg q am and 400 mg q pm for wt 37 to 49 kg; 400 mg two times per day for wt 50 to 61 kg. Use adult dose for wt greater than 61 kg. If ribavirin contraindicated, use interferon 3 to 5 million units/m² (max 3 million units/dose) SC/IM three times per week.

UNAPPROVED ADULT – Prevention of chronic hepatitis C in acute hepatitis C: 5 million units SC daily for 4 weeks then 5 million units SC three times per week for 20 weeks. Other indications: superficial bladder tumors, chronic myelogenous leukemia, cutaneous T-cell lymphoma, essential thrombocythemia, non-Hodgkin's lymphoma, and chronic granulocytic leukemia.

FORMS – Trade only: Powder/soln for injection 10, 18, 50 million units/vial. Soln for injection 18, 25 million units/multidose vial. Multidose injection pens 3, 5, 10 million units/0.2 mL (1.5 mL), 6 doses/pen.

NOTES – Monitor for depression, suicidal behavior (especially in adolescents), other severe neuropsychiatric effects. Thyroid abnormalities, hepatotoxicity, flu-like symptoms, pulmonary and cardiovascular reactions, retinal damage, neutropenia, thrombocytopenia, hypertriglyceridemia (consider monitoring). Monitor CBC, TSH, LFTs, electrolytes. Dosage adjustments for hematologic toxicity in prescribing information. Increases theophylline levels.

INTERFERON ALFA-N3 (*Alferon N*) ▶K ♀C ▶– $$$$$

WARNING – Flu-like syndrome, myalgias, alopecia. Contraindicated in egg protein allergy.

ADULT – Intralesional injection for condylomata acuminata.

PEDS – Not approved in children.

INTERFERON ALFACON-1 (*Infergen*) ▶Plasma ♀C ▶? $$$$$

WARNING – May cause or worsen serious neuropsychiatric, autoimmune, ischemic, and infectious diseases. Frequent clinical and lab monitoring required. Stop interferon if signs/symptoms of these conditions are persistently severe or worsen.

ADULT – Chronic hepatitis C, monotherapy: 9 to 15 mcg SC three times per week. Chronic

(cont.)

OVERVIEW OF BACTERIAL PATHOGENS (Selected)

By bacterial class
Gram-positive aerobic cocci: *Staph epidermidis* (coagulase negative), *Staph aureus* (coagulase positive), Streptococci: *S. pneumoniae* (pneumococcus), *S. pyogenes* (Group A), *S. agalactiae* (Group B), enterococcus **Gram-positive aerobic/facultatively anaerobic bacilli:** *Bacillus, Corynebacterium diphtheriae, Erysipelothrix rhusiopathiae, Listeria monocytogenes, Nocardia* **Gram-negative aerobic diplococci:** *Moraxella catarrhalis, Neisseria gonorrhoeae, Neisseria meningitidis* **Gram-negative aerobic coccobacilli:** *Haemophilus ducreyi, influenzae* **Gram-negative aerobic bacilli:** *Acinetobacter, Bartonella* species, *Bordetella pertussis, Brucella, Burkholderia cepacia, Campylobacter, Francisella tularensis, Helicobacter pylori, Legionella pneumophila, Pseudomonas aeruginosa, Stenotrophomonas maltophilia, Vibrio cholerae, Yersinia* **Gram-negative facultatively anaerobic bacilli:** *Aeromonas hydrophila, Eikenella corrodens, Pasteurella multocida,* Enterobacteriaceae: *E. coli, Citrobacter, Shigella, Salmonella, Klebsiella, Enterobacter, Hafnia, Serratia, Proteus, Providencia* **Anaerobes:** *Actinomyces, Bacteroides fragilis, Clostridium botulinum, Clostridium difficile, Clostridium perfringens, Clostridium tetani, Fusobacterium, Lactobacillus, Peptostreptococcus* **Defective Cell Wall Bacteria:** *Chlamydia pneumoniae, Chlamydia psittaci, Chlamydia trachomatis, Coxiella burnetii, Mycoplasma pneumoniae, Rickettsia prowazekii, Rickettsia rickettsii, Rickettsia typhi, Ureaplasma urealyticum* **Spirochetes:** *Borrelia burgdorferi, Leptospira, Treponema pallidum* **Mycobacteria:** *M. avium* complex, *M. kansasii, M. leprae, M. tuberculosis*
By bacterial name
Acinetobacter **Gram-negative aerobic bacilli** *Actinomyces* **Anaerobes** *Aeromonas hydrophila* **Gram-negative facultatively anaerobic bacilli** *Bacillus* **Gram-positive aerobic/facultatively anaerobic bacilli** *Bacteroides fragilis* **Anaerobes** *Bartonella* species **Gram-negative aerobic bacilli** *Bordetella pertussis* **Gram-negative aerobic bacilli** *Borrelia burgdorferi* **Spirochetes** *Brucella* **Gram-negative aerobic bacilli** *Burkholderia cepacia* **Gram-negative aerobic bacilli** *Campylobacter* **Gram-negative aerobic bacilli** *Chlamydia pneumoniae* **Defective cell wall bacteria** *Chlamydia psittaci* **Defective cell wall bacteria** *Chlamydia trachomatis* **Defective cell wall bacteria** *Citrobacter* **Gram-negative facultatively anaerobic bacilli** *Clostridium botulinum* **Anaerobes** *Clostridium difficile* **Anaerobes** *Clostridium perfringens* **Anaerobes** *Clostridium tetani* **Anaerobes** *Corynebacterium diphtheriae* **Gram-positive aerobic/facultatively anaerobic bacilli** *Coxiella burnetii* **Defective cell wall bacteria** *E. coli* **Gram-negative facultatively anaerobic bacilli** *Eikenella corrodens* **Gram-negative facultatively anaerobic bacilli** *Enterobacter* **Gram-negative facultatively anaerobic bacilli** *Enterobacteriaceae* **Gram-negative facultatively anaerobic bacilli** *Enterococcus* **Gram-positive aerobic cocci** *Erysipelothrix rhusiopathiae* **Gram-positive aerobic/facultatively anaerobic bacilli** *Francisella tularensis* **Gram-negative aerobic bacilli** *Fusobacterium* **Anaerobes** *Haemophilus ducreyi* **Gram-negative aerobic coccobacilli** *Haemophilus influenzae* **Gram-negative aerobic coccobacilli** *Hafnia* **Gram-negative facultatively anaerobic bacilli** *Helicobacter pylori* **Gram-negative aerobic bacilli** *Klebsiella* **Gram-negative facultatively anaerobic bacilli** *Lactobacillus* **Anaerobes** *Legionella pneumophila* **Gram-negative aerobic bacilli** *Leptospira* **Spirochetes** *Listeria monocytogenes* **Gram-positive aerobic/facultatively anaerobic bacilli** *M. avium* complex **Mycobacteria** *M. kansasii* **Mycobacteria** *M. leprae* **Mycobacteria** *M. tuberculosis* **Mycobacteria**

OVERVIEW OF BACTERIAL PATHOGENS (Selected)

By bacterial class
Moraxella catarrhalis **Gram-negative aerobic diplococci**
Myocoplasma pneumoniae **Defective cell wall bacteria**
Neisseria gonorrhoeae **Gram-negative aerobic diplococci**
Neisseria meningitidis **Gram-negative aerobic diplococci**
Nocardia **Gram-positive aerobic/facultatively anaerobic bacilli**
Pasteurella multocida **Gram-negative facultatively anaerobic bacilli**
Peptostreptococcus **Anaerobes**
Pneumococcus **Gram-positive aerobic cocci**
Proteus **Gram-negative facultatively anaerobic bacilli**
Providencia **Gram-negative facultatively anaerobic bacilli**
Pseudomonas aeruginosa **Gram-negative aerobic bacilli**
Rickettsia prowazekii **Defective cell wall bacteria**
Rickettsia rickettsii **Defective cell wall bacteria**
Rickettsia typhi **Defective cell wall bacteria**
Salmonella **Gram-negative facultatively anaerobic bacilli**
Serratia **Gram-negative facultatively anaerobic bacilli**
Shigella **Gram-negative facultatively anaerobic bacilli**
Staph aureus (coagulase positive) **Gram-positive aerobic cocci**
Staph epidermidis (coagulase negative) **Gram-positive aerobic cocci**
Stenotrophomonas maltophilia **Gram-negative aerobic bacilli**
Strep agalactiae (Group B) **Gram-positive aerobic cocci**
Strep pneumoniae (pneumococcus) **Gram-positive aerobic cocci**
Strep pyogenes (Group A) **Gram-positive aerobic cocci**
Streptococci **Gram-positive aerobic cocci**
Treponema pallidum **Spirochetes**
Ureaplasma urealyticum **Defective cell wall bacteria**
Vibrio cholerae **Gram-negative aerobic bacilli**
Yersinia **Gram-negative aerobic bacilli**

INTERFERON ALFACON-1 (*cont.*)

hepatitis C, with ribavirin: 15 mcg SC daily with wt-based PO ribavirin. Optimal therapy for chronic HCV infection is combination peginterferon alfa and ribavirin.

PEDS – Not approved in children.

FORMS – Trade only: Vials injectable soln 30 mcg/mL (0.3 mL, 0.5 mL).

NOTES – Monitor for depression, suicidal behavior, or other severe neuropsychiatric effects. Thyroid dysfunction, cardiovascular reactions, retinal damage, flu-like symptoms, thrombocytopenia, neutropenia, exacerbation of autoimmune disorders, hypertriglyceridemia (consider monitoring). Monitor CBC, thyroid function. Refrigerate injectable soln.

PALIVIZUMAB (*Synagis*) ▶L ♀C ▶? $$$$$

PEDS – Prevention of respiratory syncytial virus pulmonary disease in high-risk infants: 15 mg/kg IM monthly during RSV season with first injection before season starts (November to April in Northern hemisphere). See aappolicy.aappublications.org for eligibility criteria. Give a dose as soon as possible after cardiopulmonary bypass (due to decreased palivizumab levels) even if less than 1 month after last dose.

NOTES – Preservative-free; use within 6 h of reconstitution. Not more than 1 mL per injection site. Can interfere with immunologic- based diagnostic tests and viral culture assays for RSV, leading to false-negative diagnostic tests.

PEGINTERFERON ALFA-2A (*Pegasys*) ▶LK ♀C ▶– $$$$$

WARNING – May cause or worsen serious neuropsychiatric, autoimmune, ischemic, and infectious diseases. Frequent clinical and lab monitoring recommended. Discontinue if signs/symptoms of these conditions are persistently severe or worsen.

ADULT – Chronic hepatitis C not previously treated with alfa-interferon: 180 mcg SC in abdomen or thigh once a week for 48 weeks with or without PO ribavirin 800 to 1200 mg/day. Ribavirin dose and duration depend on genotype and body wt (see PO ribavirin entry). Hepatitis B: 180 mcg SC in abdomen or thigh once a week for 48 weeks.

PEDS – Chronic hepatitis C not previously treated with alfa-interferon, age 5 yo or older: 180 mcg/1.73 m^2 (max dose of 180 mcg) SC in abdomen or thigh once weekly. Give with PO ribavirin (see ribavirin—oral entry for dose based on wt). Treat genotypes 2 or 3 for 24 weeks; treat genotypes 1 or 4 for 48 weeks.

FORMS – Trade only: 180 mcg/1 mL soln in single-use vial, 180 mcg/0.5 mL prefilled syringe. ProClick autoinjector 135 mcg/0.5 mL and 180 mcg/0.5 mL.

(cont.)

PEGINTERFERON ALFA-2A (*cont.*)

NOTES – Contraindicated in autoimmune hepatitis; hepatic decompensation in cirrhotic patients (Child-Pugh score greater than 6 if HCV only; score greater than 5 if HIV coinfected). Monitor for depression, suicidal behavior, relapse of drug addiction, or other severe neuropsychiatric effects. Interferons can cause thrombocytopenia, neutropenia, thyroid dysfunction, hyperglycemia, hypoglycemia, cardiovascular events, colitis, pancreatitis, hypersensitivity, flu-like symptoms, pulmonary and ophthalmologic disorders. Risk of severe neutropenia/thrombocytopenia greater in HIV-infected patients. Monitor CBC, blood chemistry. Interferons increase risk of hepatic decompensation in hepatitis C/HIV coinfected patients receiving HAART with NRTI. Monitor LFTs and clinical status; discontinue peginterferon if Child-Pugh score 6 or greater. Exacerbation of hepatitis during treatment of hepatitis B; monitor LFTs more often and consider dosage reduction if ALT flares. Discontinue treatment if ALT increase is progressive despite dosage reduction or if flares accompanied by hepatic decompensation or bilirubin increase. CYP1A2 inhibitor; may increase theophylline levels (monitor). May increase methadone levels. Use cautiously if CrCl is less than 50 mL/min. Dosage adjustments for adverse effects, hepatic dysfunction, or hemodialysis in prescribing information. Store in refrigerator.

PEGINTERFERON ALFA-2B (***PEG-Intron***) ▶K? ♀C ▶– $$$$$

WARNING – May cause or worsen serious neuropsychiatric, autoimmune, ischemic, and infectious diseases. Frequent clinical and lab monitoring recommended. Discontinue if signs/symptoms of these conditions are persistently severe or worsen.

ADULT – Chronic hepatitis C not previously treated with alfa-interferon. Peginterferon alfa-2b plus ribavirin is FDA approved for use with HCV NS3/4A protease inhibitors (boceprevir, telaprevir) in adults with chronic hepatitis C. Telaprevir/boceprevir in combination with peginterferon plus weight-based ribavirin is regimen of choice for genotype 1 patients. See telaprevir or boceprevir entries for dosage regimens and duration of therapy. In combination with ribavirin for chronic hepatitis C, peginterferon is preferred over interferon alfa because of substantially higher response rate. Monotherapy (only for patients who cannot use combo therapy): 1 mcg/kg/week SC for 1 year given on same day each week. Combination therapy with oral ribavirin (see ribavirin—oral entry for ribavirin dose): 1.5 mcg/kg/week given on the same day each week. To control amount injected, use vial strength based on wt: give 50 mcg (0.5 mL, 50 mcg/0.5 mL vial) for wt less than 40 kg, give 64 mcg (0.4 mL, 80 mcg/0.5 mL vial) for 40 to 50 kg, give 80 mcg (0.5 mL, 80 mcg/0.5 mL vial) for 51 to 60 kg, give 96 mcg (0.4 mL, 120 mcg/0.5 mL vial) for 61 to 75 kg, give 120 mcg (0.5 mL, 120 mcg/0.5 mL vial) for 76 to 85 kg, give 150 mcg (0.5 mL, 150 mcg/0.5 mL vial) for 86 kg or greater. Give at bedtime or with antipyretic to minimize flu-like symptoms. Treat genotype 1 for 48 weeks. Consider stopping if HCV-RNA reduction is less than 2 $\log_{10}$ after 12 weeks or is still detectable after 24 weeks of therapy. Treat genotypes 2 and 3 for 24 weeks.

PEDS – Chronic hepatitis C not previously treated with alfa-interferon, age 3 yo or older: 60 mcg/m^2 SC once a week with ribavirin 15 mg/kg/day PO divided two times per day (see ribavirin—oral entry for dosing of Rebetol caps). Treat genotype 1 for 48 weeks. Treat genotypes 2 and 3 for 24 weeks.

FORMS – Trade only: 50, 80, 120, 150 mcg/ 0.5 mL single-use vials with diluent, 2 syringes, and alcohol swabs. Disposable single-dose Redipen 50, 80, 120, 150 mcg.

NOTES – Contraindicated in autoimmune hepatitis; hepatic decompensation in cirrhotic patients (Child-Pugh score greater than 6). Coadministration with ribavirin contraindicated if CrCl is less than 50 mL/min. Monitor for depression, suicidal behavior, exacerbation of substance use disorders, other severe neuropsychiatric effects. Thrombocytopenia, neutropenia, thyroid dysfunction, hyperglycemia, cardiovascular events, colitis, pancreatitis, hypersensitivity, flu-like symptoms, pulmonary damage. Monitor CBC, blood chemistry. May increase methadone levels. Dosage adjustments for adverse effects or renal dysfunction in prescribing information. Peginterferon should be used immediately after reconstitution, but can be refrigerated for up to 24 h.

RIBAVIRIN—INHALED (***Virazole***) ▶Lung ♀X ▶– $$$$$

WARNING – Beware of sudden pulmonary deterioration with ribavirin. Drug precipitation may cause ventilator dysfunction.

PEDS – Severe respiratory syncytial virus infection: Aerosol 12 to 18 h/day for 3 to 7 days.

(cont.)

RIBAVIRIN—INHALED (*cont.*)

NOTES – Minimize exposure to healthcare workers, especially pregnant women.

RIBAVIRIN—ORAL (*Rebetol, Copegus, Ribasphere*) ▶Cellular, K ♀X ▶– $$$$$

WARNING – Teratogen with extremely long half-life; contraindicated if pregnancy possible in patient/partner. Female patients and female partners of male patients must avoid pregnancy by using 2 forms of birth control during and for 6 months after stopping ribavirin. Obtain pregnancy test at baseline and monthly. Hemolytic anemia that may worsen cardiac disease. Assess for underlying heart disease before treatment with ribavirin. Do not use in significant/unstable heart disease. Baseline ECG if preexisting cardiac dysfunction.

ADULT – Chronic hepatitis C not previously treated with alfa-interferon: Telaprevir/boceprevir in combination with peginterferon plus weight-based ribavirin is regimen of choice for genotype 1 patients. See telaprevir or boceprevir entries for dosage regimens and duration of therapy. In combination with ribavirin for hepatitis C, peginterferon is preferred over interferon alfa-2b because of substantially higher response rate. Rebetol in combination with peginterferon alfa-2b (PegIntron): 400 mg PO two times per day for wt 65 kg or less, 400 mg PO q am and 600 mg PO q pm for 66 to 80 kg, 600 mg PO two times per day for wt 81 to 105 kg, 600 mg PO q am and 800 mg PO q pm for wt greater than 105 kg. Treat genotype 1 for 48 weeks, genotypes 2 and 3 for 24 weeks. Copegus in combination with peginterferon alfa-2a (Pegasys): For genotypes 1 and 4, treat for 48 weeks with 1000 mg/day for wt less than 75 kg, 1200 mg/day for wt 75 kg or greater. For genotypes 2 and 3, treat for 24 weeks with 800 mg/day. Divide daily dose of ribavirin two times per day and give with food. See prescribing information for dosage reductions if Hb declines.

PEDS – Chronic hepatitis C not previously treated with alfa-interferon: In combination with ribavirin for chronic hepatitis C, peginterferon is preferred over interferon alfa because of substantially higher response rate. Patients who start peginterferon plus ribavirin before their 18th birthday should continue with peds doses throughout treatment. Rebetol in combination with peginterferon alfa-2b (PegIntron), age 3 yo and older: For wt less than 47 kg or patients who cannot swallow caps: 15 mg/kg/day of soln PO divided two times per day. Caps: 400 mg two times per day for wt 47 to 59 kg, 400 mg q am and 600 mg q pm for wt 60 to 73 kg, 600 mg two times per day for wt greater than 73 kg. Take PO with food. Treat genotype 1 for 48 weeks, genotypes 2 and 3 for 24 weeks. Copegus tabs in combo with peginterferon alfa-2a (Pegasys), age 5 yo or older: 200 mg twice daily for 23 to 33 kg; 200 mg q am and 400 mg q pm for 34 to 46 kg; 400 mg twice daily for 47 to 59 kg; 400 mg q am and 600 mg q pm for 60 to 74 kg; 600 mg twice daily for 75 kg or more. Treat genotypes 2 and 3 for 24 weeks, other genotypes for 48 weeks. Take PO with food.

UNAPPROVED ADULT – In combination therapy with ribavirin for chronic hepatitis C, peginterferon is preferred over interferon alfa because of substantially higher response rate. Regimen and duration of treatment is based on genotype. Divide daily dose of ribavirin two times per day and give with food. Chronic hepatitis C, genotypes 1 and 4: Treat for 48 weeks, evaluating response after 12 weeks. Ribavirin in combination with peginterferon alfa-2b (PegIntron): 800 mg/day PO for wt 65 kg or less, 1000 mg/day for wt 66 kg to 85 kg, 1200 mg/day for wt 86 kg to 105 kg, 1400 mg/day for greater than 105 kg. Ribavirin in combination with peginterferon alfa-2a (Pegasys): 1000 mg/day PO for wt less than 75 kg, 1200 mg/day for wt 75 kg or greater. Chronic hepatitis C, genotypes 2 and 3: Treat for 24 weeks with ribavirin 800 mg/day in combo with peginterferon. Regimens provided here are from guideline for the management of chronic hepatitis C; they may vary from regimens in product labeling.

UNAPPROVED PEDS – Chronic hepatitis C, age 2 yo and older: Treat for 48 weeks with peginterferon alfa-2b (PegIntron) in combination with ribavirin 15 mg/kg/day PO divided two times per day. The regimen provided here is from guideline for the management of chronic hepatitis C; it may vary from regimens in product labeling.

FORMS – Generic/Trade: Caps 200 mg, Tabs 200, 500 mg. Generic only: Tabs 400, 600 mg. Trade only (Rebetol): Oral soln 40 mg/mL (100 mL).

NOTES – Contraindicated in hemoglobinopathies; autoimmune hepatitis; hepatic decompensation in cirrhotic patients (Child-Pugh score greater than 6 if HCV only; score greater than 5 if HIV coinfected). Get CBC at baseline, weeks 2 and 4, and periodically. Risk of anemia increased if age older than 50 yo or if renal dysfunction. Do not use if CrCl is less

(cont.)

RIBAVIRIN—ORAL (*cont.*)

than 50 mL/min. Decreased INR with warfarin; monitor INR weekly for 4 weeks after ribavirin started/stopped. May increase risk of lactic acidosis with nucleoside reverse transcriptase inhibitors. Avoid didanosine or zidovudine. Coadministration with azathioprine can cause neutropenia; monitor CBC weekly for 1st month, every other week for next 2 months, then monthly or more frequently if doses are adjusted.

TELAPREVIR (*Incivek*) ▶L ♀B ▶– $$$$$

ADULT – Chronic hepatitis C (genotype 1): 750 mg PO three times per day (q 7 to 9 h) taken with food (not low fat). Give with peginterferon and ribavirin for 12 weeks. Give peginterferon and ribavirin for additional 12 to 36 weeks based on HCV RNA levels at weeks 4 and 12, and whether patient was partial/null responder to prior therapy. Stop telaprevir if HCV RNA is greater than 1000 International units/mL at weeks 4 or 12, or detectable at week 24. Dosage adjustment for coadministration with efavirenz: 1125 mg PO q 8 h.

PEDS – Safety and efficacy not established in children.

FORMS – Trade only: 375 mg tabs in 28-day blister pack or bottle of 168 tabs.

NOTES – Not for monotherapy. Strong inhibitor of CYP3A4. Many drug interactions. Contraindicated with alfuzosin, atorvastatin, colchicine in patients with renal/hepatic impairment, most systemic corticosteroids, darunavir-ritonavir, ergot alkaloids, fosamprenavir-ritonavir, high-dose itraconazole or ketoconazole (more than 200 mg/day), lopinavir-ritonavir, lovastatin, oral midazolam, pimozide, rifabutin, rifampin, salmeterol, high-dose sildenafil or tadalafil for pulmonary hypertension, simvastatin, St. John's wort, triazolam. Reduce doses of phosphodiesterase inhibitors for erectile dysfunction to not more than sildenafil 25 mg q 48 h, tadalafil 10 mg q 72 h, or vardenafil 2.5 mg q 72 h. May increase risk of QT interval prolongation or torsades with CYP3A4 inhibitors that can prolong the QT interval (ie, clarithromycin, erythromycin, voriconazole). Inhibits p-glycoprotein. Use lowest initial dose of digoxin and monitor digoxin levels. Avoid pregnancy in female patients or female partners of male patients because of ribavirin teratogenicity. May impair efficacy of hormonal contraceptives; use 2 nonhormonal contraceptives. Can cause anemia; monitor hemoglobin at baseline and at least q 4 weeks. Monitor CBC, TSH, chemistry panel, and LFTs at weeks 2, 4, 8, and 12, and prn. Do not use in moderate to severe hepatic impairment (Child-Pugh Class B/C, score of 7 or greater). Once bottle is opened, use within 28 days.

TELBIVUDINE (*Tyzeka*, ✤*Sebivo*) ▶K ♀B ▶– $$$$$

WARNING – Nucleoside analogues can cause lactic acidosis with hepatic steatosis. Severe acute exacerbation of hepatitis B can occur after discontinuation. Monitor closely for at least 2 months after discontinuation.

ADULT – Chronic hepatitis B: 600 mg PO once daily. Refer to product labeling for baseline HBV DNA and ALT treatment criteria for HBeAg-positive and -negative patients. Choose alternate therapy if HBV DNA is detectable after 24 weeks of treatment.

PEDS – Chronic hepatitis B, age 16 yo or older: 600 mg PO once daily. Refer to product labeling for baseline HBV DNA and ALT treatment criteria for HBeAg-positive and -negative patients. Choose alternate therapy if HBV is detectable after 24 weeks of treatment.

FORMS – Trade only: Tabs 600 mg. Oral soln 100 mg/5 mL (300 mL).

NOTES – Risk of peripheral neuropathy increased by peginterferon alfa-2a; do not coadminister. No dosage adjustment needed for hepatic dysfunction. Renal dysfunction: 600 mg PO q 96 h for ESRD, q 72 h for CrCl less than 30 mL/min but not hemodialysis, q 48 h for CrCl 30 to 49 mL/min. Give dose after hemodialysis session. Contains 47 mg sodium/30 mL of oral soln.

ANTIMICROBIALS: Carbapenems

NOTE: Carbapenems can dramatically reduce valproic acid levels; use another antibiotic (preferred) or add a supplemental anticonvulsant. Possible cross-sensitivity with other beta-lactams; *C. difficile*–associated diarrhea; superinfection.

DORIPENEM (*Doribax*) ▶K ♀B ▶? $$$$$

ADULT – Complicated intra-abdominal infection: 500 mg IV q 8 h for 5 to 14 days. Complicated UTI or pyelonephritis: 500 mg IV q 8 h for 10 to 14 days.

PEDS – Not approved in children.

NOTES – Dose reduction in renal dysfunction: 250 mg q 12 h for CrCl 10 to 30 mL/min, 250 mg q 8 h for CrCl 30 to 50 mL/min.

ERTAPENEM (*Invanz*) ▶K ♀B ▶? $$$$$

ADULT – Community-acquired pneumonia, diabetic foot, complicated intra-abdominal, skin, urinary tract, acute pelvic infections: 1 g IM/IV over 30 min q 24 h for up to 14 days for IV, up to 7 days for IM. Prophylaxis, elective colorectal surgery: 1 g IV 1 h before incision.

PEDS – Community-acquired pneumonia, complicated intra-abdominal, skin, urinary tract, acute pelvic infections (3 mo to 12 yo): 15 mg/kg IV/IM q 12 h (up to 1 g/day). Use adult dose for age 13 yo or older. Infuse IV over 30 min. Can give IV for up to 14 days, IM for up to 7 days.

NOTES – Seizures (especially if renal dysfunction or CNS disorder). Not active against *Pseudomonas* and *Acinetobacter* species. IM diluted with lidocaine; contraindicated if allergic to amide-type local anesthetics. For adults with renal dysfunction: 500 mg q 24 h for CrCl 30 mL/min or less or hemodialysis. Give 150 mg supplemental dose if daily dose given within 6 h before hemodialysis session. Do not dilute in dextrose.

IMIPENEM-CILASTATIN (*Primaxin*) ▶K ♀C ▶? $$$$$

ADULT – Pneumonia, sepsis, endocarditis, polymicrobic, intra-abdominal, gynecologic, bone and joint, skin infections. Normal renal function, 70 kg or greater: mild infection: 250 to 500 mg IV q 6 h; moderate infection: 500 mg IV q 6 to 8 h or 1 g IV q 8 h; severe infection: 500 mg IV q 6 h to 1 g IV q 6 to 8 h. Complicated UTI: 500 mg IV q 6 h. See product labeling for doses in adults wt less than 70 kg. Can give up to 1.5 g/day IM for mild to moderate infections.

PEDS – Pneumonia, sepsis, endocarditis, polymicrobic, intra-abdominal, bone and joint, skin infections. 25 mg/kg IV q 12 h for age younger than 1 week old; 25 mg/kg IV q 8 h for age 1 to 4 weeks old; 25 mg/kg IV q 6 h for age 1 to 3 mo; 15 to 25 mg/kg IV q 6 h for older than 3 mo. Not for children with CNS infections, or wt less than 30 kg with renal dysfunction.

UNAPPROVED ADULT – Malignant otitis externa, empiric therapy for neutropenic fever: 500 mg IV q 6 h.

NOTES – Seizures (especially if given with ganciclovir, elderly with renal dysfunction, or cerebrovascular or seizure disorder). See product labeling for dose if CrCl is less than 70 mL/min. Not for CrCl less than 5 mL/min unless dialysis started within 48 h.

MEROPENEM (*Merrem IV*) ▶K ♀B ▶? $$$$$

ADULT – Intra-abdominal infections: 1 g IV q 8 h. Complicated skin infections: 500 mg IV q 8 h.

PEDS – Meningitis: 40 mg/kg IV q 8 h for age 3 mo or older; 2 g IV q 8 h for wt greater than 50 kg. Intra-abdominal infection: 20 mg/kg IV q 8 h for age 3 mo or older; 1 g IV q 8 h for wt greater than 50 kg. Complicated skin infections: 10 mg/kg IV q 8 h for age 3 mo or older; 500 mg IV q 8 h for wt greater than 50 kg.

UNAPPROVED ADULT – Meningitis: 40 mg/kg (max 2 g) IV q 8 h. Hospital-acquired pneumonia, complicated UTI, malignant otitis externa: 1 g IV q 8 h.

UNAPPROVED PEDS – Infant wt greater than 2 kg: 20 mg/kg IV q 12 h for age younger than 1 week old, q 8 h for 1 to 4 weeks old.

NOTES – Seizures; thrombocytopenia in renal dysfunction. For adults with renal dysfunction: Give 50% of normal dose q 24 h for CrCl less than 10 mL/min, 50% of normal dose q 12 h for CrCl 10 to 25 mL/min, normal dose q 12 h for CrCl 26 to 50 mL/min.

ANTIMICROBIALS: Cephalosporins—1st Generation

NOTE: Cephalosporins are second line to penicillins for group A strep pharyngitis, can be cross-sensitive with penicillins, and can cause *C. difficile*–associated diarrhea.

CEFADROXIL ▶K ♀B ▶+ $$$

ADULT – Simple UTI: 1 to 2 g/day PO divided one to two times per day. Other UTIs: 1 g PO two times per day. Skin infections: 1 g/day PO divided one to two times per day. Group A strep pharyngitis: 1 g/day PO divided one to two times per day for 10 days.

PEDS – UTIs, skin infections: 30 mg/kg/day PO divided two times per day. Group A streptococcal pharyngitis/tonsillitis, impetigo: 30 mg/kg/day PO divided one to two times per day. Treat pharyngitis for 10 days.

FORMS – Generic only: Tabs 1 g. Caps 500 mg. Susp 125, 250, 500 mg/5 mL.

NOTES – Dosage adjustment for renal dysfunction in adults: 500 mg PO q 36 h for CrCl less than 10 mL/min; 500 mg PO q 24 h for CrCl 11 to 25 mL/min; 1 g load then 500 mg PO q 12 h for CrCl 26 to 50 mL/min.

CEFAZOLIN ▶K ♀B ▶+ $$

ADULT – Pneumonia, sepsis, endocarditis, skin, bone and joint, genital infections. Mild infections due to Gram-positive cocci: 250 to 500 mg IM/IV q 8 h. Moderate to severe infections: 0.5 to 1 g IM/IV q 6 to 8 h. Life-threatening infections: 1 to 1.5 g IV q 6 h. Simple UTI: 1 g IM/IV q 12 h. Pneumococcal pneumonia: 500 mg IM/IV q 12 h. Surgical prophylaxis: 1 g IM/IV 30 to 60 min preop, additional 0.5 to 1 g during surgery longer than 2 h, and 0.5 to 1 g q 6 to 8 h for 24 h postop. See table for prophylaxis of bacterial endocarditis. Prevention of perinatal group B streptococcal disease: Give to mother 2 g IV at onset of labor/after membrane rupture, then 1 g IV q 8 h until delivery.

PEDS – Pneumonia, sepsis, endocarditis, skin, bone and joint infections. Mild to moderate infections: 25 to 50 mg/kg/day IM/IV divided q 6 to 8 h for age 1 mo or older. Severe infections: 100 mg/kg/day IV divided q 6 to 8 h for age 1 mo or older. See table for prophylaxis of bacterial endocarditis.

NOTES – Dose reduction for renal dysfunction in adults: Usual first dose, then 50% of usual dose q 18 to 24 h for CrCl less than 10 mL/min; 50% of usual dose q 12 h for CrCl 11 to 34 mL/min; usual dose q 8 h for CrCl 35 to 54 mL/min. Dose reduction for renal dysfunction in children: Usual first dose, then 10% of usual dose q 24 h for CrCl 5 to 20 mL/min; 25% of usual dose q 12 h for CrCl 20 to 40 mL/min; 60% of usual dose q 12 h for CrCl 40 to 70 mL/min.

CEPHALEXIN (*Keflex*) ▶K ♀B ▶? $$$

ADULT – Pneumonia, bone, GU infections. Usual dose: 250 to 500 mg PO four times per day. Max: 4 g/day. Group A strep pharyngitis, skin infections, simple UTI: 500 mg PO two times per day. Treat pharyngitis for 10 days. See table for prophylaxis of bacterial endocarditis.

PEDS – Pneumonia, GU, bone, skin infections, group A strep pharyngitis. Usual dose: 25 to 50 mg/kg/day PO in divided doses. Max dose: 100 mg/kg/day. Can give two times per day for strep pharyngitis in children older than 1 yo, skin infections. Group A strep pharyngitis, skin infections, simple UTI in patients older than 15 yo: 500 mg PO two times per day. Treat pharyngitis for 10 days. Not for otitis media, sinusitis.

FORMS – Generic/Trade: Caps 250, 500 mg. Generic only: Tabs 250, 500 mg. Susp 125, 250 mg/5 mL. Trade only: Caps 750 mg.

ANTIMICROBIALS: Cephalosporins—2nd Generation

NOTE: Cephalosporins are second line to penicillins for group A strep pharyngitis, can be cross-sensitive with penicillins, and can cause *C. difficile*-associated diarrhea.

CEFACLOR (*Ceclor*) ▶K ♀B ▶? $$$$

ADULT – Otitis media, pneumonia, group A strep pharyngitis, UTI, skin infections: 250 to 500 mg PO three times per day. Treat pharyngitis for 10 days.

PEDS – Pneumonia, group A streptococcal pharyngitis, UTI, skin infections: 20 to 40 mg/kg/day (up to 1 g/day) PO divided two times per day for pharyngitis, three times per day for other infections. Treat pharyngitis for 10 days. Otitis media: 40 mg/kg/day PO divided two times per day.

FORMS – Generic only: Caps 250, 500 mg. Susp 125, 187, 250, 375 mg per 5 mL.

CEFOTETAN ▶K/Bile ♀B ▶? $$$$$

ADULT – Usual dose: 1 to 2 g IM/IV q 12 h. UTI: 0.5 to 2 g IM/IV q 12 h or 1 to 2 g IM/IV q 24 h. Pneumonia, gynecologic, intra-abdominal, bone and joint infections: 1 to 3 g IM/IV q 12 h. Skin infections: 1 to 2 g IM/IV q 12 h or 2 g IV q 24 h. Surgical prophylaxis: 1 to 2 g IV 30 to 60 min preop. Give after cord clamp for C-section.

PEDS – Not approved in children.

UNAPPROVED PEDS – Usual dose: 40 to 80 mg/kg/day IV divided q 12 h.

NOTES – Hemolytic anemia (higher risk than other cephalosporins), clotting impairment rarely. Disulfiram-like reaction with alcohol. Dosing reduction in adults with renal dysfunction: Usual dose q 48 h for CrCl less than 10 mL/min; usual dose q 24 h for CrCl 10 to 30 mL/min.

CEFOXITIN ▶K ♀B ▶+ $$$$$

ADULT – Pneumonia, UTI, sepsis, intra-abdominal, gynecologic, skin, bone and joint infections. Uncomplicated: 1 g IV q 6 to 8 h. Moderate to severe: 1 g IV q 4 h or 2 g IV q 6 to 8 h. Infections requiring high doses: 2 g IV q 4 h or 3 g IV q 6 h. Uncontaminated GI surgery, vaginal/abdominal hysterectomy: 2 g IV 30 to 60 min preop, then 2 g IV q 6 h for 24 h. C-section: 2 g IV after cord clamped or 2 g IV q 4 h for 3 doses with 1st dose given after cord clamped.

(cont.)

CEFOXITIN (*cont.*)

PEDS – Pneumonia, UTI, sepsis, intra-abdominal, skin, bone and joint infections: 80 to 160 mg/kg/day (up to 12 g/day) IV divided into 4 to 6 doses for age 3 mo or older. Mild to moderate infections: 80 to 100 mg/kg/day IV divided into 3 to 4 doses. Surgical prophylaxis: 30 to 40 mg/kg IV 30 to 60 min preop; additional doses can be given q 6 h up to 24 h postop.

NOTES – Eosinophilia and increased AST with high doses in children. Dosing reduction in adults with renal dysfunction: Load with 1 to 2 g IV then 0.5 g IV q 24 to 48 h for CrCl less than 5 mL/min, 0.5 to 1 g IV q 12 to 24 h for CrCl 5 to 9 mL/min, 1 to 2 g IV q 12 to 24 h for CrCl 10 to 29 mL/min, 1 to 2 g IV q 8 to 12 h for CrCl 30 to 50 mL/min. Give 1 to 2 g supplemental dose after each hemodialysis.

CEFPROZIL ▶K ♀B ▶+ $$$$

ADULT – Group A strep pharyngitis: 500 mg PO once daily for 10 days. Sinusitis: 250 to 500 mg PO two times per day. Acute exacerbation of chronic/secondary infection of acute bronchitis: 500 mg PO two times per day. Skin infections: 250 to 500 mg PO two times per day or 500 mg PO once daily.

PEDS – Otitis media: 15 mg/kg/dose PO two times per day. Group A strep pharyngitis: 7.5 mg/kg/dose PO two times per day for 10 days. Sinusitis: 7.5 to 15 mg/kg/dose PO two times per day. Skin infections: 20 mg/kg PO once daily. Use adult dose for age 13 yo or older.

FORMS – Generic only: Tabs 250, 500 mg. Susp 125, 250 mg/5 mL.

NOTES – Give 50% of usual dose at usual interval for CrCl less than 30 mL/min.

CEFUROXIME (*Zinacef, Ceftin*) ▶K ♀B ▶? $$$

ADULT – Uncomplicated pneumonia, simple UTI, skin infections, disseminated Gonorrhea: 750 mg IM/IV q 8 h. Bone and joint or severe/complicated infections: 1.5 g IV q 8 h. Sepsis: 1.5 g IV q 6 h to 3 g IV q 8 h. Gonorrhea: 1.5 g IM single dose split into 2 injections, given with probenecid 1 g PO. Surgical prophylaxis: 1.5 g IV 30 to 60 min preop, then 750 mg IM/IV q 8 h for prolonged procedures. Open heart surgery: 1.5 g IV q 12 h for 4 doses with 1st dose at induction of anesthesia. Cefuroxime axetil tabs: Group A strep pharyngitis, acute sinusitis: 250 mg PO two times per day for 10 days. Acute exacerbation of chronic/secondary infection of acute bronchitis, skin infections: 250 to 500 mg PO two times per day. Lyme disease: 500 mg PO two times per day for 14 days for early disease, for 28 days for Lyme arthritis. Simple UTI: 125 to 250 mg PO two times per day. Gonorrhea: 1 g PO single dose.

PEDS – Most infections: 50 to 100 mg/kg/day IM/IV divided q 6 to 8 h. Bone and joint infections: 150 mg/kg/day IM/IV divided q 8 h (up to adult dose). Cefuroxime axetil tabs: Group A strep pharyngitis: 125 mg PO two times per day for 10 days. Otitis media, sinusitis: 250 mg PO two times per day for 10 days. Cefuroxime axetil oral susp. Group A strep pharyngitis: 20 mg/kg/day (up to 500 mg/day) PO divided two times per day for 10 days. Otitis media, sinusitis, impetigo: 30 mg/kg/day (up to 1 g/day) PO divided two times per day for 10 days. Use adult dose for age 13 yo or older.

UNAPPROVED PEDS – Lyme disease: 30 mg/kg/day PO divided two times per day (max 500 mg/dose) for 14 days for early disease, for 28 days for Lyme arthritis. Community-acquired pneumonia: 150 mg/kg/day IV divided q 8 h.

FORMS – Generic/Trade: Tabs 125, 250, 500 mg. Susp 125, 250 mg/5 mL.

NOTES – AAP recommends 5 to 7 days of therapy for children age 6 yo or older with nonsevere otitis media, and 10 days for younger children and those with severe disease. Dosage reduction for renal dysfunction in adults: 750 mg IM/IV q 24 h for CrCl less than 10 mL/min, 750 mg IM/IV q 12 h for CrCl 10 to 20 mL/min. Give supplemental dose after hemodialysis. Tabs and susp not bioequivalent on mg/mg basis. Do not crush tabs.

ANTIMICROBIALS: Cephalosporins—3rd Generation

NOTE: Cephalosporins are second line to penicillins for group A strep pharyngitis, can be cross-sensitive with penicillins, and can cause *C. difficile*–associated diarrhea.

CEFDINIR ▶K ♀B ▶? $$$$

ADULT – Community-acquired pneumonia, skin infections: 300 mg PO two times per day for 10 days. Sinusitis: 600 mg PO once daily or 300 mg PO two times per day for 10 days. Group A strep pharyngitis, acute exacerbation of chronic bronchitis: 600 mg PO once daily for 10 days or 300 mg PO two times per day for 5 to 10 days.

PEDS – Group A strep pharyngitis, otitis media: 14 mg/kg/day PO divided two times per day for 5 to 10 days or once daily for 10

(cont.)

SEXUALLY TRANSMITTED DISEASES & VAGINITIS*

Bacterial vaginosis	(1) metronidazole 5 g of 0.75% gel intravaginally daily for 5 days OR 500 mg PO two times per day for 7 days; (2) clindamycin 5 g of 2% cream intravaginally at bedtime for 7 days. In pregnancy: (1) metronidazole 500 mg PO two times per day for 7 days OR 250 mg PO three times per day for 7 days; (2) clindamycin 300 mg PO two times per day for 7 days.
Candidal vaginitis	(1) intravaginal clotrimazole, miconazole, terconazole, nystatin, tioconazole, or butoconazole; (2) fluconazole 150 mg PO single dose.
Chancroid	(1) azithromycin 1 g PO single dose; (2) ceftriaxone 250 mg IM single dose; (3) ciprofloxacin 500 mg PO two times per day for 3 days.
Chlamydia	First-line: either azithromycin 1 g PO single dose or doxycycline 100 mg PO two times per day for 7 days. Second-line: fluoroquinolones or erythromycin. In pregnancy: (1) azithromycin 1 g PO single dose; (2) amoxicillin 500 mg PO three times per day for 7 days. Repeat NAAT[‡] 3 weeks after treatment in pregnant women.
Epididymitis	(1) ceftriaxone 250 mg IM single dose + doxycycline 100 mg PO two times per day for 10 days; (2) ofloxacin 300 mg PO two times per day or levofloxacin 500 mg PO daily for 10 days if enteric organisms suspected, or negative gonococcal culture or NAAT.[†]
Gonorrhea	First-line: Single dose of ceftriaxone 250 mg IM + azithromycin 1 g PO single dose (preferred) or doxycycline 100 mg PO two times per day for 7days; Second-line: cefixime 400 mg PO (not for pharyngeal) + azithromycin (preferred)/doxycycline if ceftriaxone is not available.[†] Test-of-cure (culture and sensitivity preferred over NAAT) required for cefixime. Consult infectious disease expert if severe cephalosporin allergy.
Gonorrhea, disseminated	Initially treat with ceftriaxone 1 g IM/IV q 24 h until 24 to 48 h after improvement. Second-line alternatives: (1) cefotaxime 1 g IV q 8 h; (2) ceftizoxime 1 g IV q 8 h. Complete at least 1 week of treatment with cefixime tabs 400 mg PO two times per day.[†]
Gonorrhea, meningitis	ceftriaxone 1 to 2 g IV q 12 h for 10 to 14 days.
Gonorrhea, endocarditis	ceftriaxone 1 to 2 g IV q 12 h for at least 4 weeks.
Granuloma inguinale	doxycycline 100 mg PO two times per day for at least 3 weeks and until lesions completely healed. Alternative azithromycin 1 g PO once weekly for at least 3 weeks and until lesions completely healed.
Herpes simplex, genital, first episode	(1) acyclovir 400 mg PO three times per day for 7 to 10 days; (2) famciclovir 250 mg PO three times per day for 7 to 10 days; (3) valacyclovir 1 g PO two times per day for 7 to 10 days.
Herpes simplex, genital, recurrent	(1) acyclovir 400 mg PO three times per day for 5 days; (2) acyclovir 800 mg PO three times per day for 2 days or two times per day for 5 days; (3) famciclovir 125 mg PO two times per day for 5 days; (4) famciclovir 1 g PO two times per day for 1 day; (5) famciclovir 500 mg PO first dose, then 250 mg PO two to three times per day for 2 days; (6) valacyclovir 500 mg PO two times per day for 3 days; (7) valacyclovir 1 g PO daily for 5 days.
Herpes simplex, suppressive therapy	(1) acyclovir 400 mg PO two times per day; (2) famciclovir 250 mg PO two times per day; (3) valacyclovir 500 to 1000 mg PO daily. Valacyclovir 500 mg PO daily may be less effective than other valacyclovir/acyclovir regimens in patients who have 10 or more recurrences per year.
Herpes simplex, genital, recurrent in HIV infection	(1) acyclovir 400 mg PO three times per day for 5 to 10 days; (2) famciclovir 500 mg PO two times per day for 5 to 10 days; (3) valacyclovir 1 g PO two times per day for 5 to 10 days.
Herpes, suppressive therapy in HIV infection	(1) acyclovir 400 to 800 mg PO two to three times per day; (2) famciclovir 500 mg PO two times per day; (3) valacyclovir 500 mg PO two times per day.
Herpes simplex, prevention of transmission	For patients with not more than 9 recurrences per year: Valacyclovir 500 mg PO daily by source partner, in conjunction with safer sex practices.

Lympho-granuloma venereum	(1) doxycycline 100 mg PO two times per day for 21 days. Alternative: erythromycin base 500 mg PO four times per day for 21 days.
Pelvic inflammatory disease (PID), inpatient regimens	(1) cefoxitin 2 g IV q 6 h + doxycycline 100 mg IV/PO q 12 h; (2) clindamycin 900 mg IV q 8 h + gentamicin 2 mg/kg IM/IV loading dose, then 1.5 mg/kg IM/IV q 8 h (can substitute 3 to 5 mg/kg once-daily dosing). Can switch to PO therapy within 24 h of improvement.
Pelvic inflammatory disease (PID), outpatient treatment	ceftriaxone 250 mg IM single dose + doxycycline 100 mg PO two times per day +/– metronidazole 500 mg PO two times per day for 14 days.
Proctitis, proctocolitis, enteritis	ceftriaxone 250 mg IM single dose + doxycycline 100 mg PO two times per day for 7 days.
Sexual assault prophylaxis	ceftriaxone 250 mg IM single dose + metronidazole 2 g PO single dose + azithromycin 1 g PO single dose/doxycycline 100 mg PO two times per day for 7 days.
Syphilis, primary and secondary	(1) benzathine penicillin 2.4 million units IM single dose. (2) doxycycline 100 mg PO two times per day for 2 weeks if penicillin-allergic.
Syphilis, early latent, ie, duration less than 1 year	(1) benzathine penicillin 2.4 million units IM single dose; (2) doxycycline 100 mg PO two times per day for 2 weeks if penicillin-allergic.
Syphilis, late latent or unknown duration	(1) benzathine penicillin 2.4 million units IM q week for 3 doses; (2) doxycycline 100 mg PO two times per day for 4 weeks if penicillin-allergic.
Syphilis, tertiary	benzathine penicillin 2.4 million units IM q week for 3 doses. Consult infectious disease specialist for management of penicillin-allergic patients.
Syphilis, neuro	(1) penicillin G 18 to 24 million units/day continuous IV infusion or 3 to 4 million units IV q 4 h for 10 to 14 days; (2) if compliance can be ensured, consider procaine penicillin 2.4 million units IM daily + probenecid 500 mg PO four times per day, both for 10 to 14 days.
Syphilis in pregnancy	Treat only with penicillin regimen for stage of syphilis as noted above. Use penicillin-desensitization protocol if penicillin-allergic.
Trichomoniasis	metronidazole (can use in pregnancy) or tinidazole, each 2 g PO single dose.
Urethritis, Cervicitis	Test for chlamydia and gonorrhea with NAAT.[‡] Treat based on test results or treat presumptively if high risk of infection (Chlamydia: age 25 yo or younger, new/multiple sex partners, or unprotected sex. Gonorrhea: population prevalence greater than 5%), esp. if NAAT[‡] unavailable or patient unlikely to return for follow-up.
Urethritis, persistent/ recurrent	metronidazole/ tinidazole 2 g PO single dose + azithromycin 1 g PO single dose (if not used in first episode).

**MMWR* 2010;59:RR-12 or http://www.cdc.gov/STD/treatment/ and MMWR 2012;61(31):590. Treat sexual partners for all except herpes, candida, and bacterial vaginosis.

[†]There is a growing threat of multi drug-resistant gonorrhea, with high-level azithromycin resistance and reduced cephalosporin susceptibility reported in the US in 2011. Ceftriaxone is the most effective cephalosporin for treatment of gonorrhea. Cefixime is now second-line because of increasing risk of resistance. If cefixime treatment failure occurs, retreat with ceftriaxone 250 mg IM plus azithromycin 2 g PO both single dose and obtain infectious disease consultation. If ceftriaxone treatment failure occurs, consult infectious disease expert and CDC. Do not use azithromycin monotherapy for routine treatment of gonorrhea. If azithromycin is used in patients with cephalosporin allergy, use azithromycin 2 g PO single dose and perform culture (preferred) or NAAT in 1 week. Report treatment failure to state/local health department within 24 hours. As of April 2007, the CDC no longer recommends fluoroquinolones for gonorrhea or PID because of high resistance rates. Do not consider fluoroquinolone unless antimicrobial susceptibility can be documented by culture. If parenteral cephalosporin not feasible for PID (and NAAT is negative or culture documents fluoroquinolone susceptibility), can consider levofloxacin 500 mg PO once daily or ofloxacin 400 mg PO two times per day +/– metronidazole 500 mg PO two times per day for 14 days.

[‡]NAAT = nucleic acid amplification test.

CEFDINIR (*cont.*)

days. Sinusitis: 14 mg/kg/day PO divided once daily or two times per day for 10 days. Skin infections: 14 mg/kg/day PO divided two times per day for 10 days. Use adult dose for age 13 yo or older.

FORMS – Generic only: Caps 300 mg. Susp 125, 250 mg/5 mL.

NOTES – AAP recommends 5 to 7 days of therapy for children age 6 yo or older with non-severe otitis media, and 10 days for younger children and those with severe disease. Give iron, multivitamins with iron, or antacids at least 2 h before or after cefdinir. Complexation of cefdinir with iron may turn stools red. Reduce dose for renal dysfunction: 300 mg PO daily for adults with CrCl less than 30 mL/min. 7 mg/kg/day PO once daily up to 300 mg/day for children with CrCl less than 30 mL/min. Hemodialysis: 300 mg or 7 mg/kg PO after hemodialysis, then 300 mg or 7 mg/kg PO q 48 h.

CEFDITOREN (***Spectracef***) ▶K ♀B ▶? $$$$$

ADULT – Skin infections, group A strep pharyngitis: 200 mg PO two times per day for 10 days. Give 400 mg two times per day for 10 days for acute exacerbation of chronic bronchitis, for 14 days for community-acquired pneumonia. Take with food.

PEDS – Not approved for children younger than 12 yo. Skin infections, group A strep pharyngitis, adolescents age 12 yo or older: 200 mg PO two times per day with food for 10 days.

FORMS – Trade only: Tabs 200, 400 mg.

NOTES – Contraindicated if milk protein allergy or carnitine deficiency. Not for long-term use due to potential risk of carnitine deficiency. Do not take with drugs that reduce gastric acid (antacids, H2 blockers, etc.). Dosage adjustment for renal dysfunction: Max 200 mg two times per day if CrCl is 30 to 49 mL/min; max 200 mg once daily if CrCl is less than 30 mL/min.

CEFIXIME (***Suprax***) ▶K/Bile ♀B ▶? $$

ADULT – Simple UTI, pharyngitis, acute bacterial bronchitis, acute exacerbation of chronic bronchitis: 400 mg PO once daily. Gonorrhea: 400 mg PO single dose.

PEDS – Otitis media: 8 mg/kg/day susp PO divided one to two times per day. Pharyngitis: 8 mg/kg/day PO divided one to two times per day for 10 days. Use adult dose for wt greater than 50 kg or age 13 yo or older.

UNAPPROVED PEDS – Febrile UTI (3 to 24 mo): 16 mg/kg PO on 1st day, then 8 mg/kg PO daily to complete 14 days. Gonorrhea: 8 mg/kg (max 400 mg) PO single dose for wt less than 45 kg, 400 mg PO single dose for 45 kg or greater.

FORMS – Trade only: Susp 100, 200 mg/5 mL. Chewable tabs 100, 150, 200 mg. Tabs 400 mg. Caps 400 mg.

NOTES – Poor activity against *S. aureus*. Increased INR with warfarin. May increase carbamazepine levels. Susp stable at room temp or refrigerated for 14 days. Reduce dose in renal dysfunction: 75% of usual dose at usual interval for CrCl 21 to 60 mL/min or hemodialysis. 50% of usual dose at usual interval for CrCl less than 20 mL/min or continuous peritoneal dialysis.

CEFOTAXIME (***Claforan***) ▶KL ♀B ▶+ $$$$$

ADULT – Pneumonia, sepsis, GU and gynecologic, skin, intra-abdominal, bone and joint infections. Uncomplicated: 1 g IM/IV q 12 h. Moderate to severe: 1 to 2 g IM/IV q 8 h. Infections usually requiring high doses: 2 g IV q 6 to 8 h. Life-threatening: 2 g IV q 4 h. Meningitis: 2 g IV q 4 to 6 h. Gonorrhea: 0.5 to 1 g IM single dose.

PEDS – Pneumonia, sepsis, GU, skin, intra-abdominal, bone and joint, CNS infections. Labeled dose: 50 mg/kg/dose IV q 12 h for age younger than 1 week old; 50 mg/kg/dose IV q 8 h for age 1 to 4 weeks, 50 to 180 mg/kg/day IM/IV divided q 4 to 6 h for age 1 mo to 12 yo. AAP recommends 225 to 300 mg/kg/

(cont.)

CEPHALOSPORINS –GENERAL ANTIMICROBIAL SPECTRUM

1st generation	Gram-positive (including *Staphylococcus aureus*); basic Gram-negative coverage
2nd generation	diminished *S. aureus*, improved Gram-negative coverage compared to 1st generation; some with anaerobic coverage
3rd generation	further diminished *S. aureus*, further improved Gram-negative coverage compared to 1st and 2nd generation; some with Pseudomonal coverage and diminished Gram-positive coverage
4th generation	same as 3rd generation plus coverage against *Pseudomonas*
5th generation	Gram-negative coverage similar to 3rd generation; also active against *S. aureus* (including MRSA) and *S. pneumoniae*

CEFOTAXIME (*cont.*)
day IV divided q 6 to 8 h for *S. pneumoniae* meningitis. Mild to moderate infections: 75 to 100 mg/kg/day IV/IM divided q 6 to 8 h. Severe infections: 150 to 200 mg/kg/day IV/IM divided q 6 to 8 h.
UNAPPROVED ADULT – Disseminated gonorrhea, CDC regimen: 1 g IV q 8 h.
NOTES – Bolus injection through central venous catheter can cause arrhythmias. Decrease dose by 50% for CrCl less than 20 mL/min.

CEFPODOXIME ▶K ♀B ▶? $$$$
ADULT – Acute exacerbation of chronic bronchitis, acute sinusitis: 200 mg PO two times per day for 10 days. Community-acquired pneumonia: 200 mg PO two times per day for 14 days. Group A strep pharyngitis: 100 mg PO two times per day for 5 to 10 days. Skin infections: 400 mg PO two times per day for 7 to 14 days. Simple UTI: 100 mg PO two times per day for 7 days. Approved for treatment of gonorrhea, but CDC does not recommend. Give tabs with food.
PEDS – 5 mg/kg PO two times per day for 5 days for otitis media, for 5 to 10 days for group A strep pharyngitis, for 10 days for sinusitis. Use adult dose for age 12 yo or older.
FORMS – Generic: Tabs 100, 200 mg. Susp 50, 100 mg/5 mL.
NOTES – AAP recommends 5 to 7 days of therapy for children age 6 yo or older with nonsevere otitis media, and 10 days for younger children and those with severe disease. Do not give antacids within 2 h before and after cefpodoxime. Reduce dose in renal dysfunction: Increase dosing interval to q 24 h for CrCl less than 30 mL/min. Give 3 times per week after dialysis session for hemodialysis patients. Susp stable for 14 days refrigerated.

CEFTAZIDIME (***Fortaz, Tazicef***) ▶K ♀B ▶+ $$$$$
ADULT – Simple UTI: 250 mg IM/IV q 12 h. Complicated UTI: 500 mg IM/IV q 8 to 12 h. Uncomplicated pneumonia, mild skin infections: 500 mg to 1 g IM/IV q 8 h. Serious gynecologic, intra-abdominal, bone and joint, life-threatening infections, meningitis, empiric therapy of neutropenic fever: 2 g IV q 8 h. *Pseudomonas* lung infections in cystic fibrosis: 30 to 50 mg/kg IV q 8 h (up to 6 g/day).
PEDS – Use sodium formulations in children (Fortaz, Tazicef). UTIs, pneumonia, skin, intra-abdominal, bone and joint infections: 100 to 150 mg/kg/day (up to 6 g/day) IV divided q 8 h for age 1 mo to 12 yo. Meningitis: 150 mg/kg/day (up to 6 g/day) IV divided q 8 h for age 1 mo to 12 yo; 30 mg/kg IV q 12 h for age younger than 4 weeks old. Use adult dose and formulations for age 12 yo or older.
UNAPPROVED ADULT – *P. aeruginosa* osteomyelitis of the foot from nail puncture: 2 g IV q 8 h.
UNAPPROVED PEDS – AAP recommends 50 mg/kg IV q 8 to 12 h for age younger than 1 week old and wt greater than 2 kg, q 8 h for age 1 week old or older.
NOTES – High levels in renal dysfunction can cause CNS toxicity. Reduce dose in adults with renal dysfunction: Load with 1 g then 500 mg q 48 h for CrCl less than 5 mL/min; load with 1 g then 500 mg q 24 h for CrCl 6 to 15 mL/min; 1 g IV q 24 h for CrCl 16 to 30 mL/min; 1 g IV q 12 h for CrCl 31 to 50 mL/min. 1 g IV load in hemodialysis patients, then 1 g IV after hemodialysis sessions.

CEFTIBUTEN (***Cedax***) ▶K ♀B ▶? $$$$$
ADULT – Group A strep pharyngitis, acute exacerbation of chronic bronchitis, otitis media not due to *S. pneumoniae*: 400 mg PO once daily for 10 days.
PEDS – Group A strep pharyngitis, otitis media not due to S pneumoniae, age 6 mo or older: 9 mg/kg (up to 400 mg) PO once daily. Give susp on empty stomach.
FORMS – Trade only: Caps 400 mg. Susp 90 mg/5 mL.
NOTES – Poor activity against *S. aureus* and *S. pneumoniae*. Reduce dose in adults with renal dysfunction: 100 mg PO daily for CrCl 5 to 29 mL/min; 200 mg PO once daily for CrCl 30 to 49 mL/min. Reduce dose in children with renal dysfunction: 2.25 mg/kg PO once daily for CrCl 5 to 29 mL/min; 4.5 mg/kg PO once daily for CrCl 30 to 49 mL/min. Hemodialysis: Adults 400 mg PO and children 9 mg/kg PO after each dialysis session. Susp stable for 14 days refrigerated.

CEFTIZOXIME ▶K ♀B ▶? $$$$$
ADULT – Simple UTI: 500 mg IM/IV q 12 h. Pneumonia, sepsis, intra-abdominal, skin, bone and joint infections: 1 to 2 g IM/IV q 8 to 12 h. Pelvic inflammatory disease: 2 g IV q 8 h. Life-threatening infections: 3 to 4 g IV q 8 h. Gonorrhea: 1 g IM single dose. Split 2 g IM dose into 2 injections.
PEDS – Pneumonia, sepsis, intra-abdominal, skin, bone and joint infections: 50 mg/kg/dose IV q 6 to 8 h for age 6 mo or older. Up to 200 mg/kg/day for serious infections, not to exceed max adult dose.
UNAPPROVED PEDS – Gonorrhea, CDC regimens: 500 mg IM single dose for uncomplicated; 1 g IV q 8 h for disseminated infection.

(cont.)

CEFTIZOXIME (*cont.*)

NOTES – Can cause transient rise in eosinophils, ALT, AST, CPK in children. Not for meningitis. Dosing in adults with renal dysfunction: For less severe infection load with 500 mg to 1 g IM/IV, then 500 mg q 8 h for CrCl 50 to 79 mL/min, 250 to 500 mg q 12 h for CrCl 5 to 49 mL/min, 500 mg q 48 h or 250 mg q 24 h for hemodialysis. For life-threatening infection, give loading dose, then 750 mg to 1.5 g IV q 8 h for CrCl 50 to 79 mL/min, 500 mg to 1 g q 12 h for CrCl 5 to 49 mL/min, 500 mg to 1 g q 48 h or 500 mg q 24 h for hemodialysis. For hemodialysis patients, give dose at end of dialysis.

CEFTRIAXONE (***Rocephin***) ▶K/Bile ♀B ▶+ $$$

WARNING – Contraindicated in neonates who require (or are expected to require) IV calcium (including calcium in TPN); fatal lung/kidney precipitation of calcium ceftriaxone has been reported in neonates. In other patients, do not give ceftriaxone and calcium-containing solns simultaneously, but sequential administration is acceptable if lines are flushed with a compatible fluid between infusions. Do not dilute with Ringer's/Hartmann's soln or TPN containing calcium.

ADULT – Pneumonia, UTI, pelvic inflammatory disease (hospitalized), sepsis, meningitis, skin, bone and joint, intra-abdominal infections: Usual dose 1 to 2 g IM/IV q 24 h (max 4 g/day divided q 12 h). Gonorrhea: Single dose 250 mg IM.

PEDS – Meningitis: 100 mg/kg/day (up to 4 g/day) IV divided q 12 to 24 h. Skin, pneumonia, other serious infections: 50 to 75 mg/kg/day (up to 2 g/day) IM/IV divided q 12 to 24 h. Otitis media: 50 mg/kg (up to 1 g) IM single dose.

UNAPPROVED ADULT – Lyme disease carditis, meningitis: 2 g IV once daily for 14 days. Chancroid: 250 mg IM single dose. Disseminated gonorrhea: 1 g IM/IV q 24 h. Prophylaxis, invasive meningococcal disease: 250 mg IM single dose.

UNAPPROVED PEDS – Refractory otitis media (no response after 3 days of antibiotics): 50 mg/kg IM q 24 h for 3 doses. Lyme disease carditis, meningitis: 50 to 75 mg/kg IM/IV once daily (up to 2 g/day) for 14 days. Prophylaxis, invasive meningococcal disease: Single IM dose of 125 mg for age younger than 16 yo, 250 mg for age 16 yo or older. Gonorrhea: 125 mg IM single dose; use adult regimens provided in STD table if wt 45 kg or greater. Gonococcal bacteremia/arthritis: 50 mg/kg (max 1 g for wt 45 kg or less) IM/IV once daily for 7 days. Gonococcal ophthalmia neonatorum/gonorrhea prophylaxis in newborn: 25 to 50 mg/kg up to 125 mg IM/IV single dose at birth. Disseminated gonorrhea, infants: 25 to 50 mg/kg/day IM/IV once daily for 7 days. Typhoid fever: 50 to 75 mg/kg IM/IV once daily for 14 days.

NOTES – Can cause prolonged prothrombin time (due to vitamin K deficiency), biliary sludging/symptoms of gallbladder disease. Do not give to neonates with hyperbilirubinemia. Dilute in 1% lidocaine for IM use. Do not exceed 2 g/day in patients with both hepatic and renal dysfunction.

ANTIMICROBIALS: Cephalosporins—4th Generation

NOTE: Cross-sensitivity with penicillins possible. May cause *C. difficile*–associated diarrhea.

CEFEPIME (***Maxipime***) ▶K ♀B ▶? $$$$$

ADULT – Mild, moderate UTI: 0.5 to 1 g IM/IV q 12 h. Severe UTI, skin, complicated intra-abdominal infections: 2 g IV q 12 h. Pneumonia: 1 to 2 g IV q 12 h. Empiric therapy of febrile neutropenia: 2 g IV q 8 h.

PEDS – UTI, skin infections, pneumonia: 50 mg/kg IV q 12 h for wt 40 kg or less. Empiric therapy for febrile neutropenia: 50 mg/kg IV q 8 h for wt 40 kg or less. Do not exceed adult dose.

UNAPPROVED ADULT – *P. aeruginosa* osteomyelitis of the foot from nail puncture: 2 g IV q 12 h. Meningitis: 2 g IV q 8 h.

UNAPPROVED PEDS – Meningitis, cystic fibrosis, other serious infections: 50 mg/kg IV q 8 h (max of 6 g/day).

NOTES – An FDA safety review did not find higher mortality with cefepime than with other beta-lactams. High levels in renal dysfunction can cause CNS toxicity; dosing for CrCl less than 60 mL/min in package insert.

ANTIMICROBIALS: Cephalosporins—5th Generation

NOTE: Cephalosporins can be cross-sensitive with penicillins and can cause *C. difficile*–associated diarrhea.

CEFTAROLINE (*Teflaro*) ▶K ♀B ▶? $$$$$

ADULT – Community-acquired bacterial pneumonia, acute bacterial skin and skin structure infections: 600 mg IV q12 h infused over 1 h.

PEDS – Not approved in children.

NOTES – Direct Coombs' test seroconversion reported; hemolytic anemia is possible. Dosage reduction for renal dysfunction: 400 mg IV q 12 h for CrCl 31 to 50 mL/min; 300 mg IV q 12 h for CrCl 15 to 30 mL/min; 200 mg IV q 12 h for ESRD including hemodialysis.

ANTIMICROBIALS: Macrolides

AZITHROMYCIN (*Zithromax, Zmax*) ▶L ♀B ▶? $$

ADULT – Community-acquired pneumonia including Legionella, inpatient: 500 mg IV over 1 h daily for at least 2 days, then 500 mg PO daily for 7 to 10 days total. Pelvic inflammatory disease: 500 mg IV daily for 1 to 2 days, then 250 mg PO daily to complete 7 days. Oral for acute exacerbation of chronic bronchitis, community-acquired pneumonia, group A streptococcal pharyngitis (2nd line to penicillin), skin infections: 500 mg PO on 1st day, then 250 mg PO daily for 4 days. Acute sinusitis, alternative for acute exacerbation of chronic bronchitis: 500 mg PO daily for 3 days. Zmax for community-acquired pneumonia, acute sinusitis: 2 g PO single dose (contents of full bottle) on empty stomach. Chlamydia, chancroid: 1 g PO single dose. Gonorrhea: 2 g PO single dose (CDC does not recommend azithromycin alone for routine treatment). Get culture (preferred) or NAAT 1 week after dose. Observe patient for at least 30 min for poor GI tolerability. Prevention of disseminated *Mycobacterium avium* complex disease: 1200 mg PO once per week.

PEDS – Oral for otitis media, community-acquired pneumonia: 10 mg/kg up to 500 mg PO on 1st day, then 5 mg/kg up to 250 mg PO daily for 4 days. Acute sinusitis: 10 mg/kg PO daily for 3 days. Zmax for community-acquired pneumonia or acute sinusitis: 60 mg/kg (max 2 g) PO single dose on empty stomach for age 6 mo or older; give adult dose of 2 g for wt 34 kg or greater. Otitis media: 30 mg/kg PO single dose or 10 mg/kg PO daily for 3 days. Group A streptococcal pharyngitis (2nd line to penicillin): 12 mg/kg up to 500 mg PO daily for 5 days. Take susp on empty stomach.

UNAPPROVED ADULT – See table for prophylaxis of bacterial endocarditis. Nongonococcal urethritis: 1 g PO single dose. See STD table for recurrent/persistent urethritis. Chlamydia in pregnancy: 1 g PO single dose. *Campylobacter* gastroenteritis: 500 mg PO daily for 3 days; for HIV-infected patients, treat for 7 days for mild to moderate disease, at least 14 days for bacteremia. Traveler's diarrhea: 500 mg PO on 1st day, then 250 mg PO daily for 4 days; or 1 g PO single dose. *Mycobacterium avium* complex disease treatment in AIDS: 500 mg PO daily (use at least 2 drugs for active infection). Pertussis treatment/postexposure prophylaxis: 500 mg PO on 1st day, then 250 mg PO daily for 4 days. Cholera: 1 g PO single dose (use this regimen in pregnancy).

UNAPPROVED PEDS – Prevention of disseminated *Mycobacterium avium* complex disease: 20 mg/kg PO once per week not to exceed adult dose. *Mycobacterium avium* complex disease treatment: 5 mg/kg PO daily (use at least 2 drugs for active infection). Cystic fibrosis patients colonized with *P. aeruginosa*, age 6 yo and older: 250 mg three days per week for 24 weeks for wt less than 40 kg, 500 mg PO three days per week for 24 weeks for wt 40 kg or greater. Chlamydia trachomatis: 1 g PO single dose for age younger than 8 yo and wt greater than 44 kg, and for age 8 yo or older for any wt. Pertussis treatment/postexposure prophylaxis: 10 mg/kg PO once daily for 5 days for infants younger than 6 mo; 10 mg/kg (max 500 mg) PO single dose on day 1, then 5 mg/kg (up to 250 mg) PO once daily for 4 days for age 6 mo or older. See table for bacterial endocarditis prophylaxis. Traveler's diarrhea: 5 to 10 mg/kg PO single dose. Cholera: 20 mg/kg up to 1 g PO single dose.

FORMS – Generic/Trade: Tabs 250, 500, 600 mg. Susp 100, 200 mg/5 mL. Trade only: Packet 1000 mg. Z-Pak: #6, 250 mg tab. Tri-Pak: #3, 500 mg tab. Zmax extended-release oral susp: 2 g in 60 mL single-dose bottle.

NOTES – Severe allergic/skin reactions rarely, IV site reactions, hearing loss with prolonged

(cont.)

AZITHROMYCIN (*cont.*)

use, hepatotoxicity, exacerbation of myasthenia gravis. Can prolong QT interval and cause torsades. Try to avoid if QT interval prolonged, uncorrected hypokalemia or hypomagnesemia, clinically significant bradycardia, or coadministration of Class IA or III antiarrhythmic drug. Does not inhibit CYP enzymes. Do not take at the same time as Al/Mg antacids (except Zmax which can be taken with antacids). Monitor INR with warfarin. Single dose and 3-day regimens cause more vomiting than 5-day regimen for otitis media. Zmax: Store at room temperature and use within 12 h of reconstitution. Additional treatment required if vomiting occurs within 5 min of dose; consider for vomiting within 1 h of dose; unnecessary for vomiting more than 1 h after dose.

CLARITHROMYCIN (***Biaxin, Biaxin XL***) ▶KL ♀C ▶? $$$

ADULT – Group A streptococcal pharyngitis (2nd line to penicillin): 250 mg PO two times per day for 10 days. Acute sinusitis: 500 mg PO two times per day for 14 days. Acute exacerbation of chronic bronchitis (*S. pneumoniae/M. catarrhalis*), community-acquired pneumonia, skin infections: 250 mg PO two times per day for 7 to 14 days. Acute exacerbation of chronic bronchitis (*H. influenzae*): 500 mg PO two times per day for 7 to 14 days. *H. pylori*: See table in GI section. *Mycobacterium avium* complex disease prevention/treatment: 500 mg PO two times per day. Treat active mycobacterial infections with at least 2 drugs. Biaxin XL: Acute sinusitis: 1000 mg PO daily for 14 days. Acute exacerbation of chronic bronchitis, community-acquired pneumonia: 1000 mg PO daily for 7 days. Take Biaxin XL with food.

PEDS – Group A streptococcal pharyngitis (2nd line to penicillin), community-acquired pneumonia, sinusitis, otitis media, skin infections: 7.5 mg/kg PO two times per day for 10 days. *Mycobacterium avium* complex prevention/treatment: 7.5 mg/kg up to 500 mg PO two times per day. Two or more drugs are needed for the treatment of active mycobacterial infections.

UNAPPROVED ADULT – See table for prophylaxis of bacterial endocarditis. Pertussis treatment/postexposure prophylaxis: 500 mg PO two times per day for 7 days. Community-acquired pneumonia: 500 mg PO two times per day.

UNAPPROVED PEDS – See table for prophylaxis of bacterial endocarditis. Pertussis treatment/postexposure prophylaxis (age 1 mo or older): 7.5 mg/kg (up to 500 mg) PO two times per day for 7 days.

FORMS – Generic/Trade: Tabs 250, 500 mg. Extended-release tab 500 mg. Susp 125, 250 mg/ 5 mL. Trade only: Biaxin XL-Pak: #14, 500 mg tabs. Generic only: Extended-release tab 1000 mg.

NOTES – Can cause or exacerbate myasthenia gravis. Can prolong QT interval and cause torsades. Avoid in ongoing proarrhythmic conditions such as prolonged QT interval, uncorrected hypokalemia or hypomagnesemia, clinically significant bradycardia, or coadministration of Class IA or Class III antiarrhythmic drugs. Strong CYP3A4 inhibitor. Many drug interactions including increased levels of carbamazepine, cyclosporine, digoxin, disopyramide (monitor ECG), lovastatin (avoid), quinidine (monitor ECG), rifabutin, simvastatin (avoid), tacrolimus, theophylline. Toxicity with ergotamine, dihydroergotamine, or colchicine (reduce colchicine dose; contraindicated if renal/hepatic impairment). Reduce dose of sildenafil, tadalafil, tolterodine, vardenafil. Monitor INR with warfarin. Clarithromycin levels decreased by efavirenz (avoid concomitant use) and nevirapine enough to impair efficacy in *Mycobacterium avium* complex disease. AAP recommends 5 to 7 days of therapy for children age 6 yo or older with nonsevere otitis media, and 10 days for younger children and those with severe disease. Reduce clarithromycin dose by 50% if given with atazanavir; consider alternative for indications other than *Mycobacterium avium* complex. Dosage reduction for renal insufficiency in patients taking ritonavir, lopinavir-ritonavir (Kaletra), or ritonavir-boosted darunavir, fosamprenavir, saquinavir, or tipranavir: Decrease dose by 75% for CrCl less than 30 mL/min, decrease dose by 50% for CrCl 30 to 60 mL/min. Do not refrigerate susp.

ERYTHROMYCIN BASE (***Eryc, Ery-Tab,*** ✤ ***Erybid, P.C.E.***) ▶L ♀B ▶+ $

ADULT – Respiratory, skin infections: 250 to 500 mg PO four times per day or 333 mg PO three times per day. Pertussis, treatment/postexposure prophylaxis: 500 mg PO q 6 h for 14 days. *S. aureus* skin infections: 250 mg PO q 6 h or 500 mg PO q 12 h. Secondary prevention of rheumatic fever: 250 mg PO two times per day. Chlamydia in pregnancy, nongonococcal urethritis: 500 mg PO four times per day for 7 days. Alternative for chlamydia in pregnancy if high dose not tolerated: 250 mg PO four times per day for 14 days. Erythrasma:

(cont.)

ERYTHROMYCIN BASE (*cont.*)

250 mg PO three times per day for 21 days. Legionnaires' disease: 2 g/day PO in divided doses for 14 to 21 days.

PEDS – Usual dose: 30 to 50 mg/kg/day PO divided four times per day for 10 days. Can double dose for severe infections. Pertussis: 40 to 50 mg/kg/day PO divided four times per day for 14 days (azithromycin preferred for age younger than 1 mo due to risk of hypertrophic pyloric stenosis with erythromycin). Chlamydia: 50 mg/kg/day PO divided four times per day for 14 days for wt less than 45 kg.

UNAPPROVED ADULT – Chancroid: 500 mg PO three times per day for 7 days. *Campylobacter* gastroenteritis: 500 mg PO two times per day for 5 days.

FORMS – Generic/Trade: Tabs 250, 333, 500 mg, delayed-release cap 250 mg.

NOTES – Can prolong QT interval and cause torsades. Avoid if QT interval prolonged, uncorrected hypokalemia or hypomagnesemia, clinically significant bradycardia, or coadministration of Class IA or III antiarrhythmic drug. Incidence of sudden death may be increased when erythromycin is combined with potent CYP3A4 inhibitors. Exacerbation of myasthenia gravis. Hypertrophic pyloric stenosis in infants primarily younger than 1 mo. CYP3A4 and 1A2 inhibitor. Many drug interactions including increased levels of carbamazepine, cyclosporine, digoxin, disopyramide, tacrolimus, theophylline, some benzodiazepines and statins (avoid simvastatin and lovastatin). Monitor INR with warfarin.

ERYTHROMYCIN ETHYL SUCCINATE (***EES, EryPed***) ▶L ♀B ▶+ $

ADULT – Usual dose: 400 mg PO four times per day. Nongonococcal urethritis: 800 mg PO four times per day for 7 days. Chlamydia in pregnancy: 800 mg PO four times per day for 7 days or 400 mg PO four times per day for 14 days if high dose not tolerated. Secondary prevention of rheumatic fever: 400 mg PO two times per day. Legionnaires' disease: 3.2 g/day PO in divided doses for 14 to 21 days.

PEDS – Usual dose: 30 to 50 mg/kg/day PO divided four times per day. Maximum dose: 100 mg/kg/day. Group A streptococcal pharyngitis: 40 mg/kg/day (up to 1 g/day) PO divided two to four times per day for 10 days. Secondary prevention of rheumatic fever: 400 mg PO two times per day. Pertussis: 40 to 50 mg/kg/day (up to 2 g/day) PO divided four times per day for 14 days.

FORMS – Generic/Trade: Tabs 400. Susp 200, 400 mg/5 mL. Trade only (EryPed): Susp 100 mg/2.5 mL (50 mL).

NOTES – Can prolong QT interval and cause torsades. Avoid if QT interval prolonged, uncorrected hypokalemia or hypomagnesemia, clinically significant bradycardia, or coadministration of Class IA or III antiarrhythmic drug. Incidence of sudden death may be increased when erythromycin is combined with potent CYP3A4 inhibitors. May aggravate myasthenia gravis. Hypertrophic pyloric stenosis primarily in infants younger than 1 mo. CYP3A4 and 1A2 inhibitor. Many drug interactions including increased levels of carbamazepine, cyclosporine, digoxin, disopyramide, tacrolimus, theophylline, some benzodiazepines and statins (avoid simvastatin and lovastatin). Monitor INR with warfarin.

ERYTHROMYCIN ETHYL SUCCINATE + SULFISOXAZOLE ▶KL ♀C ▶– $$

PEDS – Otitis media: 50 mg/kg/day (based on EES dose) PO divided three to four times per day for age older than 2 mo.

FORMS – Generic only: Susp, erythromycin ethyl succinate 200 mg plus sulfisoxazole 600 mg/5 mL.

NOTES – Sulfisoxazole: Stevens-Johnson syndrome, toxic epidermal necrolysis, hepatotoxicity, blood dyscrasia, hemolysis in G6PD deficiency. Can significantly increase INR with warfarin; avoid coadministration if possible. Erythromycin: Can prolong the QT interval and cause torsades. Avoid if QT interval prolonged, uncorrected hypokalemia or hypomagnesemia, clinically significant bradycardia, or coadministration of Class IA or III antiarrhythmic drug. Incidence of sudden death may be increased when erythromycin is combined with potent CYP3A4 inhibitors. May aggravate myasthenia gravis. CYP3A4 and 1A2 inhibitor. Many drug interactions including increased levels of carbamazepine, cyclosporine, digoxin, disopyramide, tacrolimus, theophylline, some benzodiazepines and statins (avoid simvastatin and lovastatin). AAP recommends 5 to 7 days of therapy for children age 6 yo or older with nonsevere otitis media, and 10 days for younger children and those with severe disease.

ERYTHROMYCIN LACTOBIONATE (♣ ***Erythrocin IV***) ▶L ♀B ▶+ $$$$$

ADULT – For severe infections/PO not possible: 15 to 20 mg/kg/day (up to 4 g/day) IV divided q 6 h. Legionnaires' disease: 4 g/day IV divided q 6 h.

PEDS – For severe infections/PO not possible: 15 to 20 mg/kg/day (up to 4 g/day) IV divided q 6 h.

(cont.)

ERYTHROMYCIN LACTOBIONATE (*cont.*)

UNAPPROVED PEDS – 20 to 50 mg/kg/day IV divided q 6 h.

NOTES – Dilute and give slowly to minimize venous irritation. Reversible hearing loss (increased risk in elderly given 4 g or more per day), allergic reactions, exacerbation of myasthenia gravis. Can prolong QT interval and cause torsades. Avoid if QT interval prolonged, uncorrected hypokalemia or hypomagnesemia, clinically significant bradycardia, or coadministration of Class IA or III antiarrhythmic drug. Incidence of sudden death may be increased when erythromycin is combined with potent CYP3A4 inhibitors. Hypertrophic pyloric stenosis primarily in infants younger than 1 mo. CYP3A4 and 1A2 inhibitor. Many drug interactions including increased levels of carbamazepine, cyclosporine, digoxin, disopyramide, tacrolimus, theophylline, some benzodiazepines and statins (avoid simvastatin and lovastatin). Monitor INR with warfarin.

FIDAXOMICIN (*Dificid*) ▶minimal absorption ♀B ▶? $$$$$

ADULT – C. *difficile*–associated diarrhea: 200 mg PO two times per day for 10 days.

PEDS – Safety and efficacy not established in children.

FORMS – Trade only: 200 mg tabs.

NOTES – Not for systemic infections. Only treats *C. difficile*–associated diarrhea.

ANTIMICROBIALS: Penicillins—1st generation—Natural

NOTE: Anaphylaxis occurs rarely with penicillins; cross-sensitivity with cephalosporins is possible.

BENZATHINE PENICILLIN (*Bicillin L-A*) ▶K ♀B ▶? $$

WARNING – Not for IV administration, which can cause cardiorespiratory arrest and death.

ADULT – Group A streptococcal pharyngitis: 1.2 million units IM single dose. Secondary prevention of rheumatic fever: 1.2 million units IM q month (q 3 weeks for high-risk patients) or 600,000 units IM q 2 weeks. Primary, secondary, early latent syphilis: 2.4 million units IM single dose. Tertiary, late latent syphilis: 2.4 million units IM q week for 3 doses.

PEDS – Group A streptococcal pharyngitis (AHA regimen): 600,000 units IM for wt 27 kg or less; 1.2 million units IM for wt greater than 27 kg. Secondary prevention of rheumatic fever: 600,000 units IM for wt 27 kg or less; 1.2 million units IM for wt greater than 27 kg; give q month (q 3 weeks for high-risk patients). Primary, secondary, early latent syphilis: 50,000 units/kg (up to 2.4 million units) IM single dose. Late latent syphilis: 50,000 units/kg (up to 2.4 million units) IM for 3 weekly doses.

UNAPPROVED ADULT – Prophylaxis of diphtheria/treatment of carriers: 1.2 million units IM single dose.

UNAPPROVED PEDS – Prophylaxis of diphtheria/treatment of carriers: 1.2 million units IM single dose for wt 30 kg or greater; 600,000 units IM single dose for wt less than 30 kg.

FORMS – Trade only: For IM use, 600,000 units/mL; 1, 2, 4 mL syringes.

NOTES – Do not give IV. Doses last 2 to 4 weeks. Not for neurosyphilis. IM injection less painful if warmed to room temp erature before giving.

BICILLIN C-R **(procaine penicillin + benzathine penicillin)** ▶K ♀B ▶? $$$

WARNING – Not for IV administration, which can cause cardiorespiratory arrest and death.

ADULT – Scarlet fever; erysipelas; upper respiratory, skin, and soft-tissue infections due to group A strep: 2.4 million units IM single dose. Pneumococcal infections other than meningitis: 1.2 million units IM q 2 to 3 days until temperature normal for 48 h. Not for treatment of syphilis.

PEDS – Scarlet fever; erysipelas; upper respiratory, skin, and soft-tissue infections due to group A strep: 600,000 units IM for wt less than 13.6 kg; 900,000 to 1.2 million units IM for wt 13.6 to 27 kg; 2.4 million units IM for wt greater than 27 kg. Pneumococcal infections other than meningitis: 600,000 units IM q 2 to 3 days until temperature normal for 48 h. Not for treatment of syphilis.

FORMS – Trade only: For IM use 300/300 thousand units/mL procaine/benzathine penicillin; 2 mL syringe.

NOTES – Contraindicated if allergic to procaine. Do not give IV. Do not substitute Bicillin C-R for Bicillin LA in treatment of syphilis.

PENICILLIN G ▶K ♀B ▶? $$$$

ADULT – Penicillin-sensitive pneumococcal pneumonia: 8 to 12 million units/day IV divided q 4 to 6 h. Penicillin-sensitive pneumococcal meningitis: 24 million units/day IV divided q 2 to 4 h. Empiric therapy, native valve endocarditis: 20 million units/day IV continuous infusion or divided q 4 h plus nafcillin/oxacillin and gentamicin. Neurosyphilis: 18 to 24 million units/day continuous IV infusion or 3 to 4 million units IV q

(cont.)

PENICILLIN G (*cont.*)

4 h for 10 to 14 days. Bioterrorism anthrax: See www.idsociety.org/Anthrax/

PEDS – Mild to moderate infections: 25,000 to 50,000 units/kg/day IV divided q 6 h. Severe infections including pneumococcal and meningococcal meningitis: 250,000 to 400,000 units/kg/day IV divided q 4 to 6 h. Neonates age younger than 1 week and wt greater than 2 kg: 25,000 to 50,000 units/kg IV q 8 h. Neonates age 1 week or older and wt greater than 2 kg: 25,000 to 50,000 units/kg IV q 6 h. Group B streptococcal meningitis: 250,000 to 450,000 units/kg/day IV divided q 8 h for age 1 week or younger; 450,000 to 500,000 units/kg/day IV divided q 4 to 6 h for age older than 1 week. Congenital syphilis: 50,000 units/kg/dose IV q 12 h during first 7 days of life, then q 8 h thereafter to complete 10 days. Congenital syphilis or neurosyphilis: 50,000 units/kg IV q 4 to 6 h for 10 days for age older than 1 mo.

UNAPPROVED ADULT – Prevention of perinatal group B streptococcal disease: Give to mother 5 million units IV at onset of labor/after membrane rupture, then 2.5 to 3 million units IV q 4 h until delivery. Diphtheria: 100,000 to 150,000 units/kg/day IV divided q 6 h for 14 days.

UNAPPROVED PEDS – Diphtheria: 100,000 to 150,000 units/kg/day IV divided q 6 h for 14 days.

NOTES – Reduce dose in renal dysfunction.

PENICILLIN V ▶K ♀B ◗? $

ADULT – Usual dose: 250 to 500 mg PO four times per day. AHA dosing for group A streptococcal pharyngitis: 500 mg PO two to three times per day for 10 days. Secondary prevention of rheumatic fever: 250 mg PO two times per day. Vincent's infection: 250 mg PO q 6 to 8 h.

PEDS – Usual dose: 25 to 50 mg/kg/day PO divided three to four times per day. Use adult dose for age 12 yo or older. AHA dosing for group A streptococcal pharyngitis: 250 mg (for wt 27 kg or less) or 500 mg (wt greater than 27 kg) PO two or three times per day for 10 days. Secondary prevention of rheumatic fever: 250 mg PO two times per day.

UNAPPROVED PEDS – Prevention of pneumococcal infections in functional/anatomic asplenia: 125 mg PO two times per day for age younger than 3 yo; 250 mg PO two times per day for age 3 yo or older.

FORMS – Generic only: Tabs 250, 500 mg, oral soln 125, 250 mg/5 mL.

NOTES – Oral soln stable in refrigerator for 14 days.

PROCAINE PENICILLIN ▶K ♀B ◗? $$$$$

ADULT – Pneumococcal and streptococcal infections, Vincent's infection, erysipeloid: 0.6 to 1 million units IM daily. Neurosyphilis: 2.4 million units IM daily plus probenecid 500 mg PO q 6 h, both for 10 to 14 days.

PEDS – Pneumococcal and streptococcal infections, Vincent's infection, erysipeloid, for wt less than 27 kg: 300,000 units IM daily. AAP dose for mild to moderate infections, age older than 1 mo: 25,000 to 50,000 units/kg/day IM divided one to two times per day. Congenital syphilis: 50,000 units/kg IM once daily for 10 days.

FORMS – Generic: For IM use, 600,000 units/mL; 1, 2 mL syringes.

NOTES – Peak 4 h, lasts 24 h. Contraindicated if procaine allergy; skin test if allergy suspected. Transient CNS reactions with high doses.

PROPHYLAXIS FOR BACTERIAL ENDOCARDITIS*

Limited to dental or respiratory tract procedures in patients at highest risk. All regimens are single doses administered 30–60 minutes prior to procedure.	
Standard regimen	Amoxicillin 2 g PO
Unable to take oral meds	Ampicillin 2 g IM/IV; or cefazolin[†] or ceftriaxone[†] 1 g IM/IV
Allergic to penicillin	Clindamycin 600 mg PO; or cephalexin[†] 2 g PO; or azithromycin or clarithromycin 500 mg PO
Allergic to penicillin and unable to take oral meds	Clindamycin 600 mg IM/IV; or cefazolin[†] or ceftriaxone[†] 1 g IM/IV
Pediatric drug doses	Pediatric dose should not exceed adult dose. Amoxicillin 50 mg/kg, ampicillin 50 mg/kg, azithromycin 15 mg/kg, cephalexin[†] 50 mg/kg, cefazolin[†] 50 mg/kg, ceftriaxone[†] 50 mg/kg, clarithromycin 15 mg/kg, clindamycin 20 mg/kg.

*For additional details of the 2007 AHA guidelines, see http://www.americanheart.org.
[†]Avoid cephalosporins if prior penicillin-associated anaphylaxis, angioedema, or urticaria.

ANTIMICROBIALS: Penicillins—2nd generation—Penicillinase-Resistant

NOTE: Anaphylaxis occurs rarely with penicillins; cross-sensitivity with cephalosporins is possible.

DICLOXACILLIN ▶KL ♀B ▶? $$

ADULT – Usual dose: 250 to 500 mg PO four times per day. Take on empty stomach.

PEDS – Mild to moderate upper respiratory, skin, and soft-tissue infections: 12.5 mg/kg/day PO divided four times per day for age older than 1 mo. Pneumonia, disseminated infections: 25 mg/kg/day PO divided four times per day for age older than 1 mo. Follow-up therapy after IV antibiotics for Staph osteomyelitis: 50 to 100 mg/kg/day PO divided four times per day. Use adult dose for wt 40 kg or greater. Give on empty stomach.

FORMS – Generic only: Caps 250, 500 mg.

NAFCILLIN ▶L ♀B ▶? $$$$$

ADULT – Staph infections, usual dose: 500 mg IM q 4 to 6 h or 500 to 2000 mg IV q 4 h. Osteomyelitis: 1 to 2 g IV q 4 h. Empiric therapy, native valve endocarditis: 2 g IV q 4 h plus penicillin/ampicillin and gentamicin.

PEDS – Staph infections, usual dose: 25 mg/kg IM two times per day for pediatric patients who weigh less than 40 kg; give 10 mg/kg for neonates.

UNAPPROVED PEDS – Mild to moderate infections: 50 to 100 mg/kg/day IM/IV divided q 6 h. Severe infections: 100 to 200 mg/kg/day IM/IV divided q 4 to 6 h. Neonates, wt greater than 2 kg: 25 mg/kg IM/IV q 8 h for age younger than 1 week old; 25 to 35 mg/kg IM/IV q 6 h for age 1 week or older.

NOTES – Reversible neutropenia with prolonged use. Decreased INR with warfarin. Decreased cyclosporine levels.

OXACILLIN ▶KL ♀B ▶? $$$$$

ADULT – Staph infections: 250 mg to 2 g IM/IV q 4 to 6 h. Osteomyelitis: 1.5 to 2 g IV q 4 h. Empiric therapy, native valve endocarditis: 2 g IV q 4 h with penicillin/ampicillin and gentamicin.

PEDS – Mild to moderate infections: 100 to 150 mg/kg/day IM/IV divided q 6 h. Severe infections: 150 to 200 mg/kg/day IM/IV divided q 4 to 6 h. Use adult dose for wt 40 kg or greater. Newborns, wt greater than 2 kg: 25 to 50 mg/kg IV q 8 h for age younger than 1 week old, increasing to q 6 h for age 1 week or older.

NOTES – Hepatic dysfunction possible with doses greater than 12 g/day; monitor LFTs.

ANTIMICROBIALS: Penicillins—3rd generation—Aminopenicillins

NOTE: Anaphylaxis occurs rarely with penicillins; cross-sensitivity with cephalosporins is possible. *C. difficile*-associated diarrhea. High risk of rash in patients with mononucleosis or taking allopurinol.

AMOXICILLIN (*Moxatag*) ▶K ♀B ▶+ $

ADULT – ENT, skin, genitourinary infections: 250 to 500 mg PO three times per day or 500 to 875 mg PO two times per day. Pneumonia: 500 mg PO three times per day or 875 mg PO two times per day. AHA dosing for group A streptococcal pharyngitis: 50 mg/kg (max 1 g) PO once daily for 10 days. Group A streptococcal pharyngitis/tonsillitis, for age 12 yo or older: 775 mg ER tab (Moxatag) PO once daily for 10 days. Do not chew/crush Moxatag tabs. *H. pylori:* See table in GI section. See table for prophylaxis of bacterial endocarditis.

PEDS – ENT, skin, GU infections: 20 to 40 mg/kg/day PO divided three times per day or 25 to 45 mg/kg/day PO divided two times per day. See "Unapproved Peds" for AAP acute otitis media dosing. Pneumonia: 40 mg/kg/day PO divided three times per day or 45 mg/kg/day PO divided two times per day. Infants, age younger than 3 mo: 30 mg/kg/day PO divided q 12 h. AHA dosing for group A streptococcal pharyngitis: 50 mg/kg (max 1 g) PO once daily for 10 days. Group A streptococcal pharyngitis/tonsillitis, for age 12 yo or older: 775 mg ER tab (Moxatag) PO once daily for 10 days.

(cont.)

PENICILLINS—GENERAL ANTIMICROBIAL SPECTRUM

1st generation	Most streptococci; oral anaerobic coverage
2nd generation	Most streptococci; *S.aureus* (but not MRSA)
3rd generation	Most streptococci; basic Gram-negative coverage
4th generation	*Pseudomonas*

AMOXICILLIN (*cont.*)

Do not chew/crush Moxatag tabs. See table for bacterial endocarditis prophylaxis.

UNAPPROVED ADULT – High-dose for community-acquired pneumonia: 1 g PO three times per day. Lyme disease: 500 mg PO three times per day for 14 days for early disease, for 28 days for Lyme arthritis. Chlamydia in pregnancy: 500 mg PO three times per day for 7 days. Bioterrorism anthrax: See www.idsociety.org/Anthrax/

UNAPPROVED PEDS – Otitis media (AAP high-dose): 90 mg/kg/day PO divided two to three times per day. Community-acquired pneumonia: 80 to 100 mg/kg/day PO divided three to four times per day for age 4 mo to 4 yo. Lyme disease: 50 mg/kg/day (up to 1500 mg/day) PO divided three times per day for 14 days for early disease, for 28 days for Lyme arthritis. Bioterrorism anthrax: See www.idsociety.org/Anthrax/

FORMS – Generic only: Caps 250, 500 mg, Tabs 500, 875 mg, Chewable tabs 125, 200, 250, 400 mg. Susp 125, 250 mg/5 mL. Susp 200, 400 mg/5 mL. Infant gtts 50 mg/mL. Moxatag 775 mg extended-release tab.

NOTES – AAP recommends 5 to 7 days of therapy for children age 6 yo or older with nonsevere otitis media, and 10 days for younger children and those with severe disease. Reduce dose in adults with renal dysfunction: Give 250 to 500 mg PO daily for CrCl less than 10 mL/min or hemodialysis; 250 to 500 mg PO two times per day for CrCl 10 to 30 mL/min. Do not use 875 mg tab for CrCl less than 30 mL/min. Give additional dose during and at end of dialysis. Oral susp and infant gtts stable for 14 days at room temperature or in the refrigerator.

AMOXICILLIN-CLAVULANATE (***Augmentin, Augmentin ES-600, Augmentin XR,*** ✤ ***Clavulin***) ▶K ♀B ▶? $$$$

ADULT – Pneumonia, otitis media, sinusitis, skin infections, UTIs: Usual dose 500 mg PO two times per day or 250 mg PO three times per day. More severe infections: 875 mg PO two times per day or 500 mg PO three times per day. Augmentin XR: 2 tabs PO q 12 h with meals for 10 days for acute sinusitis, give 7 to 10 days for community-acquired pneumonia. See table for management of acute sinusitis.

PEDS – 200, 400 mg chewables and 200, 400 mg/5 mL susp for two times per day administration. Pneumonia, otitis media, sinusitis: 45 mg/kg/day PO divided two times per day. Less severe infections such as skin, UTIs: 25 mg/kg/day PO divided two times per day. 125, 250 mg chewables and 125, 250 mg/5 mL susp for three times per day administration. Pneumonia, otitis media, sinusitis: 40 mg/kg/day PO divided three times per day. Less severe infections such as skin, UTIs: 20 mg/kg/day PO divided three times per day. Use 125 mg/5 mL susp and give 30 mg/kg PO q 12 h for age younger than 3 mo. Give adult dose for wt 40 kg or greater. Augmentin ES-600 susp for age 3 mo or older and wt less than 40 kg. Recurrent/persistent otitis media with risk factors (antibiotics for otitis media in past 3 months and either in daycare or age 2 yo or younger): give 90 mg/kg/day PO divided two times per day with food for 10 days. See table for management of acute sinusitis.

UNAPPROVED ADULT – See table for management of acute sinusitis. Treatment of infected dog/cat bite: 875 mg PO two times per day or 500 mg PO three times per day, duration of treatment based on response.

UNAPPROVED PEDS – See table for management of acute sinusitis. IDSA recommends for community-acquired pneumonia, age older than 3 mo: 90 mg/kg/day PO divided two times per day (max dose of 2 g PO two times per day for age 5 yo and older). Treat for up to 10 days.

FORMS – Generic/Trade: (amoxicillin-clavulanate) Tabs 250/125, 500/125, 875/125 mg. Chewables, Susp 200/28.5, 400/57 mg per tab or 5 mL, 250/62.5 mg per 5 mL. (ES) Susp 600/42.9 mg per 5 mL. Trade only: Chewables, Susp 125/31.25 per tab or 5 mL, 250/62.5 mg per tab. Extended-release tabs (Augmentin XR) 1000/62.5 mg.

NOTES – Diarrhea common (less with twice daily dosing). AAP recommends 5 to 7 days of therapy for children age 6 yo or older with nonsevere otitis media, and 10 days for those with severe disease or age younger than 6 yo. Do not interchange Augmentin products with different clavulanate content. Do not use 250 mg amoxicillin plus 125 mg clavulanate tab in children with wt less than 40 kg. Suspensions stable in refrigerator for 10 days. See prescribing information for dosage reduction of Augmentin tabs if CrCl is less than 30 mL/min. Augmentin XR contraindicated if CrCl is less than 30 mL/min.

AMPICILLIN ▶K ♀B ▶? $ PO $$$$$ IV

ADULT – Usual dose: 1 to 2 g IV q 4 to 6 h or 250 to 500 mg PO four times per day. Sepsis, meningitis: 150 to 200 mg/kg/day IV divided q 3 to 4 h. Empiric therapy, native valve endocarditis: 12 g/day IV continuous infusion or divided q 4 h plus nafcillin/oxacillin

(cont.)

AMPICILLIN (*cont.*)

and gentamicin. See table for prophylaxis of bacterial endocarditis. Take oral ampicillin on an empty stomach.

PEDS – AAP recommendations: Mild to moderate infections: 100 to 150 mg/kg/day IM/IV divided q 6 h or 50 to 100 mg/kg/day PO divided four times per day. Severe infections: 200 to 400 mg/kg/day IM/IV divided q 6 h. Newborns, wt greater than 2 kg: 25 to 50 mg/kg IV given q 8 h for age younger than 1 week old, increase to q 6 h for age 1 week or older. Use adult doses for wt 40 kg or greater. Give oral ampicillin on an empty stomach. Group B streptococcal meningitis: 200 to 300 mg/kg/day IV divided q 8 h for age 7 days or younger; 300 mg/kg/day divided q 6 h for age older than 7 days. Give with gentamicin initially. See table for prophylaxis of bacterial endocarditis.

UNAPPROVED ADULT – Prevention of neonatal group B streptococcal disease: Give to mother 2 g IV at onset of labor/after membrane rupture, then 1 g IV q 4 h until delivery.

FORMS – Generic only: Caps 250, 500 mg. Susp 125, 250 mg/5 mL.

NOTES – Susp stable for 7 days at room temperature, 14 days in the refrigerator. Reduce dosing interval to q 12 to 24 h for CrCl less than 10 mL/min. Give dose after hemodialysis.

AMPICILLIN-SULBACTAM (*Unasyn*) ▶K ♀B ▶? $$$$$

ADULT – Skin, intra-abdominal, gynecologic infections: 1.5 to 3 g IM/IV q 6 h.

PEDS – Skin infections, for age 1 yo or older: 300 mg/kg/day IV divided q 6 h. Use adult dose for wt greater than 40 kg.

UNAPPROVED ADULT – Community-acquired pneumonia: 1.5 to 3 g IM/IV q 6 h with a macrolide or doxycycline.

UNAPPROVED PEDS – AAP regimens. Mild to moderate infections: 100 to 150 mg/kg/day of ampicillin IM/IV divided q 6 h. Severe infections: 200 to 400 mg/kg/day of ampicillin IM/IV divided q 6 h.

NOTES – Dosing for adults with renal impairment: Give usual dose q 24 h for CrCl 5 to 14 mL/min, q 12 h for CrCl 15 to 29 mL/min, q 6 to 8 h for adults with CrCl 30 mL/min or greater.

ANTIMICROBIALS: Penicillins—4th generation—Extended Spectrum

NOTE: Anaphylaxis occurs rarely with penicillins; cross-sensitivity with cephalosporins is possible. Hypokalemia, bleeding and coagulation abnormalities possible, especially with renal impairment.

PIPERACILLIN-TAZOBACTAM (*Zosyn*, ✤ *Tazocin*) ▶K ♀B ▶? $$$$$

ADULT – Appendicitis, peritonitis, skin infections, postpartum endometritis, pelvic inflammatory disease, moderate community-acquired pneumonia: 3.375 g IV q 6 h. Nosocomial pneumonia: 4.5 g IV q 6 h (with aminoglycoside initially and if *P. aeruginosa* is cultured).

PEDS – Appendicitis/peritonitis: 80 mg/kg of piperacillin IV q 8 h for age 2 to 9 mo; 100 mg/kg of piperacillin IV q 8 h for age older than 9 mo; use adult dose for wt greater than 40 kg.

UNAPPROVED ADULT – Serious infections: 4.5 g IV q 6 h.

UNAPPROVED PEDS – 150 to 300 mg/kg/day of piperacillin IV divided q 6 to 8 h for age younger than 6 mo, 300 to 400 mg/kg/day piperacillin IV divided q 6 to 8 h for age 6 mo or older.

NOTES – May prolong neuromuscular blockade with nondepolarizing muscle relaxants. False-positive result possible with Platelia Aspergillus EIA test (Bio-Rad Laboratories). May reduce renal excretion of methotrexate; monitor methotrexate levels and toxicity. Reduce dosing in adults with renal impairment: 2.25 g IV q 8 h for CrCl less than 20 mL/min; 2.25 g IV q 6 h for CrCl 20 to 40 mL/min. Hemodialysis: Maximum dose of 2.25 g IV q 8 h plus 0.75 g after each dialysis.

TICARCILLIN-CLAVULANATE (*Timentin*) ▶K ♀B ▶? $$$$$

ADULT – Systemic infections or UTIs: 3.1 g IV q 4 to 6 h. Gynecologic infections. Moderate: 200 mg/kg/day IV divided q 6 h. Severe: 300 mg/kg/day IV divided q 4 h. Adults with wt less than 60 kg: 200 to 300 mg/kg/day (based on ticarcillin content) IV divided q 4 to 6 h. Use q 4 h dosing interval for *Pseudomonas* infections.

PEDS – Age 3 mo or older and wt less than 60 kg: 200 mg/kg/day (based on ticarcillin content) IV divided q 6 h for mild to moderate infections, 300 mg/kg/day IV divided q 4 h for severe infections. For wt 60 kg or greater: 3.1 g IV q 6 h for mild to moderate infections; 3.1 g IV q 4 h for severe infections.

NOTES – Timentin 3.1 g is equivalent to 3 g ticarcillin and 0.1 g clavulanate. 4.75 mEq

(cont.)

ACUTE BACTERIAL SINUSITIS IN ADULTS AND CHILDREN: IDSA TREATMENT RECOMMENDATIONS

Initial therapy in patients without risk factors for resistance and infection of mild to moderate severity	
Adults: Amoxicillin-clavulanate 500 mg/125 mg PO three times per day or 875 mg/125 mg PO two times per day for 5 to 7 days	Peds: Amoxicillin-clavulanate 45 mg/kg/day PO two times per day for 10 to 14 days
Initial therapy in patients with severe infection, risk factors for resistance†, or high endemic rate of invasive penicillin-nonsusceptible S. pneumonia (≥10%)	
Adults: Treat for 5 to 7 days with: 1) Amoxicillin-clavulanate* 2000 mg/125 mg PO two times per day 2) Doxycycline 100 mg PO bid or 200 mg PO once daily	Peds: Amoxicillin-clavulanate* 90 mg/kg/day PO two times per day for 10 to 14 days
Beta-lactam allergy	
Adults: Treat for 5 to 7 days with: 1) Doxycycline 100 mg PO two times per day or 200 mg PO once daily 2) Levofloxacin 500 mg PO once daily 3) Moxifloxacin 400 mg PO once daily	Peds, type 1 hypersensitivity: Levofloxacin 10 to 20 mg/kg/day PO every 12–24 h for 10 to 14 days Peds, not type 1 hypersensitivity: Clindamycin‡ 30 to 40 mg/kg/day PO three times per day plus cefixime 8 mg/kg/day PO two times per day or cefpodoxime 10 mg/kg/day PO two times per day for 10 to 14 days
Risk factors for antibiotic resistance† or failed first-line therapy	
Adults: Treat for 5 to 7 days with: 1) Amoxicillin-clavulanate* 2000 mg/125 mg PO two times per day 2) Levofloxacin 500 mg PO once daily 3) Moxifloxacin 400 mg PO once daily	Peds: Treat for 10 to 14 days with: 1) Amoxicillin-clavulanate* 90 mg/kg/day PO two times per day 2) Clindamycin‡ 30 to 40 mg/kg/day PO three times per day plus cefixime 8 mg/kg/day PO two times per day or cefpodoxime 10 mg/kg/day PO two times per day 3) Levofloxacin 10 to 20 mg/kg/day PO every 12 to 24 h
Severe infection requiring hospitalization	
Adults: 1) Ampicillin-sulbactam 1.5 to 3 g IV every 6 h 2) Levofloxacin 500 mg PO or IV once daily 3) Moxifloxacin 400 mg PO or IV once daily 4) Ceftriaxone 1 to 2 g IV every 12 to 24 h 5) Cefotaxime 2 g IV every 4 to 6 h	Peds: 1) Ampicillin-sulbactam 200 to 400 mg/kg/day IV every 6 h 2) Ceftriaxone 50 mg/kg/day IV every 12 h 3) Cefotaxime 100 to 200 mg/kg/day IV every 6 h 4) Levofloxacin 10 to 20 mg/kg/day IV every 12 to 24 h

Adapted from Clin Infect Dis 2012;54(8):e72-e112. Available online at: http://www.idsociety.org.

*High-dose amoxicillin-clavulanate recommended for geographic regions with high endemic rates (at least 10%) of invasive penicillin-nonsusceptible *S. pneumoniae*, those with severe infection (eg, evidence of systemic toxicity with fever of 39° C or higher, and threat of suppurative complications), or risk factors for antibiotic resistance.

†Risk factors for antibiotic resistance include attendance at daycare, age <2 or >65 years, recent hospitalization, antibiotic use within the past month, or patients who are immunocompromised.

‡ Clindamycin resistance in *S. pneumoniae* common in some areas of US

TICARCILLIN-CLAVULANATE (*cont.*)

sodium per g of Timentin. Reduce dose in adults with renal dysfunction: Load with 3.1 g, then give 2 g daily for CrCl less than 10 mL/min and liver dysfunction; 2 g q 12 h for CrCl less than 10 mL/min, 2 g q 8 h for CrCl 10 to 30 mL/min; 2 g q 4 h for CrCl 30 to 60 mL/min. Peritoneal dialysis: 3.1 g q 12 h. Hemodialysis: 3.1 g load, then 2 g q 12 h and 3.1 g after each dialysis.

ANTIMICROBIALS: Quinolones—2nd Generation

NOTE: As of April 2007, the CDC no longer recommends fluoroquinolones for gonorrhea because of high resistance rates. Fluoroquinolones can cause tendon rupture (rare; risk increased by corticosteroids, age older than 60 yo, or organ transplant), phototoxicity (risk varies among agents), *C. difficile*–associated diarrhea (risk may vary among agents), QT interval prolongation (risk varies among agents; see QT drugs table), exacerbation of myasthenia gravis, CNS toxicity, peripheral neuropathy (rare), and hypersensitivity. Important quinolone drug interactions with antacids, iron, zinc, magnesium, sucralfate, buffered didanosine, caffeine, cyclosporine, phenytoin, anticoagulants, theophylline, etc.

CIPROFLOXACIN (*Cipro, Cipro XR*) ▶LK ♀C but teratogenicity unlikely ▶?+ $

WARNING – Tendon rupture (rare; risk increased by corticosteroids, age older than 60 yo, or organ transplant). Advise patients to stop fluoroquinolone, rest affected area, and seek medical advice for tendon swelling, pain, or inflammation.

ADULT – UTI: 250 to 500 mg PO two times per day or 200 to 400 mg IV q 12 h. Simple UTI: 250 mg PO two times per day for 3 days or Cipro XR 500 mg PO once daily for 3 days. Cipro XR for complicated UTI, uncomplicated pyelonephritis: 1000 mg PO once daily for 7 to 14 days. Pneumonia, skin, bone and joint infections: 400 mg IV q 8 to 12 h or 500 to 750 mg PO two times per day. Treat bone and joint infections for 4 to 6 weeks. Acute sinusitis: 500 mg PO two times per day for 10 days. Chronic bacterial prostatitis: 500 mg PO two times per day for 28 days. Infectious diarrhea: 500 mg PO two times per day for 5 to 7 days. Typhoid fever: 500 mg PO two times per day for 10 days. Nosocomial pneumonia: 400 mg IV q 8 h. Complicated intra-abdominal infection (with metronidazole): 400 mg IV q 12 h, then 500 mg PO two times per day. Empiric therapy of febrile neutropenia: 400 mg IV q 8 h with piperacillin. Bioterrorism anthrax. Inhalation or severe cutaneous anthrax treatment: 400 mg IV q 12 h with at least 1 other drug initially, then monotherapy with 500 mg PO two times per day to complete 60 days. Monotherapy for postexposure prophylaxis or treatment of less severe cutaneous anthrax: 500 mg PO two times per day for 60 days. See www.idsociety.org/Anthrax/ for more info.

PEDS – Safety and efficacy not established for most indications in children; arthropathy in juvenile animals. Still limited data, but case series of treated children show no evidence of arthropathy other than transient large-joint arthralgias. Musculoskeletal adverse events reported with ciprofloxacin treatment of complicated UTI in peds patients were mild to moderate in severity and resolved within 1 month after treatment. Complicated UTI, pyelonephritis, 1 to 17 yo: 6 to 10 mg/kg IV q 8 h, then 10 to 20 mg/kg PO q 12 h. Max of 400 mg IV or 750 mg PO per dose even for peds patients wt greater than 51 kg. Bioterrorism anthrax.

(cont.)

QUINOLONES—GENERAL ANTIMICROBIAL SPECTRUM

1st generation	1st generation quinolones are no longer available
2nd generation	Gram-negative (including *Pseudomonas*); *S. aureus* (but not MRSA or *pneumococcus*); some atypicals
3rd generation	Gram-negative (including *Pseudomonas*); Gram-positive, including *Pneumococcus* and *S aureus* (but not MRSA); expanded atypical coverage
4th generation	same as 3rd generation plus enhanced coverage of *Pneumococcus*, decreased *Pseudomonas activity*

CIPROFLOXACIN (*cont.*)

Treatment of inhalation anthrax, severe cutaneous anthrax, or cutaneous anthrax in age younger than 2 yo: 10 to 15 mg/kg IV q 12 h with at least 1 other drug initially, then monotherapy with 10 to 15 mg/kg up to 500 mg PO two times per day to complete 60 days. Monotherapy for postexposure prophylaxis or less severe cutaneous anthrax treatment: 10 to 15 mg/kg up to 500 mg PO two times per day for 60 days. See www.idsociety.org/Anthrax/ for more info.

UNAPPROVED ADULT – Acute uncomplicated pyelonephritis: 500 mg PO two times per day for 7 days. Chancroid: 500 mg PO two times per day for 3 days. Prophylaxis, high-risk GU surgery: 500 mg PO or 400 mg IV. Prophylaxis, invasive meningococcal disease: 500 mg PO single dose. Traveler's diarrhea (treatment preferred over prophylaxis). Treatment: 500 mg PO two times per day for 1 to 3 days or 750 mg PO single dose. Prophylaxis: 500 mg PO daily for no more than 3 weeks. Infectious diarrhea: 500 mg PO two times per day for 1 to 3 days for *Shigella,* for 5 to 7 days for non-typhi *Salmonella* (usually not treated). Malignant otitis externa: 400 mg IV or 750 mg PO q 12 h. TB (2nd-line treatment): 750 to 1500 mg/day IV/PO. *Salmonella* gastroenteritis in HIV infection: 500 to 750 mg PO two times per day (400 mg IV q 12 h) for 7 to 14 days if CD4 count 200 or greater, for 2 to 6 weeks if CD4 count less than 200. *Campylobacter* in HIV infection: 500 mg PO two times per day for 7 days for mild to moderate disease, at least 14 days for bacteremia.

UNAPPROVED PEDS – Usual dose: 20 to 30 mg/kg/day IV/PO divided q 12 h (max 1.5 g/day PO; max 800 mg/day IV). Acute pulmonary exacerbation of cystic fibrosis: 10 mg/kg/dose IV q 8 h for 7 days, then 20 mg/kg/dose PO q 12 h to complete 10 to 21 days of treatment. TB (2nd-line treatment): 10 to 15 mg/kg PO two times per day (max: 1.5 g/day). Cholera: 20 mg/kg up to 750 mg PO single dose for age 2 to 15 yo. Arthropathy in juvenile animals. Still limited data, but case series of treated children show no evidence of arthropathy other than transient large-joint arthralgias.

FORMS – Generic/Trade: Tabs 100, 250, 500, 750 mg. Extended-release tabs 500, 1000 mg.

NOTES – Crystalluria if alkaline urine. Ciprofloxacin inhibits CYP1A2, an enzyme that metabolizes caffeine, clozapine, tacrine, theophylline, and warfarin. Give ciprofloxacin immediate-release or Cipro XR 2 h before or 6 h after antacids, iron, sucralfate, calcium, zinc, buffered didanosine, or other highly buffered drugs. Can give with meals containing dairy products, but not with yogurt, milk, or calcium-fortified fruit juice alone. Do not give Cipro XR within 2 h of calcium doses greater than 800 mg. Watch for hypoglycemia with glyburide. Do not give oral susp in feeding or nasogastric tube. Cipro XR and immediate-release tabs are not interchangeable. Do not split, crush, or chew Cipro XR. In patients with complicated UTI or acute pyelonephritis and CrCl less than 30 mL/min, reduce dose of Cipro XR to 500 mg daily. Reduce dose of immediate-release ciprofloxacin in adults with renal dysfunction: 250 to 500 mg PO q 24 h given after dialysis session for hemodialysis/peritoneal dialysis; 250 to 500 mg PO q 18 h or 200 to 400 mg IV q 18 to 24 h for CrCl 5 to 29 mL/min; 250 to 500 mg PO q 12 h for CrCl 30 to 50 mL/min.

NORFLOXACIN (***Noroxin***) ▶LK ♀C ▶? $

WARNING – Tendon rupture (rare; risk increased by corticosteroids, age older than 60 yo, or organ transplant). Advise patients to stop fluoroquinolone, rest affected area, and seek medical advice for tendon swelling, pain, or inflammation.

ADULT – Simple UTI due to *E. coli, K. pneumoniae, P. mirabilis*: 400 mg PO two times per day for 3 days. UTI due to other organisms: 400 mg PO two times per day for 7 to 10 days. Complicated UTI: 400 mg PO two times per day for 10 to 21 days. Acute/chronic prostatitis: 400 mg PO two times per day for 28 days. Take on an empty stomach.

PEDS – Safety and efficacy not established in children; arthropathy in juvenile animals.

UNAPPROVED ADULT – Traveler's diarrhea (treatment preferred over prophylaxis). Treatment: 400 mg PO two times per day for 1 to 3 days. Prophylaxis: 400 mg PO daily for up to 3 weeks. Infectious diarrhea: 400 mg PO two times per day for 5 to 7 days for non-typhi Salmonella (usually not treated), for 1 to 3 days for *Shigella*. Prevention of spontaneous bacterial peritonitis: 400 mg PO once daily. Take on an empty stomach.

FORMS – Trade only: Tabs 400 mg.

NOTES – Crystalluria with high doses. Maintain adequate hydration. Norfloxacin inhibits CYP1A2, an enzyme that metabolizes caffeine, clozapine, ropinirole, tacrine, theophylline, tizanidine, and warfarin. Increased INR with warfarin. Do not take with dairy products. Give antacids, zinc, iron, sucralfate, multivitamins, or buffered didanosine 2 h

(cont.)

NORFLOXACIN (*cont.*)

before and after norfloxacin. Reduce dose in renal dysfunction: 400 mg PO daily for CrCl less than 30 mL/min.

OFLOXACIN (*Floxin*) ▶LK ♀C ▶?+ $$$

WARNING – Tendon rupture (rare; risk increased by corticosteroids, age older than 60 yo, or organ transplant). Advise patients to stop fluoroquinolone, rest affected area, and seek medical advice for tendon swelling, pain, or inflammation.

ADULT – Acute exacerbation of chronic bronchitis, community-acquired pneumonia, skin infections: 400 mg PO two times per day for 10 days. Simple UTI due to E. coli, K. pneumoniae: 200 mg PO two times per day for 3 days. Simple UTI due to other organisms: 200 mg PO two times per day for 7 days. Complicated UTI: 200 mg PO two times per day for 10 days. Chronic bacterial prostatitis: 300 mg PO two times per day for 6 weeks.

PEDS – Safety and efficacy not established in children; arthropathy in juvenile animals.

UNAPPROVED ADULT – Epididymitis: 300 mg PO two times per day for 10 days. Traveler's diarrhea, treatment: 300 mg PO two times per day for 1 to 3 days. Infectious diarrhea: 300 mg PO two times per day for 1 to 3 days for *Shigella,* 5 to 7 days for non-typhi *Salmonella* (usually not treated). TB (2nd-line treatment): 600 to 800 mg PO daily.

FORMS – Generic/Trade: Tabs 200, 300, 400 mg.

NOTES – May prolong QT interval; avoid using in proarrhythmic conditions or with drugs that prolong QT interval, including Class 1A and Class III antiarrhythmics. Give antacids, iron, sucralfate, multivitamins containing zinc, buffered didanosine 2 h before or after ofloxacin. May decrease metabolism of theophylline, increase INR with warfarin. Monitor glucose with antidiabetic agents. Can cause false positive on opiate urine screening immunoassay; may need confirmation test. Reduce dose in renal dysfunction: 50% of usual dose q 24 h for CrCl less than 20 mL/min; usual dose given q 24 h for CrCl 20 to 50 mL/min.

ANTIMICROBIALS: Quinolones—3rd Generation

NOTE: As of April 2007, the CDC no longer recommends fluoroquinolones for gonorrhea because of high resistance rates. Can cause tendon rupture (rare; risk increased by corticosteroids, age older than 60 yo, or organ transplant), *C. difficile*–associated diarrhea (risk may vary among agents), phototoxicity (risk varies among agents), CNS toxicity, peripheral neuropathy (rare), hypersensitivity, and QT interval prolongation (risk varies among agents; see QT drugs table). Avoid using in proarrhythmic conditions or with drugs that prolong QT including Class 1A and Class III antiarrhythmics. Important quinolone drug interactions with antacids, iron, zinc, magnesium, sucralfate, caffeine, cyclosporine, phenytoin, anticoagulants, theophylline, etc.

LEVOFLOXACIN (*Levaquin*) ▶KL ♀C ▶? $

WARNING – Tendon rupture (rare; risk increased by corticosteroids, age older than 60 yo, or organ transplant). Advise patients to stop fluoroquinolone, rest affected area, and seek medical advice for tendon swelling, pain, or inflammation.

ADULT – IV and PO doses are the same. Community-acquired pneumonia: 750 mg once daily for 5 days or 500 mg once daily for 7 to 14 days. Nosocomial pneumonia: 750 mg once daily for 7 to 14 days. Acute sinusitis: 750 mg once daily for 5 days or 500 mg once daily for 10 to 14 days. See table for management of acute sinusitis. Acute exacerbation of chronic bronchitis: 500 mg once daily for 7 days. Skin infections: 500 to 750 mg once daily for 7 to 14 days. Complicated UTI or pyelonephritis: 250 mg once daily for 10 days or 750 mg once daily for 5 days. Simple UTI: 250 mg once daily for 3 days. Chronic bacterial prostatitis: 500 mg once daily for 28 days. Postexposure prophylaxis for inhalation anthrax: 500 mg PO once daily for 60 days. See www.idsociety.org/Anthrax/ for more info. Plague: 500 mg once daily for 10 to 14 days. See www.idsociety.org/Plague/ for more info. Infuse IV doses over 60 min (250 to 500 mg) to 90 min (750 mg). Take oral soln on empty stomach.

PEDS – IV and PO doses are the same. Postexposure prophylaxis for inhalation anthrax, age 6 mo and older: Treat for 60 days with 8 mg/kg (max 250 mg/dose) two times per day if wt less than 50 kg; 500 mg once daily if wt greater than 50 kg. See www.idsociety.org/Anthrax for more info. Plague, age 6 mo and older: Treat for 10 to 14 days with 8 mg/kg (max 250 mg/dose) two times per day if wt less than 50 kg; 500 mg once daily if wt greater than 50 kg. See www.idsociety.org/

(cont.)

LEVOFLOXACIN (*cont.*)

Plague for more info. Musculoskeletal disorders (arthralgia, arthritis, tendinopathy, gait abnormality) reported in children; safety for treatment duration more than 14 days not established. Infuse IV doses over 60 min (250 to 500 mg). Take oral soln on empty stomach.

UNAPPROVED ADULT – Legionnaires' disease: 1 g IV/PO on 1st day, then 500 mg IV/PO once daily. Chlamydia, epididymitis: See STD table. TB (2nd-line treatment): 500 to 1000 mg/day IV/PO. Traveler's diarrhea, treatment: 500 mg PO once daily for 1 to 3 days. Infectious diarrhea: 500 mg PO once daily for 1 to 3 days for *Shigella*, for 5 to 7 days for *Salmonella*.

UNAPPROVED PEDS – IV and PO doses are the same. See table for management of acute sinusitis. Community-acquired pneumonia: 16 to 20 mg/kg/day divided two times per day for age 6 mo to 5 yo; 8 to 10 mg/kg/day once daily (max 750 mg once daily) for age 5 to 16 yo. Atypical pneumonia in adolescents with skeletal maturity: 500 mg PO once daily. Musculoskeletal disorders (arthralgia, arthritis, tendinopathy, gait abnormality) reported in children; safety for treatment duration more than 14 days not established. Infuse IV doses over 60 min (250 to 500 mg).

FORMS – Generic/Trade: Tabs 250, 500, 750 mg, Oral soln 25 mg/mL. Trade only: Leva-Pak: #5, 750 mg tabs.

NOTES – Give Mg/Al antacids, iron, sucralfate, multivitamins containing zinc, buffered didanosine 2 h before and after PO levofloxacin. Increased INR with warfarin. Monitor glucose with antidiabetic agents. Can cause false positive on opiate urine screening immunoassay; may need confirmation test. Dosage adjustment in renal dysfunction is based on dose used in normal renal function. For dose of 750 mg in normal renal function: Give 750 mg q 48 h for CrCl 20 to 49 mL/min; give 750 mg load, then 500 mg q 48 h for CrCl 10 to 19 mL/min, hemodialysis or CAPD. For dose of 500 mg in normal renal function: Give 500 mg load, then 250 mg q 24 h for CrCl 20 to 49 mL/min; give 500 mg load, then 250 mg q 48 h for CrCl 10 to 19 mL/min, hemodialysis or CAPD. For dose of 250 mg in normal renal function: Give 250 mg q 48 h for CrCl 10 to 19 mL/min. Dosage adjustment not necessary for uncomplicated UTI if CrCl is 10 to 19 mL/min.

ANTIMICROBIALS: Quinolones—4th Generation

NOTE: As of April 2007, the CDC no longer recommends fluoroquinolones for gonorrhea because of high resistance rates. Can cause tendon rupture (rare; risk increased by corticosteroids, age older than 60 yo, or organ transplant), C difficile-associated diarrhea (risk may vary among agents), phototoxicity (risk varies among agents), CNS toxicity, peripheral neuropathy (rare), hypersensitivity, and QT interval prolongation (risk varies among agents; see QT drugs table). Avoid using in proarrhythmic conditions or with drugs that prolong QT interval, including Class 1A and Class III antiarrhythmics. Important quinolone drug interactions with antacids, iron, zinc, magnesium, sucralfate, cimetidine, caffeine, cyclosporine, phenytoin, anticoagulants, theophylline, etc. Monitor INR with warfarin.

GEMIFLOXACIN (*Factive*) ▶Feces, K ♀C ▶– $$$$

WARNING – Tendon rupture (rare; risk increased by corticosteroids, age older than 60 yo, or organ transplant). Advise patients to stop fluoroquinolone, rest affected area, and seek medical advice for tendon swelling, pain, or inflammation.

ADULT – Acute exacerbation of chronic bronchitis: 320 mg PO daily for 5 days. Community-acquired pneumonia: 320 mg PO daily for 5 to 7 days (for 7 days for multidrug-resistant *S. pneumoniae*).

PEDS – Safety and efficacy not established in children; arthropathy in juvenile animals.

FORMS – Trade only: Tabs 320 mg.

NOTES – Maintain fluid intake to prevent crystalluria. Give 2 h before or 3 h after Al/Mg antacids, iron, multivitamins with zinc, buffered didanosine. Give at least 2 h before sucralfate. May increase INR with warfarin. Discontinue if rash develops. Reduce dose for CrCl 40 mL/min or less, hemodialysis, or CAPD: 160 mg PO daily.

MOXIFLOXACIN (*Avelox*) ▶LK ♀C ▶– $$$

WARNING – Tendon rupture (rare; risk increased by corticosteroids, age older than 60 yo, or organ transplant). Advise patients to stop fluoroquinolone, rest affected area, and seek medical advice for tendon swelling, pain, or inflammation.

ADULT – Chronic bronchitis exacerbation: 400 mg PO/IV daily for 5 days. Complicated intra-abdominal infection: (given IV initially) 400 mg PO/IV daily for 5 to 14 days. Community-acquired pneumonia, including penicillin-resistant *S. pneumoniae*: 400 mg PO/IV daily

(cont.)

MOXIFLOXACIN (*cont.*)

for 7 to 14 days. Acute sinusitis: 400 mg PO/IV daily for 10 days. See table for management of acute sinusitis. Uncomplicated skin infections: 400 mg PO/IV daily for 7 days. Complicated skin infections: 400 mg PO/IV daily for 7 to 21 days.

PEDS – Safety and efficacy not established in children; arthropathy in juvenile animals.

UNAPPROVED ADULT – TB (2nd-line treatment): 400 mg IV/PO daily.

UNAPPROVED PEDS – Atypical pneumonia in adolescents with skeletal maturity: 400 mg PO once daily. Arthropathy in juvenile animals.

FORMS – Trade only: Tabs 400 mg.

NOTES – Can prolong the QT interval and cause torsades. Avoid if QT interval prolonged, uncorrected hypokalemia or hypomagnesemia, coadministration of class IA or III antiarrhythmic drugs. Do not exceed recommended IV dose or infusion rate due to QT prolongation risk. Contraindicated with ziprasidone. Give tabs at least 4 h before or 8 h after Mg/Al antacids, iron, multivitamins with zinc, sucralfate, buffered didanosine. Dosage adjustment not required for hepatic insufficiency.

ANTIMICROBIALS: Sulfonamides

NOTE: Sulfonamides can cause Stevens-Johnson syndrome, toxic epidermal necrolysis, hepatotoxicity, blood dyscrasias, hemolysis in glucose-6-phosphate dehydrogenase (G6PD) deficiency. Avoid maternal sulfonamides when the breastfed infant is ill, stressed, premature, has hyperbilirubinemia, or has G6PD deficiency.

SULFADIAZINE ▶K ♀C ▶+ $$$$

ADULT – Usual dose: 2 to 4 g PO initially, then 2 to 4 g/day divided into 3 to 6 doses. Secondary prevention of rheumatic fever: 1 g PO daily. Toxoplasmosis treatment: 1 to 1.5 g PO four times per day with pyrimethamine and leucovorin.

PEDS – Not for infants younger than 2 mo, except as adjunct to pyrimethamine for congenital toxoplasmosis. Usual dose: Give 75 mg/kg PO initially, then 150 mg/kg/day up to 6 g/day divided into 4 to 6 doses. Secondary prevention of rheumatic fever, for wt 27 kg or less: 500 mg PO daily. Use adult dose for wt greater than 27 kg.

UNAPPROVED ADULT – CNS toxoplasmosis in AIDS. Acute therapy: For wt less than 60 kg give pyrimethamine 200 mg PO for first dose, then 50 mg PO once daily with sulfadiazine 1000 mg PO q 6 h and leucovorin 10 to 25 mg (up to 50 mg) PO once daily. For wt 60 kg or greater give pyrimethamine 200 mg PO for first dose, then 75 mg PO once daily with sulfadiazine 1500 mg PO q 6 h and leucovorin 10 to 25 mg PO once daily (up to 50 mg). Secondary prevention: Pyrimethamine 25 to 50 mg PO once daily with sulfadiazine 2000 to 4000 mg/day PO divided two to four times per day and leucovorin 10 to 25 mg PO once daily.

UNAPPROVED PEDS – Not for age younger than 2 mo, except as adjunct to pyrimethamine for congenital toxoplasmosis. AAP regimen for toxoplasmosis: 100 to 200 mg/kg/day PO with pyrimethamine and leucovorin (duration varies). Secondary prevention after CNS toxoplasmosis in HIV infection: 85 to 120 mg/kg/day PO divided in 2 to 4 doses with pyrimethamine and leucovorin.

FORMS – Generic only: Tabs 500 mg.

NOTES – Maintain fluid intake to prevent crystalluria and stone formation. Reduce dose in renal insufficiency. May increase INR with warfarin. May increase levels of methotrexate, phenytoin.

TRIMETHOPRIM-SULFAMETHOXAZOLE (***Bactrim, Septra, Sulfatrim,*** **cotrimoxazole**) ▶K ♀C ▶+ $

ADULT – UTI, shigellosis, acute exacerbation of chronic bronchitis: 1 tab PO two times per day, double strength (DS, 160 mg TMP/800 mg SMX). Travelers' diarrhea: 1 DS tab PO two times per day for 5 days. Pneumocystis pneumonia treatment: 15 to 20 mg/kg/day (based on TMP) IV divided q 6 to 8 h or PO divided three times per day for 21 days total; can use 2 DS tabs PO three times per day for mild to moderate infection. Pneumocystis pneumonia prophylaxis: 1 DS tab PO daily.

PEDS – UTI, shigellosis, otitis media: 1 mL/kg/day susp PO divided two times per day (up to 20 mL PO two times per day). Use adult dose for wt greater than 40 kg. Pneumocystis pneumonia treatment: 15 to 20 mg/kg/day (based on TMP) IV divided q 6 to 8 h or 5 mL susp/8 kg/dose PO q 6 h. Pneumocystis pneumonia prophylaxis: 150 mg/m^2/day (based on TMP) PO divided two times per day on 3 consecutive days each week. Do not use in infants younger than 2 mo; may cause kernicterus.

UNAPPROVED ADULT – Uncomplicated cystitis in women: 1 DS tab PO two times per day for

(cont.)

TRIMETHOPRIM-SULFAMETHOXAZOLE (*cont.*)

3 days. Do not use if resistance prevalence is greater than 20% or if used for UTI in previous 3 months. Bacterial prostatitis: 1 DS tab PO two times per day for 10 to 14 days for acute, for 1 to 3 months for chronic. Sinusitis: 1 DS tab PO two times per day for 10 days. *Burkholderia cepacia* pulmonary infection in cystic fibrosis: 5 mg/kg (based on TMP) IV q 6 h. Pneumocystis pneumonia prophylaxis: 1 SS tab PO daily. Primary prevention of toxoplasmosis in AIDS: 1 DS tab PO daily. Pertussis: 1 DS tab PO two times per day for 14 days (2nd line to macrolides). Community-acquired MRSA skin infections: 1 to 2 DS tabs PO two times per day for 5 to 10 days. MRSA osteomyelitis: 4 mg/kg/dose (based on TMP) PO two times per day with rifampin 600 mg PO once daily. Prevention of spontaneous bacterial peritonitis: 1 DS tab PO once daily for 5 days per week.

UNAPPROVED PEDS – Community-acquired MRSA skin infections: 1 to 1.5 mL/kg/day PO divided two times per day for 5 to 10 days. Pertussis: 1 mL/kg/day PO divided two times per day for 14 days (2nd line to macrolides).

FORMS – Generic/Trade: Tabs 80 mg TMP/400 mg SMX (SS), 160 mg TMP/800 mg SMX (DS). Susp 40 mg TMP/200 mg SMX per 5 mL. 20 mL susp = 2 SS tabs = 1 DS tab.

NOTES – Not effective for streptococcal pharyngitis. No activity against penicillin-nonsusceptible pneumococci. Bone marrow depression with high IV doses. Significantly increased INR with warfarin; avoid concomitant use if possible. Increases levels of methotrexate, phenytoin. Rifampin reduces TMP-SMX levels. Can cause hyperkalemia (risk increased by high doses of trimethoprim, renal impairment, other drugs that cause hyperkalemia). AAP recommends 5 to 7 days of therapy for children age 6 yo or older with nonsevere otitis media, and 10 days for younger children and those with severe disease. Dosing in renal dysfunction: Use 50% of usual dose for CrCl 15 to 30 mL/min. Do not use for CrCl less than 15 mL/min.

ANTIMICROBIALS: Tetracyclines

NOTE: Tetracyclines can cause photosensitivity and pseudotumor cerebri (avoid with isotretinoin which is also linked to pseudotumor cerebri). May decrease efficacy of oral contraceptives. Increased INR with warfarin. May increase risk of ergotism with ergot alkaloids. Use tetracyclines with caution in renal dysfunction; doxycycline preferred.

DEMECLOCYCLINE (*Declomycin*) ▶K, feces ♀D ▶?+ $$$$

ADULT – Usual dose: 150 mg PO four times per day or 300 mg PO two times per day on empty stomach.

PEDS – Avoid in age younger than 8 yo due to teeth staining. Usual dose: 6.6 to 13.2 mg/kg/day PO given in 2 to 4 divided doses on empty stomach.

UNAPPROVED ADULT – SIADH: 600 to 1200 mg/day PO given in 3 to 4 divided doses.

FORMS – Generic/Trade: Tabs 150, 300 mg.

NOTES – Can cause diabetes insipidus, high risk of photosensitivity. Absorption impaired by iron, calcium, Al/Mg antacids. Take with fluids (not milk) to decrease esophageal irritation. SIADH onset of action occurs within 5 to 14 days; do not increase dose more frequently than q 3 to 4 days.

DOXYCYCLINE (*Doryx, Monodox, Oracea, Periostat, Vibramycin, Vibra-Tabs,* ♣ *Doxycin*) ▶LK ♀D ▶?+ $

ADULT – Usual dose: 100 mg PO two times per day on 1st day, then 100 mg/day PO daily or divided two times per day. Severe infections: 100 mg PO two times per day. Chlamydia, nongonococcal urethritis: 100 mg PO two times per day for 7 days. Acne vulgaris: Up to 100 mg PO two times per day. Community-acquired MRSA skin infections: 100 mg PO two times per day for 5 to 10 days. Periostat for periodontitis: 20 mg PO two times per day 1 h before breakfast and dinner. Oracea for inflammatory rosacea (papules and pustules): 40 mg PO once q am on empty stomach. Cholera: 300 mg PO single dose. Primary, secondary, early latent syphilis if penicillin-allergic: 100 mg PO two times per day for 14 days. Late latent or tertiary syphilis if penicillin-allergic: 100 mg PO two times per day for 4 weeks. Not for neurosyphilis. Malaria prophylaxis: 100 mg PO daily starting 1 to 2 days before exposure until 4 weeks after. IV: 200 mg on 1st day in 1 to 2 infusions, then 100 to 200 mg/day in 1 to 2 infusions. Bioterrorism anthrax: 100 mg two times per day for 60 days. Use IV with at least 1 other drug for initial treatment of inhalation or severe cutaneous anthrax. PO monotherapy for less severe cutaneous

(cont.)

DOXYCYCLINE (*cont.*)

anthrax or postexposure prophylaxis. See www.idsociety.org/Anthrax/ for more info.

PEDS – Avoid in age younger than 8 yo due to teeth staining. Usual dose: 4.4 mg/kg/day PO divided two times per day on 1st day, then 2.2 to 4.4 mg/kg/day PO divided daily or two times per day for wt 45 kg or less. Use adult dose for wt greater than 45 kg. Malaria prophylaxis: 2 mg/kg/day up to 100 mg PO daily starting 1 to 2 days before exposure until 4 weeks after. Most PO and IV doses are equivalent. Bioterrorism anthrax: 100 mg two times per day for age older than 8 yo and wt greater than 45 kg; 2.2 mg/kg two times per day for age older than 8 yo and wt 45 kg or less, or age 8 yo or younger. Treat for 60 days. Use IV with at least 1 other drug for initial treatment of inhalation anthrax, severe cutaneous anthrax, or cutaneous anthrax in age younger than 2 yo. PO monotherapy for less severe cutaneous anthrax and postexposure prophylaxis. See www.idsociety.org/Anthrax/ for more info.

UNAPPROVED ADULT – See table for management of acute sinusitis. See STD table for granuloma inguinale, lymphogranuloma venereum, pelvic inflammatory disease treatment. Lyme disease: 100 mg PO two times per day for 14 days for early disease, for 28 days for Lyme arthritis. Prevention of Lyme disease in highly endemic area, with deer tick attachment at least 48 h: 200 mg PO single dose with food within 72 h of tick bite. Ehrlichiosis: 100 mg IV/PO two times per day for 7 to 14 days. Malaria, co-therapy with quinine/quinidine: 100 mg IV/PO two times per day for 7 days. Lymphatic filariasis: 100 mg PO two times per day for 8 weeks.

UNAPPROVED PEDS – Community-acquired MRSA skin infections: 2 mg/kg/dose PO q 12 h for wt 45 kg or less; 100 mg PO two times per day for wt greater than 45 kg. Treat for 5 to 10 days. Avoid in age younger than 8 yo due to teeth staining. Cholera: 2 to 4 mg/kg PO single dose for all ages.

FORMS – Generic/Trade: Tabs 20, 75, 100 mg. Caps 50, 100 mg. Generic only: Caps 75, 150 mg. Tabs 50, 150 mg. Susp 25 mg/5 mL (60 mL). Trade only: (Vibramycin) Syrup 50 mg/5 mL (480 mL). Delayed-release tabs (Doryx $$$$$): Generic/Trade: 75, 100, 150 mg. Delayed-release caps (Oracea $$$$$): Generic/Trade: 40 mg.

NOTES – Photosensitivity, pseudotumor cerebri, increased BUN, painful IV infusion. Do not use Oracea for treatment of infections. Do not give antacids or calcium supplements within 2 h of doxycycline. Barbiturates, carbamazepine, rifampin, and phenytoin may decrease doxycycline levels. Take with fluids to decrease esophageal irritation; can take with food/milk. Can break Doryx tabs and give immediately in a spoonful of applesauce. Do not crush or chew delayed-release pellets in tab. Maternal antimalarial prophylaxis does not harm breastfed infant or protect infant from malaria.

MINOCYCLINE (***Minocin, Dynacin, Solodyn,* ♣ *Enca***) ▶LK ♀D ▶?+ $$

ADULT – Usual dose: 200 mg IV/PO 1st dose, then 100 mg q 12 h. IV and PO doses are the same. Not more than 400 mg/day IV. Community-acquired MRSA skin infections: 200 mg PO first dose, then 100 mg PO two times per day for 5 to 10 days. Solodyn ($$$$$) for inflammatory nonnodular moderate to severe acne: 1 mg/kg PO once daily. Dose is 45 mg for wt 45 to 54 kg, 65 mg for wt 55 to 77 kg, 90 mg for 78 to 102 kg, 115 mg for wt 103 to 125 kg, 135 mg for 126 to 136 kg.

PEDS – Avoid in age younger than 8 yo due to teeth staining. Usual dose: 4 mg/kg PO 1st dose, then 2 mg/kg two times per day. Community-acquired MRSA skin infection: 4 mg/kg PO first dose, then 2 mg/kg/dose PO two times per day for 5 to 10 days. Do not exceed adult dose. IV and PO doses are the same. Solodyn ($$$$$) for inflammatory nonnodular moderate to severe acne: Give PO once daily to age 12 yo or older at dose of 45 mg for wt 45 to 54 kg, 65 mg for wt 55 to 77 kg, 90 mg for 78 to 102 kg, 115 mg for wt 103 to 125 kg, 135 mg for 126 to 136 kg.

UNAPPROVED ADULT – Acne vulgaris (traditional dosing, not for Solodyn): 50 mg PO two times per day. RA: 100 mg PO two times per day.

FORMS – Generic/Trade: Caps, Tabs 50, 75, 100 mg. Tabs, extended-release (Solodyn) 45, 90, 135 mg. Trade only: Tabs, extended-release (Solodyn) 65, 115 mg.

NOTES – Dizziness, hepatotoxicity, lupus. Do not use Solodyn for treatment of infections. Do not give antacids or calcium supplements within 2 h of minocycline. Take with fluids (not milk) to decrease esophageal irritation.

TETRACYCLINE (***Sumycin***) ▶LK ♀D ▶?+ $

ADULT – Usual dose: 250 to 500 mg PO four times per day on empty stomach. *H. pylori*: See table in GI section. Primary, secondary, early latent syphilis if penicillin-allergic: 500 mg PO four times per day for 14 days. Late latent syphilis if penicillin-allergic: 500 mg PO four times per day for 28 days.

(cont.)

TETRACYCLINE (*cont.*)

PEDS — Avoid in children younger than 8 yo due to teeth staining. Usual dose: 25 to 50 mg/kg/day PO divided in 2 to 4 doses on empty stomach.
UNAPPROVED ADULT — Malaria, cotherapy with quinine: 250 mg PO four times per day for 7 days.
UNAPPROVED PEDS — Avoid in children younger than 8 yo due to teeth staining. Malaria, cotherapy with quinine: 25 mg/kg/day PO divided four times per day for 7 days.
FORMS — Generic only: Caps 250, 500 mg.
NOTES — Increased BUN/hepatotoxicity in patients with renal dysfunction. Do not give antacids or calcium supplements within 2 h of tetracycline. Take with fluids (not milk) to decrease esophageal irritation.

ANTIMICROBIALS: Other Antimicrobials

AZTREONAM (*Azactam, Cayston*) ▸K ♀B ▸+ $$$$$

ADULT — UTI: 500 mg to 1 g IM/IV q 8 to 12 h. Pneumonia, sepsis, skin, intra-abdominal, gynecologic: Moderate infections, 1 to 2 g IM/IV q 8 to 12 h. *P. aeruginosa* or severe infections, 2 g IV q 6 to 8 h. Use IV route for doses greater than 1 g. Cystic fibrosis respiratory symptoms: 1 vial Cayston nebulized three times per day for 28 days, followed by cycle of 28 days off treatment.
PEDS — Serious gram-negative infections, usual dose: 30 mg/kg/dose IV q 6 to 8 h. Cystic fibrosis respiratory symptoms, age 7 yo and older: 1 vial Cayston nebulized three times per day for 28 days, followed by cycle of 28 days off treatment.
UNAPPROVED ADULT — Meningitis: 2 g IV q 6 to 8 h.
UNAPPROVED PEDS — *P. aeruginosa* pulmonary infection in cystic fibrosis: 50 mg/kg/dose IV q 6 to 8 h.
FORMS — Trade only: 75 mg/vial with diluent for inhalation (Cayston).
NOTES — Dosing in adults with renal dysfunction: 1 to 2 g IV load, then 50% of usual dose for CrCl 10 to 30 mL/min. 0.5 to 2 g IV load, then 25% of usual dose for CrCl less than 10 mL/min. For life-threatening infections, also give 12.5% of initial dose after each hemodialysis. Cayston: Use bronchodilator before each dose (short-acting bronchodilator 15 min to 4 h before or long-acting bronchodilator 30 min to 12 h before). Give immediately after reconstitution only with Altera nebulizer. Order of administration is bronchodilator, mucolytic, then Cayston. Stable at room temperature for 28 days.

CHLORAMPHENICOL ▸LK ♀C ▸– $$$$$

WARNING — Serious and fatal blood dyscrasias. Dose-dependent bone marrow suppression common.
ADULT — Typhoid fever, rickettsial infections: 50 mg/kg/day IV divided q 6 h. Up to 75 to 100 mg/kg/day IV for serious infections untreatable with other agents.
PEDS — Severe infections including meningitis: 50 to 100 mg/kg/day IV divided q 6 h. AAP recommends 75 to 100 mg/kg/day for invasive pneumococcal infections only in patients with life-threatening beta-lactam allergy.
NOTES — Monitor CBC q 2 days. Monitor serum levels. Therapeutic peak: 10 to 20 mcg/mL. Trough: 5 to 10 mcg/mL. Use cautiously in acute intermittent porphyria/G6PD deficiency. Gray baby syndrome in preemies and newborns. Barbiturates, rifampin decrease chloramphenicol levels. Chloramphenicol increases barbiturate, phenytoin levels and may increase INR with warfarin. Dosing in adults with hepatic dysfunction: 1 g IV load, then 500 mg q 6 h.

CLINDAMYCIN (*Cleocin,* ♣*Dalacin C*) ▸L ♀B ▸?+ $$$

WARNING — Can cause *C. difficile*-associated diarrhea.
ADULT — Serious anaerobic, streptococcal, staph infections: 600 to 900 mg IV q 8 h or 150 to 450 mg PO four times per day. Community-acquired MRSA skin infections: 300 to 450 mg PO three times per day for 5 to 10 days. Complicated MRSA skin infection: 600 mg IV/PO q 8 h for 7 to 14 days. MRSA pneumonia: 600 mg IV/PO q 8 h for 7 to 21 days. MRSA osteomyelitis: 600 mg IV/PO q 8 h. See tables for prophylaxis of bacterial endocardits and treatment of STDs (pelvic inflammatory disease).
PEDS — Serious anaerobic, streptococcal, *Staph* infections: 20 to 40 mg/kg/day IV divided q 6 to 8 h or 8 to 20 mg/kg/day (as caps) PO divided three to four times per day or 8 to 25 mg/kg/day (as palmitate oral soln) PO divided three to four times per day. MRSA pneumonia, osteomyelitis, or complicated skin infection: 40 mg/kg/day IV divided q 6 to 8 h. Do not use doses less than 37.5 mg of oral soln PO three times per day for children with

(cont.)

CLINDAMYCIN (*cont.*)

wt less than 11 kg. Infants age younger than 1 mo: 15 to 20 mg/kg/day IV divided three to four times per day. See table for prophylaxis of bacterial endocarditis.

UNAPPROVED ADULT – Bacterial vaginosis: 300 mg PO two times per day for 7 days. Oral/dental infection: 300 mg PO four times per day. Prevention of perinatal group B streptococcal disease: 900 mg IV to mother q 8 h until delivery. CNS toxoplasmosis, AIDS (with leucovorin, pyrimethamine): Acute treatment 600 mg PO/IV q 6 h; secondary prevention 300 to 450 mg PO q 6 to 8 h. AHA dose for group A streptococcal pharyngitis in penicillin-allergic patients: 20 mg/kg/day (max 1.8 g/day) PO divided three times per day for 10 days. Group A streptococcal pharyngitis, repeated culture-positive episodes: 20 mg/kg/day (max 1.8 g/day) PO divided three times per day for 10 days. Malaria, cotherapy with quinine/quinidine: 10 mg/kg base IV loading dose followed by 5 mg/kg IV q 8 h or 20 mg/kg/day base PO divided three times per day to complete 7 days.

UNAPPROVED PEDS – Community-acquired MRSA skin infections: 10 to 13 mg/kg/dose PO q 6 to 8 h for 5 to 10 days (max 40 mg/kg/day). AHA dose for group A streptococcal pharyngitis in penicillin-allergic patients: 20 mg/kg/day (max 1.8 g/day) PO divided three times per day for 10 days. Group A streptococcal pharyngitis, repeated culture-positive episodes: 20 to 30 mg/kg/day PO divided q 8 h for 10 days. Otitis media: 30 to 40 mg/kg/day PO divided three times per day. Toxoplasmosis, substitute for sulfadiazine in sulfonamide-intolerant children: 5 to 7.5 mg/kg (up to 600 mg/dose) PO/IV q 6 h plus pyrimethamine plus leucovorin. Malaria, cotherapy with quinine/quinidine: 10 mg/kg base IV loading dose followed by 5 mg/kg IV q 8 h or 20 mg/kg/day base PO divided three times per day to complete 7 days.

FORMS – Generic only: Caps 75, 150, 300 mg. Generic/Trade: Oral soln 75 mg/5 mL (100 mL).

NOTES – Not for meningitis. Not more than 600 mg/IM injection site. Avoid if lincomycin hypersensitivity. Consider D-test for MRSA inducible resistance.

COLISTIMETHATE (***Coly-Mycin M Parenteral***) ▸K ♀C ▸? $$$$$

ADULT – Gram-negative infections, especially *P. aeruginosa*: 2.5 to 5 mg/kg/day IM/IV divided q 6 to 12 h or IV continuous infusion. Inject IV slowly over 3 to 5 minutes q 12 h. For continuous infusion, inject half of daily dose over 3 to 5 minutes; give remainder as continuous infusion over 22 to 23 h, starting 1 to 2 h after first injection. Base dose on ideal body wt in obesity.

PEDS – Gram-negative infections, esp. *P. aeruginosa*: 2.5 to 5 mg/kg/day IM/IV divided q 6 to 12 h or IV continuous infusion. Inject IV slowly over 3 to 5 minutes q 12 h. For continuous infusion, inject half of daily dose over 3 to 5 minutes; give remainder as continuous infusion over 22 to 23 h, starting 1 to 2 h after first injection. Base dose on ideal body wt in obesity.

UNAPPROVED ADULT – Cystic fibrosis: Use nebulizer soln promptly after it is made. Storage for longer than 24 h increases the formation of polymyxin E1 which may cause pulmonary toxicity.

NOTES – Each vial contains 150 mg colistin activity. May enhance neuromuscular junction blockade by aminoglycosides, neuromuscular blockers. Can cause transient neurologic symptoms that can be relieved by dosage reduction. Dose-dependent, reversible nephrotoxicity. See prescribing information for dosage adjustment in adults with renal dysfunction.

DAPTOMYCIN (***Cubicin***) ▸K ♀B ▸? $$$$$

ADULT – Complicated skin infections (including MRSA): 4 mg/kg IV once daily for 7 to 14 days. *S. aureus* (including MRSA) bacteremia, including endocarditis: 6 mg/kg IV once daily for at least 2 to 6 weeks. Infuse over 30 min or inject over 2 min.

PEDS – Not approved in children.

UNAPPROVED ADULT – High dose for MRSA bacteremia/endocarditis: 8 to 10 mg/kg IV once daily. Vancomycin-resistant MRSA bacteremia: 10 mg/kg IV once daily in combo with another antibiotic. MRSA osteomyelitis: 6 mg/kg IV once daily.

UNAPPROVED PEDS – MRSA bacteremia/endocarditis: 6 to 10 mg/kg IV once daily. MRSA osteomyelitis: 6 mg/kg IV once daily.

NOTES – May cause myopathy (with doses of 6 mg/kg/day or greater), neuropathy, eosinophilic pneumonia (rare), *C. difficile*–associated diarrhea. Monitor CK levels weekly. Stop if myopathy symptoms and CK more than 5 times upper limit of normal, or no symptoms and CK at least 10 times upper limit of normal. Consider withholding statins during daptomycin treatment. Can falsely elevate PT with certain thromboplastin reagents; minimize effect by drawing PT/INR sample just before daptomycin dose or use another reagent. Not effective for pneumonia (inactivated by

(cont.)

DAPTOMYCIN (*cont.*)

surfactant). Reduce dose in adults with CrCl less than 30 mL/min: 4 mg/kg IV q 48 h for complicated skin infections; 6 mg/kg IV q 48 h for *S. aureus* bacteremia. Give dose after hemodialysis sessions. Efficacy may be reduced in patients with CrCl less than 50 mL/min. Reconstituted soln stable for up to 12 h at room temp or 48 h in refrigerator (combined time in vial and IV bag). Do not use in Readymed elastomeric infusion pump due to leaching of MBT impurity.

FOSFOMYCIN (***Monurol***) ▶K ♀B ▶? $$

ADULT – Simple UTI in women: One 3 g packet PO single dose. Dissolve granules in ½ cup of water.

PEDS – Not approved for age younger than 12 yo.

FORMS – Trade only: 3 g packet of granules.

NOTES – Metoclopramide decreases urinary excretion of fosfomycin. No additional benefit with multiple dosing. Single dose less effective than ciprofloxacin or TMP-SMX; equivalent to nitrofurantoin.

LINEZOLID (***Zyvox***, ✤ ***Zyvoxam***) ▶Oxidation/K ♀C ▶? $$$$$

ADULT – IV and PO doses are the same. Vancomycin-resistant *E. faecium* infections: 600 mg IV/PO q 12 h for 14 to 28 days. Pneumonia, complicated skin infections (including MRSA and diabetic foot): 600 mg IV/PO q 12 h for 10 to 14 days. IV infused over 30 to 120 min.

PEDS – Pneumonia, complicated skin infections (including MRSA): 10 mg/kg (up to 600 mg) IV/PO q 8 h for 10 to 14 days for age younger than 12 yo, 600 mg IV/PO q 12 h for age 12 yo or older. Vancomycin-resistant *E. faecium* infections: 10 mg/kg IV/PO q 8 h (up to 600 mg) for 14 to 28 days for age younger than 12 yo, 600 mg IV/PO q 12 h for age 12 yo or older. Uncomplicated skin infections: 10 mg/kg PO q 8 h for 10 to 14 days for age younger than 5 yo, 10 mg/kg PO q 12 h for age 5 to 11 yo, 600 mg PO q 12 h for age 12 yo or older. Preterm infants (less than 34 weeks gestational age): 10 mg/kg q 12 h, increase to 10 mg/kg q 8 h by 7 days of life. IV infused over 30 to 120 min.

UNAPPROVED ADULT – Community-acquired MRSA skin infection: 600 mg PO two times per day for 5 to 10 days.

UNAPPROVED PEDS – Community-acquired MRSA skin infection: 10 mg/kg (up to 600 mg) PO q 8 h for 5 to 10 days for age younger than 12 yo, 600 mg PO q 12 h for age 12 yo or older.

FORMS – Trade only: Tabs 600 mg. Susp 100 mg/ 5 mL.

NOTES – Myelosuppression. Monitor CBC weekly, especially if more than 2 weeks of therapy, preexisting myelosuppression, other myelosuppressive drugs, or chronic infection treated with other antibiotics. Consider stopping if myelosuppression occurs or worsens. Peripheral and optic neuropathy, primarily in those treated for more than 1 month. Ophthalmic exam recommended for visual changes at any time; monitor visual function in all patients treated for 3 months or longer. In a study comparing linezolid with vancomycin, oxacillin, or dicloxacillin for catheter-related bloodstream infections, mortality was increased in linezolid-treated patients infected only with Gram-negative bacteria. Inhibits MAO; may interact with adrenergic and serotonergic drugs, high-tyramine foods. Limit tyramine to less than 100 mg/meal. Reduce initial dose of dopamine/epinephrine. Serotonin syndrome reported with concomitant administration of serotonergic drugs (SSRIs). Rifampin can reduce linezolid exposure; clinical significance unclear. Hypoglycemia reported in diabetics treated with insulin or oral hypoglycemics. Store susp at room temperature; stable for 21 days. Gently turn bottle over 3 to 5 times before giving a dose; do not shake.

METHENAMINE HIPPURATE (***Hiprex***, ***Urex***) ▶KL ♀C ▶? $$$

ADULT – Long-term suppression of UTI: 1 g PO two times per day.

PEDS – Long-term suppression of UTI: 0.5 to 1 g PO two times per day for 6 to 12 yo, 1 g PO two times per day for older than 12 yo.

FORMS – Generic/Trade: Tab 1 g.

NOTES – Not for UTI treatment. Contraindicated if renal or severe hepatic impairment, severe dehydration. Acidify urine if *Proteus, Pseudomonas* infections. Give 1 to 2 g vitamin C PO q 4 h if urine pH is greater than 5. Avoid sulfonamides, alkalinizing foods and medications.

METRONIDAZOLE (***Flagyl***, ***Flagyl ER***, ✤ ***Florazole ER***) ▶KL ♀B ▶?– $

WARNING – Carcinogenic in animal studies; avoid unnecessary use.

ADULT – Trichomoniasis: Treat patient and sex partners with 2 g PO single dose (may be used in pregnancy per CDC), 250 mg PO three times per day for 7 days, or 375 mg PO two times per day for 7 days. Flagyl ER for bacterial vaginosis: 750 mg PO daily for 7 days on empty stomach. *H. pylori*: See table in GI section.

(cont.)

METRONIDAZOLE (*cont.*)

Anaerobic bacterial infections: Load 1 g or 15 mg/kg IV, then 500 mg or 7.5 mg/kg IV/PO q 6 to 8 h (up to 4 g/day), each IV dose over 1 h. Prophylaxis, colorectal surgery: 15 mg/kg IV completed 1 h preop, then 7.5 mg/kg IV q 6 h for 2 doses. Acute amebic dysentery: 750 mg PO three times per day for 5 to 10 days. Amebic liver abscess: 500 to 750 mg IV/PO three times per day for 10 days.

PEDS – Amebiasis: 35 to 50 mg/kg/day PO (up to 750 mg/dose) divided three times per day for 10 days.

UNAPPROVED ADULT – Bacterial vaginosis: 500 mg PO two times per day for 7 days. Bacterial vaginosis in pregnancy: 500 mg PO two times per day or 250 mg PO three times per day for 7 days. Trichomoniasis (CDC alternative to single dose): 500 mg PO two times per day for 7 days. Pelvic inflammatory disease and recurrent/persistent urethritis: See STD table. *C. difficile*-associated diarrhea, mild to moderate: 500 mg PO three times per day for 10 to 14 days. *C. difficile*-associated diarrhea, severe complicated: 500 mg IV q 8 h with PO/PR vancomycin. See table for management of *C. difficile* infection in adults. Giardia: 250 mg PO three times per day for 5 to 7 days.

UNAPPROVED PEDS – *C. difficile*-associated diarrhea: 30 mg/kg/day PO divided four times per day for 10 to 14 days (not to exceed adult dose). Trichomoniasis: 5 mg/kg PO three times per day (max 2 g/day) for 7 days. Giardia: 15 mg/kg/day PO divided three times per day for 5 to 7 days. Anaerobic bacterial infections: 30 mg/kg/day IV/PO divided q 6 h, each IV dose over 1 h (up to 4 g/day).

FORMS – Generic/Trade: Tabs 250, 500 mg, Caps 375 mg. Trade only: Tabs, extended-release 750 mg.

NOTES – Peripheral neuropathy (chronic use), seizures, encephalopathy, aseptic meningitis, optic neuropathy. Avoid long-term use.

(cont.)

C. DIFFICILE INFECTION IN ADULTS: IDSA/SHEA TREATMENT RECOMMENDATIONS

Severity	Clinical signs	Treatment
Initial episode		
Mild to moderate	Leukocytosis with WBC count 15,000 or lower AND Serum creatinine less than 1.5 times premorbid level	Metronidazole 500 mg PO q 8 h for 10 to 14 days
Severe	Leukocytosis with WBC count 15,000 or higher OR Serum creatinine at least 1.5 times greater than premorbid level	Vancomycin 125 mg PO q 6 h for 10 to 14 days
Severe complicated	Hypotension or shock, ileus, megacolon	Vancomycin 500 mg PO/NG q 6 h plus metronidazole 500 mg IV q 8 h. Consider vancomycin 500 mg/100 mL normal saline retention enema q 6 h if complete ileus.
Recurrent episodes		
First recurrence	—	Same as initial episode, stratified by severity. Use vancomycin if WBC count 15,000 or higher, or serum creatinine is increasing.
Second recurrence	—	Vancomycin taper* and/or pulsed regimen

Adapted from *Infect Control Hosp Epidemiol* 2010; 31(5). Available online at: http://www.idsociety.org.

* Example: Vancomycin 125 mg PO four times per day for 10 to 14 days, then 125 mg two times per day for 7 days, then 125 mg once daily for 7 days, then 125 mg q 2 or 3 days for 2 to 8 weeks.

METRONIDAZOLE (*cont.*)

Disulfiram reaction; avoid alcohol until at least 1 day after treatment with tabs, at least 3 days with caps/Flagyl ER. Do not give within 2 weeks of disulfiram. Interacts with barbiturates, lithium, phenytoin. Increased INR with warfarin. Darkens urine. Give iodoquinol or paromomycin after treatment for amebic dysentery or liver abscess. Can minimize infant exposure by withholding breastfeeding for 12 to 24 h after maternal single dose. Decrease dose in liver dysfunction.

NITROFURANTOIN (***Furadantin, Macrodantin, Macrobid***) ▶KL ♀B ▶+? $

WARNING – Pulmonary fibrosis with prolonged use.

ADULT – Acute uncomplicated cystitis: 50 to 100 mg PO four times per day with food/milk for 7 days or until 3 days after sterile urine. Long-term suppressive therapy: 50 to 100 mg PO at bedtime. Macrobid: 100 mg PO two times per day with food/milk for 7 days.

PEDS – UTI: 5 to 7 mg/kg/day PO divided four times per day for 7 days or until 3 days after sterile urine. Long-term suppressive therapy: Doses as low as 1 mg/kg/day PO divided one to two times per day. Give with food/milk. Macrobid, age older than 12 yo: 100 mg PO two times per day with food/milk for 7 days.

FORMS – Generic/Trade (Macrodantin): Caps 25, 50, 100 mg. Generic/Trade (Macrobid): Caps 100 mg. Generic/Trade (Furadantin): Susp 25 mg/5 mL.

NOTES – Contraindicated if CrCl less than 60 mL/min, pregnancy 38 weeks or longer, infant age younger than 1 mo. Hemolytic anemia in G6PD deficiency (including susceptible infants exposed through breastmilk), hepatotoxicity (monitor LFTs periodically), peripheral neuropathy. May turn urine brown. Do not use for complicated UTI or pyelonephritis.

RIFAXIMIN (***Xifaxan***) ▶Feces, no GI absorption ♀C ▶? $$$

ADULT – Traveler's diarrhea: 200 mg PO three times per day for 3 days. Prevention of recurrent hepatic encephalopathy ($$$$$): 550 mg PO two times per day.

PEDS – Not approved for age younger than 12 yo.

FORMS – Trade only: Tabs 200, 550 mg.

NOTES – Not effective for diarrhea complicated by fever/blood in stool or caused by pathogens other than *E. coli*. Consider switching to another agent if diarrhea persists for 24 to 48 h or worsens. Rifaximin exposure may increase in severe hepatic impairment.

SYNERCID **(quinupristin + dalfopristin)** ▶Bile ♀B ▶? $$$$$

ADULT – Complicated staphylococcal/streptococcal skin infections: 7.5 mg/kg IV q 12 h. Infuse over 1 h.

PEDS – Safety and efficacy not established in children.

UNAPPROVED ADULT – MRSA bacteremia (2nd line): 7.5 mg/kg IV q 8 h.

UNAPPROVED PEDS – Complicated staphylococcal/streptococcal skin infections: 7.5 mg/kg IV q 12 h. Infuse over 1 h.

NOTES – Indication for vancomycin-resistant *E. faecium* infections was removed from labeling because efficacy was not demonstrated in clinical trials. Venous irritation (flush with D5W after peripheral infusion; do not use normal saline/heparin), arthralgias/myalgias, hyperbilirubinemia. Infuse by central venous catheter to avoid dose-related vein irritation. CYP3A4 inhibitor. Increases levels of cyclosporine, midazolam, nifedipine, and others.

TELAVANCIN (***Vibativ***) ▶K ♀C ▶? $$$$$

WARNING – Teratogenic in animal studies. Get serum pregnancy test before use in women of child-bearing potential. Do not use in pregnancy unless potential benefit outweighs risk.

ADULT – Complicated skin infections including MRSA: 10 mg/kg IV once daily for 7 to 14 days. Infuse over 1 h.

PEDS – Safety and efficacy not established in children.

NOTES – QT interval prolongation; do not use in congenital long QT syndrome, uncompensated heart failure, or severe left ventricular hypertrophy. Nephrotoxicity; monitor renal function at least q 2 to 3 days. Efficacy may be decreased in patients with baseline CrCl of 50 mL/min or less. Cyclodextrin vehicle may accumulate in renal dysfunction. Does not interfere with coagulation, but may affect some coagulation tests. To minimize interference, draw blood for INR, aPTT, clotting time, and factor Xa right before next dose of telavancin. Use IV solution within 4 h when stored at room temp. Dosage adjustment for renal dysfunction in adults: 7.5 mg/kg IV q 24 h for CrCl 30 to 50 mL/min; 10 mg/kg q 48 h for CrCl 10 to 29 mL/min.

TELITHROMYCIN (***Ketek***) ▶LK ♀C ▶? $$$

WARNING – Contraindicated in myasthenia gravis due to reports of exacerbation, including fatal acute respiratory depression. Warn patients about exacerbation of myasthenia gravis, hepatotoxicity, visual disturbances, and loss of consciousness.

(cont.)

TELITHROMYCIN (*cont.*)

ADULT – Community-acquired pneumonia: 800 mg PO daily for 7 to 10 days. Indications for acute sinusitis and acute exacerbation of chronic bronchitis removed from labeling because potential benefit no longer justifies risk of adverse effects.

PEDS – Safety and efficacy not established in children.

FORMS – Trade only: Tabs 300, 400 mg. Ketek Pak: #10, 400 mg tabs.

NOTES – May prolong QT interval. Avoid in proarrhythmic conditions or with drugs that prolong QT interval. Life-threatening hepatotoxicity. Monitor for signs/symptoms of hepatitis. Contraindicated if history of hepatitis due to any macrolide or telithromycin. Contraindicated in myasthenia gravis. CYP3A4 substrate and inhibitor. Contraindicated with pimozide, rifampin, ergot alkaloids. Withhold simvastatin, lovastatin, or atorvastatin during course of telithromycin. Consider monitoring INR with warfarin. Give telithromycin and theophylline at least 1 h apart. Monitor for increased toxicity of digoxin, midazolam, metoprolol. CYP3A4 inducers (ie, phenytoin, carbamazepine) could reduce telithromycin levels. Dosage adjustment for CrCl less than 30 mL/min (including hemodialysis) is 600 mg once daily. On dialysis days, give after hemodialysis session. Dosage adjustment for CrCl less than 30 mL/min with hepatic dysfunction is 400 mg once daily.

TIGECYCLINE (*Tygacil*) ▶Bile, K ♀D ▶?+ $$$$$

ADULT – Complicated skin infections, complicated intra-abdominal infections, community-acquired pneumonia: 100 mg IV 1st dose, then 50 mg IV q 12 h. Infuse over 30 to 60 min.

PEDS – Not approved in children. Avoid in children age younger than 8 yo due to teeth staining.

NOTES – Consider other antibiotics for severe infection because mortality is higher with tigecycline, especially in ventilator-associated pneumonia. May decrease efficacy of oral contraceptives. Monitor INR with warfarin. Dosage adjustment for severe liver dysfunction (Child-Pugh C): 100 mg IV 1st dose, then 25 mg IV q 12 h.

TRIMETHOPRIM (*Primsol*, ♣*Proloprim*) ▶K ♀C ▶– $

ADULT – Uncomplicated UTI: 100 mg PO two times per day or 200 mg PO daily.

PEDS – Safety not established in age younger than 2 mo. Otitis media (not for *M. catarrhalis*): 10 mg/kg/day PO divided two times per day for 10 days for age 6 mo or older.

UNAPPROVED ADULT – Prophylaxis of recurrent UTI: 100 mg PO at bedtime. Pneumocystis treatment: 5 mg/kg PO three times per day with dapsone 100 mg PO daily for 21 days.

FORMS – Generic only: Tabs 100 mg. Trade only (Primsol): Oral soln 50 mg/5 mL.

NOTES – Contraindicated in megaloblastic anemia due to folate deficiency. Blood dyscrasias. Trimethoprim alone not first line for otitis media. Inhibits metabolism of phenytoin. Can cause hyperkalemia (risk increased by high doses of trimethoprim, renal impairment, or other drugs that cause hyperkalemia). Dosing in adults with renal dysfunction: 50 mg PO q 12 h for CrCl 15 to 30 mL/min. Do not use if CrCl is less than 15 mL/min.

VANCOMYCIN (*Vancocin*) ▶K ♀C ▶? $$$$$

ADULT – Severe *Staph* infections (including MRSA), endocarditis: 1 g IV q 12 h, each dose over 1 h or 30 mg/kg/day IV divided q 12 h. Empiric therapy, native valve endocarditis: 15 mg/kg (up to 2 g/day unless levels monitored) IV q 12 h with gentamicin. See table for prophylaxis of bacterial endocarditis. *C. difficile*–associated diarrhea: 125 mg PO four times per day for 10 days. IV administration ineffective for this indication. See table for management of *C. difficile* infection in adults, including higher dose of vancomycin plus metronidazole for severe complicated disease. Staphylococcal enterocolitis: 500 to 2000 mg/day PO divided three to four times per day for 7 to 10 days.

PEDS – Severe *Staph* infections (including MRSA), endocarditis: 15 mg/kg IV load, then 10 mg/kg q 12 h for age younger than 1 week, 15 mg/kg IV load, then 10 mg/kg q 8 h for age 1 week to 1 mo, 10 mg/kg IV q 6 h for age older than 1 mo. *C. difficile*–associated diarrhea: 40 mg/kg/day (up to 500 mg/day) PO divided four times per day for 10 days. IV administration ineffective for this indication.

UNAPPROVED ADULT – Usual dose: 15 to 20 mg/kg IV q 8 to 12 h. Severe infection: Consider loading dose of 25 to 30 mg/kg. Infuse over 1 h; infuse over 1.5 to 2 h if dose greater than 1 g. Base IV dose on absolute body wt. In obese patients, base initial dose on absolute body wt, then adjust dose based on trough levels. *C. difficile*–associated diarrhea: 125 mg PO four times per day for 10 to 14 days. See table for management of *C. difficile* infection in adults, including higher dose of vancomycin plus metronidazole for severe complicated disease. Prevention of perinatal group B streptococcal disease: Give to mother

(cont.)

VANCOMYCIN (*cont.*)

1 g IV q 12 h from onset of labor/after membrane rupture until delivery.

UNAPPROVED PEDS – Newborns: 10 to 15 mg/kg IV q 8 to 12 h for age younger than 1 week; 10 to 15 mg/kg IV q 6 to 8 h for age 1 week and older. Bacterial meningitis: 60 mg/kg/day IV divided q 6 h. Nonmeningeal pneumococcal infections: 40 to 45 mg/kg/day IV divided q 6 h. AAP dose for *C. difficile*–associated diarrhea: 40 mg/kg/day PO divided four times per day for at least 10 days (max 125 mg PO four times per day).

FORMS – Trade only: Caps 125, 250 mg.

NOTES – Maintain trough higher than 10 mg/L in all patients to avoid development of resistance; optimal trough for complicated infections is 15 to 20 mg/L. Draw trough just before the next dose after steady state is reached (usually after 4th dose). Monitoring of peak levels no longer recommended. "Red Neck" (or "Red Man") syndrome with rapid IV administration, vein irritation with IV extravasation, reversible neutropenia, ototoxicity, or nephrotoxicity rarely. Enhanced effects of neuromuscular blockers. Use caution with other ototoxic/nephrotoxic drugs. Individualize dose if renal dysfunction. Oral vancomycin poorly absorbed; do not use for extraluminal infections.

CARDIOVASCULAR: ACE Inhibitors

NOTE: See also Antihypertensive Combinations. Contraindicated in pregnancy. Women of child-bearing age should use reliable form of contraception; discontinue ACE inhibitor as soon as pregnancy is detected. Contraindicated with history of angioedema. Do not use with aliskerin in patients with DM or CrCl less than 60 mL/min. Hyperkalemia possible, especially if used concomitantly with other drugs that increase K+ (including K+ containing salt substitutes) and in patients with heart failure, DM, or renal impairment. An increase in serum creatinine up to 35% above baseline is acceptable and is not reason to withhold therapy unless hyperkalemia occurs. Concomitant NSAID, including selective COX-2 inhibitors, may further deteriorate renal function and decrease antihypertensive effects. Consider intestinal angioedema if abdominal pain (with or without N/V). African Americans and smokers may be at higher risk for angioedema. Swelling of tongue, glottis, or larynx may result in airway obstruction, especially with history of airway surgery. Increases risk of hypotension with volume-depleted or hyponatremic patients. African Americans may need higher dose to achieve adequate response. Renoprotection and decreased cardiovascular morbidity/mortality seen with some ACE inhibitors are most likely a class effect. Anaphylactoid reactions have been reported when ACE inhibitor patients are dialyzed with high-flux membranes (eg, AN69) or undergoing low-density lipoprotein apheresis with dextran sulfate absorption. Nitroid reactions (facial flushing, N/V, hypotension) have been reported with concomitant gold injections.

BENAZEPRIL (***Lotensin***) ▶LK ♀D ▶? $$

WARNING – Do not use in pregnancy.

ADULT – HTN: Start 10 mg PO daily, usual maintenance dose 20 to 40 mg PO daily or divided two times per day, max 80 mg/day, but added effect not apparent above 40 mg/day. Elderly, renal impairment, or concomitant diuretic therapy: Start 5 mg PO daily.

PEDS – HTN: Start 0.2 mg/kg/day (max 10 mg/day) as monotherapy; doses greater than 0.6 mg/kg/day or 40 mg/day have not been studied. Do not use if age younger than 6 yo or if glomerular filtration rate is less than 30 mL/min.

UNAPPROVED ADULT – Renoprotective dosing: 10 mg PO daily. Heart failure: Start 5 mg PO daily, usual 5 to 20 mg/day, max 40 mg/day (in 1 to 2 doses).

FORMS – Generic/Trade: Tabs unscored 5, 10, 20, 40 mg.

NOTES – Twice daily dosing may be required for 24 h BP control.

CAPTOPRIL (***Capoten***) ▶LK ♀D ▶+ $

WARNING – Do not use in pregnancy.

ADULT – HTN: Start 25 mg PO two to three times per day, usual maintenance dose 25 to 150 mg PO two to three times per day, max 450 mg/day. Elderly, renal impairment, or concomitant diuretic therapy: Start 6.25 to 12.5 mg PO two to three times per day. Heart failure: Start 6.25 to 12.5 mg PO three times per day, usual 50 to 100 mg PO three times per day, max 450 mg/day. Diabetic nephropathy: 25 mg PO three times per day.

PEDS – Not approved in children.

UNAPPROVED ADULT – Hypertensive urgency: 12.5 to 25 mg PO, repeated once or twice if necessary at intervals of 30 to 60 min.

UNAPPROVED PEDS – Neonates: 0.1 to 0.4 mg/kg/day PO divided q 6 to 8 h. Infants: Initial dose 0.15 to 0.3 mg/kg/dose, titrate to effective dose, max dose 6 mg/kg/day divided one to four times per day. Children: Initial dose 0.3

(cont.)

CAPTOPRIL (*cont.*)

to 0.5 mg/kg/dose PO q 8 h, titrate to effective dose, maximum dose 6 mg/kg/day (not to exceed 450 mg/day) divided two to four times per day.

FORMS – Generic/Trade: Tabs scored 12.5, 25, 50, 100 mg.

NOTES – A captopril soln or susp (1 mg/mL) can be made by dissolving Tabs in distilled water or flavored syrup. The soln is stable for 7 days at room temperature.

CILAZAPRIL (♣ ***Inhibace***) ▶LK ♀D ▶? $

WARNING – Do not use in pregnancy.

ADULT – Canada only. HTN: Initial dose 2.5 mg PO daily, usual maintenance dose 2.5 to 5 mg daily, max 10 mg daily. Elderly or concomitant diuretic therapy: Initiate 1.25 mg PO daily. Heart failure adjunct: Initially 0.5 mg PO daily, increase to usual maintenance of 1 to 2.5 mg daily. Renal impairment with CrCl 10 to 40 mL/min: Initiate 0.5 mg daily, max 2.5 mg/day. CrCl less than 10 mL/min 0.25 to 0.5 mg once or twice per week, adjust dose according to BP response.

PEDS – Not approved in children.

FORMS – Generic/Trade: Tabs, scored 1, 2.5, 5 mg.

NOTES – Reduce dose in hepatic/renal impairment.

ENALAPRIL (**enalaprilat,** ***Vasotec***) ▶LK ♀D ▶+ $$

WARNING – Do not use in pregnancy.

ADULT – HTN: Start 5 mg PO daily, usual maintenance dose 10 to 40 mg PO daily or divided two times per day, max 40 mg/day. If oral therapy not possible, can use enalaprilat 1.25 mg IV q 6 h over 5 min, and increase up to 5 mg IV q 6 h if needed. Renal impairment or concomitant diuretic therapy: Start 2.5 mg PO daily. Heart failure: Start 2.5 mg PO two times per day, usual dose 10 to 20 mg PO two times per day, max 40 mg/day.

PEDS – Not approved in children.

UNAPPROVED ADULT – Hypertensive crisis: Enalaprilat 1.25 to 5 mg IV q 6 h. Renoprotective dosing: 10 to 20 mg PO daily.

UNAPPROVED PEDS – HTN: Start 0.1 mg/kg/day PO daily or divided two times per day, titrate to effective dose, maximum dose 0.5 mg/kg/day; 0.005 to 0.01 mg/kg/dose IV q 8 to 24 h.

FORMS – Generic/Trade: Tabs, scored 2.5, 5 mg, unscored 10, 20 mg.

NOTES – Twice daily dosing may be required for 24 h BP control. An enalapril oral susp (0.2 mg/mL) can be made by dissolving one 2.5 mg tab in 12.5 mL sterile water, use immediately. Enalaprilat is the active metabolite of enalapril.

FOSINOPRIL (***Monopril***) ▶LK ♀D ▶? $

WARNING – Do not use in pregnancy.

ADULT – HTN: Start 10 mg PO daily, usual maintenance dose 20 to 40 mg PO daily or divided two times per day, max 80 mg/day, but added effect not apparent above 40 mg/day. Elderly, renal impairment, or concomitant diuretic therapy: Start 5 mg PO daily. Heart failure: Start 5 to 10 mg PO daily, usual 20 to 40 mg PO daily, max 40 mg/day.

(cont.)

HTN Therapy[1]

Area of Concern	BP Target	Preferred Therapy[2]	Comments
General CAD prevention	<140/90 mm Hg	ACEI, ARB, CCB, thiazide, or combination	Start 2 drugs if systolic BP ≥ 160 or diastolic BP ≥ 100
High CAD risk[3]	<130/80 mm Hg		
Stable angina, unstable angina, MI	<130/80 mm Hg	Beta-blocker[4] + (ACEI or ARB)[5]	May add dihydropyridine CCB or thiazide
Left heart failure[6,7]	<120/80 mm Hg	Beta-blocker + (ACEI or ARB) + diuretic[8] + aldosterone antagonist[9]	

[1] ACEI = angiotensin-converting enzyme inhibitor; ARB = angiotensin-receptor blocker; CCB = calcium-channel blocker; MI = myocardial infarction. Adapted from *Circulation* 2007;115:2761–2788.

[2] All patients should attempt lifestyle modifications: optimize wt, healthy diet, sodium restriction, exercise, smoking cessation, alcohol moderation.

[3] DM, chronic kidney disease, known CAD or risk equivalent (eg, peripheral artery disease, abdominal aortic aneurysm, carotid artery disease, and prior ischemic CVA/TIA), 10-year Framingham risk score ≥ 10%.

[4] Use only if hemodynamically stable. If beta-blocker contraindications or intolerable side effects (and no bradycardia or heart failure), may substitute verapamil or diltiazem.

[5] Preferred if anterior wall MI, persistent HTN, heart failure, or DM.

[6] Avoid verapamil, diltiazem, clonidine, alpha-blockers.

[7] For blacks with NYHA class III or IV HF, consider adding hydralazine/isosorbide dinitrate.

[8] Loop or thiazide.

[9] Use if NYHA class III or IV, or if clinical heart failure + LVEF < 40%.

FOSINOPRIL (*cont.*)

PEDS – HTN, age 6 to 16 yo and wt greater than 50 kg: 5 to 10 mg PO daily.

UNAPPROVED ADULT – Renoprotective dosing: 10 to 20 mg PO daily.

FORMS – Generic/Trade: Tabs scored 10 mg, unscored 20, 40 mg.

NOTES – Twice daily dosing may be required for 24 h BP control. Elimination 50% renal, 50% hepatic. Accumulation of drug negligible with impaired renal function.

LISINOPRIL (***Prinivil, Zestril***) ▸K ♀D ▸? $

WARNING – Do not use in pregnancy.

ADULT – HTN: Start 10 mg PO daily, usual maintenance dose 20 to 40 mg PO daily, max 80 mg/day, but added effect not apparent above 40 mg/day. Renal impairment or concomitant diuretic therapy: Start 2.5 to 5 mg PO daily. Heart failure, acute MI: Start 2.5 to 5 mg PO daily, usual 5 to 20 mg PO daily, max 40 mg/day.

PEDS – HTN, age older than 6 yo: 0.07 mg/kg PO daily; 5 mg/day max. Not recommended for age younger than 6 yo or with glomerular filtration rate less than 30 mL/min/1.73 m^2.

UNAPPROVED ADULT – Renoprotective dosing: 10 to 20 mg PO daily.

FORMS – Generic/Trade: Tabs unscored (Zestril) 2.5, 5, 10, 20, 30, 40 mg. Tabs scored (Prinivil) 10, 20, 40 mg.

MOEXIPRIL (***Univasc***) ▸LK ♀D ▸? $$

WARNING – Do not use in pregnancy.

ADULT – HTN: Start 7.5 mg PO daily, usual maintenance dose 7.5 to 30 mg PO daily or divided two times per day, max 30 mg/day. Renal impairment or concomitant diuretic therapy: Start 3.75 mg PO daily; max 15 mg/day with renal impairment.

PEDS – Not approved in children.

FORMS – Generic/Trade: Tabs scored 7.5, 15 mg.

NOTES – Twice daily dosing may be required for 24 h BP control.

PERINDOPRIL (***Aceon, ✤Coversyl***) ▸K ♀D ▸? $

WARNING – Do not use in pregnancy.

ADULT – HTN: Start 4 mg PO daily, usual maintenance dose 4 to 8 mg PO daily or divided two times per day, max 16 mg/day. Renal impairment or concomitant diuretic therapy: Start 2 mg PO daily or divided two times per day, max 8 mg/day. Reduction of cardiovascular events in stable CAD: Start 4 mg PO daily for 2 weeks, max 8 mg/day. Elderly (age older than 65 yo): 4 mg PO daily, max 8 mg/day.

PEDS – Not approved in children.

UNAPPROVED ADULT – Heart failure: Start 2 mg PO daily, max dose 16 mg daily. Recurrent CVA prevention: 4 mg PO daily with indapamide.

FORMS – Generic/Trade: Tabs scored 2, 4, 8 mg.

NOTES – Twice daily dosing may be required for 24 h BP control.

QUINAPRIL (***Accupril***) ▸LK ♀D ▸? $$

WARNING – Do not use in pregnancy.

ADULT – HTN: Start 10 to 20 mg PO daily (start 10 mg/day if elderly), usual maintenance dose 20 to 80 mg PO daily or divided two times per

(cont.)

ACE INHIBITOR DOSING	HTN		Heart Failure	
	Initial	Max/day	Initial	Max/day
benazepril (*Lotensin*)	10 mg daily*	80 mg	-	-
captopril (*Capoten*)	25 mg two to three times per day	450 mg	6.25 mg three times per day	450 mg
enalapril (*Vasotec*)	5 mg daily*	40 mg	2.5 mg bid twice daily	40 mg
fosinopril (*Monopril*)	10 mg daily*	80 mg	5–10 mg daily	40 mg
lisinopril (*Zestril/ Prinivil*)	10 mg daily	80 mg	2.5–5 mg daily	40 mg
moexipril (*Univasc*)	7.5 mg daily*	30 mg	-	-
perindopril (*Aceon*)	4 mg daily*	16 mg	2 mg daily	16 mg
quinapril (*Accupril*)	10–20 mg daily*	80 mg	5 mg bid	40 mg
ramipril (*Altace*)	2.5 mg daily*	20 mg	1.25–2.5 mg bid twice daily	10 mg
trandolapril (*Mavik*)	1–2 mg daily*	8 mg	1 mg daily	4 mg

bid = two times per day; tid = three times per day.
Data taken from prescribing information and *Circulation* 2009;119:e391–e479.
* May require twice daily dosing for 24-h BP control.

QUINAPRIL (*cont.*)

day, max 80 mg/day, but added effect not apparent above 40 mg/day. Renal impairment or concomitant diuretic therapy: Start 2.5 to 5 mg PO daily. Heart failure: Start 5 mg PO two times per day, usual maintenance dose 20 to 40 mg/day divided two times per day.

PEDS – Not approved in children.

FORMS – Generic/Trade: Tabs scored 5 mg, unscored 10, 20, 40 mg.

NOTES – Twice daily dosing may be required for 24 h BP control.

RAMIPRIL (*Altace*) ▶LK ♀D ▶? $$$

WARNING – Do not use in pregnancy.

ADULT – HTN: Start 2.5 mg PO daily, usual maintenance dose 2.5 to 20 mg PO daily or divided two times per day, max 20 mg/day. Renal impairment or concomitant diuretic therapy: Start 1.25 mg PO daily. Heart failure/post-MI: Start 2.5 mg PO two times per day, usual maintenance dose 5 mg PO two times per day. Reduce risk of MI, CVA, death from cardiovascular causes: Start 2.5 mg PO daily for 1 week, then 5 mg daily for 3 weeks, increase as tolerated to maintenance dose 10 mg daily.

PEDS – Not approved in children.

UNAPPROVED ADULT – Renoprotective dosing: Titrate to 10 mg PO daily.

FORMS – Generic/Trade: Caps 1.25, 2.5, 5, 10 mg.

NOTES – Twice daily dosing may be required for 24 h BP control. Cap contents can be sprinkled on applesauce and eaten or mixed with 120 mL of water or apple juice and swallowed. Mixtures are stable for 24 h at room temperature or 48 h refrigerated. Do not give with telmisartan. Hypoglycemia may occur with coadministration with insulin or hypoglycemic agents.

TRANDOLAPRIL (*Mavik*) ▶LK ♀D ▶? $$

WARNING – Do not use in pregnancy.

ADULT – HTN: Start 1 mg PO daily, usual maintenance dose 2 to 4 mg PO daily or divided two times per day, max 8 mg/day, but added effect not apparent above 4 mg/day. Heart failure/post-MI: Start 1 mg PO daily, titrate to target dose 4 mg PO daily. Renal impairment or concomitant diuretic therapy: Start 0.5 mg PO daily.

PEDS – Not approved in children.

FORMS – Generic/Trade: Tabs scored 1 mg, unscored 2, 4 mg. Twice daily dosing may be required for 24 h BP control.

NOTES – Twice daily dosing may be required for 24 h BP control.

CARDIOVASCULAR: Aldosterone Antagonists

NOTE: Hyperkalemia possible, especially if used concomitantly with other drugs that increase K+ (including K+ containing salt substitutes) and in patients with heart failure, DM, or renal impairment. Adding an aldosterone antagonist is recommended in select patients with heart failure and reduced LVEF with careful monitoring for preserved renal function and normal K+ concentration. Serum creatinine should be less than 2.5 mg/dL in men or less than 2.0 mg/dL in women and K+ should be less than 5.0 mEq/L.

EPLERENONE (*Inspra*) ▶L ♀B ▶? $$$

ADULT – HTN: Start 50 mg PO daily, increase after 4 weeks if needed to max dose 50 mg two times per day. Start 25 mg daily with concomitant moderate CYP3A4 inhibitor (eg, erythromycin, verapamil, fluconazole, saquinavir). Improve survival of stable patients with LV systolic dysfunction (LVEF 40% or less) and heart failure/post-MI: Start 25 mg PO daily; titrate to target dose 50 mg PO daily within 4 weeks, if tolerated.

PEDS – Not approved in children.

FORMS – Generic/trade: Tabs unscored 25, 50 mg.

NOTES – Contraindicated with potassium greater than 5.5 mEq/L; CrCl less than 30 mL/min; strong CYP3A4 inhibitors (ketoconazole, itraconazole, nefazodone, troleandomycin, clarithromycin, ritonavir, nelfinavir). For treatment of HTN, contraindications include Type 2 DM with microalbuminuria; serum creatinine greater than 2 mg/dL in males or greater than 1.8 mg/dL in females; CrCl less than 50 mL/min; concomitant therapy with K+ supplements, K+ sparing diuretics. Hyperkalemia more common with concomitant ACE inhibitors/ARBs. Measure serum K+ before initiating, within first week, at 1 month after starting treatment or dose adjustment, then prn. With concomitant moderate CYP3A4 inhibitor (eg, erythromycin, fluconazole, saquinavir, verapamil) check K+ and serum creatinine within 3 to 7 days of initiating eplerenone. Monitor lithium levels with concomitant lithium therapy.

SPIRONOLACTONE (*Aldactone*) ▶LK ♀D ▶+ $

WARNING – Use only for approved indications. Tumorigen in rats.

ADULT – HTN: 50 to 100 mg PO daily or divided two times per day, generally used in combination with a thiazide diuretic to

(cont.)

SPIRONOLACTONE (*cont.*)

maintain serum potassium; increase dose prn after 2 weeks based on serum potassium and BP. Edema (heart failure, hepatic disease, nephrotic syndrome): Start 100 mg PO daily or divided two times per day, maintain for 5 days, increase prn to achieve diuretic response, usual dose range 25 to 200 mg/day. Other diuretics may be needed. Diuretic-induced hypokalemia: 25 to 100 mg PO daily when potassium supplements/sparing regimens inappropriate. Severe heart failure (NYHA III or IV): Start 25 mg PO daily, max 50 mg daily. Primary hyperaldosteronism, maintenance therapy: 100 to 400 mg/day PO until surgery or indefinitely if surgery not an option.

PEDS – Edema: 3.3 mg/kg PO daily or divided two times per day.

UNAPPROVED ADULT – Hirsutism: 50 to 200 mg PO daily, maximal regression of hirsutism in 6 months. Acne: 50 to 200 mg PO daily.

UNAPPROVED PEDS – Edema/HTN: 1 to 3.3 mg/kg/day, PO daily or divided two times per day, max 200 mg/day.

FORMS – Generic/Trade: Tabs unscored 25 mg scored 50, 100 mg.

NOTES – May be helpful in patients with resistant hypertension. Contraindicated with anuria, renal insufficiency, hyperkalemia. Dosing more frequently than twice daily not necessary. Hyperkalemia more likely with doses 50 mg/day or more and with concomitant ACEIs or K+ supplements. Measure serum K+ and SrCr before initiating, after 1 week, monthly for the first 3 months, quarterly for 1 year, then q 6 months after starting treatment or dose adjustment.

CARDIOVASCULAR: Angiotensin Receptor Blockers (ARBs)

NOTE: See also Antihypertensive Combinations. Avoid concomitant ACE inhibitor use. Contraindicated in pregnancy. Women of child-bearing age should use reliable form of contraception; discontinue ARB as soon as pregnancy is detected. Do not use with aliskerin in patients with DM or CrCl less than 60 mL/min. Hyperkalemia possible, especially if used concomitantly with other drugs that increase K+ (including K+ containing salt substitutes) and in patients with heart failure, DM, or renal impairment. An increase in serum creatinine up to 35% above baseline is acceptable and is not reason to withhold therapy unless hyperkalemia occurs. Concomitant NSAID, including selective COX-2 inhibitors, may further deteriorate renal function and decrease antihypertensive effects. Rare cases of angioedema and rhabdomyolysis have been reported with ARBs. African Americans and smokers may be at higher risk for angioedema.

AZILSARTAN (*Edarbi*) ▶L – ♀D ▶? $$$

WARNING – Do not use in pregnancy.

ADULT – HTN: Start 80 mg daily, max 80 mg daily. Start 40 mg daily with concomitant high-dose diuretic therapy.

FORMS – Trade only: Tabs unscored 40, 80 mg.

CANDESARTAN (*Atacand*) ▶K ♀D ▶? $$$

WARNING – Do not use in pregnancy.

ADULT – HTN: Start 16 mg PO daily, max 32 mg/day. Volume-depleted patients: Start 8 mg PO daily. Reduce cardiovascular death and hospitalizations from heart failure (NYHA II–IV and LVEF 40% or less): Start 4 mg PO daily, may double dose q 2 weeks; max 32 mg/day.

PEDS – HTN: For age 1 to 5 yo: Start 0.20 mg/kg (oral suspension), dose range 0.05 to 0.4 mg/kg/day. For age 6 to 16 yo and wt less than 50 kg: Start 4 to 8 mg/day, range 2 to 16 mg/day. For age 6 to 16 yo, wt greater than 50 kg: Start 8 to 16 mg/day, range 4 to 32 mg/day. Doses higher than 0.4 mg/kg/day (in ages 1 to 5 yo) or 32 mg (ages 6 to 16 yo) have not been studied. For patients with possible depleted intravascular volume (eg, treated with diuretic, particularly with impaired renal function), initiate under close supervision and consider lower dose.

FORMS – Trade only: Tabs unscored 4, 8, 16, 32 mg.

EPROSARTAN (*Teveten*) ▶Fecal excretion ♀D ▶? $$$$

WARNING – Do not use in pregnancy.

ADULT – HTN: Start 600 mg PO daily, maximum 800 mg/day given daily or divided two times per day.

PEDS – Not approved in children.

FORMS – Generic/Trade: Tabs unscored 400, 600 mg.

IRBESARTAN (*Avapro*) ▶L ♀D ▶? $$$

WARNING – Do not use in pregnancy.

ADULT – HTN: Start 150 mg PO daily, max 300 mg/day. Volume-depleted patients: Start 75 mg PO daily. Type 2 diabetic nephropathy: Start 150 mg PO daily, target dose 300 mg daily.

PEDS – Not approved in children.

FORMS – Generic/Trade: Tabs unscored 75, 150, 300 mg.

LOSARTAN (*Cozaar*) ▶L ♀D ▶? $$$
WARNING – Do not use in pregnancy.
ADULT – HTN: Start 50 mg PO daily, max 100 mg/day given daily or divided two times per day. Volume-depleted patients or history of hepatic impairment: Start 25 mg PO daily. CVA risk reduction in patients with HTN and LV hypertrophy (may not be effective in black patients): Start 50 mg PO daily. If need more BP reduction add HCTZ 12.5 mg PO daily; then increase losartan to 100 mg/day, then increase HCTZ to 25 mg/day. Type 2 diabetic nephropathy: Start 50 mg PO daily, target dose 100 mg daily.
PEDS – HTN: Start 0.7 mg/kg/day (up to 50 mg), doses greater than 1.4 mg/kg/day or above 100 mg have not been studied. Do not use for age younger than 6 yo or if glomerular filtration rate is less than 30 mL/min.
UNAPPROVED ADULT – Heart failure: Start 12.5 mg PO daily, target dose 50 mg daily. Renoprotective dosing: Start 50 mg PO daily, increase to 100 mg daily prn for BP control.
FORMS – Generic/Trade: Tabs unscored 25, 50, 100 mg.
NOTES – Monitor BP control when adding or discontinuing rifampin, fluconazole, or erythromycin.

OLMESARTAN (*Benicar*) ▶K ♀D ▶? $$$
WARNING – Do not use in pregnancy.
ADULT – HTN: Start 20 mg PO daily, maximum 40 mg/day.
PEDS – HTN, 6 to 16 yo: Weight 20 to less than 35 kg: Start 10 mg PO daily, max 20 mg/day. Weight 35 kg or more: Start 20 mg PO daily, max 40 mg/day. Contraindicated in children younger than 1 yo.
FORMS – Trade only: Tabs unscored 5, 20, 40 mg.

TELMISARTAN (*Micardis*) ▶L ♀D ▶? $$$
WARNING – Do not use in pregnancy.
ADULT – HTN: Start 40 mg PO daily, maximum 80 mg/day. Cardiovascular risk reduction in patients older than 55 yo unable to take ACE inhibitors: Start 80 mg PO daily, max 80 mg/day.
PEDS – Not approved in children.
FORMS – Trade only: Tabs unscored 20, 40, 80 mg.
NOTES – Swallow tabs whole, do not break or crush. May increase digoxin level.

VALSARTAN (*Diovan*) ▶L ♀D ▶? $$$
WARNING – Do not use in pregnancy.
ADULT – HTN: Start 80 to 160 mg PO daily, max 320 mg/day. Heart failure: Start 40 mg PO two times per day, target dose 160 mg two times per day; there is no evidence of added benefit when used with adequate dose of ACE inhibitor. Reduce mortality/morbidity post-MI with LV systolic dysfunction/failure: Start 20 mg PO two times per day, increase to 40 mg PO two times per day within 7 days, target dose 160 mg two times per day.
PEDS – HTN: Start 1.3 mg/kg/day (up to 40 mg), max 2.7 mg/kg/day (or 160 mg). Do not use if younger than 6 yo.
UNAPPROVED ADULT – Renoprotective dosing: 80 to 160 mg PO daily.
FORMS – Trade only: Tabs scored 40 mg, unscored 80, 160, 320 mg.

CARDIOVASCULAR: Anti-Dysrhythmics/Cardiac Arrest

ADENOSINE (*Adenocard*) ▶Plasma ♀C ▶? $$$
ADULT – PSVT conversion (not A-fib): 6 mg rapid IV and flush, preferably through a central line. If no response after 1 to 2 min then 12 mg. A 3rd dose of 12 mg may be given prn.
PEDS – PSVT conversion wt less than 50 kg: Initial dose 50 to 100 mcg/kg IV, give subsequent doses q 1 to 2 min prn and increase the dose 50 to 100 mcg/kg each time, up to a max single dose of 300 mcg/kg or 12 mg (whichever is less). PST coversion wt 50 kg or greater: Use adult dosage.
NOTES – Half-life is less than 10 sec. Give doses by rapid IV push followed by NS flush. Need higher dose if on theophylline or caffeine, lower dose if on dipyridamole or carbamazepine. May cause respiratory collapse in patients with asthma, COPD. Use in setting with cardiac resuscitation readily available. Do not confuse with adenosine phosphate used for the symptomatic relief of varicose vein complications.

AMIODARONE (*Cordarone, Pacerone*) ▶L ♀D ▶– $$$$
WARNING – May cause potentially fatal toxicities, including pulmonary toxicity, hepatic injury, and worsened arrhythmia. Only use for adults with life-threatening ventricular arrhythmias when other treatments ineffective or not tolerated.
ADULT – Life-threatening ventricular arrhythmia without cardiac arrest: Load 150 mg IV over 10 min, then 1 mg/min for 6 h, then 0.5 mg/min for 18 h. Mix in D5W. Oral loading dose 800 to 1600 mg PO daily for 1 to 3

(cont.)

AMIODARONE (*cont.*)

weeks, reduce dose to 400 to 800 mg daily for 1 month when arrhythmia is controlled or adverse effects are prominent, then reduce to lowest effective dose, usually 200 to 400 mg daily.

PEDS – Not approved in children.

UNAPPROVED ADULT – Atrial fibrillation (refractory or with accessory pathway): Loading dose 600 to 800 mg PO daily for 7 to 14 days, then 200 to 400 mg daily. Maintain sinus rhythm with A-fib: 100 to 400 mg PO daily. Shock-refractory VF/pulseless VT: 300 mg or 5 mg/kg IV bolus followed by unsynchronized shock, additional 150 mg bolus may be given if serious arrhythmias recur. Stable monomorphic ventricular tachycardia: 150 mg IV over 10 min, repeat q 10 to 15 min prn.

UNAPPROVED PEDS – May cause death or other serious side effects in children (see NOTES); do not use in infants younger than 30 days of age and use only if medically warranted if 30 days of age or older. Ventricular arrhythmia: IV therapy limited data; 5 mg/kg IV over 30 min; followed by 5 mcg/kg/min infusion; increase infusion prn up to max 10 mcg/kg/min or 20 mg/kg/day. Give loading dose in 1 mg/kg aliquots with each aliquot given over 5 to 10 min; do not exceed 30 mg/min.

FORMS – Trade only (Pacerone): Tabs unscored 100 mg. Generic/Trade: Tabs scored 200, 400 mg.

NOTES – Proarrhythmic. Contraindicated in cardiogenic shock; severe sinus-node dysfunction with marked sinus bradycardia; 2nd/3rd degree heart block; bradycardia without pacemaker that has caused syncope. Consider inpatient rhythm monitoring during initiation of therapy, especially when treating life-threatening arrhythmias. Consult cardiologist before using with other antiarrhythmic agents. Do not use with iodine allergy. Photosensitivity and skin discoloration (blue/gray color) with oral therapy. Hypo- or hyperthyroidism possible. Monitor LFTs, TFTs, and PFTs. Baseline and regular eye exams. Prompt ophthalmic examination needed with changes in visual acuity or decreased peripheral vision. Most manufacturers of laser refractive devices contraindicate eye laser surgery when taking amiodarone. Long elimination half-life, approximately 26 to 107 days. Drug interactions may persist after discontinuance due to long half-life. May increase levels of substrates of p-glycoprotein and drugs metabolized by CYP450 enzymes (CYP1A2, CYP2C9, CYP2D6, CYP3A4). Coadministration of fluoroquinolones, macrolides, loratadine, trazodone, azoles, or Class IA and III antiarrhythmic drugs may prolong QTc. May double or triple phenytoin level. May increase cyclosporine level. May increase digoxin level; discontinue digoxin or reduce dose by 50%. May increase INR with warfarin therapy; reduce warfarin dose by 33 to 50%. Do not use with simvastatin doses greater than 20 mg/day, lovastatin doses greater than 40 mg/day; may increase atorvastatin level (use lower dose); increases risk of myopathy and rhabdomyolysis. Coadministration with clopidogrel may result in ineffective platelet inhibition. Do not use with grapefruit juice. Use cautiously with beta-blockers and calcium channel blockers. Protease inhibitors, cimetidine may increase levels. Give two times per day if intolerable GI effects occur with once daily dosing. IV therapy may cause hypotension and bradycardia in adults. Administer IV infusion using a nonevacuated glass bottle and in-line IV filter. Use central line when concentration exceeds 2 mg/mL. May cause congenital hypothyroidism and hyperthyroidism if given during pregnancy. Avoid use in children younger than 1 mo: IV form contains benzyl alcohol, which may cause gasping syndrome (gasping respirations, hypotension, bradycardia, and cardiovascular collapse). In children 1 mo to 15 yo may cause life-threatening hypotension, bradycardia, and AV block. May adversely affect male reproductive tract development in infants and toddlers from plasticizer exposure from IV tubing; use syringes instead of IV tubing to administer doses to infants and toddlers.

ATROPINE (*AtroPen*) ▶K ♀C ▶– $

ADULT – Bradyarrhythmia/CPR: 0.5 to 1 mg IV q 3 to 5 min, max 0.04 mg/kg (3 mg). Treatment of muscarinic symptoms of insecticide or nerve agent poisonings: Mild symptoms: 1 injection of 2 mg auto-injector pen, 2 additional injections after 10 min may be given in rapid succession if severe symptoms develop. Severe symptoms: 3 injections of 2 mg pen in rapid succession. Administer in mid-lateral thigh. Max 3 injections.

PEDS – CPR: 0.02 mg/kg/dose IV q 5 min for 2 to 3 doses prn (max single dose 0.5 mg); minimum single dose, 0.1 mg; max cumulative dose 1 mg. Treatment of muscarinic symptoms of insecticide or nerve agent poisonings: Follow adult dosing instructions, but if wt less than 7 kg use 0.25 mg pen, if wt 7 to 18 kg use 0.5 mg pen, if wt 18 to 41 kg use 1 mg pen, if wt greater than 41 kg use 2 mg pen.

(cont.)

ATROPINE (*cont.*)

UNAPPROVED ADULT – ET administration prior to IV access: 2 to 2.5 times the recommended IV dose in 10 mL of NS or distilled water.

FORMS – Trade only: Prefilled auto-injector pen: 0.25 mg (yellow), 0.5 mg (blue), 1 mg (dark red), 2 mg (green).

NOTES – Injector should be used by someone who has adequate training in recognizing and treating nerve agent or insecticide intoxication. Seek immediate medical attention after injection(s).

DIGOXIN (*Lanoxin, Lanoxicaps, Digitek,* ✤ *Toloxin*) ▸KL ♀C ▸+ $

ADULT – Systolic heart failure, rate control of chronic A-fib: Age younger than 70 yo: 0.25 mg PO daily; age 70 yo or older: 0.125 mg PO daily; impaired renal function: 0.0625 to 0.125 mg PO daily; titrate based on response. Rapid A-fib: Total loading dose (TLD), 10 to 15 mcg/kg IV/PO, give in 3 divided doses q 6 to 8 h; give ~50% TLD for 1 dose, then ~25% TLD for 2 doses (eg, 70 kg with normal renal function: 0.5 mg, then 0.25 mg q 6 to 8 h for 2 doses). Impaired renal function, 6 to 10 mcg/kg IV/PO TLD, given in 3 divided doses q 6 to 8 h. Titrate to minimum effective dose. Other agents (ie, beta blockers, diltiazem, verapamil) more effective in controlling ventricular rate in A-fib.

PEDS – Heart failure with normal sinus rhythm: IV loading based on age: premature neonate: 15 to 25 mcg/kg; full-term neonate: 20 to 30 mcg/kg; age 1 to 24 mo: 30 to 50 mcg/kg; age 2 to 5 yo: 25 to 35 mcg/kg; age 5 to 10 yo: 15 to 30 mcg/kg; age older than 10 yo: 8 to 12 mcg/kg. Start by administering half of the total loading dose and then reassess in 4 to 8 h to determine need for second half of loading dose. Daily IV maintenance: Use 20 to 30% of actual IV loading dose for premature neonate; use 25 to 35% of actual IV loading dose for ages full-term to older than 10 yo; use divided two times per day for age younger than 10 yo. Daily PO maintenance: age 2 to 5 yo: 10 to 15 mcg/kg; age 6 to 10 yo: 7 to 10 mcg/kg; age older than 10 yo: 3 to 5 mcg/kg. Caution: Pediatric doses are in mcg, elixir product is labeled in mg/mL. Atrial fibrillation: Titrate to minimum dose needed to achieve desired ventricular rate without undesirable side effects.

UNAPPROVED ADULT – Reentrant PSVT (after carotid massage, IV adenosine, IV beta-blocker, IV diltiazem): 8 to 15 mcg/kg (based on ideal body wt) IV, give 50% of total dose initially, 25% 4 to 6 h later, and then the final 25% 4 to 6 h later.

FORMS – Generic/Trade: Tabs, scored (Lanoxin, Digitek) 0.125, 0.25 mg; elixir 0.05 mg/mL. Trade only: Caps (Lanoxicaps), 0.1, 0.2 mg.

NOTES – Proarrhythmic. Consider patient-specific characteristics (lean/ideal wt, CrCl, age, concomitant disease states, concomitant medications, and factors likely to alter pharmacokinetic/dynamic profile of digoxin) when dosing; see prescribing information for alterations based on wt and renal function. Assess electrolytes, renal function, levels periodically. Elimination prolonged with renal impairment. Maintain normal potassium, magnesium, and calcium levels. Adjust dose based on response and therapeutic serum levels (range from 0.8 to 2 ng/mL); about one-third of patients have clinical toxicity with concentrations less than 2 ng/mL. Lower serum trough levels (0.5 to 1 ng/mL) may be appropriate for heart failure; A-fib may need higher levels. 100 mcg Lanoxicaps are equivalent to 125 mcg tabs or elixir. Avoid administering IM due to severe local irritation. Many drug and herb interactions. See prescribing information for full information before using in patients with sinus node disease, AV block, accessory AV pathway, certain heart failure disorders with preserved LV function, hypermetabolic states, thyroid disease, beriberi heart disease, or planned cardioversion. Do not use with acute MI or myocarditis. Therapeutic doses may cause EKG changes (PR interval prolongation, ST segment depression) and false positive ST-T changes during exercise testing; these are expected and do not indicate toxicity.

DIGOXIN IMMUNE FAB (*Digibind, DigiFab*) ▸K ♀C ▸? $$$$$

ADULT – Digoxin toxicity: Acute ingestion of known amount: 1 vial binds approximately 0.5 mg digoxin. Acute ingestion of unknown amount: 10 vials IV, may repeat once. Toxicity during chronic therapy: 6 vials usually adequate; one formula is: Number vials = (serum dig level in ng/mL) × (kg)/100.

PEDS – Digoxin toxicity: Dose varies. Acute ingestion of known amount: One vial binds approximately 0.5 mg digoxin. Acute ingestion of unknown amount: 10 vials IV, may repeat once; monitor for volume overload. Toxicity during chronic therapy: 1 vial usually adequate for infants and small children (less than 20 kg); one formula is: Number vials = (serum dig level in ng/mL) × (kg)/100.

NOTES – After digoxin immune fab infusion, use free digoxin level to guide therapy. Total serum digoxin concentration will be falsely elevated for several days.

DISOPYRAMIDE (*Norpace, Norpace CR,* ♣ *Rythmodan*) ▶KL ♀C ▶+ $$$$

WARNING – Proarrhythmic. Contraindicated in preexisting/congenital QT prolongation, history of torsades de pointes, cardiogenic shock; 2nd/3rd degree heart block without pacemaker Only use for adults with life-threatening ventricular arrhythmias; increased mortality in patients with non-life-threatening ventricular arrhythmias and structural heart disease (ie, MI, LV dysfunction).

ADULT – Rarely indicated, consult cardiologist. Ventricular arrhythmia: 400 to 800 mg PO daily in divided doses (immediate-release is divided q 6 h; extended-release is divided q 12 h). With cardiomyopathy or possible cardiac decompensation, limit initial dose to 100 mg of immediate-release q 6 to 8 h; do not give a loading dose. With liver disease or moderate renal impairment (CrCl greater than 40 mg/dL): 400 mg/day PO in divided doses. Use immediate-release form when CrCl is less than 40 mg/dL: Give 100 mg q 8 h for CrCl 30 to 40 mg/dL, give 100 mg q 12 h for CrCl 15 to 30 mg/dL, give 100 mg q 24 h for CrCl less than 15 mg/dL.

PEDS – Ventricular arrhythmia: Divide all doses q 6 h. Younger than 1 yo: 10 to 30 mg/kg/day; age 1 to 4 yo: 10 to 20 mg/kg/day; age 4 to 12 yo:10 to 15 mg/kg/day; age 12 to 18 yo: 6 to 15 mg/kg/day.

UNAPPROVED ADULT – Maintain sinus rhythm with A-fib: 400 to 750 mg/day in divided doses.

FORMS – Generic/Trade: Caps immediate-release 100, 150 mg; extended-release 150 mg. Trade only: Caps, extended-release 100 mg.

NOTES – Proarrhythmic. Consider inpatient rhythm monitoring during initiation of therapy, especially when treating life-threatening arrhythmias. Anticholinergic side effects (dry mouth, constipation, blurred vision, urinary hesitancy) commonly occur. Reduce dose in patients with CrCl less than 40 mL/min. Initiate as an outpatient with extreme caution. May start 6 to 12 h after last dose of quinidine, or 3 to 6 h after last dose of procainamide. May start extended-release form 6 h after last dose of immediate-release form.

DOFETILIDE (*Tikosyn*) ▶KL ♀C ▶– $$$$

WARNING – Available only to hospitals and prescribers who have received appropriate dosing and treatment initiation education. Must be initiated or re-initiated in a facility that can provide CrCl calculation, ECG monitoring, and cardiac resuscitation. Monitor on telemetry for a minimum of 3 days.

ADULT – Conversion of A-fib/flutter: Specialized dosing based on CrCl and QTc interval.

PEDS – Not approved in children.

FORMS – Trade only: Caps, 0.125, 0.25, 0.5 mg.

NOTES – Proarrhythmic. Rarely indicated. Contraindicated in acquired/congenital QT prolongation; CrCl less than 20 mL/min; baseline QTc interval more than 440 msec or more than 500 msec in patients with ventricular conduction abnormalities; or with concomitant HCTZ, verapamil, cimetidine, ketoconazole, megestrol, prochlorperazine, or trimethoprim. Use with heart rate below 50 bpm has not been studied. Serum K+, Mg++ should be within normal range prior to initiating and during therapy. Monitor K+ and Mg++ (low levels increase risk of arrhythmias). Assess CrCl and QTc prior to first dose. Continuously monitor ECG during hospital initiation and adjust dose based on QTc interval. Do not discharge within 12 h after conversion to normal sinus rhythm. Effects may be increased by known CYP3A4 inhibitors and drugs that inhibit renal elimination. Using with phenothiazines, cisapride, TCAs, macrolides, fluoroquinolones may increase QTc.

DRONEDARONE (*Multaq*) ▶L ♀X $$$$

WARNING – Contraindicated with NYHA Class IV heart failure, symptomatic heart failure with recent decompensation requiring hospitalization, or atrial fibrillation who will not or cannot be cardioverted into normal sinus rhythm. Increases risk of death, stroke, and heart failure in patients with decompensated heart failure or permanent atrial fibrillation.

ADULT – Reduce hospitalization risk for patients with atrial fib who are in sinus rhythm and have a history of paroxysmal or persistent atrial fib: 400 mg PO two times per day with morning and evening meals.

PEDS – Not approved in children.

FORMS – Trade: Tabs unscored 400 mg.

NOTES – Proarrhythmic. Do not use with 2nd or 3rd degree AV block or sick sinus syndrome without functioning pacemaker; bradycardia less than 50 bpm; QTc Bazett interval greater than 500 ms; liver or lung toxicity related to previous amiodarone use; severe hepatic impairment; pregnancy; lactation; grapefruit juice; drugs or herbals that increase QT interval; Class I or III antiarrhythmic agents; potent inhibitors of CYP3A4 enzyme system (clarithromycin, itraconazole, ketoconazole, nefazodone, ritonavir, voriconazole); or inducers of CYP3A4 enzyme system (carbamazepine, phenytoin, phenobarbital, rifampin, St. John's wort). Correct hypo/

(cont.)

DRONEDARONE (*cont.*)

hyperkalemia and hypomagnesium before giving. Monitor EKG q 3 months; if in atrial fib, then either stop dronedarone or cardiovert. May initiate or exacerbate heart failure symptoms; teach patients to report symptoms of new or worsening heart failure (eg, wt gain, edema, SOB). May be associated with hepatic injury; teach patients to report symptoms of hepatic injury (eg, anorexia, nausea, vomiting, fatigue, malaise, right upper quadrant discomfort, jaundice, dark urine); discontinue if hepatic injury is suspected. Serum creatinine and/or BUN may increase during first weeks, but does not reflect change in renal function; reversible when discontinued. Give with appropriate antithrombotic therapy. May increase INR when used with warfarin. May increase dabigatran or other P-glycoprotein substrates level. May increase digoxin level; discontinue digoxin or reduce dose by 50%; monitor for digoxin toxicity. Use cautiously with beta-blockers (BB) and calcium channel blockers (CCB); initiate lower doses of BB or CCB; initiate at low dose and monitor EKG. Do not use with more than 10 mg of simvastatin. May increase level of sirolimus, tacrolimus, or CYP3A4 substrates with narrow therapeutic index.

FLECAINIDE (*Tambocor*) ▶K ♀C ▶– $$$$

WARNING – Proarrhythmic. Increased mortality in patients with non-life-threatening ventricular arrhythmias with history of MI; not recommended for use with chronic atrial fibrillation.

ADULT – Prevention of paroxysmal atrial fib/flutter or PSVT, with symptoms and no structural heart disease: Start 50 mg PO q 12 h, may increase by 50 mg two times per day q 4 days, max 300 mg/day. Life-threatening ventricular arrhythmias without structural heart disease: Start 100 mg PO q 12 h, may increase by 50 mg two times per day q 4 days, max 400 mg/day. With CrCl less than 35 mL/min: Start 50 mg PO two times per day.

PEDS – Consult pediatric cardiologist.

UNAPPROVED ADULT – Cardioversion of recent onset atrial fib: 200 to 300 mg PO single dose. Maintain sinus rhythm with A-fib: 200 to 300 mg/day in divided doses.

FORMS – Generic/Trade: Tabs unscored 50 mg, scored 100, 150 mg.

NOTES – Contraindicated in cardiogenic shock; sick sinus syndrome or significant conduction delay; 2nd/3rd degree heart block or bundle brand block without pacemaker; acquired/congenital QT prolongation; or patients with history of torsades de pointes. Consider inpatient rhythm monitoring during initiation of therapy, especially when treating life-threatening arrhythmias. Use with AV nodal slowing agent (beta-blocker, verapamil, diltiazem) to minimize risk of 1:1 atrial flutter. Reduce dose if QRS widening more than 20% from baseline or if 2nd/3rd degree AV block. Correct hypo/hyperkalemia before giving. Increases digoxin level 13 to 19%. Consult cardiologist before using with other antiarrhythmic agents. Reduce dose of flecainide 50% when used with amiodarone. Quinidine, cimetidine may increase levels. Use cautiously with disopyramide, verapamil, or impaired hepatic function. Use cautiously with impaired renal function; will take more than 4 days to reach new steady-state level. Target trough level 0.2 to 1 mcg/mL.

IBUTILIDE (*Corvert*) ▶K ♀C ▶? $$$$$

WARNING – Proarrhythmic; only administer by trained personnel with continuous ECG monitoring, capable of identifying and treating acute ventricular arrhythmias. Potentially fatal ventricular arrhythmias may occur with/without QT prolongation and can lead to torsades de pointes.

ADULT – Recent onset A-fib/flutter: Give 0.01 mg/kg over 10 min for wt less than 60 kg, may repeat if no response after 10 min. Give 1 mg (10 mL) IV over 10 min for wt 60 kg or greater, may repeat once if no response after 10 min. Useful in combination with DC cardioversion if DC cardioversion alone is unsuccessful.

PEDS – Not approved in children.

NOTES – Proarrhythmic. Serum K+, Mg++ should be within normal range prior to initiating and during therapy. Monitor K+ and Mg++ (low levels increase risk of arrhythmias). Keep on cardiac monitor at least 4 h. Use with caution, if at all, when QT interval is greater than 500 ms, severe LV dysfunction, or in patients already using class Ia or III antiarrhythmics. Stop infusion when arrhythmia is terminated.

ISOPROTERENOL (*Isuprel*) ▶LK ♀C ▶? $$$

ADULT – Refractory bradycardia or 3rd degree AV block: Bolus method: 0.02 to 0.06 mg IV; infusion method, dilute 2 mg in 250 mL D5W (8 mcg/mL), a rate of 37.5 mL/h delivers 5 mcg/min. General dose range 2 to 20 mcg/min.

PEDS – Refractory bradycardia or 3rd degree AV block: Dilute 2 mg in 250 mL D5W (8 mcg/mL). Start IV infusion 0.05 mcg/kg/min, increase q 5 to 10 min by 0.1 mcg/kg/min until desired effect or onset of toxicity, max 2 mcg/kg/min. For a 10 kg child, a rate of 8 mL/h delivers 0.1 mcg/kg/min.

LIDOCAINE (*Xylocaine, Xylocard*) ▶LK ♀B ▶? $

ADULT – Ventricular arrhythmia: Load 1 mg/kg IV, then 0.5 mg/kg IV q 8 to 10 min prn to max 3 mg/kg. IV infusion: 4 g in 500 mL D5W (8 mg/mL) at 1 to 4 mg/min.

PEDS – Ventricular arrhythmia: Loading dose 1 mg/kg IV/intraosseous slowly; may repeat for 2 doses 10 to 15 min apart; max 3 to 5 mg/kg in 1 h. ET tube: Use 2 to 2.5 times IV dose. IV infusion: 4 g in 500 mL D5W (8 mg/mL) at 20 to 50 mcg/kg/min. For a 10 kg child a rate of 3 mL/h delivers 40 mcg/kg/min.

UNAPPROVED ADULT – ET administration prior to IV access: 2 to 2.5 times the recommended IV dose in 10 mL of NS or distilled water. Shock-refractory VF/pulseless VT: 1 to 1.5 mg/kg IV push once, then 0.5 to 0.75 mg/kg IV push q 5 to 10 min prn to max 3 mg/kg.

NOTES – Reduce infusion in heart failure, liver disease, elderly. Not for routine use after acute MI. Monitor for CNS side effects with prolonged infusions.

MEXILETINE (*Mexitil*) ▶L ♀C ▶– $$$

WARNING – Proarrhythmic. Increased mortality in patients with non-life-threatening ventricular arrhythmias and structural heart disease (ie, MI, LV dysfunction).

ADULT – Rarely indicated, consult cardiologist. Ventricular arrhythmia: Start 200 mg PO q 8 h with food or antacid, max dose 1200 mg/day. Patients responding to q 8 h dosing may be converted to q 12 h dosing with careful monitoring, max 450 mg/dose q 12 h.

PEDS – Not approved in children.

FORMS – Generic only: Caps 150, 200, 250 mg.

NOTES – Patients may require decreased dose with severe liver disease. CNS side effects may limit dose titration. Monitor level when given with phenytoin, rifampin, phenobarbital, cimetidine, fluvoxamine. May increase theophylline level.

PROCAINAMIDE (*Pronestyl*) ▶LK ♀C ▶? $

WARNING – Proarrhythmic. Increased mortality in patients with non-life-threatening ventricular arrhythmias and structural heart disease (ie, MI, LV dysfunction). Contraindicated with systemic lupus erythematosus. Has been associated with blood dyscrasias.

ADULT – Ventricular arrhythmia: Loading dose: 100 mg IV q 10 min or 20 mg/min (150 mL/h) until QRS widens more than 50%, dysrhythmia suppressed, hypotension, or total of 17 mg/kg or 1000 mg delivered. Infusion: Dilute 2 g in 250 mL D5W (8 mg/mL) run at rate of 15 to 45 mL/h to deliver 2 to 6 mg/min. If rhythm unresponsive, guide therapy by serum procainamide/NAPA levels.

PEDS – Not approved in children.

UNAPPROVED ADULT – Maintenance of sinus rhythm with A-fib: 1000 to 4000 mg/day in divided doses. Restoration of sinus rhythm in atrial fibrillation with accessory pathway (preexcitation): 100 mg IV q 10 min or 20 mg/min until QRS widens more than 50%, dysrhythmia suppressed, hypotension, or total of 17 mg/kg or 1000 mg delivered.

UNAPPROVED PEDS – Arrhythmia: 2 to 6 mg/kg IV over 5 min, max loading dose 100 mg, repeat loading dose q 5 to 10 min prn up to max 15 mg/kg; 20 to 80 mcg/kg/min IV infusion, max dose 2 g/day. Consult pediatric cardiologist or intensivist.

NOTES – Proarrhythmic. Use lower dose or longer dosing interval with liver disease. Use cautiously with renal impairment or failure. Avoid with preexisting peripheral neuropathy. If positive antinuclear antibody (ANA) test develops, weigh risk/benefit of continued therapy. Evaluate complete blood count, including white cell, differential, and platelet counts, weekly for first 12 weeks of therapy and periodically afterward, and if patient develops unusual bleeding/bruising or signs of infection. If hematologic disorders are identified, discontinue therapy.

PROPAFENONE (*Rythmol, Rythmol SR*) ▶L ♀C ▶? $$$$

WARNING – Proarrhythmic. Increased mortality in patients with non-life-threatening ventricular arrhythmias and structural heart disease (ie, MI, LV dysfunction).

ADULT – Prevention of paroxysmal atrial fib/flutter or PSVT, with symptoms and no structural heart disease; or life-threatening ventricular arrhythmias: Start (immediate-release) 150 mg PO q 8 h; may increase after 3 to 4 days to 225 mg PO q 8 h; max 900 mg/day. Prolong time to recurrence of symptomatic atrial fib without structural heart disease: 225 mg SR PO q 12 h, may increase after 5 days to 325 mg PO q 12 h, max 425 mg q 12 h.

PEDS – Not approved in children.

UNAPPROVED ADULT – Cardioversion of recent onset atrial fib: 600 mg PO single dose. Outpatient prn therapy for recurrent atrial fib in highly select patients ("pill-in-the-pocket"): Single dose PO of 450 mg for wt less than 70 kg, 600 mg for wt 70 kg or greater.

FORMS – Generic/Trade: Tabs immediate-release scored 150, 225, 300 mg. Trade only: SR, Caps 225, 325, 425 mg.

(cont.)

PROPAFENONE (*cont.*)

NOTES – Consider inpatient rhythm monitoring during initiation of therapy, especially when treating life-threatening arrhythmias. Do not use with structural heart disease or for ventricular rate control during atrial fib. Consider using with AV nodal blocking agent (beta-blocker, verapamil, diltiazem) to minimize risk of 1:1 atrial flutter. Reduce dose if QRS widening more than 20% from baseline or if 2nd/3rd degree AV block. Correct hypo/hyperkalemia and hypomagnesium before giving. Consult cardiologist before using with other antiarrhythmic agents. May increase digoxin level 35 to 85%. May increase beta-blocker, cyclosporine, desipramine, haloperidol, imipramine, theophylline, venlafaxine levels. May increase INR when used with warfarin. Amiodarone, cimetidine, desipramine, erythromycin, ketoconazole, paroxetine, ritonavir, saquinavir, sertraline may increase level and risk of QT prolongation. Instruct patient to report any changes in OTC, prescription, supplement use and symptoms that may be associated with altered electrolytes (prolonged/excessive diarrhea, sweating, vomiting, thirst, appetite loss). Reduce dose 70 to 80% with impaired hepatic function. Use cautiously with impaired renal function. Bioavailability of 325 mg SR two times per day is equivalent to 150 mg immediate-release three times per day. Poorly metabolized by 10% population; reduce dose and monitor for toxicity.

QUINIDINE ▶LK ♀C ▶+ $$$– gluconate, $–sulfate

WARNING – Proarrhythmic. Associated with QT prolongation and torsades de pointes. Contraindicated with complete AV block or left bundle branch block. Increased mortality in patients with non-life-threatening arrhythmias and structural heart disease (ie, MI, LV dysfunction).

ADULT – Arrhythmia: Gluconate, extended-release: 324 to 648 mg PO q 8 to 12 h; sulfate, immediate-release: 200 to 400 mg PO q 6 to 8 h; sulfate, extended-release: 300 to 600 mg PO q 8 to 12 h. Consider inpatient rhythm and QT monitoring during initiation of therapy. Life-threatening malaria: Load with 10 mg/kg (max 600 mg) IV over 1 to 2 h, then 0.02 mg/kg/min for at least 24 h. Dose given as quinidine gluconate. When parasitemia is less than 1% and PO meds tolerated, convert to PO quinine to complete 3 days (Africa/South America) or 7 days (Southeast Asia). Also give doxycycline, tetracycline, or clindamycin.

PEDS – Not approved in children.

UNAPPROVED PEDS – Arrhythmia: Test dose (oral sulfate or IM/IV gluconate) 2 mg/kg (max 200 mg). Sulfate: 15 to 60 mg/kg/day PO divided q 6 h. Life-threatening malaria: Load with 10 mg/kg IV over 1 to 2 h, then 0.02 mg/kg/min for at least 24 h. Dose given as quinidine gluconate. When parasitemia is less than 1% and PO meds tolerated, convert to PO quinine to complete 3 days (Africa/South America) or 7 days (Southeast Asia). Also give doxycycline, tetracycline, or clindamycin.

FORMS – Generic gluconate: Tabs, extended-release unscored 324 mg. Generic sulfate: Tabs, scored immediate-release 200, 300 mg, Tabs, extended-release 300 mg.

NOTES – Proarrhythmic. QRS widening, QT interval prolongation (risk increased by hypokalemia, hypomagnesemia, or bradycardia), hypotension, hypoglycemia. Use cautiously with renal impairment/failure or hepatic disease. Use extreme caution with history of QT prolongation or torsades de pointes. Contraindicated with ziprasidone. Monitor ECG and BP. Drug interactions with some antiarrhythmics, digoxin, phenytoin, phenobarbital, rifampin, verapamil. Do not chew, break, or crush extended-release tabs. Do not use with digitalis toxicity, hypotension, AV/bundle branch block, or myasthenia gravis. Quinidine gluconate 267 mg = quinidine sulfate 200 mg.

SODIUM BICARBONATE ▶K ♀C ▶? $

ADULT – Cardiac arrest: 1 mEq/kg dose IV initially, followed by repeat doses up to 0.5 mEq/kg at 10-min intervals during continued arrest. Severe acidosis: 2 to 5 mEq/kg dose IV administered as a 4 to 8 h infusion. Repeat dosing based on lab values.

PEDS – Cardiac arrest: Neonates or infants age younger than 2 yo, 1 mEq/kg dose IV slow injection initially, followed by repeat doses up to 1 mEq/kg at 10-min intervals during continued arrest. To avoid intracranial hemorrhage due to hypertonicity, use a 1:1 dilution of 8.4% (1 mEq/mL) sodium bicarbonate and dextrose 5% or use the 4.2% (0.5 mEq/mL) product.

UNAPPROVED ADULT – Prevention of contrast-induced nephropathy: Administer 154 mEq/L soln at 3 mL/kg/h IV for 1 h before contrast, followed by infusion of 1 mL/kg/h for 6 h post procedure. If wt greater than 110 kg then dose based on 110 kg wt.

NOTES – Full correction of bicarbonate deficit should not be attempted during the first 24 h. May exacerbate intracellular acidosis.

SOTALOL (***Betapace, Betapace AF*** ▶K ♀B ▶– $$$$

WARNING – Initiate or reinitiate this product in a facility with cardiac resuscitation capacity, continuous EKG and CrCl monitoring. Do not substitute Betapace for Betapace AF.

ADULT – Ventricular arrhythmia (Betapace), symptomatic A-fib/A-flutter (Betapace AF): Start 80 mg PO two times per day, usual maintenance dose 160 to 320 mg/day divided two times per day, max 640 mg/day. Adjust dose if CrCl is less than 60 mL/min.

PEDS – Not approved in children.

FORMS – Generic/Trade: Tabs, scored 80, 120, 160, 240 mg, Tabs, scored (Betapace AF) 80, 120, 160 mg.

NOTES – Proarrhythmic. Caution, higher incidence of torsades de pointes with doses higher than 320 mg/day, in women, or heart failure.

CARDIOVASCULAR: Anti-Hyperlipidemic Agents—Bile Acid Sequestrants

CHOLESTYRAMINE (***Questran, Questran Light, Prevalite, LoCHOLEST, LoCHOLEST Light***) ▶Not absorbed ♀C ▶+ $$$

ADULT – Elevated LDL-C: Start 4 g PO daily to two times per day before meals, usual maintenance 12 to 24 g/day in divided doses two to four times per day before meals, max 24 g/day.

PEDS – Not approved in children.

UNAPPROVED ADULT – Cholestasis-associated pruritus: 4 to 8 g two to three times per day. Diarrhea: 4 to 16 g/day.

UNAPPROVED PEDS – Elevated LDL-C: Start 240 mg/kg/day PO divided three times per day before meals, usual maintenance 8 to 16 g/day divided three times per day.

FORMS – Generic/Trade: Powder for oral susp, 4 g cholestyramine resin/9 g powder (Questran, LoCHOLEST), 4 g cholestyramine resin/5 g powder (Questran Light), 4 g cholestyramine resin/5.5 g powder (Prevalite, LoCHOLEST Light). Each available in bulk powder and single-dose packets.

NOTES – Administer other drugs at least 2 h before or 4 to 6 h after cholestyramine to avoid decreased absorption of the other agent. May divide up to 6 times per day. Mix powder with 60 to 180 mL of water, milk, fruit juice, or drink. Avoid carbonated liquids for mixing. GI problems common, mainly constipation. May cause elevated triglycerides; do not use when triglycerides exceed 400 mg/dL.

COLESEVELAM (***Welchol***) ▶Not absorbed ♀B ▶+ $$$$$

ADULT – LDL-C reduction or glycemic control of type 2 DM: 3.75 g once daily or 1.875 g PO two times per day, max 3.75 g/day. Give with meal and 4 to 8 ounces of water, fruit juice, or diet soft drink. 3.75 g are equivalent to 6 tabs; 1.875 g are equivalent to 3 tabs.

PEDS – Hyperlipidemia, 10 yo or older: 3.75 g once daily or 1.875 g PO two times per day, max 3.75 g/day. Give with meal and 4 to 8 ounces of water, fruit juice, or diet soft drink. 3.75 g are equivalent to 6 tabs; 1.875 g are equivalent to 3 tabs.

FORMS – Trade only: Tabs unscored 625 mg. Powder single-dose packets 1.875, 3.75 g

NOTES – GI problems common, mainly constipation. May cause elevation of triglycerides. Do not use with triglyderides above 500 mg/dL, or history of bowel obstruction or hypertriglyceridemia-induced pancreatitis. May decrease levels of cyclosporine, glyburide, levothyroxine, oral contraceptives containing ethinyl estradiol and norethindrone, phenytoin, warfarin.

COLESTIPOL (***Colestid, Colestid Flavored***) ▶Not absorbed ♀B ▶+ $$$$

ADULT – Elevated LDL-C: Tabs: Start 2 g PO daily to two times per day with full glass of liquid, max 16 g/day. Granules: Start 5 g PO one to two times per day, increase by 5-g increments as tolerated at 1- to 2-month intervals, max 30 g/day. Mix granules in at least 90 mL of noncarbonated liquid.

PEDS – Not approved in children.

UNAPPROVED PEDS – 125 to 250 mg/kg/day PO in divided doses two to four times per day, dosing range 10 to 20 g/day.

FORMS – Generic/Trade: Tabs 1 g. Granules for oral susp, 5 g/7.5 g powder.

NOTES – Administer other drugs at least 1 h before or 4 to 6 h after colestipol to avoid decreased absorption of the other agent. Swallow tabs whole. GI problems common, mainly constipation. May increase triglycerides; do not use when triglycerides are above 400 mg/dL.

CARDIOVASCULAR: Anti-Hyperlipidemic Agents—HMG-CoA Reductase Inhibitors ("Statins") and combinations

NOTE: Each statin has restricted maximum doses that are lower than typical maximum doses when used with certain interacting medications; see prescribing information for complete information. Muscle issues: Measure creatine kinase before starting therapy. Evaluate muscle symptoms before starting therapy, 6 to 12 weeks after starting/increasing therapy, and at each follow-up visit. Risk of muscle issues increase with advanced age (65 yo or older), female gender, uncontrolled hypothyroidism, renal impairment, higher statin doses, and concomitant use of certain medicines (eg, fibrates, niacin 1 g or more, colchicine, or ranolazine). Teach patients to report promptly unexplained muscle pain, tenderness, or weakness; rule out common causes; discontinue if myopathy diagnosed or suspected. Obtain creatine kinase, TSH, vitamin D level when patient complains of muscle soreness, tenderness, weakness, or pain. With tolerable muscle complaints or asymptomatic creatine kinase increase to less than 10 times upper limit of normal, continue statin at same or reduced dose; use symptoms to guide continuing/discontinuing statin. With intolerable muscle symptoms with/without creatine kinase elevation, discontinue statin; when asymptomatic, may restart same/different statin at same/lower dose. With rhabdomyolysis, discontinue statin, provide IV hydration; weigh risk/benefit of statin therapy when recovered. Hepatotoxicity: Rare. Monitor LFTs before initiating statin therapy and as clinically indicated thereafter. May initiate, continue, or increase dose of statin with modest LFT elevation (less than 3 times upper limit of normal). Repeat LFTs and rule out other causes with isolated, asymptomatic LFT elevation less than 3 times upper limit of normal. Consider continuing vs discontinuing statin or reducing statin dose. Discontinue statin with objective evidence of liver injury; seek cause; consider referral to gastroenterologist or hepatologist. Statins may increase the risk of hyperglycemia (and type 2 DM) or transient memory problems; benefits usually outweigh risks.

ADVICOR **(lovastatin + niacin)** ▶LK ♀X ▶– $$$$

ADULT – Hyperlipidemia: 1 tab PO at bedtime with a low-fat snack, max 40/2000 mg/day. Establish dose using extended-release niacin first. If already on lovastatin, substitute combo product with lowest niacin dose. If therapy is discontinued more than 7 days, reinstitute therapy with lowest dose. See component drugs for other dosing restrictions.

PEDS – Not approved in children.

FORMS – Trade only: Tabs, unscored extended-release lovastatin/niacin 20/500, 20/750, 20/1000, 40/1000 mg.

NOTES – Swallow whole; do not break, chew, or crush. Immediate-release aspirin or NSAID 30 min prior may decrease niacin flushing reaction. Niacin may worsen glucose control, peptic ulcer disease, gout, headaches, and menopausal flushing.

ATORVASTATIN (***Lipitor***) ▶L ♀X ▶– $$$$

ADULT – Hyperlipidemia, prevention of cardiovascular events, including Type 2 DM: Start 10 mg PO daily, 40 mg daily for LDL-C reduction greater than 45%, increase at intervals of 4 weeks or more to a max of 80 mg/day. Do not give with cyclosporine, tipranavir plus ritonavir, or telaprevir. Use with caution and lowest dose necessary with lopinavir plus ritonavir. Do not exceed 20 mg/day when given with clarithromycin, itraconazole, other protease inhibitors (saquinavir plus ritonavir, darunavir plus ritonavir, fosamprenavir, or fosamprenavir plus ritonavir). Do not exceed 40 mg/day when given with nelfinavir.

PEDS – Hyperlipidemia, 10 yo or older: Start 10 mg daily, max 20 mg/day. See prescribing information for more information.

FORMS – Generic/Trade Tabs unscored 10, 20, 40, 80 mg.

NOTES – Metabolized by CYP3A4 enzyme system. May give any time of day. May increase digoxin level. Take concomitant rifampin at the same time with atorvastatin to avoid reduction of atorvastatin level. May increase levels or norethindrone and ethinyl estradiol. Patients with recent CVA/TIA and no CHD who received atorvastatin 80 mg/day had a higher incidence of hemorrhagic stroke and nonfatal hemorrhagic stroke than placebo group in the posthoc analysis of the SPARCL trial.

CADUET **(amlodipine + atorvastatin)** ▶L ♀X ▶– $$$$

ADULT – Simultaneous treatment of HTN and hypercholesterolemia: Establish dose using component drugs first. Dosing interval: Daily.

PEDS – Not approved in children.

FORMS – Trade only: Tabs, 2.5/10, 2.5/20, 2.5/40, 5/10, 5/20, 5/40, 5/80, 10/10, 10/20, 10/40, 10/80 mg.

FLUVASTATIN (***Lescol, Lescol XL***) ▶L ♀X ▶– $$$

ADULT – Hyperlipidemia: Start 20 mg PO at bedtime for LDL-C reduction of less than 25%,

(cont.)

FLUVASTATIN (*cont.*)

40 to 80 mg at bedtime for LDL-C reduction of 25% or more, max 80 mg/day, give 80 mg daily (Lescol XL) or 40 mg two times per day. Prevention of cardiac events post-percutaneous coronary intervention: 80 mg of extended-release PO daily, max 80 mg daily. Do not exceed 20 mg/day when given with cylosporine or fluconazole.

PEDS – Hyperlipidemia: Start 20 mg PO at bedtime, max 80 mg daily (XL) or divided two times per day. See prescribing information for more information.

FORMS – Trade only: Caps 20, 40 mg. Tabs extended-release unscored 80 mg.

NOTES – Mainly metabolized by CYP2C9, so less potential for drug interactions. Monitor blood sugar levels when given with glyburide and the dose of fluvastatin is changed. Monitor phenytoin levels when given with phenytoin and fluvastatin is initiated or the dose is changed. Monitor INR when given with warfarin and fluvastatin is initiated, discontinued, or the dose is changed.

LOVASTATIN (***Mevacor, Altoprev***) ▶L ♀X ▶– $

ADULT – Hyperlipidemia, prevention of cardiovascular events: Start 20 mg PO daily with the evening meal, increase at intervals of 4 weeks or more to max 80 mg/day (daily or divided two times per day). Altoprev dosed daily with max dose 60 mg/day. Do not use with boceprevir, clarithromycin, cyclosporine, erythromycin, gemfibrozil, more than 1 quart/day grapefruit juice, HIV protease inhibitors, itraconazole, ketoconazole, nefazodone, posaconazole, telaprevir, or telithromycin; increases risk of myopathy. Do not exceed 20 mg/day when given with danazol, diltiazem, verapamil, or CrCl less than 30 mL/min. Do not exceed 40 mg/day when used with amiodarone.

PEDS – Hyperlipidemia, 10 yo or older: Start 10 mg PO q pm, max 40 mg/day. See prescribing information for more information.

FORMS – Generic/Trade: Tabs unscored 20, 40 mg. Trade only: Tabs extended-release (Altoprev) 20, 40, 60 mg.

NOTES – Metabolized by CYP3A4 enzyme system.

PITAVASTATIN (***Livalo***) ▶L – ♀X ▶– $$$$

ADULT – Hyperlipidemia: Start 2 mg PO at bedtime, max 4 mg daily. CrCl 15 to 59 mL/min or end-stage renal disease receiving hemodialysis: Max start 1 mg PO daily, max 2 mg daily. Do not use with cyclosporine. Do not exceed 1

(cont.)

LDL CHOLESTEROL GOALS[1]

Risk Category	LDL Goal	Lifestyle Changes[2]	Also Consider Meds at LDL (mg/dL)[3]
High risk: CHD or equivalent risk,[4,5,6] 10-year risk > 20%	<100 (optional <70)[7]	LDL ≥100[8]	≥100 (<100: consider Rx options)[9]
Moderately high risk: 2+ risk factors,[10] 10-year risk 10–20%	<130 (optional <100)	LDL ≥130[8]	≥130 (100–129: consider Rx options)[11]
Moderate risk: 2+ risk factors,[10] 10-year risk <10%	<130 mg/dL	LDL ≥130	≥160
Lower risk: 0 to 1 risk factor[5]	<160 mg/dL	LDL ≥160	≥190 (160–189: Rx optional)

[1]CHD = coronary heart disease. LDL = low density lipoprotein. Adapted from NCEP: *JAMA* 2001; 285:2486; NCEP Report: *Circulation* 2004;110:227–239. All 10-year risks based upon Framingham stratification; calculator available at: http://hin.nhlbi.nih.gov/atpiii/calculator.asp?usertype = prof.

[2]Dietary modification, wt reduction, exercise.

[3]When using LDL-lowering therapy, achieve at least 30 to 40% LDL reduction.

[4]Equivalent risk defined as DM other atherosclerotic disease (peripheral artery disease, abdominal aortic aneurysm, symptomatic carotid artery disease, CKD, or prior ischemic CVA/TIA), or ≥ 2 risk factors such that 10-year risk >20%.

[5]History of ischemic CVA or transient ischemic attack = CHD risk equivalents (*Stroke* 2006;37:577-617).

[6]Chronic kidney disease = CHD risk equivalent [*Am J Kidney Dis* 2003 Apr;41(4 suppl 3):I-IV,S1-91].

[7]For any patient with atherosclerotic disease, may treat to LDL < 70 mg/dL (*Circulation* 2011;124:2458-73).

[8]Regardless of LDL, lifestyle changes are indicated when lifestyle-related risk factors (obesity, physical inactivity, ↑ TG, ↓ HDL, or metabolic syndrome) are present.

[9]If baseline LDL < 100, starting LDL-lowering therapy is an option based on clinical trials. With ↑ TG or ↓ HDL, consider combining fibrate or nicotinic acid with LDL-lowering drug.

[10]Risk factors: Cigarette smoking, HTN (BP ≥140/90 mmHg or on antihypertensive meds), low HDL (< 40 mg/dL), family history of CHD (1° relative: ♂ < 55 yo, ♀ < 65 yo), age (♂ ≥45 yo, ♀ ≥55 yo).

[11]At baseline or after lifestyle changes, initiating therapy to achieve LDL < 100 is an option based on clinical trials.

PITAVASTATIN (*cont.*)

mg/day when given with erythromycin. Do not exceed 2 mg/day when given with rifampin.

PEDS – Not approved in children.

FORMS – Trade only: Tabs 1, 2, 4 mg.

NOTES – Mainly metabolized by CYP2C9.

PRAVASTATIN (*Pravachol*) ▶L ♀X ▶– $

ADULT – Hyperlipidemia/prevention of cardiovascular events: Start 40 mg PO daily, increase at intervals of 4 weeks or more to max 80 mg/day. Renal or hepatic impairment: Start 10 mg PO daily. Do not exceed 20 mg/day when given with cyclosporine. Do not exceed 40 mg/day when given with clarithromycin.

PEDS – Hyperlipidemia, 8 to 13 yo: 20 mg PO daily; 14 to 18 yo: 40 mg PO daily. See prescribing information for more information.

FORMS – Generic/Trade: Tabs unscored 10, 20, 40, 80 mg.

NOTES – Not metabolized substantially by the CYP isoenzyme system, less potential for drug interactions.

ROSUVASTATIN (*Crestor*) ▶L ♀X ▶– $$$$

ADULT – Hyperlipidemia, slow progression of atherosclerosis, primary prevention of cardiovascular disease: Start 10 to 20 mg daily, may adjust dose after 2 to 4 weeks, max 40 mg/day. Do not start with 40 mg; use 40 mg only when treatment goal not achieved with 20 mg/day. Renal impairment (CrCl less than 30 mL/min and not on hemodialysis): Start 5 mg PO daily, max 10 mg/day. Asians: Start 5 mg PO daily. When given with atazanavir with or without ritonavir or lopinavir with ritonavir, do not exceed 10 mg/day. When given with cyclosporine, do not exceed 5 mg/day. Avoid using with gemfibrozil; if used concomitantly, do not exceed 10 mg/day.

PEDS – Hyperlipidemia, 10 yo or older: Start 5 to 20 mg PO daily, max 20 mg/day. See prescribing information for more information. Canada only: May use with age older than 8 yo with homozygous familial hypercholesterolemia.

UNAPPROVED ADULT – Primary prevention of major cardiovascular events in patients with LDL-C less than 130 mg/dL and high-sensitivity CRP 2 mg/dL or greater: 20 mg PO daily.

FORMS – Trade only: Tabs unscored 5, 10, 20, 40 mg.

NOTES – Partially metabolized by CYP2C9 enzyme system. Potentiates effects of warfarin; monitor INR. Give aluminum- and magnesium-containing antacids more than 2 h after rosuvastatin. Proteinuria, with unknown clinical significance, reported with 40 mg/day; consider dose reduction when using 40 mg/day with unexplained persistent proteinuria.

LIPID REDUCTION BY CLASS/AGENT[1]

Drug class/agent	*LDL*	*HDL*	*TG*
Bile acid sequestrants[2]	↓ 15–30%	↑ 3–5%	No change or ↑
Cholesterol absorption inhibitor[3]	↓ 18%	↑ 1%	↓ 8%
Fibrates[4]	↓ 5–20%	↑ 10–20%	↓ 20–50%
Lovastatin+ext'd release niacin[5]*	↓ 30–42%	↑ 20–30%	↓ 32–44%
Niacin[6]*	↓ 5–25%	↑ 15–35%	↓ 20–50%
Omega 3 fatty acids[7]	↓ 5% or ↑ 44%	↓ 4% or ↑ 9%	↓ 27-45
Statins[8]	↓ 18–63%	↑ 5–15%	↓ 7–35%
Simvastatin+ezetimibe[9]	↓ 45–59%	↑ 6–10%	↓ 23–31%

[1]LDL = low density lipoprotein. HDL = high density lipoprotein. TG = triglycerides. Adapted from NCEP: *JAMA* 2001; 285:2486 and prescribing information.
[2]Cholestyramine (4–16 g), colestipol (5–20 g), colesevelam (2.6–3.8 g).
[3]Ezetimibe (10 mg). When added to statin therapy, will ↓ LDL 25%, ↑ HDL 3%, ↓ TG 14% in addition to statin effects.
[4]Fenofibrate (145–200 mg), gemfibrozil (600 mg two times per day).
[5]Advicor® (20/1000–40/2000 mg).
[6]Extended release nicotinic acid (Niaspan® 1–2 g), immediate release (crystalline) nicotinic acid (1.5–3 g), sustained release nicotinic acid (Slo-Niacin® 1–2 g).
[7]Lovaza (4 g), Vascepa (4 g)
[8]Atorvastatin (10–80 mg), fluvastatin (20–80 mg), lovastatin (20–80 mg), pravastatin (20–80 mg), rosuvastatin (5–40 mg), simvastatin (20–40 mg).
[9]Vytorin® (10/10–10/40 mg).
*Lowers lipoprotein a.

SIMCOR **(simvastatin + niacin)** ▶LK ♀X ▶– $$$

ADULT – Hyperlipidemia: 1 tab PO at bedtime with a low-fat snack, max 40/2000 mg/day. If niacin-naive or switching from immediate-release niacin, start: 20/500 mg PO q pm. If receiving extended-release niacin, do not start with more than 40/2000 mg PO q pm. Do not use with boceprevir, clarithromycin, cyclosporine, danazol, diltiazem, erythromycin, fenofibrate, gemfibrozil, grapefruit juice more than 1 quart/day, HIV protease inhibitors, itraconazole, ketoconazole, nefazodone, posaconazole, telaprevir, telithromycin, verapamil; increases risk of myopathy. Do not exceed 20/1000 mg/day when used in Chinese patients or with amiodarone, amlodipine, or ranolazine.

PEDS – Not approved in children.

FORMS – Trade only: Tabs, unscored extended-release simvastatin/niacin 20/500, 20/750, 20/1000 mg.

NOTES – Swallow whole; do not break, chew, or crush. Immediate-release aspirin or NSAID 30 min prior may decrease niacin flushing reaction. Niacin may worsen glucose control, peptic ulcer disease, gout, headaches, and menopausal flushing. May increase INR when given with warfarin.

SIMVASTATIN (*Zocor*) ▶L ♀X ▶– $$$$

ADULT – Do not initiate therapy with or titrate to 80 mg/day; only use 80 mg/day in patients who have taken this dose for more than 12 months without evidence of muscle toxicity. Hyperlipidemia: Start 10 to 20 mg PO q pm, max 40 mg/day. Reduce cardiovascular mortality/events in high risk for coronary heart disease event: Start 40 mg PO q pm, max 40 mg/day. Severe renal impairment: Start 5 mg/day, closely monitor. Chinese patients: Do not exceed 20 mg/day with niacin 1 g or more daily. Do not use with boceprevir, clarithromycin, cyclosporine, danazol, erythromycin, gemfibrozil, grapefruit juice more than 1 quart/day, HIV protease inhibitors, itraconazole, ketoconazole, nefazodone, posaconazole, telaprevir, telithromycin; increases risk of myopathy. Do not exceed 10 mg/day when used with diltiazem, dronedarone, or verapamil. Do not exceed 20 mg/day when used with amiodarone, amlodipine, or ranolazine.

PEDS – Hyperlipidemia, 10 yo or older: Start 10 mg PO q pm, max 40 mg/day. See prescribing information for more information.

FORMS – Generic/Trade: Tabs unscored 5, 10, 20, 40, 80 mg.

NOTES – May increase INR when given with warfarin.

VYTORIN **(ezetimibe + simvastatin)** ▶L ♀X ▶– $$$$

ADULT – Hyperlipidemia: Start 10/10 or 10/20 mg PO q pm, max 10/40 mg/day. Restrict the use of the 10/80 mg dose to patients who have taken it at least 12 months without muscle toxicity. See simvastatin monograph for other dose restrictions.

PEDS – Not approved in children.

UNAPPROVED ADULT – Reduce risk of CV events in patients with CKD, not on dialysis: 10/20 mg/day.

FORMS – Trade only: Tabs, unscored ezetimibe/simvastatin 10/10, 10/20, 10/40, 10/80 mg.

NOTES – Give at least 2 h before or 4 h after colestipol or cholestyramine. May increase INR when given with warfarin.

CARDIOVASCULAR: Anti-Hyperlipidemic Agents—Other

BEZAFIBRATE (♣ *Bezalip*) ▶K ♀D ▶– $$$

ADULT – Canada only. Hyperlipidemia/hypertriglyceridemia: 200 mg of immediate-release PO two to three times per day, or 400 mg of sustained-release PO q am or q pm with or after food. Reduce dose in renal insufficiency or dialysis. The 400 mg SR tab should not be used if CrCl is less than 60 mL/min or creatinine greater than 1.5 mg/dL.

PEDS – Not approved in children.

FORMS – Canada Trade only: Sustained-release tab 400 mg.

NOTES – Increased risk of myopathy and rhabdomyolysis when used with a statin. May increase serum creatinine level without changing estimated glomerular filtration rate (eGFR). May increase INR with warfarin; reduce warfarin dose by 50%; monitor INR. Do not use in primary biliary cirrhosis. Take either at least 2 h before or 4 h after colestipol or cholestyramine.

EZETIMIBE (*Zetia*, ♣ *Ezetrol*) ▶L ♀C ▶? $$$$

WARNING – May increase cyclosporine levels.

ADULT – Hyperlipidemia: 10 mg PO daily alone or in combination with statin or fenofibrate.

PEDS – Not approved in children.

UNAPPROVED PEDS – Hyperlipidemia, 10 yo or older: 10 mg PO daily coadministered with simvastatin.

FORMS – Trade only: Tabs, unscored 10 mg.

(cont.)

EZETIMIBE (*cont.*)

NOTES – Take either at least 2 h before or 4 h after colestipol or cholestyramine. Monitor cyclosporine levels (may increase). When used with statin, monitor LFTs before initiating and as clinically indicated thereafter.

FENOFIBRATE (*TriCor, Antara, Fenoglide, Lipofen, Triglide,* ✤ *Lipidil Micro, Lipidil Supra, Lipidil EZ*) ▶LK ♀C ◗– $$$

ADULT – Hypertriglyceridemia: Tricor tabs: Start 48 to 145 mg PO daily, max 145 mg/day. Antara: 43 to 130 mg PO daily; max 130 mg daily. Fenoglide: 40 to 120 mg PO daily; max 120 mg daily. Lipofen: 50 to 150 mg PO daily, max 150 mg daily. Triglide: 50 to 160 mg PO daily, max 160 mg daily. Generic tabs: 54 to 160 mg, max 160 mg daily. Generic caps: 67 to 200 mg PO daily, max 200 mg daily. Hypercholesterolemia, mixed dyslipidemia: Tricor tabs: 145 mg PO daily. Antara: 130 mg PO daily. Fenoglide: 120 mg daily. Lipofen: 150 mg daily. Triglide: 160 mg daily. Generic tabs: 160 mg daily. Generic caps: 200 mg PO daily. Renal impairment, elderly: Tricor tabs: Start 48 mg PO daily; Antara: Start 43 mg PO daily; Fenoglide: 40 mg daily/Lipofen: Start 50 mg daily; Triglide: Start 50 mg PO daily; generic tabs: Start 40 to 54 mg PO daily; generic caps 43 mg PO daily.

PEDS – Not approved in children.

FORMS – Generic only: Tabs unscored 54, 160 mg. Generic caps 67, 134, 200 mg. Trade only: Tabs (TriCor) unscored 48, 145 mg. Caps (Antara) 43, 130 mg. Tabs (Fenoglide) unscored 40, 120 mg. Tabs (Lipofen) unscored 50, 100, 150 mg. Tabs (Triglide) unscored 50, 160 mg.

NOTES – All formulations, except Antara, Tricor, and Triglide, should be taken with food to increase plasma concentrations. Conversion between forms: Generic 200 mg cap with food is equivalent to 145 mg Tricor; Lipofen 150 mg with food is equivalent to Tricor 160 mg with food. Monitor LFTs, dose-related hepatotoxicity. Increased risk of myopathy and rhabdomyolysis when used with a statin. May increase INR with warfarin. Contraindicated with active liver disease, gall bladder disease, and/or CrCl less than 30 mL/min. May increase serum creatinine level without changing estimated glomerular filtration rate (eGFR).

FENOFIBRIC ACID (*Fibricor, TriLipix*) ▶LK ♀C ◗– $$$

ADULT – Mixed dyslipidemia and CHD or CHD risk equivalent in combination with optimal statin therapy: TriLipix: 135 mg PO daily. Hypertriglyceridemia: Fibricor: 35 to 105 mg PO daily, max 105 mg daily. TriLipix: 45 to 135 mg PO daily, max 135 mg daily. Hypercholesterolemia, mixed dyslipidemia: Fibricor: 105 mg PO daily. TriLipix: 135 mg PO daily. Renal impairment: Fibricor: 35 mg PO daily. TriLipix: 45 mg PO daily.

PEDS – Not approved in children.

FORMS – Trade only: Caps (TriLipix) delayed-release 45, 135 mg. Tabs (Fibricor) 35, 105 mg.

NOTES – Monitor LFTs, dose-related hepatotoxicity. Increased risk of myopathy and rhabdomyolysis when used with a statin. May increase the INR with warfarin. Contraindicated with active liver disease, gall bladder disease, and/or CrCl less than 30 mL/min. Give bile acid sequestrants more than 1 h before or at least 4 to 6 h after fenofibric acid administration. Coadministration of immunosuppressant or other potentially nephrotoxic medications may increase the risk of nephrotoxicity. May increase serum creatinine level without changing estimated glomerular filtration rate (eGFR).

STATINS

Minimum Dose for 30-40% LDL	LDL*
atorvastatin 10 mg	–39%
fluvastatin 40 mg two times per day	–36%
fluvastatin XL 80 mg	–35%
lovastatin 40 mg	–31%
pitavastatin 2 mg	–36%
pravastatin 40 mg	–34%
rosuvastatin 5 mg	–45%
simvastatin 20 mg	–38%

LDL = low-density lipoprotein. Will get ~6% decrease in LDL with every doubling of dose.
*Adapted from *Circulation* 2004;110:227-239.

GEMFIBROZIL (*Lopid*) ▶LK ♀C ▶? $$$

ADULT – Hypertriglyceridemia, primary prevention of artery heart disease: 600 mg PO two times per day 30 min before meals.

PEDS – Not approved in children.

FORMS – Generic/Trade: Tabs scored 600 mg.

NOTES – Not as safe as fenofibrate or fenofibric acid when used in combination with a statin; increases risk of myopathy and rhabdomyolysis. May increase INR with warfarin. Do not use with repaglinide; increases risk of hypoglycemia. Do not give bile acid sequestrants within 2 h of gemfibrozil administration. Consider alternative therapy when baseline serum creatinine is greater than 2 mg/dL. May increase serum creatinine level without changing estimated glomerular filtration rate (eGFR).

CARDIOVASCULAR: Antiadrenergic Agents

CLONIDINE (*Catapres, Catapres-TTS, Jenloga, Kapvay,* ✣ *Dixarit*) ▶LK ♀C ▶? $$

ADULT – Immediate-release, HTN: Start 0.1 mg PO two times per day, may increase by 0.1 mg/day each week, usual maintenance dose 0.2 to 0.6 mg/day in 2 to 3 divided doses, max 2.4 mg/day. Extended-release (Jenloga), HTN: Start 0.1 mg daily at bedtime, may increase by 0.1 mg/day each week, max 0.6 mg daily. Transdermal (Catapres-TTS), HTN: Start 0.1 mg/24 h patch q week, titrate to desired effect, max effective dose 0.6 mg/24 h (two 0.3 mg/24 h patches).

PEDS – HTN: Start 5 to 7 mcg/kg/day PO divided q 6 to 12 h, titrate at 5- to 7-day intervals to 5 to 25 mcg/kg/day divided q 6 h; max 0.9 mg/day. Transdermal therapy not recommended in children. Extended release (Kapvay), ADHD (6 to 17 yo): Start 0.1 mg PO at bedtime; may increase by 0.1 mg/day each week; give twice daily with equal or higher dose at bedtime, max 0.4 mg daily.

UNAPPROVED ADULT – HTN urgency: Initially 0.1 to 0.2 mg PO, followed by 0.1 mg q 1 h prn up to a total dose of 0.5 to 0.7 mg. Menopausal flushing: 0.1 to 0.4 mg/day PO divided two to three times per day; transdermal applied weekly 0.1 mg/day. Tourette syndrome: 3 to 5 mcg/kg/day PO divided two to four times per day. Opioid withdrawal, adjunct: 0.1 to 0.3 mg PO three to four times per day or 0.1 to 0.2 mg PO q 4 h tapering off over days 4 to 10. Alcohol withdrawal, adjunct: 0.1 to 0.2 mg PO q 4 h prn. Smoking cessation: Start 0.1 mg PO two times per day, increase 0.1 mg/day at weekly intervals to 0.75 mg/day as tolerated; transdermal (Catapres-TTS): 0.1 to 0.2 mg/24 h patch q week for 2 to 3 weeks after cessation. ADHD: 5 mcg/kg/day PO for 8 weeks. Posttraumatic stress disorder: Start 0.1 mg PO at bedtime, max 0.6 mg/day in divided doses.

UNAPPROVED PEDS – ADHD: Start 0.05 mg PO at bedtime, titrate based on response over 8 weeks to max 0.2 mg/day (for wt less than 45 kg) or to max 0.4 mg/day (wt 45 kg or greater) in 2 to 4 divided doses. Tourette syndrome: 3 to 5 mcg/kg/day PO divided two to four times per day.

FORMS – Generic/Trade: Tabs immediate-release unscored (Catapres) 0.1, 0.2, 0.3 mg. Transdermal weekly patch 0.1 mg/day (TTS-1), 0.2 mg/day (TTS-2), 0.3 mg/day (TTS-3). Generic only: Oral Susp, Extended-release, 0.09 mg/mL (118 mL). Tabs extended-release unscored (Jenloga, Kapvay) 0.1, 0.2 mg.

NOTES – The sympatholytic action of clonidine may worsen sinus node dysfunction and atrioventricular block, especially in patients taking other sympatholytic drugs. Monitor for bradycardia when taking concomitant digoxin, nondihydropyridine calcium channel blockers, or beta blockers. Use lower initial dose with renal impairment. Rebound HTN with abrupt discontinuation of tabs, especially at doses that exceed 0.7 mg/day. Taper therapy slowly q 3 to 7 days to avoid rebound HTN. Dispose of used patches carefully, keep away from children. Remove patch before defibrillation, cardioversion, or MRI to avoid skin burns. Transdermal therapy should not be interrupted during the surgical period. Oral therapy should be continued within 4 h of surgery and restarted as soon as possible afterward. May potentiate the CNS depressive effects of alcohol, barbiturates, or other sedating drugs. Concomitant TCAs may reduce the BP-lowering effects. Concomitant neuroleptics may induce or exacerbate orthostatic regulation disturbances (eg, orthostatic hypotension, dizziness, fatigue). With alcoholic delirium, high intravenous doses of clonidine may increase the arrhythmogenic potential (QT prolongation, ventricular fibrillation) of high IV doses of haloperidol. Do not crush, chew, or break extended-release tabs. Monitor response and side effects when interchanging between clonidine products; many are not equivalent on mg:mg basis.

DOXAZOSIN (*Cardura, Cardura XL*) ▶L ♀C ▶? $$

WARNING – Not first-line agent for HTN. Increased risk of heart failure in patients who used doxazosin compared to diuretic in treating HTN.

ADULT – BPH, immediate-release: Start 1 mg PO at bedtime, titrate by doubling the dose over at least 1- to 2-week intervals up to max 8 mg PO at bedtime. Extended-release (not approved for HTN): Start 4 mg PO q am with breakfast, titrate dose in 3 to 4 weeks to max dose 8 mg PO q am. HTN: Start 1 mg PO at bedtime, max 16 mg/day. Avoid use of doxazosin alone to treat combined HTN and BPH.

PEDS – Not approved in children.

UNAPPROVED ADULT – Promote spontaneous passage of ureteral calculi: 4 mg (XL formulation only) PO daily usually combined with an NSAID, antiemetic, and opioid of choice.

(cont.)

SELECTED DRUGS THAT MAY PROLONG THE QT INTERVAL

alfuzosin	erythromycin*†	levofloxacin	quetiapine‡
amantadine	escitalopram	lithium	quinidine*†
amiodarone*†	famotidine	methadone*†	ranolazine
arsenic trioxide*	felbamate	moexipril/HCTZ	risperidone‡
atazanavir	fingolimod	moxifloxacin*	sertindole
azithromycin*	flecainide*	nicardipine	sotalol*†
chloroquine*	foscarnet	nilotinib	sunitinib
chlorpromazine*	fosphenytoin	octreotide	tacrolimus
cisapride*	gatifloxacin	ofloxacin	tamoxifen
citalopram*	gemifloxacin	ondansetron	telithromycin
clarithromycin*	granisetron	oxytocin	thioridazine*
clozapine	halofantrine*†	paliperidone	tizanidine
disopyramide*†	haloperidol*‡	pentamidine*†	tolterodine
dofetilide*†	ibutilide*†	perflutren lipid microspheres	vandetanib*
dolasetron	iloperidone		vardenafil
dronedarone	indapamide	phenothiazines‡	venlafaxine
droperidol*	isradipine	pimozide*†	voriconazole
eribulin	lapatinib	procainamide*	ziprasidone‡

NOTE: This table may not include all drugs that prolong the QT interval or cause torsades. Risk of drug-induced QT prolongation may be increased in women, elderly, hypokalemia, hypomagnesemia, bradycardia, starvation, CHF, & CNS injuries. Hepatorenal dysfunction and drug interactions can increase the concentration of QT interval-prolonging drugs. Coadministration of QT interval-prolonging drugs can have additive effects. Avoid these (and other) drugs in congenital prolonged QT syndrome (www.qtdrugs.org).

*Torsades reported in product labeling/case reports.

†Increased in women.

‡QT prolongation: thioridazine > ziprasidone > risperidone, quetiapine, haloperidol.

DOXAZOSIN (*cont.*)

FORMS – Generic/Trade: Tabs scored 1, 2, 4, 8 mg. Trade only (Cardura XL): Tabs extended-release 4, 8 mg.

NOTES – Orthostatic hypotension is common. Bedtime dosing may minimize side effects. Initial 1 mg dose is used to decrease postural hypotension that may occur after the 1st few doses. If therapy is interrupted for several days, restart at the 1 mg dose. Increased risk of hypotension when used with erectile dysfunction medication (eg, sildenafil, tadalafil, vardenafil); use lowest dose of erectile dysfunction medication. Use caution with concomitant strong CYP3A4 inhibitor (eg, clarithromycin, itraconazole, ketoconazole, nefazodone, protease inhibitor, telithromycin, or voriconazole). Intraoperative floppy iris syndrome may occur during cataract surgery, if patient is on or previously taken alpha-1 blocker.

GUANABENZ (***Wytensin***) ▶LK ♀C ▶– $$$

WARNING – Sedation, rebound HTN with abrupt discontinuation especially with high doses.

ADULT – HTN: Start 2 to 4 mg PO two times per day, max 32 mg two times per day.

PEDS – Children older than 12 yo: Initial dose 0.5 to 2 mg/day divided two times per day, usual maintenance dose 4 to 24 mg/day divided two times per day.

FORMS – Generic only: Tabs, 4, 8 mg.

NOTES – Sedation. Rebound HTN with abrupt discontinuation, especially at higher doses (32 mg/day). Taper therapy over 4 to 7 days to avoid rebound HTN.

GUANFACINE (***Tenex***) ▶K ♀B ▶? $

ADULT – HTN: Start 1 mg PO at bedtime, increase to 2 to 3 mg at bedtime if needed after 3 to 4 weeks, max 3 mg/day.

PEDS – HTN age 12 yo and older: Use adult dosage.

UNAPPROVED PEDS – ADHD: Start 0.5 mg PO daily, titrate by 0.5 mg q 3 to 4 days as tolerated to 0.5 mg PO three times per day.

FORMS – Generic/Trade: Tabs unscored 1, 2 mg.

NOTES – Most of antihypertensive effect is seen at 1 mg/day. Rebound HTN with abrupt discontinuation.

METHYLDOPA (***Aldomet***) ▶LK ♀B ▶+ $

ADULT – HTN: Start 250 mg PO two to three times per day usual maintenance dose 500 to 3000 mg/day divided two to four times per day, max 3000 mg/day. Hypertensive crisis: 250 to 500 mg IV q 6 h, max 1 g IV q 6 h, max 4000 mg/day.

PEDS – HTN: 10 mg/kg/day PO divided two to four times per day, titrate dose to max dose 65 mg/kg/day or 3000 mg/day, whichever is less.

FORMS – Generic only: Tabs unscored 125, 250, 500 mg.

NOTES – May be used to manage BP during pregnancy. IV form has a slow onset of effect and other agents preferred for rapid reduction of BP. Hemolytic anemia possible.

PRAZOSIN (***Minipress***) ▶L ♀C ▶? $$

WARNING – Not first-line agent for HTN. Increased risk of heart failure in patients who used related drug doxazosin compared to diuretic in treating HTN.

ADULT – HTN: Start 1 mg PO two to three times per day, usual maintenance dose 20 mg/day divided two to three times per day, max 40 mg/day, but doses higher than 20 mg/day usually do not increase efficacy.

PEDS – Not approved in children.

UNAPPROVED ADULT – Posttraumatic stress disorder nightmares: Start 1 mg PO at bedtime, increase weekly by 1 to 2 mg/day to max dose of 20 mg/day. Doses greater than 10 mg/day are divided early evening and at bedtime.

UNAPPROVED PEDS – HTN: Start 0.005 mg/kg PO single dose; increase slowly prn up to maintenance dose 0.025 to 0.150 mg/kg/day divided q 6 h; max dose 0.4 mg/kg/day.

FORMS – Generic/Trade: Caps 1, 2, 5 mg.

NOTES – Othostatic hypotension common; to avoid, start with 1 mg at bedtime, and increase dose gradually. Increased risk of hypotension when used with erectile dysfunction medication (eg, sildenafil, tadalafil, verdenafil); use lowest dose of erectile dysfunction medication. Intraoperative floppy iris syndrome may occur during cataract surgery, if patient is on or previously taken alpha-1 blocker.

RESERPINE (***Serpasil***) ▶LK ♀C ▶– $

ADULT – HTN: Start 0.05 to 0.1 mg PO daily or 0.1 mg PO every other day, max dose 0.25 mg/day.

PEDS – Not approved in children.

FORMS – Generic only: Tabs, scored 0.1, 0.25 mg.

NOTES – Should be used in combination with a diuretic to counteract fluid retention and augment BP control. May cause depression at higher doses, avoid use in patients with uncontrolled depression or active peptic ulcer disease.

TERAZOSIN (***Hytrin***) ▶LK ♀C ▶? $$

WARNING – Not first-line for HTN. Increased risk of heart failure in patients who used related drug doxazosin compared to diuretic in treating HTN.

(cont.)

TERAZOSIN (*cont.*)

ADULT – HTN: Start 1 mg PO at bedtime usual effective dose 1 to 5 mg PO daily or divided two times per day, max 20 mg/day. BPH: Start 1 mg PO at bedtime; titrate dose in a stepwise fashion to 2, 5, or 10 mg PO at bedtime to desired effect. Treatment with 10 mg PO at bedtime for 4 to 6 weeks may be needed to assess benefit. Maximum 20 mg/day.

PEDS – Not approved in children.

FORMS – Generic/Trade: Tabs Caps 1, 2, 5, 10 mg.

NOTES – Orthostatic hypotension is common. Bedtime dosing may minimize side effects. Initial 1 mg dose is used to decrease postural hypotension that may occur after the first few doses. If therapy is interrupted for several days, restart at the 1 mg dose. Increased risk of hypotension when used with erectile dysfunction medication (eg, sildenafil, tadalafil, verdenafil); use lowest dose of erectile dysfunction medication. Intraoperative floppy iris syndrome may occur during cataract surgery, if patient is on or previously taken alpha-1 blocker.

CARDIOVASCULAR: Antihypertensive Combinations

NOTE: Dosage should first be adjusted by using each drug separately. See component drugs for metabolism, pregnancy, and lactation.

ACCURETIC **(quinapril + hydrochlorothiazide)** ▶See component drugs ♀See component drugs ◗See component drugs $$

WARNING – Do not use in pregnancy.

ADULT – HTN: Establish dose using component drugs first. Dosing interval: Daily.

PEDS – Not approved in children.

FORMS – Generic/Trade: Tabs, scored 10/12.5, 20/12.5, unscored 20/25 mg.

ALDACTAZIDE **(spironolactone + hydrochlorothiazide)** ▶See component drugs ♀See component drugs ◗See component drugs $$

WARNING – Spironolactone is a tumorigen in rats. Use only for approved indications and only if necessary. Should not be used for initial therapy of edema or HTN; these conditions require individualized dosing. Treatment of HTN and edema should be reevaluated as patient's condition warrants.

ADULT – HTN: Establish dose using component drugs first. Dosing interval: Daily to two times per day.

PEDS – Not approved in children.

FORMS – Generic/Trade: Tabs, unscored 25/25. Trade only: Tabs, scored 50/50 mg.

ALDORIL **(methyldopa + hydrochlorothiazide)** ▶See component drugs ♀See component drugs ◗See component drugs $$

WARNING – Titrate component drugs first to avoid hypotension.

ADULT – HTN: Establish dose using component drugs first. Dosing interval: two times per day.

PEDS – Not approved in children.

FORMS – Generic only: Tabs, unscored, 250/15, 250/25 mg.

AMTURNIDE **(aliskiren + amlodipine + hydrochlorothiazide)** ▶See component drugs – ♀D ◗– $$$

WARNING – Do not use in pregnancy.

ADULT – HTN: Establish dose using component drugs first, max 300/10/25 mg daily. Dosing interval: daily.

PEDS – Not approved in children.

FORMS – Trade only: Tabs, unscored 150/5/12.5, 300/5/12.5, 300/5/25, 300/10/12.5, 300/10/25 mg.

APRESAZIDE **(hydralazine + hydrochlorothiazide)** ▶See component drugs ♀See component drugs ◗See component drugs $$

ADULT – HTN: Establish dose using component drugs first. Dosing interval: two times per day.

PEDS – Not approved in children.

FORMS – Generic only: Caps 25/25, 50/50 mg.

ATACAND HCT **(candesartan + hydrochlorothiazide,** ✦ ***Atacand Plus*****)** ▶See component drugs ♀See component drugs ◗See component drugs $$$

WARNING – Do not use in pregnancy.

ADULT – HTN: Establish dose using component drugs first. Dosing interval: Daily.

PEDS – Not approved in children.

FORMS – Trade only: Tabs, unscored 16/12.5, 32/12.5, 32/25 mg.

AVALIDE **(irbesartan + hydrochlorothiazide)** ▶See component drugs ♀See component drugs ◗See component drugs $$$

WARNING – Do not use in pregnancy.

ADULT – HTN: Establish dose using component drugs first. Dosing interval: Daily. HTN, initial therapy for patients needing multiple medications: Start 150/12.5 PO daily, may increase after 1 to 2 weeks, max 300/25 daily.

PEDS – Not approved in children.

FORMS – Generic/Trade: Tabs, unscored 150/12.5. Trade only: 300/12.5, 300/25 mg.

AZOR **(amlodipine + olmesartan)** ▶See component drugs ♀See component drugs ▶See component drugs $$$
WARNING – Do not use in pregnancy.
ADULT – HTN: Establish dose using component drugs first. Dosing interval: Daily. HTN, initial therapy for patients needing multiple medications: Start 5/20 mg PO daily, may increase after 1 to 2 weeks, max 10/40 daily.
PEDS – Not approved in children.
FORMS – Trade only: Tabs, unscored 5/20, 5/40, 10/20, 10/40 mg.

BENICAR HCT **(olmesartan + hydrochlorothiazide)** ▶See component drugs ♀See component drugs ▶See component drugs $$$$
WARNING – Do not use in pregnancy.
ADULT – HTN: Establish dose using component drugs first. Dosing interval: Daily.
PEDS – Not approved in children.
FORMS – Trade only: Tabs, unscored 20/12.5, 40/12.5, 40/25 mg.

CAPOZIDE **(captopril + hydrochlorothiazide)** ▶See component drugs ♀See component drugs ▶See component drugs $$
WARNING – Do not use in pregnancy.
ADULT – HTN: Establish dose using component drugs first. Dosing interval: two to three times per day.
PEDS – Not approved in children.
FORMS – Generic/Trade: Tabs, scored 25/15, 25/25, 50/15, 50/25 mg.

CLORPRES **(clonidine + chlorthalidone)** ▶See component drugs ♀See component drugs ▶See component drugs $$$$
ADULT – HTN: Establish dose using component drugs first. Dosing interval: two to three times per day.
PEDS – Not approved in children.
FORMS – Trade only: Tabs, scored 0.1/15, 0.2/15, 0.3/15 mg.

CORZIDE **(nadolol + bendroflumethiazide)** ▶See component drugs ♀See component drugs ▶See component drugs $$$
WARNING – Avoid abrupt cessation in ischemic heart disease or HTN; may exacerbate angina and MI. Warn patients against interruption or discontinuation without physician's advice.
ADULT – HTN: Establish dose using component drugs first. Dosing interval: Daily.
PEDS – Not approved in children.
FORMS – Generic/Trade: Tabs 40/5, 80/5 mg.

DIOVAN HCT **(valsartan + hydrochlorothiazide)** ▶See component drugs ♀See component drugs ▶See component drugs $$$
WARNING – Do not use in pregnancy.
ADULT – HTN: Establish dose using component drugs first. Dosing interval: Daily. May be used as add-on/switch therapy when HTN not adequately controlled by valsartan or HCTZ.
PEDS – Not approved in children.
FORMS – Trade only: Tabs, unscored 80/12.5, 160/12.5, 320/12.5, 160/25, 320/25 mg.

DUTOPROL **(metoprolol succinate + hydrochlorothiazide)** ▶See component drugs – ♀See component drugs. $
WARNING – Avoid abrupt cessation in coronary heart disease or HTN.
ADULT – HTN: Establish dose using component drugs first. Dosing interval: Daily.
FORMS – Trade only: Tabs, unscored 25/12.5, 50/12.5, 100/12.5.

DYAZIDE **(triamterene + hydrochlorothiazide)** ▶See component drugs ♀See component drugs ▶See component drugs $
ADULT – HTN: Establish dose using component drugs first. Dosing interval: Daily.
PEDS – Not approved in children.
FORMS – Generic/Trade: Caps, (Dyazide) 37.5/25 mg. Generic only: Caps, 50/25 mg.
NOTES – Dyazide 37.5/25 cap same combination as Maxzide-25 tab.

EDARBYCLOR **(azilsartan + chlorthalidone)** ▶See component drugs – See component drugs ♀D ▶? $$$$
WARNING – Do not use in pregnancy.
ADULT – HTN: Establish dose using component drugs first. Dosing interval: Daily. HTN, intial therapy for patients needing multiple medications: Start 40/12.5 PO daily, may increase after 2 to 4 weeks, max 40/25 daily.
FORMS – Trade only: Tabs, unscored 40/12.5, 40/25 mg.

EXFORGE **(amlodipine + valsartan)** ▶See component drugs ♀See component drugs ▶See component drugs $$$
WARNING – Do not use in pregnancy.
ADULT – HTN: Establish dose using component drugs first. Dosing interval: Daily. HTN, initial therapy for patients needing multiple medications: Start 5/160 PO daily, may increase after 1 to 2 weeks, max 10/320 daily.
PEDS – Not approved in children.
FORMS – Trade only: Tabs, unscored 5/160, 5/320, 10/160, 10/320 mg.

EXFORGE HCT **(amlodipine + valsartan + hydrochlorothiazide)** ▶See component drugs ♀See component drugs ▶See component drugs $$$
WARNING – Do not use in pregnancy.
ADULT – HTN: Establish dose using component drugs first. Dosing interval: Daily. May be used as add-on/switch therapy when HTN not adequately controlled on any two

(cont.)

EXFORGE HCT *(cont.)*
of the following classes: calcium channel blockers, angiotensin receptor blockers, and diuretics.
PEDS – Not approved in children.
FORMS – Trade only: Tabs, unscored 5/160/12.5, 5/160/25, 10/160/12.5, 10/160/25, 10/320/25 mg.

HYZAAR **(losartan + hydrochlorothiazide)** ▶See component drugs ♀See component drugs ▶See component drugs $$$
WARNING – Do not use in pregnancy.
ADULT – HTN: Establish dose using component drugs first. Dosing interval: Daily. Severe HTN: Start 50/12.5 PO daily, may increase to 100/25 PO daily after 2 to 4 weeks. CVA risk reduction in HTN and LV hypertrophy (CVA risk reduction may not occur in patients of African descent): Establish dose using component drugs first. Dosing interval: Daily.
PEDS – Not approved in children.
FORMS – Generic/Trade: Tabs, unscored 50/12.5, 100/12.5, 100/25 mg.

INDERIDE **(propranolol + hydrochlorothiazide)** ▶See component drugs ♀See component drugs ▶See component drugs $$
ADULT – HTN: Establish dose using component drugs first. Dosing interval: Daily to two times per day.
PEDS – Not approved in children.
FORMS – Generic/Trade: Tabs, scored 40/25, 80/25 mg.
NOTES – Do not crush or chew cap contents. Swallow whole.

INHIBACE PLUS **(cilazapril + hydrochlorothiazide)** ▶See component drugs ♀See component drugs ▶See component drugs $$
WARNING – Do not use in pregnancy.
ADULT – Canada only, HTN: Establish dose using component drugs first. Dosing interval daily.
PEDS – Not approved in children.
FORMS – Trade: Tabs, scored 5/12.5 mg.

LEXXEL **(enalapril + felodipine)** ▶See component drugs ♀See component drugs ▶See component drugs $$
WARNING – Do not use in pregnancy.
ADULT – HTN: Establish dose using component drugs first. Dosing interval: Daily.
PEDS – Not approved in children.
FORMS – Trade only: Tabs, unscored 5/2.5, 5/5 mg.
NOTES – Do not crush or chew, swallow whole.

LOPRESSOR HCT **(metoprolol + hydrochlorothiazide)** ▶See component drugs ♀See component drugs ▶See component drugs $$$
WARNING – Abrupt cessation may exacerbate angina pectoris and MI. Warn patients against interruption or discontinuation without physician's advice.
ADULT – HTN: Establish dose using component drugs first. Dosing interval: Daily to two times per day.
PEDS – Not approved in children.
FORMS – Generic/Trade: Tabs, scored 50/25, 100/25, 100/50 mg.

LOTENSIN HCT **(benazepril + hydrochlorothiazide)** ▶See component drugs ♀See component drugs ▶See component drugs $$
WARNING – Do not use in pregnancy.
ADULT – HTN: Establish dose using component drugs first. Dosing interval: Daily.
PEDS – Not approved in children.
FORMS – Generic/Trade: Tabs, scored 5/6.25, 10/12.5, 20/12.5, 20/25 mg.

LOTREL **(amlodipine + benazepril)** ▶See component drugs ♀See component drugs ▶See component drugs $$$
WARNING – Do not use in pregnancy.
ADULT – HTN: Establish dose using component drugs first. Dosing interval: Daily.
PEDS – Not approved in children.
FORMS – Generic/Trade: Caps, 2.5/10, 5/10, 5/20, 10/20 mg. Trade only: Caps, 5/40, 10/40 mg.

MAXZIDE **(triamterene + hydrochlorothiazide,** ✤***Triazide*****)** ▶See component drugs ♀See component drugs ▶See component drugs $
ADULT – HTN: Establish dose using component drugs first. Dosing interval: Daily.
PEDS – Not approved in children.
FORMS – Generic/Trade: Tabs, scored 75/50 mg.

MAXZIDE-25 **(triamterene + hydrochlorothiazide)** ▶See component drugs ♀See component drugs ▶See component drugs $
ADULT – HTN: Establish dose using component drugs first. Dosing interval: Daily.
PEDS – Not approved in children.
FORMS – Generic/Trade: Tabs, scored 37.5/25 mg.

MICARDIS HCT **(telmisartan + hydrochlorothiazide,** ✤***Micardis Plus*****)** ▶See component drugs ♀See component drugs ▶See component drugs $$$
WARNING – Do not use in pregnancy.
ADULT – HTN: Establish dose using component drugs first. Dosing interval: Daily.
PEDS – Not approved in children.
FORMS – Trade only: Tabs, unscored 40/12.5, 80/12.5, 80/25 mg.
NOTES – Swallow tabs whole, do not break or crush. Caution in hepatic insufficiency.

MINIZIDE **(prazosin + polythiazide)** ▶See component drugs ♀See component drugs ◗See component drugs $$$

ADULT – HTN: Establish dose using component drugs first. Dosing interval: two to three times per day.

PEDS – Not approved in children.

FORMS – Trade only: Caps, 1/0.5, 2/0.5, 5/0.5 mg.

MODURETIC **(amiloride + hydrochlorothiazide,** ✦ ***Moduret*****)** ▶See component drugs ♀See component drugs ◗See component drugs $

ADULT – HTN: Establish dose using component drugs first. Dosing interval: Daily.

PEDS – Not approved in children.

FORMS – Generic only: Tabs, scored 5/50 mg.

MONOPRIL HCT **(fosinopril + hydrochlorothiazide)** ▶See component drugs ♀See component drugs ◗See component drugs $$

WARNING – Do not use in pregnancy.

ADULT – HTN: Establish dose using component drugs first. Dosing interval: Daily.

PEDS – Not approved in children.

FORMS – Generic/Trade: Tabs, unscored 10/12.5, scored 20/12.5 mg.

PRINZIDE **(lisinopril + hydrochlorothiazide)** ▶See component drugs ♀See component drugs ◗See component drugs $$

WARNING – Do not use in pregnancy.

ADULT – HTN: Establish dose using component drugs first. Dosing interval: Daily.

PEDS – Not approved in children.

FORMS – Generic/Trade: Tabs, unscored 10/12.5, 20/12.5, 20/25 mg.

TARKA **(trandolapril + verapamil)** ▶See component drugs ♀See component drugs ◗See component drugs $$$

WARNING – Do not use in pregnancy.

ADULT – HTN: Establish dose using component drugs first. Dosing interval: Daily.

PEDS – Not approved in children.

FORMS – Trade only: Tabs, unscored 2/180, 1/240, 2/240, 4/240 mg.

NOTES – Contains extended-release form of verapamil. Do not chew or crush, swallow whole. Hypotension, bradyarrhythmias, and lactic acidosis have occurred in patients receiving concurrent erythromycin or clarithromycin.

TEKAMLO **(aliskiren + amlodipine)** ▶See component drugs – ♀D ◗– $$$$

WARNING – Do not use in pregnancy.

ADULT – HTN, initial or add-on therapy: Start 150/5 mg daily, may increase after 1 to 2 weeks, max 300/10 mg daily.

FORMS – Trade only: Tabs unscored 150/5, 150/10, 300/5, 300/10 mg.

TEKTURNA HCT **(aliskiren + hydrochlorothiazide)** ▶See component drugs ♀See component drugs ◗See component drugs $$$

WARNING – Avoid in pregnancy.

ADULT – HTN: Establish dose using component drugs first. Dosing interval: Daily. HTN, initial therapy for patients needing multiple medications: Start 150/12.5 PO daily, may increase after 1 to 2 weeks, max 300/25 daily.

PEDS – Not approved in children.

FORMS – Trade only: Tabs, unscored 150/12.5, 150/25, 300/12.5, 300/25 mg.

TENORETIC **(atenolol + chlorthalidone)** ▶See component drugs ♀See component drugs ◗See component drugs $

WARNING – Avoid abrupt cessation in coronary heart disease or HTN.

ADULT – HTN: Establish dose using component drugs first. Dosing interval: Daily.

PEDS – Not approved in children.

FORMS – Generic/Trade: Tabs, scored 50/25, unscored 100/25 mg.

TEVETEN HCT **(eprosartan + hydrochlorothiazide)** ▶See component drugs ♀See component drugs ◗See component drugs $$$

WARNING – Do not use in pregnancy.

ADULT – HTN: Establish dose using component drugs first. Dosing interval: Daily.

PEDS – Not approved in children.

FORMS – Trade only: Tabs, unscored 600/12.5, 600/25 mg.

TRIBENZOR **(amlodipine + olmesartan + hydrochlorothiazide)** ▶See component drugs – ♀D ◗– $$$$

WARNING – Do not use in pregnancy.

ADULT – HTN: Establish dose using component drugs first. Dosing interval: Daily. May increase after 2 weeks, max 10/40/25 mg daily.

PEDS – Not approved in children.

FORMS – Trade only: Tabs, unscored 5/20/12.5, 5/40/12.5, 5/40/25, 10/40/12.5, 10/40/25 mg.

TWYNSTA **(amlodipine + telmisartan)** ▶See component drugs $$$$

WARNING – Do not use in pregnancy.

ADULT – HTN: Establish dose using component drugs first. Dosing interval: Daily. HTN, initial therapy for patients needing multiple medications: Start 5/40 to 5/80 mg PO daily, may increase after 2 weeks, max 10/80 mg daily. Do not use as initial therapy in patients 75 yo or older or with hepatic impairment.

PEDS – Not approved in children.

FORMS – Trade only: Tabs, unscored 5/40, 5/80, 10/40, 10/80 mg.

UNIRETIC **(moexipril + hydrochlorothiazide)** ▶See component drugs ♀See component drugs ▶See component drugs $$

WARNING – Do not use in pregnancy.

ADULT – HTN: Establish dose using component drugs first. Dosing interval: Daily to two times per day.

PEDS – Not approved in children.

FORMS – Generic/Trade: Tabs, scored 7.5/12.5, 15/12.5, 15/25 mg.

VASERETIC **(enalapril + hydrochlorothiazide)** ▶See component drugs ♀See component drugs ▶See component drugs $$

WARNING – Do not use in pregnancy.

ADULT – HTN: Establish dose using component drugs first. Dosing interval: Daily to two times per day.

PEDS – Not approved in children.

FORMS – Generic/Trade: Tabs, unscored 5/12.5, 10/25 mg.

ZESTORETIC **(lisinopril + hydrochlorothiazide)** ▶See component drugs ♀See component drugs ▶See component drugs $$

WARNING – Do not use in pregnancy.

ADULT – HTN: Establish dose using component drugs first. Dosing interval: Daily.

PEDS – Not approved in children.

FORMS – Generic/Trade: Tabs, unscored 10/12.5, 20/12.5, 20/25 mg.

ZIAC **(bisoprolol + hydrochlorothiazide)** ▶See component drugs ♀See component drugs ▶See component drugs $$

WARNING – Avoid abrupt cessation.

ADULT – HTN: Establish dose using component drugs first. Dosing interval: Daily.

PEDS – Not approved in children.

FORMS – Generic/Trade: Tabs, unscored 2.5/6.25, 5/6.25, 10/6.25 mg.

CARDIOVASCULAR: Antihypertensives—Other

ALISKIREN (*Tekturna,* ♣ *Rasilez*) ▶LK ♀D ▶–? $$$

WARNING – Avoid in pregnancy.

ADULT – HTN: 150 mg PO daily, max 300 mg/day.

PEDS – Not approved in children.

FORMS – Trade only: Tabs unscored 150, 300 mg.

NOTES – Women of child bearing age should use reliable form of contraception; discontinue aliskerin as soon as pregnancy is detected. Do not use with ACE inhibitors or angiotensin receptor blockers in patients with DM or CrCl <60 mL/min. Do not use with cyclosporine or itraconazole. Concomitant NSAID, including selective COX-2 inhibitors, may further deteriorate renal function (usually reversible) and decrease antihypertensive effects. Hyperkalemia possible, especially if used concomitantly with other drugs that increase K+ (including K+ containing salt substitutes) and in patients with heart failure, DM, or renal impairment. Monitor potassium and renal function periodically. May increase creatine kinase, uric acid levels. Best absorbed on empty stomach; high-fat meals decrease absorption.

FENOLDOPAM (***Corlopam***) ▶LK ♀B ▶? $$$

ADULT – Severe HTN: Dilute 10 mg in 250 mL D5W (40 mcg/mL), rate at 11 mL/h delivers 0.1 mcg/kg/min for 70 kg adult, titrate q 15 min, usual effective dose 0.1 to 1.6 mcg/kg/min. Lower initial doses (0.03 to 0.1 mcg/kg/min) associated with less reflex tachycardia.

PEDS – Reduce BP: Start 0.2 mcg/kg/min, increase by up to 0.3 to 0.5 mcg/kg/min q 20 to 30 min. Max infusion 0.8 mcg/kg/min. Administer in hospital by continuous infusion pump; use max 4 h; monitor BP and HR continuously. Refer to prescribing information for dilution instructions and infusion rates.

UNAPPROVED ADULT – Prevention of contrast nephropathy in those at risk (conflicting evidence of efficacy): Start 0.03 mcg/kg/min infusion 60 min prior to dye. Titrate infusion q 15 min up to 0.1 mcg/kg/min if BP tolerates. Maintain infusion (with concurrent saline) up to 4 to 6 h after procedure.

NOTES – Avoid concomitant beta-blocker use due to hypotension. Use cautiously with glaucoma or increased intraocular HTN.

HYDRALAZINE (***Apresoline***) ▶LK ♀C ▶+ $

ADULT – HTN: Start 10 mg PO two to four times per day for 2 to 4 days, increase to 25 mg two to four times per day, then 50 mg two to four times per day if necessary, max 300 mg/day. Hypertensive emergency: 10 to 20 mg IV; if no IV access, 10 to 50 mg IM. Use lower doses initially and repeat prn to control BP. Preeclampsia/eclampsia: 5 to 10 mg IV initially, followed by 5 to 10 mg IV q 20 to 30 min prn to control BP.

PEDS – Not approved in children.

UNAPPROVED ADULT – Heart failure: Start 10 to 25 mg PO three times per day, target dose 75 mg three times per day, max 100 mg three times per day. Use in combination with isosorbide dinitrate for patients intolerant to ACE inhibitors.

(cont.)

HYDRALAZINE (*cont.*)

UNAPPROVED PEDS – HTN: Start 0.75 to 1 mg/kg/day PO divided two to four times per day, increase slowly over 3 to 4 weeks up to 7.5 mg/kg/day; initial IV dose 1.7 to 3.5 mg/kg/day divided in 4 to 6 doses. HTN urgency: 0.1 to 0.2 mg/kg IM/IV q 4 to 6 h prn. Max single dose, 25 mg PO and 20 mg IV.

FORMS – Generic only: Tabs unscored 10, 25, 50, 100 mg.

NOTES – Headache, nausea, dizziness, tachycardia, peripheral edema, systemic lupus erythematosus-like syndrome. Usually used in combination with diuretic and beta-blocker to counter side effects.

METYROSINE (***Demser***) ▶K ♀C ▶? $$$$$

ADULT – Pheochromocytoma: Start 250 mg PO four times per day, increase by 250 to 500 mg/day prn, max dose 4 g/day.

PEDS – Pheochromocytoma age older than 12 yo: Use adult dosage.

FORMS – Trade only: Caps, 250 mg.

MINOXIDIL (***Loniten***) ▶K ♀C ▶+ $$

WARNING – Potent vasodilator; may produce serious complications from hypotension and reflex tachycardia. Relatively contraindicated in patients with coronary disease (ie, recent/acute MI, CAD, angina). May increase pulmonary artery pressure. Has been associated with development of pericardial effusion and tamponade; more likely to occur in patients with renal disease.

ADULT – Refractory HTN: Start 2.5 to 5 mg PO daily, increase at no less than 3-day intervals, usual dose 10 to 40 mg daily, max 100 mg/day.

PEDS – Not approved in children younger than 12 yo.

UNAPPROVED PEDS – HTN: Start 0.2 mg/kg PO daily, increase q 3 days prn up to 0.25 to 1 mg/kg/day daily or divided two times per day; max 50 mg/day.

FORMS – Generic only: Tabs, scored 2.5, 10 mg.

NOTES – Edema, wt gain, hypertrichosis, may exacerbate heart failure. Usually used in combination with a diuretic and a beta-blocker to counteract side effects.

NITROPRUSSIDE (***Nitropress***) ▶RBCs ♀C ▶– $

WARNING – May cause significant hypotension. Reconstituted soln must be further diluted before use. Cyanide toxicity may occur, especially with high infusion rates (10 mcg/kg/min), hepatic/renal impairment, and prolonged infusions (longer than 3 to 7 days). Protect from light.

ADULT – Hypertensive emergency: 50 mg in 250 mL D5W (200 mcg/mL), start at 0.3 mcg/kg/min (for 70 kg adult give 6 mL/h) via IV infusion, titrate slowly, usual range 0.3 to 10 mcg/kg/min, max 10 mcg/kg/min.

PEDS – Severe HTN: Use adult dosage.

NOTES – Discontinue if inadequate response to 10 mcg/kg/min after 10 min. Cyanide toxicity with high doses, hepatic/renal impairment, and prolonged infusions, check thiocyanate levels. Protect IV infusion minibag from light.

PHENOXYBENZAMINE (***Dibenzyline***) ▶KL ♀C ▶? $$$$$

ADULT – Pheochromocytoma: Start 10 mg PO two times per day, increase slowly every other day prn, usual dose 20 to 40 mg two to three times per day, max 120 mg/day.

PEDS – Not approved in children.

UNAPPROVEDPEDS – Pheochromocytoma: 0.2 mg/kg/day PO daily in divided doses two to three times per day; initial dose no more than 10 mg, increase slowly every other day prn, usual dose 0.4 to 1.2 mg/kg/day.

FORMS – Trade only: Caps, 10 mg.

NOTES – Patients should be observed after each dosage increase for symptomatic hypotension and other adverse effects. Do not use for essential HTN.

PHENTOLAMINE (***Regitine, Rogitine***) ▶Plasma ♀C ▶? $$$

ADULT – Diagnosis of pheochromocytoma: 5 mg IV/IM. Rapid IV administration is preferred. An immediate, marked decrease in BP should occur, typically, 60 mmHg SBP and 25 mmHg DBP decrease in 2 min. HTN during pheochromocytoma surgery: 5 mg IV/IM 1 to 2 h preop, 5 mg IV during surgery prn.

PEDS – Diagnosis of pheochromocytoma: 0.05 to 0.1 mg/kg IV/IM, up to 5 mg/dose. Rapid IV administration is preferred. An immediate, marked decrease in BP should occur, typically, 60 mmHg SBP and 25 mmHg DBP decrease in 2 min. HTN during pheochromocytoma surgery: 0.05 to 0.1 mg/kg IV/IM 1 to 2 h preop, repeat q 2 to 4 h prn.

UNAPPROVED ADULT – IV extravasation of catecholamines: 5 to 10 mg in 10 mL NS, inject 1 to 5 mL SC (in divided doses) around extravasation site. Hypertensive crisis: 5 to 15 mg IV.

UNAPPROVED PEDS – IV extravasation of catecholamines: Neonates, 2.5 to 5 mg in 10 mL NS, inject 1 mL SC (in divided doses) around extravasation site; children, use adult dosage.

NOTES – Weakness, flushing, hypotension; priapism with intracavernous injection. Use within 12 h of extravasation. Distributed to hospital pharmacies, at no charge, only for use in life-threatening situations. Call (888) 669-6682 for ordering.

CARDIOVASCULAR: Antiplatelet Drugs

ABCIXIMAB (*ReoPro*) ▶Plasma ♀C ▶? $$$$$

ADULT – Platelet aggregation inhibition, prevention of acute cardiac ischemic events associated with PTCA: 0.25 mg/kg IV bolus over 1 min via separate infusion line 10 to 60 min before procedure, then 0.125 mcg/kg/min up to 10 mcg/min infusion for 12 h. Unstable angina not responding to standard therapy when percutaneous coronary intervention (PCI) is planned within 24 h: 0.25 mg/kg IV bolus over 1 min via separate infusion line, followed by 10 mcg/min IV infusion for 18 to 24 h, concluding 1 h after PCI.

PEDS – Not approved in children.

NOTES – Thrombocytopenia possible. Discontinue abciximab, heparin, and aspirin if uncontrollable bleeding occurs.

AGGRENOX **(acetylsalicylic acid + dipyridamole)** ▶LK ♀D ▶? $$$$

ADULT – Prevention of CVA after TIA/CVA: 1 cap PO two times per day. Headaches are common adverse effect.

PEDS – Not approved in children.

FORMS – Trade only: Caps, 25 mg aspirin/200 mg extended-release dipyridamole.

NOTES – Do not crush or chew Caps. May need supplemental aspirin for prevention of MI. Concomitant anticoagulants, NSAIDs, or antiplatelet agents increase bleeding risk.

CLOPIDOGREL (*Plavix*) ▶LK ♀B ▶? $$$$

WARNING – Requires activation to an active metabolite by the CYP system, mainly CYP2C19. When treated at recommended doses, poor metabolizers have higher cardiovascular event rates after acute coronary syndrome or percutaneous coronary intervention than patients with normal CYP2C19 function. Tests to determine a patient's CYP2C19 genotype may aid in determining therapeutic strategy. Consider alternative treatment or treatment strategies in patients identified as CYP2C19 poor metabolizers.

ADULT – Reduction of thrombotic events after recent acute MI, recent CVA, established peripheral arterial disease: 75 mg PO daily. Non-ST segment elevation acute coronary syndrome: 300 mg loading dose, then 75 mg PO daily in combination with aspirin PO daily. ST segment elevation MI: Start with/without 300 mg loading dose, then 75 mg PO daily in combination with aspirin, with/without thrombolytic.

PEDS – Not approved in children.

UNAPPROVED ADULT – Medical treatment, without stent, of unstable angina/non-ST segment elevation MI: 300 to 600 mg loading dose, then 75 mg daily in combination with aspirin for at least 1 month and up to 1 year. Medical treatment, without stent and with/without thrombolytics, of ST segment elevation MI: 300 mg loading dose, then 75 mg daily in combination with aspirin for at least 14 days and up to 1 year. When early percutaneous coronary intervention is planned: 600 mg loading dose; consider using 300 mg if patient received thrombolytic within 12 to 24 h, then 150 mg once a day for 6 days, then 75 mg daily for at least 1 year. Post bare metal stent placement or post drug-eluting stent placement: 75 mg daily in combination with aspirin for at least 1 year (in patients not at high risk for bleeding). Post-percutaneous coronary brachytherapy: 75 mg daily in combination with aspirin for at least 1 year. Acute coronary syndrome with aspirin allergy or reduction of thrombotic events in high-risk patient after TIA: 75 mg PO daily.

FORMS – Generic/Trade Tabs unscored 75, 300 mg.

NOTES – Effectiveness is reduced with impaired CYP2C19 function; avoid drugs that are strong or moderate CYP2C19 inhibors (eg, omeprazole, esomeprazole, cimetidine, etravirine, felbamate, fluconazole, fluoxetine, fluvoxamine, ketoconazole, voriconazole). Contraindicated with active pathologic bleeding (peptic ulcer or intracranial bleed). Prolongs bleeding time. Discontinue use 5 days before elective surgery, except in 1st year post coronary stent implantation; premature discontinuation increases risk of cardiovascular events. Concomitant aspirin increases bleeding risk. Cardiovascular (but not CVA) patients may receive additional benefit when given with aspirin. Should not be used with aspirin for primary prevention of cardiovascular events.

DIPYRIDAMOLE (*Persantine*) ▶L ♀B ▶? $$$

ADULT – Prevention of thromboembolic complications of cardiac valve replacement: 75 to 100 mg PO four times per day in combination with warfarin.

PEDS – Not approved in children younger than 12 yo.

UNAPPROVED ADULT – Platelet aggregation inhibition: 150 to 400 mg/day PO divided three to four times per day.

FORMS – Generic/Trade: Tabs unscored 25, 50, 75 mg.

NOTES – May cause chest pain when used in CAD.

EPTIFIBATIDE (*Integrilin*) ▶K ♀B ▶? $$$$$

ADULT – Acute coronary syndrome (unstable angina/non-ST segment elevation MI): Load 180 mcg/kg IV bolus, then IV infusion 2 mcg/kg/min for up to 72 h. If percutaneous coronary intervention (PCI) occurs during the infusion, continue infusion for 18 to 24 h after procedure. PCI: Load 180 mcg/kg IV bolus just before procedure, followed by infusion 2 mcg/kg/min and a second 180 mcg/kg IV bolus 10 min after the first bolus. Continue infusion for up to 18 to 24 h (minimum 12 h) after the procedure. Renal impairment (CrCl less than 50 mL/min): No change in bolus dose; decrease infusion to 1 mcg/kg/min. For obese patient (greater than 121 kg): max bolus dose 22.6 mg; max infusion rate 15 mg/h. Renal impairment and obese: max bolus dose 22.6 mg; max infusion rate 7.5 mg/h.

PEDS – Not approved in children.

NOTES – Discontinue infusion prior to CABG. Give with aspirin and heparin/enoxaparin, unless contraindicated. Contraindicated in patients on dialysis, with a history of bleeding diathesis or active abnormal bleeding within past 30 days, severe hypertension (SBP greater than 200 mmHg or DBP greater than 110 mmHg) not controlled on antihypertensive therapy; major surgery within past 6 weeks; stroke within 30 days or any history of hemorrhagic stroke. Thrombocytopenia possible; monitor platelets. If profound thrombocytopenia occurs or platelets decrease to less than 100,000 mm^3, discontinue eptifibatide and heparin and monitor serial platelet counts, assess for drug-dependent antibodies, and treat as appropriate.

PRASUGREL (*Effient*) ▶LK ♀B ▶? $$$$

WARNING – May cause significant, fatal bleeding. Do not use with active bleeding or history of TIA or CVA. Generally not recommend for patients 75 yo and older. Do not start in patients likely to need urgent CABG. When possible, discontinue 7 days prior to any surgery. Risk factors for bleeding: Body wt less than 60 kg, propensity to bleed, concomitant medications that increase bleeding risk. Suspect bleeding with hypotension and recent coronary angiography, PCI, CABG, or other surgical procedure. Premature discontinuation increases risk of stent thrombosis, MI, and death.

ADULT – Reduction of thrombotic events, including stent thrombosis, after acute coronary syndrome managed with percutaneous coronary intervention (PCI): 60 mg loading dose, then 10 mg PO daily in combination with aspirin. Wt less than 60 kg: Consider lower maintenance dose, 5 mg PO daily.

PEDS – Not approved in children.

FORMS – Trade: Tabs unscored 5, 10 mg.

NOTES – Concomitant warfarin or NSAID increases bleeding risk.

TICAGRELOR (*Brilinta*) ▶L – ♀C ▶? $$$$$

WARNING – May cause significant, fatal bleeding. Do not use with active bleeding or history of intracranial hemorrhage. Do not start in patients likely to need urgent CABG. When possible, discontinue 5 days prior to any surgery. Suspect bleeding with hypotension and recent coronary angiography, PCI, CABG, or other surgical procedure. If possible, manage bleeding without discontinuing ticagrelor; discontinuation increases risk of cardiovascular events. After the initial dose of aspirin, use with aspirin 75 to 100 mg daily; doses of aspirin greater than 100 mg daily reduce the effectiveness of ticagrelor.

ADULT – Reduction of thrombotic events in patients with acute coronary syndrome (MI or unstable angina): 180 mg loading dose, then 90 mg PO two times daily in combination with aspirin. After the initial dose of aspirin, do not use more than 100 mg of aspirin daily with ticagrelor.

PEDS – Not approved in children.

FORMS – Trade only: Tabs, unscored 90 mg.

NOTES – Do not use with strong CYP3A inhibitors (eg, clarithromycin, HIV protease inhibitors, itraconazole, ketoconazole, nefazodone, telithromycin, voriconazole), CYP3A inducers (eg, carbamazepine, dexamethasone, phenobarbital, phenytoin, rifampin), or severe hepatic impairment. Monitor digoxin levels when initiating or changing ticagrelor therapy. Increases risk of statin-related side effects when used concomitantly with more than 40 mg daily of simvastatin or lovastatin.

TICLOPIDINE (*Ticlid*) ▶L ♀B ▶? $$$$

WARNING – May cause life-threatening neutropenia, agranulocytosis, and thrombotic thrombocytopenia purpura (TTP). During 1st 3 months of treatment, monitor patient clinically and hematologically for neutropenia or TTP; discontinue if evidence is seen.

ADULT – Due to adverse effects, other antiplatelet agents preferred. Platelet aggregation inhibition, reduction of thrombotic CVA: 250 mg PO twice daily with food. Prevention of cardiac stent occlusion: 250 mg PO twice daily in combination with aspirin 325 mg PO daily for up to 30 days post-stent implantation.

PEDS – Not approved in children.

UNAPPROVED ADULT – Prevention of graft occlusion with CABG: 250 mg PO two times per day.

(cont.)

TICLOPIDINE (*cont.*)

FORMS – Generic/Trade: Tabs unscored 250 mg.
NOTES – Check CBC q 2 weeks during the first 3 months of therapy. Neutrophil counts usually return to normal within 1 to 3 weeks following discontinuation. Loading dose 500 mg PO on day 1 may be used for prevention of cardiac stent occlusion.

TIROFIBAN (*Aggrastat*) ▶K ♀B ▶? $$$$$

ADULT – Acute coronary syndromes (unstable angina and non-Q-wave MI): Start 0.4 mcg/kg/min IV infusion for 30 min, then decrease to 0.1 mcg/kg/min for 48 to 108 h or until 12 to 24 h after coronary intervention.
PEDS – Not approved in children.
NOTES – Thrombocytopenia possible. Concomitant aspirin and heparin/enoxaparin use recommended, unless contraindicated. Dose heparin to keep PTT 2 times normal. Decrease bolus dose and rate of infusion by 50% in patients with CrCl less than 30 mL/min. Dilute concentrate soln before using.

CARDIOVASCULAR: Beta-Blockers

NOTE: See also antihypertensive combinations. Not first line for HTN (unless concurrent angina, post-MI, or heart failure). Nonselective beta-blockers, including carvedilol and labetalol, are contraindicated with asthma; use agents with beta-1 selectivity and monitor cautiously; beta-1 selectivity diminishes at high doses. Contraindicated with acute decompensated heart failure, sick sinus syndrome without pacer, cardiogenic shock, heart block greater than first degree, or severe bradycardia. Agents with intrinsic sympathomimetic activity (eg, pindolol) are contraindicated post acute MI. Abrupt cessation may precipitate angina, MI, arrhythmias, tachycardia, rebound HTN; or with thyrotoxicosis, thyroid storm; discontinue by tapering over 1 to 2 weeks. Do not routinely stop chronic beta-blocker therapy prior to surgery. Discontinue beta-blocker several days before discontinuing concomitant clonidine to minimize the risk of rebound HTN. Some inhalation anesthetics may increase the cardiodepressant effect of beta-blockers. With pheochromocytoma, give beta-blocker only after initiating alpha-blocker; using beta-blocker alone may increase BP due to the attenuation of beta-mediated vasodilatation in skeletal muscle (unopposed alpha stimulation). Patients actively using cocaine should avoid beta-blockers with unopposed alpha-adrenergic vasoconstriction, because this will promote coronary artery vasoconstriction/spasm (carvedilol or labetalol have additional alpha-1-blocking effects and are safer). Concomitant amiodarone, disopyramide, clonidine, digoxin, or nondihydropyridine calcium channel blockers may increase risk of bradycardia. Monitor for heart failure exacerbation and hypotension (particularly orthostatic) when titrating dose. May increase blood sugar or mask tachycardia occurring with hypoglycemia. May aggravate psoriasis or symptoms of arterial insufficiency. Intraoperative floppy iris syndrome may occur during cataract surgery, if patient is on or has previously taken agents with alpha-1 blocking activity. Cross-sensitivity between beta-blockers can occur.

ACEBUTOLOL (*Sectral*) ▶LK ♀B ▶– $$

WARNING – Avoid abrupt cessation in coronary heart disease or HTN.
ADULT – HTN: Start 400 mg PO daily or 200 mg PO two times per day, usual maintenance 400 to 800 mg/day, max 1200 mg/day. Twice daily dosing appears to be more effective than daily dosing.
PEDS – Not approved in children age younger than 12 yo.
UNAPPROVED ADULT – Angina: Start 200 mg PO two times per day, increase prn up to 800 mg/day.
FORMS – Generic/Trade: Caps 200, 400 mg.
NOTES – Beta-1 receptor selective; has mild intrinsic sympathomimetic activity.

ATENOLOL (*Tenormin*) ▶K ♀D ▶– $

WARNING – Avoid abrupt cessation in coronary heart disease or HTN.
ADULT – Acute MI: 50 to 100 mg PO daily or in divided doses. HTN: Start 25 to 50 mg PO daily or divided two times per day, max 100 mg/day. Renal impairment, elderly: Start 25 mg PO daily, increase prn. Angina: Start 50 mg PO daily or divided two times per day, increase prn to max of 200 mg/day.
PEDS – Not approved in children.
UNAPPROVED ADULT – Reduce perioperative cardiac events (death) in high-risk patients undergoing noncardiac surgery: Start 5 to 10 mg IV prior to anesthesia, then 50 to 100 mg PO daily during hospitalization (max 7 days). Maintain HR between 55 to 65 bpm. Hold dose for HR less than 55 bpm and SBP less than 100 mmHg. Reentrant PSVT associated with ST-elevation MI (after carotid massage, IV adenosine): 2.5 to 5 mg over 2 min to 10 mg max over 10 to 15 min. Rate control of atrial fibrillation/flutter: Start 25 mg PO daily, titrate to desired heart rate.
UNAPPROVED PEDS – HTN: 1 to 1.2 mg/kg/dose PO daily, max 2 mg/kg/day.

(cont.)

ATENOLOL (*cont.*)

FORMS – Generic/Trade: Tabs unscored 25, 100 mg; scored, 50 mg.

NOTES – Beta-1 receptor selective. Doses greater than 100 mg/day usually do not provide further BP lowering. Risk of hypoglycemia to neonates born to mothers using atenolol at parturition or while breastfeeding. May be less effective for HTN and lowering CV event risk than other beta-blockers.

BETAXOLOL (***Kerlone***) ▶LK ♀C ▶? $$

WARNING – Avoid abrupt cessation in coronary heart disease or HTN.

ADULT – HTN: Start 5 to 10 mg PO daily, max 20 mg/day. Renal impairment, elderly: Start 5 mg PO daily, increase prn.

PEDS – Not approved in children.

FORMS – Generic: Tabs scored 10 mg, unscored 20 mg.

NOTES – Beta-1 receptor selective.

BISOPROLOL (***Zebeta***, ***✤Monocor***) ▶LK ♀C ▶? $$

WARNING – Avoid abrupt cessation in coronary heart disease or HTN.

ADULT – HTN: Start 2.5 to 5 mg PO daily, max 20 mg/day. Renal impairment: Start 2.5 mg PO daily, increase prn.

PEDS – Not approved in children.

UNAPPROVED ADULT – Compensated heart failure: Start 1.25 mg PO daily, double dose q 2 weeks as tolerated to goal 10 mg/day. Reduce perioperative cardiac events (death, MI) in high-risk patients undergoing noncardiac surgery: Start 5 mg PO daily, at least 1 week prior to surgery, increase to 10 mg daily to maintain HR less than 60 bpm, continue for 30 days postop. Hold dose for HR less than 50 bpm or SBP less than 100 mmHg.

FORMS – Generic/Trade: Tabs scored 5 mg, unscored 10 mg.

NOTES – Monitor closely for heart failure exacerbation and hypotension when titrating dose. Avoid in decompensated heart failure (ie, NYHA class IV heart failure or pulmonary edema). Stabilize dose of digoxin, diuretics, and ACE inhibitor before starting bisoprolol. Highly beta-1 receptor selective.

CARVEDILOL (***Coreg***, ***Coreg CR***) ▶L ♀C ▶? $$$$

WARNING – Avoid abrupt cessation in coronary heart disease or HTN.

ADULT – Heart failure: Immediate-release: Start 3.125 mg PO two times per day, double dose q 2 weeks as tolerated up to max of 25 mg two times per day (for wt 85 kg or less) or 50 mg two times per day (for wt 85 kg or greater). Heart failure, sustained-release: Start 10 mg PO daily, double dose q 2 weeks as tolerated up to max of 80 mg/day. Reduce cardiovascular risk in post-MI with LV dysfunction, immediate-release: Start 3.125 to 6.25 mg PO two times per day, double dose q 3 to 10 days as tolerated to max of 25 mg two times per day. LV dysfunction post-MI, sustained-release: Start 10 to 20 mg PO daily, double dose q 3 to 10 days as tolerated to max of 80 mg/day. HTN, immediate-release: Start 6.25 mg PO two times per day, double dose q 7 to 14 days as tolerated to max 50 mg/day. HTN, sustained-release: Start 20 mg PO daily, double dose q 7 to 14 days as tolerated to max 80 mg/day.

PEDS – Not approved in children.

FORMS – Generic/Trade: Tabs immediate-release unscored 3.125, 6.25, 12.5, 25 mg. Trade only: Caps extended-release 10, 20, 40, 80 mg.

NOTES – Alpha-1, beta-1, and beta-2 receptor blocker. Avoid in hepatic impairment. May reversibly elevate LFTs. Amiodarone may increase carvedilol levels. May increase digoxin levels. Reduce the dose with bradycardia (less than 55 bpm). Take with food to decrease orthostatic hypotension. Separate Coreg CR and alcohol (including medications containing alcohol) by at least 2 h. Give Coreg CR in the morning. The contents of Coreg CR may be sprinkled over applesauce and consumed immediately. Dosing conversion from immediate-release to sustained-release: 3.125 mg two times per day is equivalent to 10 mg CR; 6.25 mg two times per day is equivalent to 20 mg CR; 12.5 mg two times per day is equivalent to 40 mg CR; 25 mg two times per day is equivalent to 80 mg CR.

ESMOLOL (***Brevibloc***) ▶K ♀C ▶? $

ADULT – SVT/HTN emergency: Load 500 mcg/kg over 1 min, dilute 5 g in 500 mL (10 mg/mL), and give 3.5 mL to deliver 35 mg bolus for 70 kg patient) then start infusion 50 to 200 mcg/kg/min (40 mL/h delivers 100 mcg/kg/min for 70 kg patient). If optimal response is not attained, repeat IV load and increase IV infusion to 100 mcg/kg/min for 4 min. If necessary, additional boluses (500 mcg/kg/min over 1 min) may be given followed by IV infusion with increased dose by 50 mcg/kg/min for 4 min. Max IV infusion rate 200 mcg/kg/min.

PEDS – Not approved in children.

(cont.)

ESMOLOL (*cont.*)

UNAPPROVED PEDS – Same schedule as adult except loading dose 100 to 500 mcg/kg IV over 1 min and IV infusion 25 to 100 mcg/kg/min. IV infusions may be increased by 25 to 50 mcg/kg/min q 5 to 10 min. Titrate dose based on response.

NOTES – Hypotension. Beta-1 receptor selective. Half-life is 9 min.

LABETALOL (*Trandate*) ▶LK ♀C ▶+ $$$

WARNING – Avoid abrupt cessation in coronary heart disease or HTN.

ADULT – HTN: Start 100 mg PO two times per day, usual maintenance dose 200 to 600 mg two times per day, max 2400 mg/day. HTN emergency: Start 20 mg slow IV injection, then 40 to 80 mg IV q 10 min prn up to 300 mg total cumulative dose or start 0.5 to 2 mg/min IV infusion, adjust rate prn up to total cumulative dose 300 mg.

PEDS – Not approved in children.

UNAPPROVED PEDS – HTN: 4 mg/kg/day PO divided two times per day, increase prn up to 40 mg/kg/day. IV: Start 0.3 to 1 mg/kg/dose (max 20 mg) slow IV injection q 10 min or 0.4 to 1 mg/kg/h IV infusion up to 3 mg/kg/h.

FORMS – Generic/Trade: Tabs scored 100, 200, 300 mg.

NOTES – Alpha-1, beta-1, and beta-2 receptor blocker. May be used to manage BP during pregnancy.

METOPROLOL (*Lopressor, Toprol-XL,* ✤ *Betaloc*) ▶L ♀C ▶? $$

WARNING – Avoid abrupt cessation in coronaryheart disease or HTN.

ADULT – Acute MI: 50 to 100 mg PO q 12 h; or 5 mg IV q 5 to 15 min up to 15 mg, then start 50 mg PO q 6 h for 48 h, then 100 mg PO two times per day as tolerated. HTN (immediate-release): Start 100 mg PO daily or in divided doses, increase prn up to 450 mg/day; may require multiple daily doses to maintain 24-h BP control. HTN (extended-release): Start 25 to 100 mg PO daily, increase prn q week up to 400 mg/day. Heart failure: Start 12.5 to 25 mg (extended-release) PO daily, double dose q 2 weeks as tolerated up to max 200 mg/day. Angina: Start 50 mg PO two times per day (immediate-release) or 100 mg PO daily (extended-release), increase prn up to 400 mg/day. Take with food.

PEDS – HTN 6 yo or older: Start 1 mg/kg, max 50 mg/daily. Not recommended for younger than 6 yo.

UNAPPROVED ADULT – Atrial tachyarrhythmia, except with Wolff-Parkinson-White syndrome: 2.5 to 5 mg IV q 2 to 5 min prn to control rapid ventricular response, max 15 mg over 10 to 15 min. Reentrant PSVT (after carotid massage, IV adenosine): 2.5 to 5 mg q 2 to 5 min to 15 mg max over 10 to 15 min. Reduce perioperative cardiac events (death) in high-risk patients undergoing noncardiac surgery: Start 100 mg (extended-release) 2 h prior to anesthesia, then 50 to 100 mg (extended-release) PO daily or 2.5 to 5 mg IV q 6 h during hospitalization (max 7 days). Maintain HR between 55 and 65 bpm. Hold dose for HR less than 55 bpm and SBP less than 100 mmHg. Rate control of atrial fibrillation/flutter: Start 25 mg PO two times per day, titrate to desired heart rate.

FORMS – Generic/Trade: Tabs scored 50, 100 mg, extended-release 25, 50, 100, 200 mg. Generic only: Tabs scored 25 mg.

NOTES – Beta-1 receptor selective. Immediate-release form is metoprolol tartrate; extended-release form is metoprolol succinate. When switching from immediate-release to extended-release product, use same total daily dose. The immediate- and extended-release products may not give same clinical response on mg:mg basis; monitor response and side effects when interchanging between metoprolol products. Do not start high-dose extended-release form in patients undergoing noncardiac surgery. Monitor closely for heart failure exacerbation and hypotension when titrating dose. Stabilize dose of diuretics and ACE inhibitor before starting metoprolol. May need lower doses in elderly and in patients with liver impairment. Extended-release tabs may be broken in half, but do not chew or crush.

NADOLOL (*Corgard*) ▶K ♀C ▶– $$

WARNING – Avoid abrupt cessation in coronary heart disease or HTN.

ADULT – HTN: Start 20 to 40 mg PO daily, usual maintenance dose 40 to 80 mg/day, max 320 mg/day. Renal impairment: Start 20 mg PO daily, adjust dosage interval based on severity of renal impairment: For CrCl < 10 mL/min give q 40 to 60 h; for CrCl 10 to 30 mL/min give q 24 to 48 h; for CrCl 31 to 50 mL/min give q 24 to 36 h. Angina: Start 40 mg PO daily, usual maintenance dose 40 to 80 mg/day, max 240 mg/day.

PEDS – Not approved in children.

UNAPPROVED ADULT – Prevent rebleeding esophageal varices: 40 to 160 mg/day PO. Titrate dose to reduce heart rate to 25% below baseline.

FORMS – Generic/Trade: Tabs scored 20, 40, 80, 120, 160 mg.

NOTES – Beta-1 and beta-2 receptor blocker.

NEBIVOLOL (*Bystolic*) ▶L ♀C ▶– $$$

WARNING – Avoid abrupt cessation in coronary heart disease or HTN.

ADULT – HTN: Start 5 mg PO daily, max 40 mg/day. Severe renal impairment (CrCl < 30 mL/min), moderate hepatic impairment: Start 2.5 mg PO daily, increase cautiously.

PEDS – Not approved in children.

FORMS – Trade only: Tabs unscored 2.5, 5, 10, 20 mg.

NOTES – Do not use with severe liver impairment.

PENBUTOLOL (*Levatol*) ▶LK ♀C ▶? $$$$

WARNING – Avoid abrupt cessation in coronary heart disease or HTN.

ADULT – HTN: Start 20 mg PO daily, usual maintenance dose 20 to 40 mg, max 80 mg/day.

PEDS – Not approved in children.

FORMS – Trade only: Tabs, scored 20 mg.

NOTES – Beta-1 and beta-2 receptor blocker; has mild intrinsic sympathomimetic activity.

PINDOLOL (♣ *Visken*) ▶K ♀B ▶? $$$

WARNING – Avoid abrupt cessation in coronary heart disease or HTN.

ADULT – HTN: Start 5 mg PO two times per day, usual maintenance dose 10 to 30 mg/day, max 60 mg/day.

PEDS – Not approved in children.

UNAPPROVED ADULT – Angina: 15 to 40 mg/day PO in divided doses three to four times per day.

FORMS – Generic only: Tabs, scored 5, 10 mg.

NOTES – Has intrinsic sympathomimetic activity (partial beta-agonist activity); beta-1 and beta-2 receptor blocker.

PROPRANOLOL (*Inderal, Inderal LA, InnoPran XL*) ▶L ♀C ▶+ $$

WARNING – Avoid abrupt cessation in coronary heart disease or HTN.

ADULT – HTN: Start 20 to 40 mg PO two times per day, usual maintenance dose 160 to 480 mg/day, max 640 mg/day; extended-release (Inderal LA): Start 60 to 80 mg PO daily, usual maintenance dose 120 to 160 mg/day, max 640 mg/day; extended-release (InnoPran XL): Start 80 mg at bedtime (10 pm), max 120 mg at bedtime. Angina: Start 10 to 20 mg PO three to four times per day, usual maintenance 160 to 240 mg/day, max 320 mg/day; extended-release (Inderal LA): Start 80 mg PO daily, same usual dosage range and max for HTN. Migraine prophylaxis: Start 40 mg PO two times per day or 80 mg PO daily (extended-release), max 240 mg/day. Supraventricular tachycardia or rapid atrial fibrillation/flutter: 10 to 30 mg PO three to four times per day. MI: 180 to 240 mg/day PO in divided doses two to four times per day. Pheochromocytoma surgery: 60 mg PO in divided doses two to three times per day beginning 3 days before surgery, use in combination with an alpha-blocking agent. IV: Reserved for life-threatening arrhythmia, 1 to 3 mg IV, repeat dose in 2 min if needed, additional doses only after 4 h. Not for use in hypertensive emergency. Essential tremor: Start 40 mg PO two times per day, titrate prn to 120 to 320 mg/day.

PEDS – HTN: Start 1 mg/kg/day PO divided two times per day, usual maintenance dose 2 to 4 mg/kg/day PO divided two times per day, max 16 mg/kg/day.

UNAPPROVED ADULT – Prevent rebleeding esophageal varices: 20 to 180 mg PO two times per day. Titrate dose to reduce heart rate to 25% below baseline. Control heart rate with A-fib: 80 to 240 mg/day daily or in divided doses. Thyrotoxicosis: 60 to 80 mg q 4 h; or IV 0.5 to 1 mg over 10 min q 3 h.

UNAPPROVED PEDS – Arrhythmia: 0.01 to 0.1 mg/kg/dose (max 1 mg/dose) by slow IV push. Manufacturer does not recommend IV propranolol in children.

FORMS – Generic/Trade: Tabs, scored 40, 60, 80 mg. Caps, extended-release 60, 80, 120, 160 mg. Generic only: Soln 20, 40 mg/5 mL. Tabs, 10, 20 mg. Trade only: (InnoPran XL at bedtime) 80, 120 mg.

NOTES – Beta-1 and beta-2 receptor blocker. The immediate- and extended-release products may not give same clinical response on mg:mg basis; monitor response and side effects when interchanging between products. Extended-release caps (Inderal LA) may be opened, and the contents sprinkled on food for administration, cap contents should be swallowed whole without crushing or chewing. InnoPran XL is a chronotherapeutic product; give at bedtime to blunt early morning surge in BP. Acute alcohol use may increase propranolol level; chronic alcohol use may decrease propranolol level.

TIMOLOL (*Blocadren*) ▶LK ♀C ▶+ $$$

WARNING – Avoid abrupt cessation in coronary heart disease or HTN.

ADULT – HTN: Start 10 mg PO two times per day, usual maintenance 20 to 40 mg/day, max 60 mg/day. MI: 10 mg PO two times per day, started 1 to 4 weeks post MI. Migraine headaches: Start 10 mg PO two times per day, use 20 mg/day daily or divided two times per day for prophylaxis, increase prn

(cont.)

TIMOLOL (*cont.*)

up to max 60 mg/day; stop therapy if satisfactory response not obtained after 6 to 8 weeks of max dose.

PEDS – Not approved in children.

UNAPPROVED ADULT – Angina: 15 to 45 mg/day PO divided three to four times per day.

FORMS – Generic only: Tabs, 5, 10, 20 mg.

NOTES – Beta-1 and beta-2 receptor blocker.

CARDIOVASCULAR: Calcium Channel Blockers (CCBs)—Dihydropyridines

NOTE: See also antihypertensive combination. Avoid in decompensated heart failure. May increase proteinuria, edema. Extended-/controlled-/sustained-release forms: Swallow whole; do not chew/crush.

AMLODIPINE (***Norvasc***) ▶L ♀C ▶? $

ADULT – HTN, CAD: Start 5 mg PO daily, max 10 mg/day. Elderly, small, frail, or with hepatic insufficiency: Start 2.5 mg PO daily.

PEDS – HTN (6 to 17 yo): 2.5 to 5 mg PO daily.

UNAPPROVED PEDS – HTN: Start 0.1 to 0.2 mg/kg/day PO daily, max 0.3 mg/kg/day (max 10 mg daily).

FORMS – Generic/Trade: Tabs unscored 2.5, 5, 10 mg.

NOTES – Do not use with more than 20 mg of simvastatin.

CLEVIDIPINE (***Cleviprex***) ▶KL ♀C ▶? $$$

ADULT – HTN: Start 1 to 2 mg/h IV, double dose q 1.5 min as approaches BP goal, then titrate at smaller increments q 5 to 10 min to desired BP, usual maintenance dose 4 to 6 mg/h, max 32 mg/h IV. An increase of 1 to 2 mg/h will decrease SBP approximately 2 to 4 mmHg.

PEDS – Not approved in children.

NOTES – Contraindicated with egg or soy allergy, defective lipid metabolism, or severe aortic stenosis. May exacerbate heart failure.

FELODIPINE (***Plendil, ✤Renedil***) ▶L ♀C ▶? $$

ADULT – HTN: Start 2.5 to 5 mg PO daily, usual maintenance dose 5 to 10 mg/day, max 10 mg/day.

PEDS – Not approved in children.

FORMS – Generic/Trade: Tabs extended-release, unscored 2.5, 5, 10 mg.

NOTES – Extended-release tab. May increase tacrolimus level. Concomitant CYP3A4 inhibitors (eg, ketoconazole, itraconazole, erythromycin, grapefruit juice, cimetidine) may increase felodipine level.

ISRADIPINE (***DynaCirc, DynaCirc CR***) ▶L ♀C ▶? $$$$

ADULT – HTN: Start 2.5 mg PO tow times per day, usual maintenance 5 to 10 mg/day, max 20 mg/day divided two times per day (max 10 mg/day in elderly). Controlled-release (DynaCirc CR): Start 5 mg PO daily, usual maintenance dose 5 to 10 mg/day, max 20 mg/day.

PEDS – Not approved in children.

FORMS – Trade only: Tabs controlled-release 5, 10 mg. Generic only: Immediate-release caps 2.5, 5 mg.

NICARDIPINE (***Cardene, Cardene SR***) ▶L ♀C ▶? $$

ADULT – HTN: Sustained-release (Cardene SR): Start 30 mg PO two times per day, usual maintenance dose 30 to 60 mg PO two times per day, max 120 mg/day; immediate-release: Start 20 mg PO three times per day, usual maintenance dose 20 to 40 mg PO three times per day, max 120 mg/day. Angina: Immediate-release: Start 20 mg PO three times per day, usual maintenance dose 20 to 40 mg three times per day. Short-term management of HTN, patient not receiving PO nicardipine: Begin IV infusion at 5 mg/h, titrate infusion rate by 2.5 mg/h q 5 to 15 min prn, max 15 mg/h. Short-term management of HTN, patient receiving PO nicardipine: If using 20 mg PO q 8 h, give 0.5 mg/h IV; if using 30 mg PO q 8 h, give 1.2 mg/h IV; if using 40 mg PO q 8 h, give 2.2 mg/h. When discontinuing IV nicardipine and transitioning to an oral BP regimen: Administer first dose of nicardipine PO 1 h prior to discontinuing IV infusion; or initiate BP-lowering agent other than nicardipine upon discontinuation of IV infusion.

PEDS – Not approved in children.

UNAPPROVED PEDS – HTN: 0.5 to 3 mcg/kg/min IV infusion.

FORMS – Generic/Trade: Caps immediate-release 20, 30 mg. Trade only: Caps sustained-release 30, 45, 60 mg.

NOTES – Hypotension, especially with immediate-release caps and IV. Decrease dose if hepatically impaired. Titrate carefully if renally impaired. Use sustained-release caps for HTN only, not for angina. May increase cyclosporine level. Concomitant cimetidine may increase nicardipine level.

NIFEDIPINE (*Procardia, Adalat, Procardia XL, Adalat CC, Afeditab CR,* ♣ *Adalat XL, Adalat PA*) ▶L ♀C ▶– $$

ADULT – HTN: Extended-release: Start 30 to 60 mg PO daily, max 120 mg/day. Angina: Extended-release: Start 30 to 60 mg PO daily, max 120 mg/day; immediate-release: Start 10 mg PO three times per day, usual maintenance dose 10 to 20 mg three times per day, max 120 mg/day.

PEDS – Not approved in children.

UNAPPROVED ADULT – Preterm labor: Loading dose 10 mg PO q 20 to 30 min if contractions persist up to 40 mg within the first h. After contractions are controlled, maintenance dose: 10 to 20 mg PO q 4 to 6 h or 60 to 160 mg extended-release PO daily. Duration of treatment has not been established. Promotes spontaneous passage of ureteral calculi: Extended-release, 30 mg PO daily for 10 to 28 days.

UNAPPROVED PEDS – HTN: 0.25 to 0.5 mg/kg/dose PO q 4 to 6 h prn, max 10 mg/dose or 3 mg/kg/day. Doses less than 0.25 mg/kg may be effective.

FORMS – Generic/Trade: Caps 10, 20 mg. Tabs extended-release (Adalat CC, Afeditab CR, Procardia XL) 30, 60 mg, (Adalat CC, Procardia XL) 90 mg.

NOTES – Do not use immediate-release caps for treating HTN, hypertensive emergencies, or ST-elevation MI. Immediate-release caps should not be chewed and swallowed or given sublingually; may cause excessive hypotension, CVA. Extended-release tabs can be substituted for immediate-release caps at the same dose in patients whose angina is controlled. Extended-release tabs have been associated with gastrointestinal obstruction; use extended-release tabs cautiously in patients with preexisting severe gastrointestinal narrowing. Metabolized by the CYP3A4 enzyme system. Use alternative BP-lowering medication when patient on carbamazepine, phenobarbital, phenytoin, rifampin, or St. John's wort; these reduce levels of nifidepine significantly. Concomitant clarithromycin, erythromycin, fluconazole, fluoxetine, grapefruit, HIV protease inhibitors, ketoconazole, itraconazole, or nefazodone increases nifedipine level. Increases tacrolimus level. Stop grapefruit juice intake at least 3 days prior to starting nifedipine. Severe hypotension and/or increased fluid volume requirements may occur when used with beta-blocker for patient who had surgery using high-dose fentanyl anesthesia; when appropriate, discontinue nifedipine at least 36 h prior to surgery that may require high-dose fentanyl anesthesia.

NISOLDIPINE (*Sular*) ▶L ♀C ▶? $$$

ADULT – HTN: Start 17 mg PO daily, may increase by 8.5 mg weekly, max 34 mg/day. Impaired hepatic function, elderly: Start 8.5 mg PO daily, titrate prn.

PEDS – Not approved in children.

FORMS – Trade only: Tabs extended-release 8.5, 17, 25.5, 34 mg. These replace the former 10, 20, 30, 40 mg tabs. Generic only: Tabs extended-release 20, 30, 40 mg.

NOTES – Take on an empty stomach. Sular 8.5, 17, 25.5, 34 mg replace 10, 20, 30, 40 mg respectively.

CARDIOVASCULAR: Calcium Channel Blockers (CCBs)—Non-Dihydropyridines

NOTE: See also Antihypertensive Combinations. Avoid in decompensated heart failure; sick sinus syndrome or 2nd/3rd degree heart block without pacemaker; acute MI and pulmonary congestion; or systolic blood pressure less than 90 mmHg systolic.

DILTIAZEM (*Cardizem, Cardizem LA, Cardizem CD, Cartia XT, Dilacor XR, Diltiazem CD, Diltzac, Diltia XT, Tiazac, Taztia XT*) ▶L ♀C ▶+ $$

ADULT – Atrial fibrillation/flutter, PSVT: 20 mg (0.25 mg/kg) IV bolus over 2 min. If needed and patient tolerated IV bolus with no hypotension, rebolus 15 min later with 25 mg (0.35 mg/kg). IV infusion: Start 10 mg/h, increase by 5 mg/h (usual range 5 to 15 mg/h). Once a day, extended-release (Cardizem CD, Cartia XT, Dilacor XR, Diltia XT, Taztia XT, Tiazac), HTN: Start 120 to 240 mg PO daily, usual maintenance range 240 to 360 mg/day, max 540 mg/day. Once a day, graded extended-release (Cardizem LA), HTN: Start 180 to 240 mg, max 540 mg/day. Twice a day, sustained-release (Cardizem SR), HTN: Start 60 to 120 mg PO two times per day, max 360 mg/day. Immediate-release, angina: Start 30 mg PO four times per day, max 360 mg/day divided three to four times per day. Extended-release, angina: 120 to 180 mg PO daily, max 540 mg/day. Once a day, graded extended-release (Cardizem LA), angina: Start 180 mg PO daily, doses greater than 360 mg may provide no additional benefit.

PEDS – Not approved in children. Diltiazem injection should be avoided in neonates due

(cont.)

DILTIAZEM (*cont.*)

to potential toxicity from benzyl alcohol in the injectable product.

UNAPPROVED ADULT – Control heart rate with chronic A-fib: 120 to 360 mg/day daily or in divided doses.

UNAPPROVED PEDS – HTN: Start 1.5 to 2 mg/kg/day PO divided three to four times per day, max 3.5 mg/kg/day.

FORMS – Generic/Trade: Tabs immediate-release, unscored (Cardizem) 30, scored 60, 90, 120 mg; Caps extended-release (Cardizem CD, Cartia XT daily) 120, 180, 240, 300, 360 mg, (Diltzac, Taztia XT, Tiazac daily) 120, 180, 240, 300, 360, 420 mg, (Dilacor XR, Diltia XT) 120, 180, 240 mg. Trade only: Tabs extended-release graded (Cardizem LA daily) 120, 180, 240, 300, 360, 420 mg.

NOTES – Sinus bradycardia resulting in hospitalization and pacemaker insertion has been reported with concomitant clonidine; monitor heart rate. May increase levels of buspirone, lovastatin, quinidine, simvastatin. Do not use with more than 10 mg of simvastatin or 20 mg of lovastatin. Contents of extended-release caps may be sprinkled over food. Do not chew or crush cap contents. May accumulate with hepatic impairment. Monitor response and side effects when interchanging between diltiazem products; many are not equivalent on mg:mg basis. Cardizem LA is a chronotherapeutic product; give at bedtime to blunt early morning surge in BP.

VERAPAMIL (***Isoptin SR, Calan, Covera-HS, Verelan, Verelan PM***) ▶L ♀C ▶– $$

ADULT – SVT: 5 to 10 mg (0.075 to 0.15 mg/kg) IV over 2 min; a 2nd dose of 10 mg IV may be given 15 to 30 min later if needed. PSVT, rate control with atrial fibrillation: 240 to 480 mg/day PO divided three to four times per day. Angina: Start 40 to 80 mg PO three to four times per day, max 480 mg/day; sustained-release (Isoptin SR, Calan SR, Verelan): Start 120 to 240 mg PO daily, max 480 mg/day (use twice daily dosing for doses greater than 240 mg/day with Isoptin SR and Calan SR); extended-release (Covera-HS): Start 180 mg PO at bedtime max 480 mg/day. HTN: Same as angina, except (Verelan PM): Start 100 to 200 mg PO at bedtime max 400 mg/day; (Covera-HS) start 180 mg PO at bedtime max 480 mg/day; immediate-release tabs should be avoided in treating HTN.

PEDS – SVT age 1 to 15 yo: 2 to 5 mg (0.1 to 0.3 mg/kg) IV, max dose 5 mg. Repeat dose once in 30 min if needed, max second dose 10 mg. Immediate-release and sustained-release tabs not approved in children.

FORMS – Generic/Trade: Tabs, immediate-release, scored (Calan) 40, 80, 120 mg; Tabs, sustained-release, unscored (Isoptin SR) 120, scored 180, 240 mg; Caps, sustained-release (Verelan) 120, 180, 240, 360 mg; Caps, extended-release (Verelan PM) 100, 200, 300 mg. Trade only: Tabs, extended-release (Covera-HS) 180, 240 mg.

NOTES – Contraindicated in severe LV dysfunction, A-fib/flutter conducted via accessory pathway (ie, Wolff-Parkinson-White). Grapefruit juice may increase level. Do not use with more than 10 mg of simvastatin or 20 mg of lovastatin. Hypotension, bradyarrhythmias, and lactic acidosis have been reported with concomitant telithromycin. Sinus bradycardia resulting in hospitalization and pacemaker insertion has been reported with concomitant clonidine; monitor heart rate. May increase digoxin level 50 to 75%. May increase doxorubicin level. May change the level of certain chemotherapeutic agents; may get reduced absorption of verapamil with some chemotherapeutic regimens; see prescribing information for complete list. Scored, sustained-release tabs (Calan SR, Isoptin SR) may be broken and each piece swallowed whole, do not chew or crush. Other extended-release tabs (Covera-HS) should be swallowed whole. Monitor response and side effects when interchanging between verapamil products; many are not equivalent on mg:mg basis. Contents of sustained-release caps may be sprinkled on food (eg, applesauce). Do not chew or crush cap contents. Use cautiously with impaired renal/hepatic function. Covera-HS and Verelan PM are chronotherapeutic products; give at bedtime to blunt early morning surge in BP.

CARDIOVASCULAR: Diuretics—Carbonic Anhydrase Inhibitors

ACETAZOLAMIDE (***Diamox, Diamox Sequels***) ▶LK ♀C ▶+ $

ADULT – Glaucoma: 250 mg PO up to four times per day (immediate-release) or 500 mg PO up to two times per day (sustained-release). Max 1 g/day. Acute glaucoma: 250 mg IV q 4 h or 500 mg IV initially with 125 to 250 mg q 4 h, followed by oral therapy. Mountain sickness prophylaxis:

(cont.)

ACETAZOLAMIDE (*cont.*)

125 to 250 mg PO two to three times per day, beginning 1 to 2 days prior to ascent and continuing at least 5 days at higher altitude. Edema: Rarely used, start 250 to 375 mg IV/PO q am given intermittently (every other day or 2 consecutive days followed by none for 1 to 2 days) to avoid loss of diuretic effect.

PEDS – Diuretic: 5 mg/kg PO/IV q am.

UNAPPROVED ADULT – Urinary alkalinization: 5 mg/kg IV, may repeat two or three times daily prn to maintain an alkaline diuresis.

UNAPPROVED PEDS – Glaucoma: 8 to 30 mg/kg/day PO, divided three times per day. Acute glaucoma: 5 to 10 mg/kg IV q 6 h.

FORMS – Generic only: Tabs 125, 250 mg. Generic/Trade: Caps extended-release 500 mg.

NOTES – A susp (250 mg/5 mL) can be made by crushing and mixing tabs in flavored syrup. The susp is stable for 7 days at room temperature. 1 tab may be softened in 2 teaspoons of hot water, then add to 2 teaspoons of honey or syrup, and swallowed at once. Use cautiously in sulfa allergy. Prompt descent is necessary if severe forms of high-altitude sickness occur (eg, pulmonary or cerebral edema). Test the drug for tolerance/allergies 1 to 2 weeks before initial dosing prior to ascent.

METHAZOLAMIDE (*methazolamide*) ▶LK – ♀C ◗? $$

ADULT – Glaucoma: 50 to 100 mg PO two to three times per day.

PEDS – Not approved in children.

UNAPPROVED ADULT – Mountain sickness prophylaxis: 150 to 200 mg PO daily.

FORMS – Generic only: Tabs, unscored 25 mg, scored 50 mg.

NOTES – Contraindicated with uncorrected electrolyte imbalance, metabolic acidosis, acidemia, adrenal insufficiency, renal failure, anuria, or severe hepatic impairment. Monitor electrolytes at baseline and periodically. May potentiate acidosis and neurologic side effects in patients on dialysis. May increase blood sugar.

CARDIOVASCULAR: Diuretics—Loop

NOTE: Give second dose of twice daily schedule in mid-afternoon to avoid nocturia when treating edema. Thiazides are preferred diuretics for HTN. With decreased renal function (CrCl less than 30 mL/min), loop diuretics may be more effective than thiazides for HTN. Rare hypersensitivity in patients allergic to sulfa-containing drugs, except ethacrynic acid.

BUMETANIDE (*Bumex*, ✤*Burinex*) ▶K ♀C ◗? $

ADULT – Edema: 0.5 to 2 mg PO daily, repeat doses at 4- to 5-h intervals prn until desired response is attained, max 10 mg/day; 0.5 to 1 mg IV/IM, repeat doses at 2- to 3-h intervals prn until desired response is attained, max 10 mg/day. Dosing for 3 to 4 consecutive days followed by no drug for 1 to 2 days is acceptable. Twice daily dosing may enhance diuretic effect. IV injections should be over 1 to 2 min. An IV infusion may be used, change bag q 24 h.

PEDS – Not approved in children.

UNAPPROVED PEDS – Edema: 0.015 to 0.1 mg/kg/dose PO/IV/IM daily or every other day, max 0.1 mg/kg/day or 10 mg/day.

FORMS – Generic/Trade: Tabs scored 0.5, 1, 2 mg.

NOTES – 1 mg bumetanide is roughly equivalent to 40 mg oral furosemide. IV administration is preferred when GI absorption is impaired.

ETHACRYNIC ACID (*Edecrin*) ▶K ♀B ◗? $$$

ADULT – Edema: 0.5 to 1 mg/kg IV, max 100 mg/dose; 25 mg PO daily on day 1, followed by 50 mg PO two times per day on day 2, followed by 100 mg PO in the morning and 50 to 100 mg PO in the evening depending on the response to the morning dose, max 400 mg/day.

PEDS – Not approved in children.

UNAPPROVED ADULT – HTN: 25 mg PO daily, max 100 mg/day divided two to three times per day.

UNAPPROVED PEDS – Edema: 1 mg/kg IV; 25 mg PO daily, increase slowly by 25 mg increments prn. Ethacrynic acid should not be administered to infants.

FORMS – Trade only: Tabs scored 25 mg.

NOTES – Ototoxicity possible. Does not contain a sulfonamide group; can be safely used in patients with true sulfa allery. Do not administer SC or IM due to local irritation. IV ethacrynic acid should be reconstituted to a concentration of 50 mg/mL and given slowly by IV infusion over 20 to 30 min. May increase lithium levels.

FUROSEMIDE (*Lasix*) ▶K ♀C ◗? $

ADULT – HTN: Start 10 to 40 mg PO twice daily, max 600 mg daily. Edema: Start 20 to 80 mg

(cont.)

FUROSEMIDE (*cont.*)

IV/IM/PO, increase dose by 20 to 40 mg in 6 to 8 h until desired response is achieved, max 600 mg/day. Give maintenance dose daily or divided two times per day. IV infusion: 0.05 mg/kg/h, titrate rate to desired response.
PEDS – Edema: 0.5 to 2 mg/kg/dose IV/IM/PO q 6 to 12 h, max 6 mg/kg/dose. IV infusion: 0.05 mg/kg/h, titrate rate to achieve desired response.
UNAPPROVED ADULT – Ascites: 40 mg PO daily in combination with spironolactone; may increase dose after 2 to 3 days if no response.
FORMS – Generic/Trade: Tabs unscored 20, scored 40, 80 mg. Generic only: Oral soln 10 mg/mL, 40 mg/5 mL.
NOTES – Oral absorption may decrease in acute heart failure exacerbation. Bioequivalence of oral form is 50% of IV dose. Monitor renal function in elderly. Do not use with lithium. Increases risk of ototoxicity when used with other drugs associated with ototoxicity, especially with renal dysfunction. May potentiate renal dysfunction when used with other drugs associated with renal dysfunction. May antagonize the muscle-relaxing effects of tubocurarine. Ototoxicity is associated with rapid IV administration (more than 4mg/min).

TORSEMIDE (***Demadex***) ▶LK ♀B ▶? $
ADULT – HTN: Start 5 mg PO daily, increase prn q 4 to 6 weeks, max 10 mg daily. Edema: Start 10 to 20 mg IV/PO daily, double dose prn, max 200 mg IV/PO daily. Ascites: 5 to 10 mg IV/PO daily, double dose prn, max 40 mg daily.
PEDS – Not approved in children.
FORMS – Generic/Trade: Tabs scored 5, 10, 20, 100 mg.

CARDIOVASCULAR: Diuretics—Potassium Sparing

NOTE: See also Antihypertensive Combinations and Aldosterone Antagonists. May cause hyperkalemia; greater incidence with renal impairment, DM, or elderly. Monitor potassium levels before initiating therapy, when adjusting diuretic doses, and with illness that may alter renal function. Use cautiously with other agents that may cause hyperkalemia (eg, ACE inhibitors, ARBs, aliskiren).

AMILORIDE (***Midamor***) ▶LK ♀B ▶? $$$
WARNING – May cause hyperkalemia.
ADULT – Diuretic-induced hypokalemia: Start 5 mg PO daily, increase prn, max 20 mg/day. Edema/HTN: Start 5 mg PO daily in combination with another diuretic, usually a thiazide for HTN, increase prn, max 20 mg/day. Other diuretics may need to be added when treating edema.
PEDS – Not approved in children.
UNAPPROVED ADULT – Hyperaldosteronism: 10 to 40 mg PO daily. Do not use combination product (Moduretic) for treatment of primary hyperaldosteronism.
UNAPPROVED PEDS – Edema: 0.625 mg/kg daily for children weighing 6 to 20 kg.
FORMS – Generic only: Tabs, unscored 5 mg.
NOTES – Spironolactone is generally preferred for treating primary hyperaldosteronism.

TRIAMTERENE (***Dyrenium***) ▶LK ♀B ▶– $$$
WARNING – May cause hyperkalemia. Incidence is greater with renal impairment, DM, or elderly. Monitor potassium frequently, before initiation, when adjusting diuretic doses, and with illness that may alter renal function.
ADULT – Edema (cirrhosis, nephrotic syndrome, heart failure): Start 100 mg PO two times per day, max 300 mg/day. Most patients can be maintained on 100 mg PO daily or every other day after edema is controlled. Other diuretics may be needed.
PEDS – Not approved in children.
UNAPPROVED PEDS – Edema: 4 mg/kg/day divided two times per day after meals, increase to 6 mg/kg/day if needed, max 300 mg/day.
FORMS – Trade only: Caps 50, 100 mg.
NOTES – Combination product with HCTZ (eg, Dyazide, Maxzide) available for HTN.

CARDIOVASCULAR: Diuretics—Thiazide Type

NOTE: See also Antihypertensive Combinations. Possible hypersensitivity in sulfa allergy. Should be used for most patients with HTN, alone or combined with other antihypertensive agents. Thiazides are not recommended for gestational HTN. Coadministration with NSAIDs, including selective COX-2 inhibitors, may reduce the antihypertensive, diuretic, and natriuretic effects of thiazides. Thiazide-induced hypokalemia is associated with increased fasting blood glucose and new onset DM; keep potassium 4.0 mg/dL or greater to minimize risk; may use thiazide in combination with oral potassium supplementation, ACE inhibitor, ARB, or potassium-sparing diuretic to maintain K+ level.

CHLOROTHIAZIDE (*Diuril*) ▶L ♀C, D if used in pregnancy-induced HTN ▶+ $

ADULT – HTN: Start 125 to 250 mg PO daily or divided two times per day, max 1000 mg/day divided two times per day. Edema: 500 to 2000 mg PO/IV daily or divided two times per day. Dosing on alternate days or for 3 to 4 consecutive days followed by no drug for 1 to 2 days is acceptable.

PEDS – Edema: Infants: Start 10 to 20 mg/kg/day PO daily or divided two times per day, up to 30 mg/kg/day divided two times per day. Children 6 mo to 2 yo: 10 to 20 mg/kg/day PO daily or divided two times per day, max 375 mg/day. Children 2 to 12 yo: Start 10 to 20 mg/kg/day PO daily or divided two times per day, up to 1 g/day. IV formulation not recommended for infants or children.

FORMS – Trade only: Susp 250 mg/5 mL. Generic only: Tabs, scored 250, 500 mg.

NOTES – Do not administer SC or IM.

CHLORTHALIDONE (*Thalitone*) ▶L ♀B, D if used in pregnancy-induced HTN ▶+ $

ADULT – HTN: For generic, start 12.5 to 25 mg PO daily, usual maintenance dose 12.5 to 50 mg/day, max 50 mg/day. For Thalitone, start 15 mg PO daily, usual maintenance 30 to 45 mg/day, max 50 mg/day. Edema: For generic, start 50 to 100 mg PO daily or 100 mg every other day or 100 mg 3 times a week, usual maintenance dose 150 to 200 mg/day, max 200 mg/day. For Thalitone, start 30 to 60 mg PO daily or 60 mg every other day, usual maintenance dose 90 to 120 mg PO daily or every other day.

PEDS – Not approved in children.

UNAPPROVED ADULT – Nephrolithiasis: 25 to 50 mg PO daily.

UNAPPROVED PEDS – Edema: 2 mg/kg PO 3 times a week.

FORMS – Trade only: Tabs unscored (Thalitone) 15 mg. Generic only: Tabs unscored 25, 50 mg.

NOTES – Thalitone has greater bioavailability than generic forms, do not interchange. Doses greater than 50 mg/day for HTN are usually associated with hypokalemia with little added BP control.

HYDROCHLOROTHIAZIDE (*HCTZ, Oretic, Microzide*) ▶L ♀B, D if used in pregnancy-induced HTN ▶+ $

ADULT – HTN: Start 12.5 to 25 mg PO daily, usual maintenance dose 25 mg/day, max 50 mg/day. Edema: 25 to 100 mg PO daily or in divided doses or 50 to 100 mg PO every other day or 3 to 5 days/week, max 200 mg/day.

PEDS – Edema: 1 to 2 mg/kg/day PO daily or divided two times per day, max 37.5 mg/day in infants up to 2 yo, max 100 mg/day in children 2 to 12 yo.

UNAPPROVED ADULT – Nephrolithiasis: 50 to 100 mg PO daily.

FORMS – Generic/Trade: Tabs scored 25, 50 mg; Caps 12.5 mg.

NOTES – Doses 50 mg/day or greater may cause hypokalemia with little added BP control.

INDAPAMIDE (*Lozol*, ♣ *Lozide*) ▶L ♀B, D if used in pregnancy-induced HTN ▶? $

ADULT – HTN: Start 1.25 to 2.5 mg PO daily, max 5 mg/day. Edema, heart failure: 2.5 to 5 mg PO q am.

PEDS – Not approved in children.

FORMS – Generic only: Tabs unscored 1.25, 2.5 mg.

METHYCLOTHIAZIDE (*Enduron*) ▶L ♀B, D if used in pregnancy-induced HTN ▶? $

ADULT – HTN: Start 2.5 mg PO daily, usual maintenance dose 2.5 to 5 mg/day. Edema: Start 2.5 mg PO daily, usual maintenance dose 2.5 to 10 mg/day.

PEDS – Not approved in children.

FORMS – Generic/Trade: Tabs, scored, 2.5, 5 mg.

METOLAZONE (*Zaroxolyn*) ▶L ♀B, D if used in pregnancy-induced HTN ▶? $$$

ADULT – Edema (heart failure, renal disease): 5 to 10 mg PO daily, max 10 mg/day in heart failure, 20 mg/day in renal disease. If used with loop diuretic, start with 2.5 mg PO daily. Reduce to lowest effective dose as edema resolves. May be given every other day as edema resolves.

(cont.)

CARDIAC PARAMETERS AND FORMULAS

Cardiac output (CO) = heart rate × CVA volume [normal 4 to 8 L/min]
Cardiac index (CI) = CO/BSA [normal 2.8 to 4.2 L/min/m^2]
MAP (mean arterial press) = [(SBP – DBP)/3] + DBP [normal 80 to 100 mmHg]
SVR (systemic vasc resis) = (MAP – CVP) × (80)/CO [normal 800 to 1200 dyne × sec/cm^5]
PVR (pulm vasc resis) = (PAM – PCWP) × (80)/CO [normal 45 to 120 dyne × sec/cm^5]
QTc = QT/square root of RR [normal 0.38 to 0.42]
Right atrial pressure (central venous pressure) [normal 0 to 8 mmHg]
Pulmonary artery systolic pressure (PAS) [normal 20 to 30 mmHg]
Pulmonary artery diastolic pressure (PAD) [normal 10 to 15 mmHg]
Pulmonary capillary wedge pressure (PCWP) [normal 8 to 12 mmHg (post-MI ~16 mmHg)]

METOLAZONE (*cont.*)

PEDS – Not approved in children.
UNAPPROVED PEDS – Edema: 0.2 to 0.4 mg/kg/day daily or divided two times per day.
FORMS – Generic/Trade: Tabs 2.5, 5, 10 mg.
NOTES – Generally used for diuretic resistance, not HTN. When used with furosemide or other loop diuretics, administer metolazone 30 min before IV loop diuretic. Correct electrolyte imbalances before initiating therapy. Combination diuretic therapy may increase the risk of electrolyte disturbances.

CARDIOVASCULAR: Nitrates

NOTE: Avoid if systolic BP is less than 90 mmHg or greater than 30 mmHg below baseline; heart rate less than 50 or greater than 100 beats per minute; or right ventricular infarction. Avoid in those who have received erectile dysfunction therapy, with sildenafil or vardenafil, in the last 24 h. Only with close medical supervision and hemodynamic monitoring, may give nitrate 12 h after avanafil or 48 h after tadalafil.

AMYL NITRITE ▶Lung ♀X ▶- $
ADULT – Angina: 0.3 mL inhaled prn.
PEDS – Not approved in children.
NOTES – Flammable. Avoid use in areas with open flames. To avoid syncope, use only when lying down.

ISOSORBIDE DINITRATE (*Isordil, Dilatrate-SR*) ▶L ♀C ▶? $
ADULT – Acute angina: 2.5 to 10 mg SL or chewed immediately, repeat prn q 5 to 10 min up to 3 doses in 30 min. SL and chew tabs may be used prior to events likely to provoke angina. Angina prophylaxis: Start 5 to 20 mg PO three times per day (7 am, noon, and 5 pm), max 40 mg three times per day. Sustained-release (Dilatrate SR): Start 40 mg PO two times per day, max 80 mg PO two times per day (8 am and 2 pm).
PEDS – Not approved in children.
UNAPPROVED ADULT – Heart failure: 10 to 40 mg PO three times per day, max 80 mg three times per day. Use in combination with hydralazine.
FORMS – Generic/Trade: Tabs, scored 5, 10, 20, 30 mg. Trade only: Tabs, (Isordil) 40 mg, Caps, extended-release (Dilatrate-SR) 40 mg. Generic only: Tabs, sustained-release 40 mg, Tabs, sublingual 2.5, 5 mg.
NOTES – Use SL or chew tabs for an acute angina attack. Extended-release tabs may be broken, but do not chew or crush, swallow whole; do not use for acute angina. Allow for a nitrate-free period of 10 to 14 h each day to avoid nitrate tolerance.

ISOSORBIDE MONONITRATE (*ISMO, Monoket, Imdur*) ▶L ♀C ▶? $$
ADULT – Angina: 20 mg PO two times per day (8 am and 3 pm). Extended-release (Imdur): Start 30 to 60 mg PO daily, max 240 mg/day.
PEDS – Not approved in children.
FORMS – Generic/Trade: Tabs unscored (ISMO, twice daily dosing) 20 mg, scored (Monoket, twice daily dosing) 10, 20 mg extended-release, scored (Imdur, daily dosing) 30, 60, unscored 120 mg.
NOTES – Extended-release tab may be broken, but do not chew or crush, swallow whole. Do not use for acute angina.

NITROGLYCERIN INTRAVENOUS INFUSION ▶L ♀C ▶? $
ADULT – Perioperative HTN, acute MI/heart failure, acute angina: Mix 50 mg in 250 mL D5W (200 mcg/mL), start at 10 to 20 mcg/min IV (3 to 6 mL/h), then titrate upward by 10 to 20 mcg/min q 3 to 5 min until desired effect is achieved.
PEDS – Not approved in children.
UNAPPROVED ADULT – Hypertensive emergency: Start 10 to 20 mcg/min IV infusion, titrate up to 100 mcg/min. Antihypertensive effect is usually evident in 2 to 5 min. Effect may persist for only 3 to 5 min after infusion is stopped.
UNAPPROVED PEDS – IV infusion: Start 0.25 to 0.5 mcg/kg/min, increase by 0.5 to 1 mcg/kg/min q 3 to 5 min prn, max 5 mcg/kg/min.
NOTES – Nitroglycerin migrates into polyvinyl chloride (PVC) tubing. Use lower initial doses (5 mcg/min) with non-PVC tubing. Use with caution in inferior/right ventricular MI.

NITROGLYCERIN OINTMENT (*Nitro-BID*) ▶L ♀C ▶? $
ADULT – Angina prophylaxis: Start 0.5 inch q 8 h applied to nonhairy skin area, maintenance 1 to 2 inch q 8 h, maximum 4 inch q 4 to 6 h.
PEDS – Not approved in children.
FORMS – Trade only: Ointment, 2%, tubes 1, 30, 60 g (Nitro-BID).
NOTES – Do not use for acute angina attack. One inch ointment contains about 15 mg nitroglycerin. Allow for a nitrate-free period of 10 to 14 h each day to avoid nitrate tolerance. Generally change to oral tabs or transdermal patch for long-term therapy.

NITROGLYCERIN SPRAY (*Nitrolingual, NitroMist*) ▶L ♀C ▶? $$$$

ADULT – Acute angina: 1 to 2 sprays under the tongue at the onset of attack, repeat prn, max 3 sprays in 15 min. A dose may be given 5 to 10 min before activities that might provoke angina.

PEDS – Not approved in children.

FORMS – Trade only: Nitrolingual soln, 4.9, 12 mL. 0.4 mg/spray (60 or 200 sprays/canister); NitroMist aerosol 0.4 mg/spray (230 sprays/canister).

NOTES – AHA guidelines recommend calling 911 if chest pain not relieved or gets worse after using 1 dose of nitroglycerin. May be preferred over SL tabs in patients with dry mouth. Patient can see how much medicine is left in the upright bottle. Nitrolingual: Replace bottle when fluid is below level of center tube; NitroMist: Replace bottle when fluid reaches the bottom of the hole in the side of the container. Before initial use, prime pump: Nitrolingual, spray 5 times into air (away from self and others); NitroMist, spray 10 times into air (away from self and others). Prime at least once q 6 weeks if not used: Nitrolingual spray 1 time into the air (away from self and others); NitroMist spray twice into the air (away from self and others). Do not shake NitroMist before using.

NITROGLYCERIN SUBLINGUAL (*Nitrostat, NitroQuick*) ▶L ♀C ▶? $

ADULT – Acute angina: 0.4 mg under tongue or between the cheek and gum, repeat dose q 5 min prn up to 3 doses in 15 min. A dose may be given 5 to 10 min before activities that might provoke angina.

PEDS – Not approved in children.

FORMS – Generic/Trade: Sublingual tabs unscored 0.3, 0.4, 0.6 mg; in bottles of 100 or package of 4 bottles with 25 tabs each.

NOTES – AHA guidelines recommend calling 911 if chest pain not relieved or gets worse after using 1 dose of nitroglycerin. May produce a burning/tingling sensation when administered, although this should not be used to assess potency. Store in original glass bottle to maintain potency/stability. Traditionally, unused tabs should be discarded 6 months after the original bottle is opened; however, the Nitrostat product is stable for 24 months after the bottle is opened or until the expiration date on the bottle, whichever is earlier. If used rarely, prescribe package with 4 bottles with 25 tabs each.

NITROGLYCERIN SUSTAINED RELEASE ▶L ♀C ▶? $

ADULT – Angina prophylaxis: Start 2.5 mg PO two to three times per day, then titrate upward prn.

PEDS – Not approved in children.

FORMS – Generic only: Caps, extended-release 2.5, 6.5, 9 mg.

NOTES – Do not use for acute angina attack. Swallow whole, do not chew or crush. Allow for a nitrate-free period of 10 to 14 h each day to avoid nitrate tolerance.

NITROGLYCERIN TRANSDERMAL (*Minitran, Nitro-Dur, ✤ Trinipatch, Transderm-Nitro*) ▶L ♀C ▶? $$

ADULT – Angina prophylaxis: Start with lowest dose and apply 1 patch for 12 to 14 h each day to nonhairy skin.

PEDS – Not approved in children.

FORMS – Generic/Trade: Transdermal system 0.1, 0.2, 0.4, 0.6 mg/h. Trade only: (Nitro-Dur) 0.3, 0.8 mg/h.

NOTES – Do not use for acute angina attack. Allow for a nitrate-free period of 10 to 14 h each day to avoid nitrate tolerance.

CARDIOVASCULAR: Pressors/Inotropes

DOBUTAMINE ▶Plasma ♀D ▶– $

ADULT – Inotropic support in cardiac decompensation (heart failure, cardiogenic shock, surgical procedures): 2 to 20 mcg/kg/min. Mix 250 mg in 250 mL D5W (1 mg/mL); a rate of 21 mL/h delivers 5 mcg/kg/min for a 70 kg patient. Alternatively, mix 200 mg in 100 mL D5W (2 mg/mL); a rate of 10.5 mL/h delivers 5 mcg/kg/min for a 70 kg patient.

PEDS – Not approved in children.

UNAPPROVED ADULT – Refractory septic shock: 2 to 20 mcg/kg/min.

UNAPPROVED PEDS – Use adult dosage. Use lowest effective dose.

NOTES – For short-term use, up to 72 h.

DOPAMINE ▶Plasma ♀C ▶– $

WARNING – Avoid extravasation; peripheral ischemia, necrosis, gangrene may occur. If extravasation occurs, infiltrate the area as soon as possible with a soln of phentolamine and normal saline.

ADULT – Pressor: Start 5 mcg/kg/min, increase prn by 5 to 10 mcg/kg/min increments at 10-min intervals, max 50 mcg/kg/min. Mix 400 mg in 250 mL D5W (1600 mcg/mL); a rate of 13 mL/h delivers 5 mcg/kg/min in a 70 kg patient. Alternatively, mix 320 mg in 100 mL

(cont.)

DOPAMINE (*cont.*)

D5W (3200 mcg/mL); a rate of 6.5 mL/h delivers 5 mcg/kg/min in a 70 kg patient.

PEDS – Not approved in children.

UNAPPROVED ADULT – Symptomatic bradycardia unresponsive to atropine: 5 to 20 mcg/kg/min IV infusion.

UNAPPROVED PEDS – Pressor: Use adult dosage.

NOTES – Doses in mcg/kg/min: 2 to 4 is the traditional renal dose; recent evidence suggests ineffective and active at dopaminergic receptors; 5 to 10 is the cardiac dose: Active at dopaminergic and beta-1 receptors; greater than 10 is active at the dopaminergic, beta-1, and alpha-1 receptors.

EPHEDRINE ▶K ♀C ▶? $

ADULT – Pressor: 10 to 25 mg IV slow injection, with repeat doses q 5 to 10 min prn, max 150 mg/day. Orthostatic hypotension: 25 mg PO daily to four times per day. Bronchospasm: 25 to 50 mg PO q 3 to 4 h prn.

PEDS – Not approved in children.

UNAPPROVED PEDS – Pressor: 3 mg/kg/day SC or IV in 4 to 6 divided doses.

FORMS – Generic only: Caps, 50 mg.

EPINEPHRINE (***EpiPen, EpiPen Jr, Twinject,*** **adrenalin**) ▶Plasma ♀C ▶– $

ADULT – Cardiac arrest: 1 mg (1:10,000 soln) IV, repeat q 3 to 5 min if needed; infusion 1 mg in 250 mL D5W (4 mcg/mL) at rate of 15 to 60 mL/h delivers 1 to 4 mcg/min. Anaphylaxis: 0.1 to 0.5 mg SC/IM (1:1000 soln), may repeat SC dose q 10 to 15 min for anaphylactic shock. Acute asthma and hypersensitivity reactions: 0.1 to 0.3 mg of 1:1000 soln SC or IM. Hypersensitivity reactions: 0.01 mg/kg SC autoinjector.

PEDS – Cardiac arrest: 0.01 mg/kg IV/intraosseous (IO) (max 1 mg/dose) or 0.1 mg/kg ET (max 10 mg/dose), repeat 0.1 to 0.2 mg/kg IV/IO/ET q 3 to 5 min if needed. Neonates: 0.01 to 0.03 mg/kg IV (preferred) or up to 0.1 mg/kg ET, repeat q 3 to 5 min if needed; IV infusion start 0.1 mcg/kg/min, increase in increments of 0.1 mcg/kg/min if needed, max 1 mcg/kg/min. Anaphylaxis: 0.01 mg/kg (0.01 mL/kg of 1:1000 injection) SC, may repeat SC dose at 20-min to 4-h intervals depending on severity of condition. Acute asthma: 0.01 mL/kg (up to 0.5 mL) of 1:1000 soln SC or IM; repeat q 15 min for 3 to 4 doses prn. Hypersensitivity reactions: 0.01 mg/kg SC autoinjector.

UNAPPROVED ADULT – Symptomatic bradycardia unresponsive to atropine: 2 to 10 mcg/min IV infusion. ET administration prior to IV access: 2 to 2.5 times the recommended IV dose in 10 mL of NS or distilled water.

FORMS – Soln for injection: 1:1000 (1 mg/mL in 1 mL amps or 10 mL vial). Trade only: EpiPen Auto-injector delivers one 0.3 mg (1:1000, 0.3 mL) IM dose. EpiPen Jr. Autoinjector delivers one 0.15 mg (1:2000, 0.3 mL) IM dose. Twinject auto-injector delivers one 0.15 mg (1:1000, 0.15 mL) or 0.3 mg (1:1000, 0.3 mL) IM/SQ dose.

NOTES – Cardiac arrest: Adult: Use the 1:10,000 injectable soln for IV use in cardiac arrest (10 mL = 1 mg). Peds: Use 1:10,000 for initial IV dose, then 1:1000 for subsequent dosing or ET doses. Anaphylaxis: Use the 1:1000 injectable soln for SC/IM (0.1 mL = 0.1 mg);. consider EpiPen Jr. in patients weighing less than 30 kg. Directions for Epi-Pen: Remove cap. Place black tip end on thigh and push down to inject. Hold in place for 10 sec. May be injected directly through clothing.

INAMRINONE ▶K ♀C ▶? $$$$$

ADULT – Heart failure (NYHA class III, IV): 0.75 mg/kg bolus IV over 2 to 3 min, then infusion 100 mg in 100 mL NS (1 mg/mL); a rate of 21 mL/h delivers 5 mcg/kg/min for a 70 kg patient. An additional IV bolus of 0.75 mg/kg may be given 30 min after initiating therapy if needed. Total daily dose should not exceed 10 mg/kg.

PEDS – Not approved in children.

UNAPPROVED ADULT – CPR: 0.75 mg/kg bolus IV over 2 to 3 min, followed by 5 to 15 mcg/kg/min.

UNAPPROVED PEDS – Inotropic support: 0.75 mg/kg IV bolus over 2 to 3 min, followed by 3 to 5 mcg/kg/min (neonates) or 5 to 10 mcg/kg/min (children) maintenance infusion.

NOTES – Thrombocytopenia possible. Name changed from "amrinone" to avoid medication errors.

MIDODRINE (✤ ***Amatine***) ▶LK ♀C ▶? $$$$$

WARNING – May cause significant supine HTN. Contraindicated with severe cardiac disease or persistent/excessive supine HTN.

ADULT – The last daily dose should be no later than 6 pm to avoid supine HTN during sleep. Orthostatic hypotension: Start 10 mg PO three times per day, increase dose prn to max 40 mg/day. Renal impairment: Start 2.5 mg three times per day.

PEDS – Not approved in children.

FORMS – Generic: Tabs, scored 2.5, 5, 10 mg.

NOTES – The last daily dose should be no later than 6 pm to avoid supine HTN during sleep.

MILRINONE (*Primacor*) ▶K ♀C ▶? $$

ADULT – Systolic heart failure (NYHA class III, IV): Load 50 mcg/kg IV over 10 min, then begin IV infusion of 0.375 to 0.75 mcg/kg/min. Renal impairment: Infusion rate for CrCl 5 mL/min or less: 0.2 mcg/kg/min; CrCl 6 to 10 mL/min: 0.23 mcg/kg/min; CrCl 11 to 20 mL/min: 0.28 mcg/kg/min; CrCl 21 to 30 mL/min: 0.33 mcg/kg/min; CrCl 31 to 40 mL/min: 0.38 mcg/kg/min; CrCl 41 to 50 mL/min: 0.43 mcg/kg/min."

PEDS – Not approved in children.

UNAPPROVED PEDS – Inotropic support: Limited data, 50 mcg/kg IV bolus over 10 min, followed by 0.5 to 1 mcg/kg/min IV infusion, titrate to effect within dosing range.

NOREPINEPHRINE (*Levophed*) ▶Plasma ♀C ▶? $

WARNING – Tissue ischemia, necrosis, gangrene may occur with extravasation. If extravasation occurs, infiltrate affected area with a soln of phentolamine in NS as soon as possible.

ADULT – Acute hypotension: Start 8 to 12 mcg/min, adjust to maintain BP, average maintenance rate 2 to 4 mcg/min, mix 4 mg in 500 mL D5W (8 mcg/mL); a rate of 22.5 mL/h delivers 3 mcg/min. Ideally through central line.

PEDS – Not approved in children.

UNAPPROVED PEDS – Acute hypotension: Start 0.05 to 0.1 mcg/kg/min IV infusion, titrate to desired effect, max dose 2 mcg/kg/min.

NOTES – Avoid extravasation, do not administer IV push or IM.

PHENYLEPHRINE—INTRAVENOUS ▶Plasma ♀C ▶– $

WARNING – Avoid with severe cardiac disease, including CAD and dilated cardiomyopathy. Tissue ischemia, necrosis, gangrene may occur with extravasation. If extravasation occurs, infiltrate affected area with a soln of phentolamine in NS as soon as possible.

ADULT – Mild to moderate hypotension: 0.1 to 0.2 mg slow IV injection, do not exceed 0.5 mg in initial dose, repeat dose prn no less than q 10 to 15 min; 1 to 10 mg SC/IM, initial dose should not exceed 5 mg. Infusion for severe hypotension: 20 mg in 250 mL D5W (80 mcg/mL), start 100 to 180 mcg/min (75 to 135 mL/h), usual dose once BP is stabilized 40 to 60 mcg/min.

PEDS – Not approved in children.

UNAPPROVED PEDS – Mild to moderate hypotension: 5 to 20 mcg/kg IV bolus q 10 to 15 min prn; 0.1 to 0.5 mcg/kg/min IV infusion, titrate to desired effect.

NOTES – Avoid SC or IM administration during shock, use IV route to ensure drug absorption.

CARDIOVASCULAR: Pulmonary Arterial Hypertension

AMBRISENTAN (*Letairis*) ▶L ♀X ▶– $$$$$

WARNING – Contraindicated in pregnancy. Women of childbearing age need pregnancy test prior to starting therapy and monthly thereafter. Prevent pregnancy during treatment and for 1 month after stopping treatment with two acceptable methods of contraception, unless the patient had tubal sterilization or uses Copper T 380A IUD or LNg 20 IUS. Only available through restricted program; prescribers, pharmacies, patients must enroll.

ADULT – Pulmonary arterial hypertension: Start 5 mg PO daily; if tolerated, may increase to 10 mg/day.

PEDS – Not approved in children.

FORMS – Trade only: Tabs, unscored 5, 10 mg.

NOTES – Monitor hemoglobin at initiation, after 1 month of therapy, then periodically. If acute pulmonary edema develops during therapy initiation, consider underlying pulmonary veno-occlusive disease and discontinue treatment if necessary. Not recommended with moderate or severe hepatic impairment. Do not give more than cyclosporine 5 mg with concomitant ambrisentan. May reduce sperm count. Do not split, crush, or chew tablets.

BOSENTAN (*Tracleer*) ▶L ♀X ▶–? $$$$$

WARNING – Hepatotoxicity; monitor LFTs prior to starting therapy and monthly thereafter. Contraindicated in pregnancy due to birth defects; women of childbearing age must use reliable contraception and have monthly pregnancy tests. Oral, injectable, transdermal, and implanted contraception must be supplemented with another method. Women of childbearing age need pregnancy test before each refill.

ADULT – Pulmonary arterial hypertension: Start 62.5 mg PO two times per day for 4 weeks, increase to 125 mg two times per day maintenance dose. With low body wt (less than 40 kg) and older than 12 yo: 62.5 mg PO two times per day. Stop bosentan more than 36 h prior

(cont.)

BOSENTAN (*cont.*)

to initiating ritonavir; when on ritonavir more than 10 days, give bosentan 62.5 mg PO daily or every other day.

PEDS – Not approved in children.

FORMS – Trade only: Tabs, unscored 62.5, 125 mg.

NOTES – Available only through access program by calling 866-228-3546. Concomitant glyburide or cyclosporine is contraindicated. Induces metabolism of other drugs (eg, contraceptives, simvastatin, lovastatin, atorvastatin). Do not use with both CYP2C9 inhibitor (eg, amiodarone, fluconazole) and strong CYP3A4 inhibitor (eg, ketoconazole, itraconazole, ritonavir) or moderate CYP3A4 inhibitor (eg, amprenavir, erythromycin, fluconazole, diltiazem); will increase levels of bosentan. May decrease warfarin plasma concentration; monitor INR. Rifampin alters bosentan levels; monitor LFTs weekly for 4 weeks, followed by normal monitoring. Discontinue with signs of pulmonary edema. Monitor hemoglobin after 1 and 3 months of therapy, then q 3 months. May reduce sperm count in some men.

EPOPROSTENOL (*Flolan*) ▶Plasma ♀B ▶? $$$$$

ADULT – Pulmonary arterial hypertension (PAH): Acute dose ranging, 2 ng/kg/min increments via IV infusion until the patient develops symptomatic intolerance (mean maximal dose without symptoms 8.6 ng/kg/min), start continuous IV infusion at 4 ng/kg/min or less than the patient's maximum-tolerated infusion (MTI) rate for acute dose ranging. If the MTI rate is less than 5 ng/kg/min, start chronic IV infusion at ½ the MTI.

PEDS – Not approved in children.

NOTES – Administer by continuous IV infusion via a central venous catheter. Temporary peripheral IV infusions may be used until central access is established. Inhibits platelet aggregation; may increase bleeding risk.

ILOPROST (*Ventavis*) ▶L ♀C ▶? $$$$$

ADULT – Pulmonary arterial hypertension: Start 2.5 mcg/dose by inhalation (as delivered at mouthpiece); if well tolerated increase to 5 mcg/dose by inhalation (as delivered at mouthpiece). Use 6 to 9 times a day (minimum of 2 h between doses) during waking h.

PEDS – Not approved in children.

NOTES – Only administer with Prodose or I-neb AAD Systems. Each single-use ampule delivers 20 mcg to medication chamber of nebulizer and 2.5 or 5 mcg to the mouthpiece; discard remaining soln after each inhalation. Do not mix with other medications. Avoid contact with skin/eyes or oral ingestion. Monitor vital signs when initiating therapy. Do not initiate therapy if SBP is less than 85 mmHg. With Child-Pugh Class B or C hepatic impairment, consider increasing the dosing interval (eg, 3 to 4 h between doses) depending on patient's response at end of dosing interval. Do not use in patients with moderate to severe hepatic impairment and/or 3 times the upper limit of transaminase or patients on dialysis. May potentiate bleeding risk for patients on anticoagulants. May potentiate hypotensive effects of other medications. Discontinue therapy if pulmonary edema occurs; this may be sign of pulmonary venous hypertension. May induce bronchospasm; carefully monitor patients with COPD, severe asthma, or acute pulmonary infection. Epistaxis and gingival bleeding may occur during first month of therapy.

SILDENAFIL (*Revatio*) ▶LK ♀B ▶– $$$$

ADULT – Pulmonary arterial hypertension: 20 mg PO three times per day, approximately 4 to 6 h apart; or 10 mg IV three times per day.

PEDS – Not approved in children.

FORMS – Trade only (Revatio): Tabs 20 mg.

NOTES – Contraindicated with nitrates. Coadministration is not recommended with ritonavir, potent CYP3A inhibitors, or other phosphodiesterase-5 inhibitors. Alpha-blockers may potentiate hypotension. Use not recommended for patients with pulmonary veno-occlusive disease. Sudden vision loss due to nonarteritic ischemic optic neuropathy has been reported. Discontinue with sudden decrease/loss of hearing. Teach patients to seek medical attention for vision loss, hearing loss, or erections lasting longer than 4 h.

TADALAFIL (*Adcirca*) ▶L ♀B ▶– $$$$

ADULT – Pulmonary arterial hypertension: 40 mg PO daily, 20 mg if CrCl less than 80 mL/min or mild to moderate hepatic impairment. Avoid with CrCl less than 30 mL/min or severe hepatic impairment.

PEDS – Not approved in children.

FORMS – Trade only (Adcirca): Tabs 20 mg.

NOTES – Contraindicated with nitrates; If nitrates needed and had tadalafil in last 48 h, give nitrate under close medical supervision with hemodynamic monitoring. Coadministration is not recommended with potent CYP3A inhibitors (itraconazole,

(cont.)

TADALAFIL (*cont.*)

ketoconazole), potent CYP3A inducers (rifampin), or other phosphodiesterase-5 inhibitors. Caution with ritonavir, see prescribing info for specific dose adjustments. Alpha-blockers or alcohol may potentiate hypotension. Use not recommended for patients with pulmonary veno-occlusive disease. Sudden vision loss due to nonarteritic ischemic optic neuropathy has been reported. Retinal artery occlusion has been reported. Discontinue with sudden decrease/loss of hearing. Transient global amnesia. Teach patients to seek medical attention for vision loss, hearing loss, or erections lasting longer than 4 h.

TREPROSTINIL (*Tyvaso*) ▸KL – ♀B ▸? $$$$$

ADULT – Pulmonary arterial hypertension: Start 3 breaths (18 mcg) per treatment session four times per day during waking hours; treatments should be at least 4 h apart; may reduce initial dose to 1 to 2 breaths per treatment session if 3 breaths not tolerated. May increase by 3 breaths q 1 to 2 weeks as tolerated, max 9 breaths (54 mcg) per treatment four times per day.

PEDS – Not approved in children.

FORMS – 1.74 mg in 2.9 mL inhalation solution.

NOTES – Administer undiluted with the Tyvaso inhalation system. A single breath delivers about 6 mcg treprostinil; discard remaining solution at the end of each day. Do not mix with other medications. Avoid contact with skin/eyes or oral ingestion. Safety and efficacy not established with existing lung disease (asthma, COPD). Carefully monitor patients with acute pulmonary infection. May need to adjust doses if CYP2C8 inducers (rifampin) or CYP2C8 inhibitors (gemfibrozil). Use cautiously in the elderly and those with liver or renal dysfunction. May potentiate bleeding risk for patients on anticoagulants. May potentiate hypotensive effects of other medications.

TREPROSTINIL SODIUM (***Remodulin***) ▸KL ♀B ▸? $$$$$

ADULT – Pulmonary arterial hypertension: Continuous SC (preferred) or central IV infusion. Start 1.25 ng/kg/min based on ideal body wt. Reduce to 0.625 ng/kg/min if initial dose not tolerated. Dose based on clinical response and tolerance. Increase by no more than 1.25 ng/kg/min/week in first 4 weeks, then increase by no more than 2.5 ng/kg/min/week. Max 40 ng/kg/min. Mild to moderate hepatic insufficiency: Start 0.625 ng/kg/min based on ideal body wt; increase cautiously. Not studied with severe hepatic insufficiency. Transitioning from epoprostenol: Must be done in hospital; initiate at 10% epoprostenol dose; gradually increase dose as epoprostenol dose is decreased (see chart in prescribing information).

PEDS – Not approved in children.

NOTES – Use cautiously in the elderly and those with liver or renal dysfunction. Initiate in setting with personnel and equipment for physiological monitoring and emergency care. Administer by continuous infusion using infusion pump. Patient must have access to backup infusion pump and infusion sets. Must dilute prior to giving IV; see prescribing information for details. May potentiate bleeding risk for patients on anticoagulants. May potentiate hypotensive effects of other medications.

CARDIOVASCULAR: Thrombolytics

ALTEPLASE (***tpa, t-PA, Activase, Cathflo,*** ✤***Activase rt-PA***) ▸L ♀C ▸? $$$$$

ADULT – Acute MI: wt 67 kg or less, give 15 mg IV bolus, then 0.75 mg/kg (max 50 mg) over 30 min, then 0.5 mg/kg (max 35 mg) over the next 60 min; wt greater than 67 kg, give 15 mg IV bolus, then 50 mg over 30 min, then 35 mg over the next 60 min. Acute ischemic CVA with symptoms 3 h or less: 0.9 mg/kg (max 90 mg); give 10% of total dose as an IV bolus, and the remainder IV over 60 min. Multiple exclusion criteria. Select patients may receive with symtoms 4.5 h or less (age younger than 80 yo; baseline NIHSS score 25 or less; no anticoagulant use; or no combination of prior stroke and DM). Acute pulmonary embolism: 100 mg IV over 2 h, then restart heparin when PTT twice normal or less. Occluded central venous access device: 2 mg/mL in catheter for 2 h. May use second dose if needed.

PEDS – Occluded central venous access device: Wt at least 10 kg but less than 30 kg: Dose equal to 110% of the internal lumen volume, not to exceed 2 mg/2 mL. Other uses not approved in children.

NOTES – Must be reconstituted. Soln must be used within 8 h after reconstitution.

RETEPLASE (***Retavase***) ▶L ♀C ▶? $$$$$

ADULT – Acute MI: 10 units IV over 2 min; repeat 1 dose in 30 min.

PEDS – Not approved in children.

NOTES – Must be reconstituted with sterile water for injection to 1 mg/mL concentration. Soln must be used within 4 h after reconstitution.

STREPTOKINASE (***Streptase, Kabikinase***) ▶L ♀C ▶? $$$$$

ADULT – Acute MI: 1.5 million units IV over 60 min. Pulmonary embolism: 250,000 units IV loading dose over 30 min, followed by 100,000 units/h IV infusion for 24 h (maintain infusion for 72 h if concurrent DVT suspected). DVT: 250,000 units IV loading dose over 30 min, followed by 100,000 units/h IV infusion for 24 h. Occluded arteriovenous catheter: 250,000 units instilled into the catheter, remove soln containing 250,000 units of drug from catheter after 2 h using a 5 mL syringe.

PEDS – Not approved in children.

NOTES – Must be reconstituted. Soln must be used within 8 h of reconstitution. Do not shake vial. Do not repeat use in less than 1 year. Do not use with history of severe allergic reaction.

TENECTEPLASE (***TNKase***) ▶L ♀C ▶? $$$$$

ADULT – Acute MI: Single IV bolus dose over 5 sec based on body wt: wt less than 60 kg: 30 mg; wt 60 to 69 kg: 35 mg; wt 70 to 79 kg: 40 mg; wt 80 to 89 kg: 45 mg; wt 90 kg or more: 50 mg.

PEDS – Not approved in children.

NOTES – Must be reconstituted. Soln must be used within 8 h after reconstitution.

UROKINASE (***Kinlytic***) ▶L ♀B ▶? $$$$$

ADULT – Pulmonary embolism: 4400 units/kg IV loading dose over 10 min, followed by IV infusion 4400 units/kg/h for 12 h. Occluded IV catheter: 5000 units instilled into the catheter with a tuberculin syringe, remove soln containing 5000 units of drug from catheter after 5 min using a 5 mL syringe. Aspiration attempts may be repeated q 5 min. If unsuccessful, cap catheter and allow 5000 units of soln to remain in catheter for 30 to 60 min before again attempting to aspirate soln and residual clot.

PEDS – Not approved in children.

UNAPPROVED ADULT – Acute MI: 2 to 3 million units IV infusion over 45 to 90 min. Give ½ the total dose as a rapid initial IV injection over 5 min.

UNAPPROVED PEDS – Arterial or venous thrombosis: 4400 units/kg IV loading dose over 10 min, followed by 4400 units/kg/h for 12 to 72 h. Occluded IV catheter: 5000 units in catheter for 1-4 h.

NOTES – Must be reconstituted. Do not shake vial.

CARDIOVASCULAR: Volume Expanders

ALBUMIN (***Albuminar, Buminate, Albumarc,*** ✦ ***Plasbumin***) ▶L ♀C ▶? $$$$$

ADULT – Shock, burns: 500 mL of 5% soln (50 mg/mL) infused as rapidly as tolerated. Repeat infusion in 30 min if response is inadequate. 25% soln may be used with or without dilution. Undiluted 25% soln should be infused at 1 mL/min to avoid too rapid plasma volume expansion.

PEDS – Shock, burns: 10 to 20 mL/kg IV infusion at 5 to 10 mL/min using 50 mL of 5% soln.

UNAPPROVED PEDS – Shock/hypovolemia: 1 g/kg/dose IV rapid infusion. Hypoproteinemia: 1 g/kg/dose IV infusion over 30 to 120 min.

NOTES – Fever, chills. Monitor for plasma volume overload (dyspnea, fluid in lungs, abnormal increase in BP or CVP). Less likely to cause hypotension than plasma protein fraction, more purified. In treating burns, large volumes of crystalloid solns (0.9% sodium chloride) are used to maintain plasma volume with albumin. Use 5% soln in pediatric hypovolemic patients. Use 25% soln in pediatric patients with volume restrictions.

DEXTRAN (***Rheomacrodex, Gentran, Macrodex***) ▶K ♀C ▶? $$

ADULT – Shock/hypovolemia: Dextran 40, Dextran 70 and 75, up to 20 mL/kg during the first 24 h, up to 10 mL/kg/day thereafter, do not continue for longer than 5 days. The first 500 mL may be infused rapidly with CVP monitoring. DVT/PE prophylaxis during surgery: Dextran 40, 50 to 100 g IV infusion the day of surgery, continue for 2 to 3 days postop with 50 g/day. 50 g/day may be given every 2nd or 3rd day thereafter up to 14 days.

PEDS – Total dose should not exceed 20 mL/kg.

UNAPPROVED ADULT – DVT/PE prophylaxis during surgery: Dextran 70 and 75 solns have been used. Other uses: To improve circulation with sickle cell crisis, prevention of nephrotoxicity with radiographic contrast media, toxemia of late pregnancy.

(cont.)

THROMBOLYTIC THERAPY FOR ACUTE MI

Indications (if high-volume cath lab unavailable)	Clinical history and presentation strongly suggestive of MI within 12 h plus at least 1 of the following: 1 mm ST elevation in at least 2 contiguous leads; new left BBB; or 2 mm ST depression in V1–4 suggestive of true posterior MI.
Absolute contraindications	Previous cerebral hemorrhage, known cerebral aneurysm or arteriovenous malformation, known intracranial neoplasm, recent (<3 months) ischemic CVA (except acute ischemic CVA <3 h), aortic dissection, active bleeding or bleeding diathesis (excluding menstruation), significant closed head or facial trauma (<3 months).
Relative contraindications	Severe uncontrolled HTN (>180/110 mm Hg) on presentation or chronic severe HTN; prior ischemic CVA (>3 months), dementia, other intracranial pathology; traumatic/prolonged (>10 min) cardiopulmonary resuscitation; major surgery (<3 weeks); recent (within 2–4 weeks) internal bleeding; puncture of noncompressible vessel; pregnancy; active peptic ulcer disease; current use of anticoagulants. For streptokinase/anistreplase: prior exposure (>5 days ago) or prior allergic reaction.

Reference: *Circulation* 2004;110:588-636

DEXTRAN (*cont.*)

NOTES – Monitor for plasma volume overload (dyspnea, fluid in lungs, abnormal increase in BP or CVP) and anaphylactoid reactions. May impair platelet function. Less effective than other agents for DVT/PE prevention.

HETASTARCH (***Hespan, Hextend***) ▶K ♀C ▶? $$

ADULT – Shock/hypovolemia: 500 to 1000 mL IV infusion, total daily dose usually should not exceed 20 mL/kg (1500 mL). Renal impairment: CrCl less than 10 mL/min, usual initial dose followed by 20 to 25% of usual dose.

PEDS – Not approved in children.

UNAPPROVED PEDS – Shock/hypovolemia: 10 mL/kg/dose; do not exceed 20 mL/kg/day.

NOTES – Monitor for volume overload. Little or no antigenic properties compared to dextran.

PLASMA PROTEIN FRACTION (***Plasmanate, Protenate, Plasmatein***) ▶L ♀C ▶? $$$

ADULT – Shock/hypovolemia: Adjust initial rate according to clinical response and BP, but rate should not exceed 10 mL/min. As plasma volume normalizes, infusion rate should not exceed 5 to 8 mL/min. Usual dose 250 to 500 mL. Hypoproteinemia: 1000 to 1500 mL/day IV infusion.

PEDS – Shock/hypovolemia: Initial dose 6.6 to 33 mL/kg infused at a rate of 5 to 10 mL/min.

NOTES – Fever, chills, hypotension with rapid infusion. Monitor for volume overload. Less pure than albumin products.

CARDIOVASCULAR: Other

BIDIL **(hydralazine + isosorbide dinitrate)** ▶LK ♀C ▶? $$$$$

ADULT – Heart failure (adjunct to standard therapy in black patients): Start 1 tab PO three times per day, increase as tolerated to max 2 tabs three times per day. May decrease to ½ tab three times per day with intolerable side effects; try to increase dose when side effects subside.

PEDS – Not approved in children.

FORMS – Trade only: Tabs, scored 37.5/20 mg.

NOTES – See component drugs.

CILOSTAZOL (***Pletal***) ▶L ♀C ▶? $$$$

WARNING – Contraindicated in heart failure of any severity due to decreased survival.

ADULT – Intermittent claudication: 100 mg PO twice daily on empty stomach. 50 mg PO twice daily with CYP3A4 inhibitors (eg, ketoconazole, itraconazole, erythromycin, diltiazem) or CYP2C19 inhibitors (like omeprazole). Beneficial effect may take up to 12 weeks.

PEDS – Not approved in children.

FORMS – Generic/Trade: Tabs 50, 100 mg.

NOTES – Caution with moderate/severe liver impairment or CrCl less than 25 mL/min. Give with other antiplatelet therapy (aspirin or clopidogrel) when treating peripheral arterial disease to reduce cardiovascular risk. Grapefruit juice may increase levels and the risk of side effects.

ISOXSUPRINE ▶KL ♀C ▶? $$
ADULT – Adjunctive therapy for cerebral vascular insufficiency and PVD: 10 to 20 mg PO three to four times per day.
PEDS – Not approved in children.
FORMS – Generic: Tabs, 10, 20 mg.
NOTES – Drug has questionable therapeutic effect.

NESIRITIDE (*Natrecor*) ▶K, plasma ♀C ▶? $$$$$
ADULT – Hospitalized patients with decompensated heart failure with dyspnea at rest: 2 mcg/kg IV bolus over 1 min, then 0.01 mcg/kg/min IV infusion for up to 48 h. Do not initiate at higher doses. Limited experience with increased doses: 0.005 mcg/kg/min increments, preceded by 1 mcg/kg bolus, no more frequently than q 3 h up to max infusion dose 0.03 mcg/kg/min. Mix 1.5 mg vial in 250 mL D5W (6 mcg/mL). A bolus of 23.3 mL is 2 mcg/kg for a 70 kg patient, infusion set at rate 7 mL/h delivers a 0.01 mcg/kg/min for a 70 kg patient.
PEDS – Not approved in children.
NOTES – May increase mortality; meta-analysis showed nonstatistically significant increased risk of death within 30 days post treatment compared with noninotropic control group. Not indicated for outpatient infusion, for scheduled repetitive use, to improve renal function, or to enhance diuresis. Contraindicated as primary therapy for cardiogenic shock and when SBP less than 90 mm Hg. Discontinue if dose-related symptomatic hypotension occurs and support BP prn. May restart infusion with dose reduced by 30% (no bolus dose) once BP stabilized. Do not shake reconstituted vial, and dilute vial prior to administration. Incompatible with most injectable drugs; administer agents using separate IV lines. Do not measure BNP levels while infusing; may measure BNP at least 2 to 6 h after infusion completion.

PAPAVERINE ▶LK ♀C ▶? $
ADULT – Cerebral and peripheral ischemia: Start 150 mg PO two times per day, increase to max 300 mg two times per day if needed. Start 30 mg IV/IM, dose range 30 to 120 mg q 3 h prn. Give IV doses over 1 to 2 min.
PEDS – Not approved in children.
FORMS – Generic only: Caps, extended-release, 150 mg.

PENTOXIFYLLINE (*Trental*) ▶L ♀C ▶? $$$
ADULT – Intermittent claudication: 400 mg PO three times per day with meals. With CNS/GI adverse effects, may decrease to two times per day. Beneficial effect may take up to 8 weeks. May be less effective in relieving cramps, tiredness, tightness, and pain during exercise.
PEDS – Not approved in children.
FORMS – Generic/Trade: Tabs, extended-release 400 mg.
NOTES – Contraindicated with recent cerebral/retinal bleed. Increases theophylline levels. Increases INR with warfarin.

RANOLAZINE (*Ranexa*) ▶LK ♀C ▶? $$$$$
ADULT – Chronic angina: 500 mg PO two times per day, increase to 1000 mg PO two times per day prn based on clinical symptoms, max 2000 mg daily. Max 500 mg two times per day, if used with diltiazem, verapamil, or moderate CYP3A inhibitors.
PEDS – Not approved in children.
FORMS – Trade only: Tabs extended-release 500, 1000 mg.
NOTES – Baseline and follow-up ECGs; may prolong QT interval. Contraindicated with hepatic cirrhosis, potent CYP3A4 inhibitors (eg, clarithromycin, protease inhibitors, itraconazole, ketoconazole, nefazodone), CYP3A inducers (eg, carbamazepine, phenobarbital, phenytoin, rifabutin, rifapentin, rifampin, St. John's wort). Limit dose of ranolazine to max 500 mg two times per day with moderate CYP3A inhibitors (eg, diltiazem, erythromycin, fluconazole, grapefruit juice-containing products, verapamil). Limit simvastatin to 20 mg when used with ranolazine. P-glycoprotein inhibitors (eg, cyclosporine) increase ranolazine levels; titrate ranolazine based on clinical response. Increases levels of CYP3A substrates (eg, lovastatin, simvastatin), cyclosporine, tacrolimus, sirolimus, antipsychotics, TCA(s), drugs transported by P-glycoprotein, drugs metabolized by CYP2D6 (eg, digoxin). Swallow whole; do not crush, break, or chew. May be less effective in women. Teach patients to report palpitations or fainting spells.

CONTRAST MEDIA: MRI Contrast—Gadolinium-based

NOTE: Black Box Warning for all drugs in this class. Avoid gadolinium-based contrast agents if severe renal insufficiency (GFR less than 30 mL/min/1.73 m^2) due to risk of nephrogenic systemic fibrosis/nephrogenic fibrosing dermopathy. Similarly avoid in acute renal insufficiency of any severity due to hepatorenal syndrome or during the perioperative phase of liver transplant.

GADOBENATE (*MultiHance*) ▶K ♀C ▶? $$$$
ADULT – Noniodinated, nonionic IV contrast for MRI.
PEDS – Not approved in children.

GADOBUTROL (*Gadavist*, ♣*Gadavist*) ▶K - ♀C ▶?©V $$$$
ADULT – 0.1 mL/kg for age 2 yo or older up to a maximum of 14 mL.
PEDS – 0.1 mL/kg for age 2 yo or older.
NOTES – Formulated at a higher concentration (1 mmol/mL) compared to certain other gadolinium-based contrast agents, resulting in a lower volume of administration.

GADODIAMIDE (*Omniscan*) ▶K ♀C ▶? $$$$
ADULT – Noniodinated, nonionic IV contrast for MRI.
PEDS – Noniodinated, nonionic IV contrast for MRI.
NOTES – Use caution if renal disease. May falsely lower serum calcium. Not for intrathecal use.

GADOPENTETATE (*Magnevist*) ▶K ♀C ▶? $$$
ADULT – Noniodinated IV contrast for MRI.
PEDS – Age older than 2 yo: Noniodinated IV contrast for MRI.
NOTES – Use caution in sickle cell and renal disease.

GADOTERIDOL (*Prohance*) ▶K ♀C ▶? $$$$
ADULT – Noniodinated, nonionic IV contrast for MRI.
PEDS – Age older than 2 yo: Noniodinated, nonionic IV contrast for MRI.
NOTES – Use caution in sickle cell and renal disease.

GADOVERSETAMIDE (*OptiMARK*) ▶K ♀C ▶– $$$$
ADULT – Noniodinated IV contrast for MRI.
PEDS – Not approved in children.
NOTES – Use caution in sickle cell and renal disease.

CONTRAST MEDIA: MRI Contrast—Other

FERUMOXIDES (*Feridex*) ▶L ♀C ▶? $$$$
ADULT – Noniodinated, nonionic, iron-based IV contrast for hepatic MRI.
PEDS – Not approved in children.
NOTES – Contains dextran.

FERUMOXSIL (*GastroMARK*) ▶L ♀B ▶? $$$$
ADULT – Noniodinated, nonionic, iron-based, oral GI contrast for MRI.
PEDS – Not approved in children younger than 16 yo.

MANGAFODIPIR (*Teslascan*) ▶L ♀– ▶– $$$$
ADULT – Noniodinated IV contrast for MRI.
PEDS – Not approved in children.
NOTES – Contains manganese.

CONTRAST MEDIA: Other

INDIGOTINDISULFONATE (*Indigo Carmine*) ▶K ♀C ▶? $
ADULT – Identification of ureteral tears during surgery: 5 mL IV.
PEDS – Identification of ureteral tears during surgery: Use less than the adult dose.
FORMS – Trade only: 40 mg/5 mL vial.

ISOSULFAN BLUE (*Lymphazurin*) ▶LK ♀? ▶? $$$$$
ADULT – Lymphography, identification of lymphatics during cancer surgery: 0.5 to 3 mL SC.
PEDS – Optimal dosing not defined.
FORMS – Trade only: 1% (10 mg/ mL) 5 mL vial.

PENTETATE INDIUM (*Indium DTPA*) ▶K ♀C ▶? $$$$$
ADULT – Radionuclide cisternography.
PEDS – Not approved in children.
FORMS – 1 mCi/mL, 1.5 mL vial.

CONTRAST MEDIA: Radiography Contrast

NOTE: Beware of allergic or anaphylactoid reactions. Avoid IV contrast in renal insufficiency or dehydration. Hold metformin (Glucophage) prior to or at the time of iodinated contrast dye use and for 48 h after procedure. Restart after procedure only if renal function is normal.

BARIUM SULFATE ▶Not absorbed ♀? ▶+ $
ADULT – Noniodinated GI (eg, oral, rectal) contrast.
PEDS – Noniodinated GI (eg, oral, rectal) contrast.
NOTES – Contraindicated if suspected esophageal, gastric, or intestinal perforation. Use with caution in GI obstruction. May cause abdominal distention, cramping, and constipation with oral use.

DIATRIZOATE (*Cystografin, Gastrografin, Hypaque, MD-Gastroview, RenoCal, Reno-DIP, Reno-60, Renografin*) ▶K ♀C ▶? $
WARNING – Not for intrathecal or epidural use.
ADULT – Iodinated, ionic, high osmolality IV, or GI contrast.
PEDS – Iodinated, ionic, high osmolality IV, or GI contrast.

(cont.)

DIATRIZOATE (*cont.*)

NOTES – High osmolality contrast may cause tissue damage if infiltrated/extravasated. IV: Hypaque, Renografin, Reno-DIP, RenoCal. GI: Gastrografin, MD-Gastroview.

IODIXANOL (*Visipaque*) ▶K ♀B ▶? $$$

ADULT – Iodinated, nonionic, iso-osmolar IV contrast.

PEDS – Iodinated, nonionic, iso-osmolar IV contrast.

NOTES – Not for intrathecal use.

IOHEXOL (*Omnipaque*) ▶K ♀B ▶? $$$

ADULT – Iodinated, nonionic, low osmolality IV, and oral/body cavity contrast.

PEDS – Iodinated, nonionic, low osmolality IV, and oral/body cavity contrast.

IOPAMIDOL (*Isovue*) ▶K ♀? ▶? $$

ADULT – Iodinated, nonionic, low osmolality IV contrast.

PEDS – Iodinated, nonionic, low osmolality IV contrast.

IOPROMIDE (*Ultravist*) ▶K ♀B ▶? $$$

ADULT – Iodinated, nonionic, low osmolality IV contrast.

PEDS – Iodinated, nonionic, low osmolality IV contrast.

IOTHALAMATE (*Conray*, *♣Vascoray*) ▶K ♀B ▶– $

ADULT – Iodinated, ionic, high osmolality IV contrast.

PEDS – Iodinated, ionic, high osmolality IV contrast.

NOTES – High osmolality contrast may cause tissue damage if infiltrated/extravasated.

IOVERSOL (*Optiray*) ▶K ♀B ▶? $$

ADULT – Iodinated, nonionic, low osmolality IV contrast.

PEDS – Iodinated, nonionic, low osmolality IV contrast.

IOXAGLATE (*Hexabrix*) ▶K ♀B ▶– $$$

ADULT – Iodinated, ionic, low osmolality IV contrast.

PEDS – Iodinated, ionic, low osmolality IV contrast.

IOXILAN (*Oxilan*) ▶K ♀B ▶– $$$

ADULT – Iodinated, nonionic, low osmolality IV contrast.

PEDS – Iodinated, nonionic, low osmolality IV contrast.

DERMATOLOGY: Acne Preparations

NOTE: For topical agents, wash area prior to application. Wash hands before and after application; avoid eye area.

ACANYA **(clindamycin + benzoyl peroxide)** ▶K ♀C ▶+ $$$$

ADULT – Acne: Apply once daily.

PEDS – Not approved in children 12 yo or younger.

FORMS – Trade only: Gel (clindamycin 1.2% + benzoyl peroxide 2.5%) 50 g.

NOTES – Expires 2 months after mixing.

ADAPALENE (*Differin*) ▶Bile ♀C ▶? $$$$

ADULT – Acne: Apply at bedtime.

PEDS – Not approved in children.

UNAPPROVED PEDS – Acne: Apply at bedtime.

FORMS – Generic/Trade: Gel 0.1%. Cream 0.1% (45 g). Trade only: Gel 0.3% (45 g). Soln 0.1% (30 mL). Swabs 0.1% (60 ea).

NOTES – During early weeks of therapy, acne exacerbation may occur. May cause erythema, scaling, dryness, pruritus, and burning in up to 40% of patients. Therapeutic results take 8 to 12 weeks.

AZELAIC ACID (*Azelex, Finacea, Finevin*) ▶K ♀B ▶? $$$$

ADULT – Acne (Azelex, Finevin): Apply two times per day. Rosacea (Finacea): Apply two times per day.

PEDS – Not approved in children.

UNAPPROVED ADULT – Melasma: Apply two times per day.

UNAPPROVED PEDS – Acne: Apply at bedtime.

FORMS – Trade only: Cream 20%, 30, 50 g (Azelex). Gel 15% 50 g (Finacea).

NOTES – Improvement of acne occurs within 4 weeks. Monitor for hypopigmentation especially in patients with dark complexions. Avoid use of occlusive dressings.

BENZACLIN **(clindamycin + benzoyl peroxide)** ▶K ♀C ▶+ $$$$

ADULT – Acne: Apply two times per day.

PEDS – Not approved in children.

UNAPPROVED PEDS – Acne: Apply at bedtime.

FORMS – Generic/Trade: Gel (clindamycin 1% + benzoyl peroxide 5%) 50 g (jar). Trade only: 25, 35 g (jar) and 50 g (pump).

NOTES – Expires 10 weeks after mixing.

BENZAMYCIN **(erythromycin base + benzoyl peroxide)** ▶LK ♀C ▶? $$$

ADULT – Acne: Apply two times per day.

PEDS – Not approved in children.

UNAPPROVED PEDS – Acne: Apply at bedtime.

FORMS – Generic/Trade: Gel (erythromycin 3% + benzoyl peroxide 5%) 23.3, 46.6 g. Trade only: Benzamycin Pak, #60 gel pouches.

NOTES – Must be refrigerated, expires 3 months after pharmacy dispensing.

BENZOYL PEROXIDE (*Benzac, Benzagel 10%, Desquam, Clearasil,* ✤ *Solugel*) ▶LK ♀C ▶? $

ADULT – Acne: Cleansers: Wash one to two times per day. Creams/gels/lotion: Apply daily initially, gradually increase to two to three times per day if needed.

PEDS – Not approved in children.

UNAPPROVED PEDS – Acne: Cleansers: Wash one to two times per day. Creams/gels/lotion: Apply daily initially, gradually increase to two to three times per day if needed.

FORMS – OTC and Rx generic: Liquid 2.5, 5, 10%. Bar 5, 10%. Mask 5%. Lotion 4, 5, 8, 10%. Cream 5, 10%. Gel 2.5, 4, 5, 6, 10, 20%. Pad 3, 4, 6, 8, 9%. Other strengths available.

NOTES – If excessive drying or peeling occurs, reduce frequency of application. Use with PABA-containing sunscreens may cause transient skin discoloration. May bleach fabric.

CLENIA **(sulfacetamide + sulfur)** ▶K ♀C ▶? $$$

ADULT – Acne, rosacea, seborrheic dermatitis: Apply cream/lotion daily to three times per day, foaming wash daily to two times per day.

PEDS – Not approved in children.

FORMS – Generic only: Lotion (sodium sulfacetamide 10%/sulfur 5%) 25, 30, 45, 60 g. Trade only: Cream (sodium sulfacetamide 10%/sulfur 5%) 28 g. Generic/Trade: Foaming Wash 170, 340 g.

NOTES – Avoid with sulfa allergy, renal failure.

CLINDAMYCIN—TOPICAL (*Cleocin T, Clindagel, ClindaMax, Evoclin,* ✤ *Dalacin T*) ▶L ♀B ▶– $

ADULT – Acne: Apply daily (Evoclin, Clindagel) or two times per day (Cleocin T).

PEDS – Not approved in children.

UNAPPROVED ADULT – Rosacea: Apply lotion two times per day.

UNAPPROVED PEDS – Acne: Apply two times per day.

FORMS – Generic/Trade: Gel 1% 30, 60 g. Lotion 1% 60 mL. Soln 1% 30, 60 mL. Trade only: Foam 1% 50, 100 g (Evoclin). Gel 1% 40, 75 mL (Clindagel).

NOTES – Concomitant use with erythromycin may decrease effectiveness. Most common adverse effects dryness, erythema, burning, peeling, oiliness, and itching. *C. difficile*-associated diarrhea has been reported with topical use.

✤ ***DIANE-35*** **(cyproterone + ethinyl estradiol)** ▶L ♀X ▶– $$

WARNING – Not recommended in women who smoke. Increased risk of thromboembolism, CVA, MI, hepatic neoplasia, and gallbladder disease. Nausea, breast tenderness, and breakthrough bleeding are common, transient side effects. Nighttime dosing may minimize nausea. Effectiveness is reduced by hepatic enzyme-inducing drugs such as certain anticonvulsants and barbiturates, rifampin, rifabutin, griseofulvin, and protease inhibitors. Antibiotics or products that contain St. John's wort may reduce efficacy.

ADULT – Canada only. In women, severe acne unresponsive to oral antibiotics and other treatments, with associated symptoms of androgenization, including seborrhea and mild hirsutism: 1 tab PO daily for 21 consecutive days, stop for 7 days, repeat cycle.

PEDS – Not approved in children.

FORMS – Canada Generic/Trade: Blister pack of 21 tabs 2 mg cyproterone acetate/0.035 mg ethinyl estradiol.

NOTES – Higher thromboembolic risk than other oral contraceptives, therefore only indicated for acne, and not solely for contraception (although effective for the latter). Same warnings, precautions, and contraindications as other oral contraceptives.

DUAC **(clindamycin + benzoyl peroxide,** ✤ ***Clindoxyl*****)** ▶K ♀C ▶+ $$$$

ADULT – Acne: Apply at bedtime.

PEDS – Not approved in children.

UNAPPROVED PEDS – Acne: Apply at bedtime.

FORMS – Trade only: Gel (clindamycin 1% + benzoyl peroxide 5%) 45 g.

NOTES – Expires 2 months after pharmacy dispensing.

EPIDUO **(adapalene + benzoyl peroxide)** ▶Bile, K ♀C ▶? $$$$$

ADULT – Acne: Apply daily.

PEDS – Not approved in children.

FORMS – Trade only: Gel (0.1% adapalene + benzoyl peroxide 2.5%) 45 g.

NOTES – During early weeks of therapy, acne exacerbation may occur. May cause erythema, scaling, dryness, pruritus, and burning.

ERYTHROMYCIN—TOPICAL (*Eryderm, Erycette, Erygel, A/T/S,* ✤ *Sans-Acne, Erysol*) ▶L ♀B ▶? $

ADULT – Acne: Apply two times per day.

PEDS – Not approved in children.

UNAPPROVED PEDS – Acne: Apply two times per day.

FORMS – Generic/Trade: Soln 2% 60 mL. Pads 2%. Gel 2% 30, 60 g. Ointment 2% 25 g. Generic only: Soln 1.5% 60 mL.

NOTES – May be more irritating when used with other acne products. Concomitant use with clindamycin may decrease effectiveness.

ISOTRETINOIN (*Amnesteem, Claravis, Sotret,* ♣ *Clarus*) ▶LK ♀X ▶– $$$$$

WARNING – Contraindicated in pregnant women or in women who may become pregnant. If used in a woman of childbearing age, patient must have severe, disfiguring acne, be reliable, comply with mandatory contraceptive measures, receive written and oral instructions about hazards of taking during pregnancy, have 2 negative pregnancy tests prior to beginning therapy. Must use 2 forms of effective contraception from 1 month prior until 1 month after discontinuation of therapy, unless absolute abstinence is chosen or patient has undergone a hysterectomy. Men should not father children. May cause depression, suicidal thoughts, and aggressive or violent behavior; monitor for symptoms. Obtain written informed consent. Write prescription for no more than a 1-month supply. Informed consent documents available from the manufacturer.

ADULT – Severe, recalcitrant cystic acne: 0.5 to 2 mg/kg/day PO divided two times per day for 15 to 20 weeks. Typical target dose is 1 mg/kg/day. May repeat 2nd course of therapy after at least 2 months off therapy.

PEDS – Not approved in children.

UNAPPROVED ADULT – Prevention of 2nd primary tumors in patients treated for squamous cell carcinoma of the head and neck: 50 to 100 mg/m²/day PO. Also been used in keratinization disorders.

UNAPPROVED PEDS – Severe, recalcitrant cystic acne: 0.5 to 2 mg/kg/day PO divided two times per day for 15 to 20 weeks. Typical target dose is 1 mg/kg/day. Maintenance therapy for neuroblastoma: 100 to 250 mg/m²/day PO in 2 divided doses.

FORMS – Generic: Caps 10, 20, 40 mg. Generic only (Sotret and Claravis): Caps 30 mg.

NOTES – Prescription can be for a maximum of a 1-month supply. May cause headache; cheilitis; drying of mucous membranes including eyes, nose, mouth; hair loss; abdominal pain; pyuria; joint and muscle pain/stiffness; conjunctivitis; elevated ESR; and changes in serum lipids and LFTs. Effect on bone loss unknown; use caution in patients predisposed to osteoporosis. In children in whom skeletal growth is not complete, do not exceed the recommended dose for the recommended duration of treatment. Pseudotumor cerebri has occurred during therapy; avoid concomitant vitamin A, tetracycline, minocycline. May cause corneal opacities, decreased night vision, and inflammatory bowel disease. May decrease carbamazepine concentrations. Avoid excessive exposure to sunlight.

SALICYLIC ACID (*Akurza, Clearasil Cleanser, Stridex Pads*) ▶Not absorbed ♀? ▶? $

ADULT – Acne (OTC): Apply/wash area up to 3 times a day. Removal of excessive keratin in hyperkeratotic disorders (Rx): Apply to affected area at bedtime and cover. Hydrate skin before application.

PEDS – Acne: Apply/wash area up to 3 times a day.

FORMS – OTC Generic/Trade: Pads, Gel, Lotion, Liquid, Mask scrub, 0.5%, 1%, 2%. Rx Trade only (Akurza): Cream 6% 340 g. Lotion 6%, 355 mL.

♣ ***SULFACET-R*** (**sulfacetamide + sulfur**) ▶K ♀C ▶? $$$

ADULT – Canada only: Acne, rosacea, seborrheic dermatitis: Apply cream/gel one to three times per day, foaming wash one to two times per day.

PEDS – Not approved in children.

FORMS – Generic/Trade: Lotion (sodium sulfacetamide 10%/sulfur 5%) 25 g.

NOTES – Avoid with sulfa allergy or renal failure.

SULFACETAMIDE—TOPICAL (*Klaron*) ▶K ♀C ▶? $$$$

ADULT – Acne: Apply two times per day.

PEDS – Not approved in children.

FORMS – Generic/Trade: Lotion 10% 118 mL.

NOTES – Cross-sensitivity with sulfa or sulfite allergy.

TAZAROTENE (*Tazorac, Avage*) ▶L ♀X ▶? $$$$

ADULT – Acne (Tazorac): Apply 0.1% cream at bedtime. Palliation of fine facial wrinkles, mottled hyper- and hypopigmentation, benign facial lentigines (Avage): Apply at bedtime. Psoriasis: Apply 0.05% cream at bedtime, increase to 0.1% prn.

PEDS – Not approved in children.

UNAPPROVED PEDS – Acne: Apply 0.1% cream at bedtime. Psoriasis: Apply 0.05% cream at bedtime.

FORMS – Trade only (Tazorac): Cream 0.05% and 0.1% 30, 60 g. Gel 0.05% and 0.1% 30, 100 g. Trade only (Avage): Cream 0.1% 15, 30 g.

NOTES – Avoid using gel formulation with other medications or cosmetics that are considered drying. In psoriasis, may reduce irritation and improve efficacy by using topical corticosteroid in morning and tazarotene at bedtime. Desquamation, burning, dry skin, erythema, pruritus may occur in up to 30% of patients. May cause photosensitivity.

TRETINOIN—TOPICAL (*Retin-A, Retin-A Micro, Renova, Retisol-A,* ✤ *Stieva-A, Rejuva-A, Vitamin A Acid Cream*) ▶LK ♀C ▶? $$$

ADULT – Acne (Retin A, Retin-A Micro): Apply at bedtime. Wrinkles, hyperpigmentation, tactile roughness (Renova): Apply at bedtime.

PEDS – Not approved in children.

UNAPPROVED ADULT – Used in skin cancer and lamellar ichthyosis, mollusca contagiosa, verrucae plantaris, verrucae planae juvenilis, hyperpigmented lesions in black individuals, ichthyosis vulgaris, and pityriasis rubra pilaris.

FORMS – Generic/Trade: Cream 0.025% 20, 45 g, 0.05% 20, 45 g, 0.1% 20, 45 g. Gel 0.025% 15, 45 g, 0.1% 15, 45 g. Trade only: Renova cream 0.02% 40, 60 g. Retin-A Micro gel 0.04%, 0.1% 20, 45, 50 g.

NOTES – May induce erythema, peeling. Minimize sun exposure. Concomitant use with sulfur, resorcinol, benzoyl peroxide, or salicylic acid may result in skin irritation. Gel preps are flammable.

VELTIN **(clindamycin + tretinoin)** ▶LK – ♀C ▶? $$$$

WARNING – Clindamycin has been reproted to cause severe colitis.

ADULT – Acne: Apply at bedtime.

PEDS – Has not been studied in children younger than 12 yo.

FORMS – Trade: Gel clindamycin 1.2% + tretinoin 0/025%, 30 g.

ZIANA **(clindamycin + tretinoin)** ▶LK ♀C ▶? $$$$

ADULT – Acne: Apply at bedtime.

PEDS – Use adult dose for age 12 yo or older.

FORMS – Trade only: Gel clindamycin 1.2% + tretinoin 0.025% 30, 60 g.

NOTES – May induce erythema, peeling. Minimize sun exposure.

DERMATOLOGY: Actinic Keratosis Preparations

AMINOLEVULINIC ACID (*Levulan Kerastick*) ▶Not absorbed ♀C ▶? $$$$

ADULT – Non-hyperkeratotic actinic keratoses: Apply soln to lesions on scalp or face; expose to special light source 14 to 18 h later.

PEDS – Not approved in children.

FORMS – Trade only: 20% soln, single-use applicator stick.

NOTES – Soln should be applied by healthcare personnel. Advise patients to avoid sunlight during 14 to 18 h period before blue light illumination.

DICLOFENAC—TOPICAL (*Solaraze, Voltaren*) ▶L ♀B ▶? $$$$$

ADULT – Solaraze: Actinic/solar keratoses: Apply two times per day to lesions for 60 to 90 days. Voltaren: OA of areas amenable to topical therapy: 2 g (upper extremities) to 4 g (lower extremities) four times per day.

PEDS – Not approved in children.

FORMS – Trade only: Gel 3% 50 g (Solaraze), 100 g (Solaraze, Voltaren).

NOTES – Avoid exposure to sun and sunlamps. Use caution in aspirin-sensitive patients. When using for OA (Voltaren), maximum daily dose 16 g to any single lower extremity joint, 8 g to any single upper extremity joint.

FLUOROURACIL—TOPICAL (*5-FU, Carac, Efudex, Fluoroplex*) ▶L ♀X ▶– $$$

WARNING – Contraindicated in pregnant women or women who plan to get pregnant during therapy. Avoid application to mucous membranes.

ADULT – Actinic or solar keratoses: Apply two times per day to lesions for 2 to 6 weeks. Superficial basal cell carcinomas: Apply 5% cream/soln two times per day.

PEDS – Not approved in children.

UNAPPROVED ADULT – Condylomata acuminata: 1% soln in 70% ethanol and the 5% cream has been used.

FORMS – Trade only: Cream 0.5% 30 g (Carac), 5% 25 g (Efudex), 1% 30 g (Fluoroplex). Generic/Trade: Soln 2%, 5% 10 mL (Efudex). Cream 5% 40 g.

NOTES – May cause severe irritation and photosensitivity. Contraindicated in women who are or who may become pregnant during therapy. Avoid application to mucous membranes.

INGENOL (*Picato*) ▶not absorbed – ♀C ▶? $$$

ADULT – Actinic keratosis on face and scalp: Apply 0.015% gel to affected areas once daily for 3 days. Actinic keratosis on trunk and extremities: Apply 0.05% gel to affected areas once daily for 2 days.

PEDS – Not approved in children.

FORMS – Trade: Gel 0.015% 0.25 g, 0.05% 0.25g.

NOTES – Avoid contact with the periocular area.

METHYLAMINOLEVULINATE (*Metvix, Metvixia*) ▶Not absorbed ♀C ▶? ?

ADULT – Non-hyperkeratotic actinic keratoses of face/scalp: Apply cream 1 mm thick (max

(cont.)

METHYLAMINOLEVULINATE (*cont.*)

1 g) to lesion and 5 mm surrounding area; cover with dressing for 3 h; remove dressing and cream and perform illumination therapy. Repeat in 7 days.

PEDS – Not approved in children.

FORMS – Trade only: Cream 16.8%, 2 g tube.

NOTES – Use in immunocompetent individuals. Lesion debridement should be performed prior to application of cream. Formulated in peanut and almond oil; has not been tested in patients allergic to peanuts.

DERMATOLOGY: Antibacterials (Topical)

BACITRACIN ▶Not absorbed ♀C ▶? $

ADULT – Minor cuts, wounds, burns, or skin abrasions: Apply one to three times per day.

PEDS – Not approved in children.

UNAPPROVED PEDS – Minor cuts, wounds, burns, or skin abrasions: Apply one to three times per day.

FORMS – OTC Generic/Trade: Ointment 500 units/g 1, 15, 30 g.

NOTES – May cause contact dermatitis or anaphylaxis.

FUSIDIC ACID—TOPICAL (✤ *Fucidin*) ▶L ♀? ▶? $

ADULT – Skin infections: Apply three to four times per day.

PEDS – Canada only. Skin infections: Apply three to four times per day.

FORMS – Canada trade only: Cream 2% fusidic acid 5, 15, 30 g. Ointment 2% sodium fusidate 5, 15, 30 g.

NOTES – Contains lanolin; possible hypersensitivity.

GENTAMICIN—TOPICAL (*Garamycin*) ▶K ♀D ▶? $

ADULT – Skin infections: Apply three to four times per day.

PEDS – Skin infections in children older than 1 yo: Apply three to four times per day.

FORMS – Generic only: Ointment 0.1% 15, 30 g. Cream 0.1% 15, 30 g.

MAFENIDE (*Sulfamylon*) ▶LK ♀C ▶? $$

ADULT – Adjunctive treatment of burns: Apply one to two times per day.

PEDS – Adjunctive treatment of burns: Apply one to two times per day.

FORMS – Trade only: Cream 5% 57, 114, 454 g. Topical soln 50 g packets.

NOTES – Can cause metabolic acidosis. Contains sulfonamides.

METRONIDAZOLE—TOPICAL (***Noritate, MetroCream, MetroGel, MetroLotion,*** ✤ ***Rosasol***) ▶KL ♀B(– in 1st trimester) ▶– $$$

ADULT – Rosacea: Apply daily (1%) or two times per day (0.75%).

PEDS – Not approved in children.

UNAPPROVED ADULT – A 1% soln prepared from the oral tabs has been used in the treatment of infected decubitus ulcers.

FORMS – Trade only: Gel (MetroGel) 1% 45, 60 g. Cream (Noritate) 1% 60 g. Generic/Trade: Gel 0.75% 45 g. Cream 0.75% 45 g. Lotion (MetroLotion) 0.75% 59 mL.

NOTES – Results usually noted within 3 weeks, with continuing improvement through 9 weeks. Avoid using vaginal prep on face due to irritation because of formulation differences.

MUPIROCIN (***Bactroban, Centany***) ▶Not absorbed ♀B ▶? $$

ADULT – Impetigo: Apply three times per day for 3 to 5 days. Infected wounds: Apply three times per day for 10 days. Nasal MRSA eradication: 0.5 g in each nostril two times per day for 5 days.

PEDS – Impetigo (mupirocin cream/ointment): Apply three times per day. Infected wounds: Apply three times per day for 10 days. Nasal form not approved in children younger than 12 yo.

FORMS – Generic/Trade: Ointment 2% 22 g. Nasal ointment 2% 1 g single-use tubes (for MRSA eradication). Trade only: Cream 2% 15, 30 g.

NEOSPORIN CREAM **(neomycin + polymyxin + bacitracin)** ▶K ♀C ▶? $

ADULT – Minor cuts, wounds, burns, or skin abrasions: Apply one to three times per day.

PEDS – Not approved in children.

UNAPPROVED PEDS – Minor cuts, wounds, burns, or skin abrasions: Apply one to three times per day.

FORMS – OTC Trade only: neomycin 3.5 mg/g + polymyxin 10,000 units/g 15 g and unit dose 0.94 g.

NOTES – Neomycin component can cause contact dermatitis.

NEOSPORIN OINTMENT **(bacitracin + neomycin + polymyxin)** ▶K ♀C ▶? $

ADULT – Minor cuts, wounds, burns, or skin abrasions: Apply one to three times per day.

PEDS – Not approved in children.

UNAPPROVED PEDS – Minor cuts, wounds, burns, or skin abrasions: Apply one to three times per day.

FORMS – OTC Generic/Trade: bacitracin 400 units/g + neomycin 3.5 mg/g + polymyxin 5000 units/g 15, 30 g and "to go" 0.9 g packets.

NOTES – Also known as triple antibiotic ointment. Neomycin component can cause contact dermatitis.

POLYSPORIN **(bacitracin + polymyxin, ♣ *Polytopic*)** ▶K ♀C ◗? $

ADULT – Minor cuts, wounds, burns, or skin abrasions: Apply one to three times per day.

PEDS – Not approved in children.

UNAPPROVED PEDS – Minor cuts, wounds, burns, or skin abrasions: Apply one to three times per day.

FORMS – OTC Trade only: Ointment 15, 30 g and unit dose 0.9 g. Powder 10 g.

NOTES – May cause allergic contact dermatitis and rarely contact anaphylaxis.

RETAPAMULIN (***Altabax***) ▶Not absorbed ♀B ◗? $$$

ADULT – Impetigo: Apply two times per day for 5 days.

PEDS – Impetigo (9 mo or older): Apply two times per day for 5 days.

FORMS – Trade only: Ointment 1% 5, 10, 15 g.

NOTES – Do not apply to nasal mucosa.

SILVER SULFADIAZINE (***Silvadene, Flamazine***) ▶LK ♀B ◗– $$

ADULT – Burns: Apply one to two times per day.

PEDS – Not approved in children.

UNAPPROVED ADULT – Has been used for pressure ulcers.

UNAPPROVED PEDS – Burns: Apply one to two times per day.

FORMS – Generic/Trade: Cream 1% 20, 50, 85, 400, 1000 g.

NOTES – Avoid in sulfa allergy. Leukopenia, primarily decreased neutrophil count in up to 20% of patients. Significant absorption may occur and serum sulfa concentrations approach therapeutic levels. Avoid in G6PD deficiency. Use caution in pregnancy nearing term, premature infants, infants 2 mo or younger and in patients with renal or hepatic dysfunction.

DERMATOLOGY: Antifungals (Topical)

BUTENAFINE (***Lotrimin Ultra, Mentax***) ▶L ♀B ◗? $

ADULT – Tinea pedis: Apply daily for 4 weeks or two times per day for 7 days. Tinea corporis, tinea versicolor, or tinea cruris: Apply daily for 2 weeks.

PEDS – Not approved in children.

FORMS – Rx Trade only: Cream 1% 15, 30 g (Mentax). OTC Trade only: Cream 1% 12, 24 g (Lotrimin Ultra).

NOTES – Most common adverse effects include contact dermatitis, burning, and worsening of condition. If no improvement in 4 weeks, reevaluate diagnosis.

CICLOPIROX (***Loprox, Penlac,*** ♣ ***Stieprox shampoo***) ▶K ♀B ◗? $$$$

ADULT – Tinea pedis, cruris, corporis, and versicolor, candidiasis (cream, lotion): Apply two times per day. Onychomycosis of fingernails/toenails (nail soln): Apply daily to affected nails; apply over previous coat; remove with alcohol q 7 days. Seborrheic dermatitis (Loprox shampoo): Shampoo twice weekly for 4 weeks.

PEDS – Onychomycosis of fingernails/toenails in children age 12 yo or older (nail soln): Apply daily to affected nails; apply over previous coat; remove with alcohol q 7 days (Penlac). Not approved in children younger than 12 yo.

FORMS – Trade only: Shampoo (Loprox) 1% 120 mL. Generic/Trade: Gel 0.77% 30, 45, 100 g. Nail soln (Penlac) 8% 6.6 mL. Cream (Loprox) 0.77% 15, 30, 90 g. Lotion (Loprox TS) 0.77% 30, 60 mL.

NOTES – Clinical improvement of tinea usually occurs within 1st week. Patients with tinea versicolor usually exhibit clinical and mycological clearing after 2 weeks. If no improvement in 4 weeks, reevaluate diagnosis. Do not get shampoo in eyes. No safety information available in diabetes or immunocompromise. Shampoo may affect hair color in those with light-colored hair. For nail soln, infected portion of each nail should be removed by healthcare professional as frequently as monthly. Oral antifungal therapy is more effective for onychomycosis than Penlac.

CLOTRIMAZOLE—TOPICAL (***Lotrimin AF, Mycelex,*** ♣ ***Canesten, Clotrimaderm***) ▶L ♀B ◗? $

ADULT – Tinea pedis, cruris, corporis, and versicolor, and cutaneous candidiasis: Apply two times per day.

PEDS – Tinea pedis, cruris, corporis, versicolor, cutaneous candidiasis: Apply two times per day.

FORMS – Note that Lotrimin brand cream, lotion, soln are clotrimazole, while Lotrimin powders and liquid spray are miconazole. Rx Generic only: Cream 1% 15, 30, 45 g. Soln 1% 10, 30 mL. OTC Trade only (Lotrimin AF): Cream 1% 12, 24 g. Soln 1% 10 mL.

NOTES – If no improvement in 4 weeks, reevaluate diagnosis.

ECONAZOLE ▶Not absorbed ♀C ◗? $$

ADULT – Tinea pedis, cruris, corporis, and versicolor: Apply daily. Cutaneous candidiasis: Apply two times per day.

(cont.)

ECONAZOLE (*cont.*)

PEDS – Not approved in children.

FORMS – Generic only: Cream 1% 15, 30, 85 g.

NOTES – Treat candidal infections, tinea cruris, and tinea corporis for 2 weeks and tinea pedis for 1 month to reduce risk of recurrence.

KETOCONAZOLE—TOPICAL (***Extina, Nizoral, Xolegel, ♣ Ketoderm***) ▶L ♀C ▶? $$

ADULT – Shampoo (2%): Tinea versicolor: Apply to affected area, leave on for 5 min, rinse. Cream: Cutaneous candidiasis, tinea corporis, tinea cruris, and tinea versicolor: Apply daily. Seborrheic dermatitis: Apply cream (2%) two times per day for 4 weeks or gel daily for 2 weeks or foam two times per day for 4 weeks. Dandruff: Apply shampoo (1%) twice a week.

PEDS – Not approved in children younger than 12 yo.

UNAPPROVED ADULT – Seborrheic dermatitis: Apply cream (2%) daily.

UNAPPROVED PEDS – Shampoo (2%): Tinea versicolor: Apply to affected area, leave on for 5 min, rinse. Cream: Cutaneous candidiasis, tinea corporis, tinea cruris, and tinea versicolor: Apply daily. Seborrheic dermatitis: Apply cream (2%) two times per day. Dandruff: Apply shampoo (1%) twice a week.

FORMS – Generic/Trade: Cream 2% 15, 30, 60 g. Shampoo 2% 120 mL. Trade only: Shampoo 1% 120, 210 mL (OTC Nizoral). Gel 2% 15 g (Xolegel). Foam 2% 50, 100 g (Extina).

NOTES – Treat candidal infections, tinea cruris, tinea corporis, and tinea versicolor for 2 weeks. Treat seborrheic dermatitis for 4 weeks. Treat tinea pedis for 6 weeks.

MICONAZOLE—TOPICAL (***Micatin, Lotrimin AF, ZeaSorb AF***) ▶L ♀+ ▶? $

ADULT – Tinea pedis, cruris, corporis, and versicolor, cutaneous candidiasis: Apply two times per day.

PEDS – Not approved in children.

UNAPPROVED PEDS – Tinea pedis, cruris, corporis, and versicolor, cutaneous candidiasis: Apply two times per day.

FORMS – Note that Lotrimin brand cream, lotion, soln are clotrimazole, while Lotrimin powders and liquid spray are miconazole. OTC Trade only: Powder 2% 70, 160 g. Spray powder 2% 90, 100, 140 g. Spray liquid 2% 90, 105 mL. Gel 2% 24 g.

NOTES – Symptomatic relief generally occurs in 2 to 3 days. Treat Candida, tinea cruris, tinea corporis for 2 weeks, tinea pedis for 1 month to reduce risk of recurrence.

NAFTIFINE (***Naftin***) ▶LK ♀B ▶? $$$

ADULT – Tinea pedis, cruris, and corporis: Apply daily (cream) or two times per day (gel).

PEDS – Not approved in children.

FORMS – Trade only: Cream 1% 15, 30, 60, 90 g. Gel 1% 20, 40, 60, 90 g.

NOTES – If no improvement in 4 weeks, reevaluate diagnosis.

NYSTATIN—TOPICAL (***Mycostatin, ♣ Nilstat, Nyaderm, Candistatin***) ▶Not absorbed ♀C ▶? $

ADULT – Cutaneous or mucocutaneous Candida infections: Apply two to three times per day.

PEDS – Cutaneous or mucocutaneous Candida infections: Apply two to three times per day.

FORMS – Generic/Trade: Cream, Ointment 100,000 units/g 15, 30 g. Powder 100,000 units/g 15, 30, 60 g.

NOTES – Ineffective for dermatophytes/tinea. For fungal infections of the feet, dust feet and footwear with powder.

OXICONAZOLE (***Oxistat, Oxizole***) ▶? ♀B ▶? $$$

ADULT – Tinea pedis, cruris, and corporis: Apply one to two times per day. Tinea versicolor (cream only): Apply daily.

PEDS – Cream: Tinea pedis, cruris, and corporis: Apply one to two times per day. Tinea versicolor: Apply daily.

FORMS – Trade only: Cream 1% 15, 30, 60 g. Lotion 1% 30 mL.

SERTACONAZOLE (***Ertaczo***) ▶Not absorbed ♀C ▶? $$$

ADULT – Tinea pedis: Apply two times per day.

PEDS – Not approved for children younger than 12 yo.

FORMS – Trade only: Cream 2% 30, 60 g.

TERBINAFINE—TOPICAL (***Lamisil, Lamisil AT***) ▶L ♀B ▶? $

ADULT – Tinea pedis: Apply two times per day. Tinea cruris and corporis: Apply one to two times per day. Tinea versicolor (soln): Apply two times per day.

PEDS – Not approved in children.

UNAPPROVED ADULT – Cutaneous candidiasis.

UNAPPROVED PEDS – Tinea pedis: Apply two times per day. Tinea cruris and corporis: Apply one to two times per day. Tinea versicolor (soln): Apply two times per day.

FORMS – OTC Trade only (Lamisil AT): Cream 1% 12, 24 g. Spray pump soln 1% 30 mL. Gel 1% 6, 12 g.

NOTES – In many patients, improvement noted within 3 to 4 days, but therapy should continue for a minimum of 1 week, maximum of 4 weeks. Topical therapy not effective for nail fungus.

TOLNAFTATE (*Tinactin*) ▶? ♀? ▶? $

ADULT – Tinea pedis, tinea cruris, tinea corporis, and tinea versicolor: Apply two times per day. Prevention of tinea pedis (powder and aerosol): Apply prn.

PEDS – Tinea pedis, tinea cruris, tinea corporis, and tinea versicolor: Apply two times per day for older than 2 yo. Prevention of tinea pedis (powder and aerosol): Apply prn.

FORMS – OTC Generic/Trade: Cream 1% 15, 30 g. Soln 1% 10 mL. Powder 1% 45 g. OTC Trade only: Gel 1% 15 g. Powder 1% 90 g. Spray powder 1% 100, 133, 150 g. Spray liquid 1% 100, 113 mL.

DERMATOLOGY: Antiparasitics (Topical)

A-200 **(pyrethrins + piperonyl butoxide,** ***✤R&C*****)** ▶L ♀C ▶? $

ADULT – Head lice: Apply shampoo, wash after 10 min. Reapply in 5 to 7 days.

PEDS – Head lice: Apply shampoo, wash after 10 min. Reapply in 5 to 7 days.

FORMS – OTC Generic/Trade: Shampoo (0.33% pyrethrins, 4% piperonyl butoxide) 60, 120 mL.

NOTES – Use caution if allergic to ragweed. Avoid contact with mucous membranes.

BENZYL ALCOHOL (***Ulesfia***) ▶not absorbed – ♀B ▶? $$$$

ADULT – Head Lice: Apply to dry hair to saturate scalp and hair. Amount depends on hair length. Rinse after 10 minutes. Reapply in 7 days, if necessary.

PEDS – 6 mo or older: Apply to dry hair to saturate scalp and hair. Rinse after 10 minutes. Reapply in 7 days, if necessary.

FORMS – Lotion 5% 60 mL.

CROTAMITON (***Eurax***) ▶? ♀C ▶? $$

ADULT – Scabies: Massage cream/lotion into entire body from chin down, repeat 24 h later, bathe 48 h later. Pruritus: Massage into affected areas prn.

PEDS – Not approved in children.

UNAPPROVED PEDS – Scabies: Massage cream/lotion into entire body from chin down, repeat 24 h later, bathe 48 h later. Pruritus: Massage into affected areas prn.

FORMS – Trade only: Cream 10% 60 g. Lotion 10% 60, 480 mL.

NOTES – Patients with scabies should change bed linen and clothing in am after 2nd application and bathe 48 h after last application. Consider treating entire family if treating scabies.

LINDANE ▶L ♀B ▶? $

WARNING – For use only in patients who have failed other agents. Seizures and deaths have been reported with repeat or prolonged use. Use caution with infants, children, elderly, those who weigh less than 50 kg. Contraindicated in premature infants and patients with uncontrolled seizures.

ADULT – Head/crab lice: Lotion: Apply 30 to 60 mL to affected area, wash off after 12 h. Shampoo: Apply 30 to 60 mL, wash off after 4 min. Scabies (lotion): Apply 30 to 60 mL to total body from neck down, wash off after 8 to 12 h.

PEDS – Lindane penetrates human skin and has potential for CNS toxicity. Studies indicate potential toxic effects of topical lindane are greater in young. Maximum dose for age younger than 6 yo is 30 mL.

FORMS – Generic only: Lotion 1% 60, 480 mL. Shampoo 1% 60, 480 mL.

NOTES – For lice, reapply if living lice noted after 7 days. After shampooing, comb with fine-tooth comb to remove nits. Consider treating entire family if treating scabies.

MALATHION (***Ovide***) ▶? ♀B ▶? $$$$

ADULT – Head lice: Apply to dry hair, let dry naturally, wash off in 8 to 12 h.

PEDS – Head lice in children: Apply to dry hair, let dry naturally, wash off in 8 to 12 h for 6 yo or older.

FORMS – Generic/Trade only: Lotion 0.5% 59 mL.

NOTES – Do not use hair dryer; flammable. Avoid contact with eyes. Use a fine-tooth comb to remove nits and dead lice. Application may be repeated in 7 to 9 days.

PERMETHRIN (***Elimite, Acticin, Nix, ✤ Kwellada-P***) ▶L ♀B ▶? $$

ADULT – Scabies (cream): Massage cream into entire body (avoid mouth, eyes, nose), wash off after 8 to 14 h. 30 g is typical adult dose. Head lice (liquid): Apply to clean, towel-dried hair, saturate hair and scalp, wash off after 10 min.

PEDS – Scabies (cream) age older than 2 mo: Massage cream into entire body (avoid mouth, eyes, nose), wash off after 8 to 14 h. Head lice (liquid) in age older than 2 yo: Saturate hair and scalp, wash off after 10 min.

FORMS – Generic/Trade: Cream (Elimite, Acticin) 5% 60 g. OTC Generic/Trade: Liquid creme rinse (Nix) 1% 60 mL.

NOTES – If necessary, may repeat application in 7 days. Consider treating entire family if treating scabies.

RID **(pyrethrins + piperonyl butoxide)** ▶L ♀C ▶? $

ADULT – Head Lice: Apply shampoo/mousse, wash after 10 min. Reapply in 5 to 10 days prn.

PEDS – Head Lice: Apply shampoo/mousse, wash after 10 min. Reapply in 5 to 10 days prn.

FORMS – OTC Generic/Trade: Shampoo 60, 120, 240 mL. OTC Trade only: Mousse 5.5 oz.

NOTES – Use caution if allergic to ragweed. Avoid contact with mucus membranes. Available alone or as part of a RID 1-2-3 kit containing shampoo, egg, and nit comb-out gel and home lice control spray for nonwashable items.

SKLICE (***ivermectin***) ▶minimal absorption - ♀C ▶? $$$$

ADULT – Head Lice: Apply to dry hair. Rinse after 10 min. Second application not necessary.

PEDS – Not approved in children younger than 6 mo. In children 6 mo and older, use adult dosing.

FORMS – Trade: Lotion 0.5%, 120 mL.

SPINOSAD (***Natroba***) ▶not absorbed – ♀B ▶? $$$$$

ADULT – Head Lice: Apply to dry hair/scalp to cover. Leave on 10 min then rinse. Retreat if live lice seen after 7 days.

PEDS – 4 yo and older: Head Lice: Apply to dry hair/scalp to cover. Leave on 10 min then rinse. Retreat if live lice seen after 7 days.

FORMS – Topical susp, 0.9%, 120 mL.

DERMATOLOGY: Antipsoriatics

ACITRETIN (***Soriatane***) ▶L ♀X ▶– $$$$$

WARNING – Contraindicated in pregnancy and avoid pregnancy for 3 years following medication discontinuation. Major human fetal abnormalities have been reported. Females of child-bearing age must avoid alcohol while on medication and for 2 months following therapy since alcohol prolongs elimination of a teratogenic metabolite. Use in reliable females of reproductive potential only if they have severe, unresponsive psoriasis, have received written and oral warnings of the teratogenic potential, are using 2 reliable forms of contraception, and have 2 negative pregnancy tests within 1 week prior to starting therapy. Contraception should start at least 1 month prior to therapy and continue for 3 years following discontinuation. Must have negative monthly pregnancy test during treatment. Therefore, prescribe limited amount and do not allow refill until documented negative pregnancy test. Following discontinuation, repeat pregnancy test q 3 months. It is unknown whether residual acitretin in seminal fluid poses a risk to the fetus while a male patient is taking the drug or after it is discontinued.

ADULT – Severe psoriasis: Initiate at 25 to 50 mg PO daily.

PEDS – Not approved in children.

UNAPPROVED ADULT – Lichen planus: 30 mg/day PO for 4 weeks, then titrate to 10 to 50 mg/day for 12 weeks total. Sjögren-Larsson syndrome: 0.47 mg/kg/day PO. Also used in Darier's disease, palmoplantar pustulosis, nonbullous and bullous ichthyosiform erythroderma, lichen sclerosus et atrophicus of the vulva, palmoplantar lichen nitidus, and chemoprevention for high-risk immunosuppressed patients with history of squamous cell carcinomas of the skin.

UNAPPROVED PEDS – Has been used in children with lamellar ichthyosis. Pediatric use is not recommended. Adverse effects on bone growth are suspected.

FORMS – Trade only: Caps 10, 25 mg.

NOTES – Transient worsening of psoriasis may occur, and full benefit may take 2 to 3 months. Elevated LFTs may occur in one-third of patients; monitor LFTs at 1- to 2-week intervals until stable and then periodically thereafter. Monitor serum lipid concentrations q 1 to 2 weeks until response to drug is established. May decrease tolerance to contact lenses due to dry eyes. Avoid prolonged exposure to sunlight. May cause hair loss. May cause depression. May cause bone changes, especially with use more than 6 months. Many adverse drug reactions.

ALEFACEPT (***Amevive***) ▶? ♀B ▶? $$$$$

ADULT – Moderate to severe psoriasis: 7.5 mg IV or 15 mg IM once a week for 12 doses. May repeat with 1 additional 12 weeks course after 12 weeks have elapsed from last dose.

PEDS – Not approved in children.

NOTES – Monitor CD4+ T lymphocyte cells weekly; withhold therapy if count less than 250/mcL and stop altogether if less than 250/mcL for 1 month. Do not give to HIV-positive patients or with other immunosuppressive or phototherapy.

ANTHRALIN (***Drithocreme***) ▶? ♀C ▶– $$$

ADULT – Chronic psoriasis: Apply daily.

(cont.)

ANTHRALIN (*cont.*)

PEDS – Not approved in children.
UNAPPROVED PEDS – Chronic psoriasis: Apply daily.
FORMS – Trade only: Cream 0.5, 1% 50 g.
NOTES – Short contact periods (ie, 15 to 20 min) followed by removal with an appropriate solvent (soap or petrolatum) may be preferred. May stain fabric, skin, or hair.

CALCIPOTRIENE (***Dovonex, Sorilux***) ▸L ♀C ▸? $$$$

ADULT – Moderate plaque psoriasis: Apply two times per day.
PEDS – Not approved in children.
UNAPPROVED ADULT – Has been used for vitiligo.
UNAPPROVED PEDS – Moderate plaque psoriasis: Apply two times per day. Has been used for vitiligo.
FORMS – Trade only: Ointment 0.005% 30, 60, 100 g (Dovonex). Cream 0.005% 30, 60, 100 g (Dovonex). Foam 0.005%60, 120 g (Sorilux). Generic/Trade: Scalp soln 0.005% 60 mL.
NOTES – Avoid contact with face. Do not exceed 100 g/week to minimize risk of hypercalcemia, hypercalciuria. Burning, itching, and skin irritation may occur in 10 to 15% of patients.

METHOXSALEN (***8-MOP, Oxsoralen-Ultra***) ▸Skin ♀C ▸? $$$$$

WARNING – Should only be perscribed by physicians who have special training. For the treatment of patients with psoriasis, restrict to severe cases. Possibility of ocular damage, aging of the skin, and skin cancer (including melanoma).
ADULT – Psoriasis: Dose based on wt (0.4 mg/kg/dose), 1½ to 2 h before ultraviolet light exposure.
PEDS – Not approved in children.
FORMS – Soft gelatin cap 10 mg (Oxsoralen-Ultra). Hard gelatin cap 10 mg (8-MOP).
NOTES – Oxsoralen-Ultra (soft gelatin cap) cannot be interchanged with 8-MOP (hard gelatin cap) due to significant bioavailability differences and photosensitization onset times. Take with food or milk. Wear ultraviolet light–blocking glasses and avoid sun exposure after ingestion and for remainder of day.

TACLONEX **(calcipotriene + betamethasone,** ✤ ***Dovobet, Xamiol***) ▸L ♀C ▸? $$$$$

ADULT – Psoriasis: Apply daily for up to 4 weeks.
PEDS – Not approved in children.
FORMS – Calcipotriene 0.005% + betamethasone dipropionate. Trade only: Ointment 15, 30, 60, 100 g. Topical susp 15, 30, 60 g.
NOTES – Do not exceed 100 g/week. Do not use on more than 30% of body surface area. Do not apply to face, groin, or axillae.

USTEKINUMAB (***Stelara***) ▸L– ♀B ▸? $$$$$

WARNING – Can cause serious infections. Discontinue if serious infection. Caution if high risk of malignancy. Theoretical risk of infection from *Mycobacterium, Salmonella,* and BCG vaccine. Evaluate patients for TB prior to therapy. Risk of reversible posterior leukoencephalopathy syndrome.
ADULT – Severe plaque psoriasis: Less than 100 kg/45 mg initially and 4 weeks later, followed by 45 mg q 12 weeks. Greater than 100 kg/90 mg initially and 4 weeks later, followed by 90 mg q 12 weeks.
PEDS – Not approved in children.
FORMS – Trade only: 45 and 90 mg prefilled syringe and vial.

DERMATOLOGY: Antivirals (Topical)

ACYCLOVIR—TOPICAL (***Zovirax***) ▸K ♀C ▸? $$$$$

ADULT – Initial episodes of herpes genitalis: Apply ointment q 3 h (6 times per day) for 7 days. Non-life-threatening mucocutaneous herpes simplex in immunocompromised patients: Apply ointment q 3 h (6 times per day) for 7 days. Recurrent herpes labialis: Apply cream 5 times per day for 4 days.
PEDS – Recurrent herpes labialis: Apply cream 5 times per day for 4 days for age 12 yo or older.
UNAPPROVED PEDS – Initial episodes of herpes genitalis: Apply ointment q 3 h (6 times per day) for 7 days. Non-life-threatening mucocutaneous herpes simplex in immunocompromised patients: Apply ointment q 3 h (6 times per day) for 7 days.
FORMS – Trade only: Ointment 5% 15 g. Cream 5% 2, 5 g.
NOTES – Use finger cot or rubber glove to apply ointment to avoid dissemination. Burning/stinging may occur in up to 28% of patients. Oral form more effective than topical for herpes genitalis.

DOCOSANOL (***Abreva***) ▸Not absorbed ♀B ▸? $

ADULT – Oral-facial herpes (cold sores): Apply 5 times per day until healed.
PEDS – Oral-facial herpes (cold sores): Use adult dose for age 12 yo or older.
FORMS – OTC Trade only: Cream 10% 2 g.

IMIQUIMOD (*Aldara, Zyclara, ✤ Vyloma*) ▶Not absorbed ♀C ▶? $$$$$
ADULT – External genital and perianal warts, 3.75% cream: Apply 3 times a week at bedtime for up to 16 weeks. Wash off after 8 h. Non-hyperkeratotic, non-hypertrophic actinic keratoses on face/scalp in immunocompetent adults, 2.5% or 3.75% cream: Apply to face or scalp (but not both) twice a week for up to 16 weeks (Aldara) or once daily for two 2-week periods separated by a 2-week break (Zyclara). Wash off after 8 h. Primary superficial basal cell carcinoma: Apply 5 times per week for 6 weeks (Aldara). Wash off after 8 h.
PEDS – External genital and perianal warts: Apply 3 times per week at bedtime and wash off after 6 to 10 h for age 12 yo or older (Aldara) or once daily for two 2-week periods separated by a 2-week break (Zyclara).
UNAPPROVED ADULT – Molluscum contagiosum: Apply 3 times per week for 6 to 10 h.
UNAPPROVED PEDS – Molluscum contagiosum.
FORMS – Generic/Trade: Cream 5% (Aldara) single-use packets, 3.75% (Zyclara) 7.5 g and 15 g pump, 2.5% 7.5 g and 15 g pump.
NOTES – May weaken condoms and diaphragms. Avoid sexual contact while cream is on when used for genital/perianal warts. Most common adverse effects include erythema, itching, erosion, burning, excoriation, edema, and pain. Discard partially used packets.

PENCICLOVIR (*Denavir*) ▶Not absorbed ♀B ▶? $$
ADULT – Recurrent herpes labialis (cold sores): Apply q 2 h while awake for 4 days.
PEDS – Not approved in children.
UNAPPROVED PEDS – Recurrent herpes labialis: Apply q 2 h while awake for 4 days.
FORMS – Trade only: Cream 1% tube 1.5 g.
NOTES – Start therapy as soon as possible during prodrome. For moderate to severe cases of herpes labialis, systemic treatment with famciclovir or acyclovir may be preferred.

PODOFILOX (*Condylox, ✤ Condyline, Wartec*) ▶? ♀C ▶? $$$$
ADULT – External genital warts (gel and soln) and perianal warts (gel only): Apply two times per day for 3 consecutive days of a week and repeat for up to 4 weeks.
PEDS – Not approved in children.
FORMS – Generic/Trade: Soln 0.5% 3.5 mL. Trade only: Gel 0.5% 3.5 g.

PODOPHYLLIN (*Podocon-25, Podofin, Podofilm*) ▶? ♀– ▶– $$$
ADULT – Genital wart removal: Initial application: Apply to wart and leave on for 30 to 40 min to determine patient's sensitivity. Thereafter, use minimum contact time necessary (1 to 4 h depending on result). Remove dried podophyllin with alcohol or soap and water.
PEDS – Not approved in children.
FORMS – Not to be dispensed to patients. For hospital/clinic use; not intended for outpatient prescribing. Trade only: Liquid 25% 15 mL.
NOTES – Not to be dispensed to patients. Do not treat large areas or numerous warts all at once. Contraindicated in diabetics, pregnancy, patients using steroids or with poor circulation, and on bleeding warts.

SINECATECHINS (*Veregen*) ▶Unknown ♀C ▶? $$$$$
ADULT – Apply three times per day to external genital warts for up to 16 weeks.
PEDS – Not approved in children.
FORMS – Trade only: Ointment 15% 15, 30 g.
NOTES – Botanical drug product. Contains a partially purified fraction of the water extract of green tea leaves. Do not use on open wounds. Do not use in immunocompromised patients. Generic name used to be kunecatechins.

DERMATOLOGY: Atopic Dermatitis Preparations

NOTE: Potential risk of cancer. Should only be used as second-line agent for short-term and intermittent treatment of atopic dermatitis in those unresponsive to or intolerant of other treatments. Long-term safety has not been established. Avoid use in immunocompromised patients and in children younger than 2 yo. Use minimum amount to control symptoms.

PIMECROLIMUS (*Elidel*) ▶L ♀C ▶? $$$$
ADULT – Atopic dermatitis: Apply two times per day.
PEDS – Atopic dermatitis: Apply two times per day for age 2 yo or older.
FORMS – Trade only: Cream 1% 30, 60, 100 g.
NOTES – Long-term safety unclear.

TACROLIMUS—TOPICAL (*Protopic*) ▶Minimal absorption ♀C ▶? $$$$$
ADULT – Atopic dermatitis: Apply two times per day.

(cont.)

TACROLIMUS—TOPICAL (*cont.*)

PEDS – Atopic dermatitis: Apply 0.03% ointment two times per day for age 2 to 15 yo.

UNAPPROVED ADULT – Vitiligo: Apply 0.1% two times per day. Chronic allergic contact dermatitis (ie, nickel-induced): Apply 0.1% ointment two times per day.

FORMS – Trade only: Ointment 0.03%, 0.1% 30, 60, 100 g.

NOTES – Do not use with an occlusive dressing. Continue treatment for 1 week after clearing of symptoms.

DERMATOLOGY: Corticosteroid/Antimicrobial Combinations

CORTISPORIN **(neomycin + polymyxin + hydrocortisone)** ▶LK ♀C ▶? $$$

ADULT – Corticosteroid-responsive dermatoses with secondary infection: Apply two to four times per day.

PEDS – Not approved in children.

UNAPPROVED PEDS – Corticosteroid-responsive dermatoses with secondary infection: Apply two to four times per day.

FORMS – Trade only: Cream 7.5 g. Ointment 15 g.

NOTES – Due to concerns about nephrotoxicity and ototoxicity associated with neomycin, do not use over wide areas or for prolonged periods of time.

♣ ***FUCIDIN H*** **(fusidic acid + hydrocortisone)** ▶L ♀? ▶? $$

ADULT – Canada only. Atopic dermatitis: Apply three times per day.

PEDS – Canada only. Atopic dermatitis: Apply three times per day for age 3 yo or older.

FORMS – Canada Trade only: Cream (2% fusidic acid, 1% hydrocortisone acetate) 30 g.

♣ ***LOCACORTEN VIOFORM*** **(flumethasone + clioquinol)** ▶? ♀? ▶? $$

ADULT – Canada only. Skin: Apply two to three times per day. Otic gtts: 2 to 3 gtts two times per day.

PEDS – Canada only. Skin: Apply two to three times per day for age 2 yo or older. Otic gtts: 2 to 3 gtts two times per day.

FORMS – Canada trade only: Cream 0.02% flumethasone, 3% clioquinol 15, 50 g. Otic gtts 0.02% flumethasone, 1% clioquinol, 10 mL.

NOTES – May stain clothing.

LOTRISONE **(clotrimazole + betamethasone,** ♣ ***Lotriderm*****)** ▶L ♀C ▶? $$$

ADULT – Tinea pedis, cruris, and corporis: Apply two times per day.

PEDS – Not approved in children.

FORMS – Generic/Trade: Cream (clotrimazole 1% + betamethasone 0.05%) 15, 45 g. Lotion (clotrimazole 1% + betamethasone 0.05%) 30 mL.

NOTES – Treat tinea cruris and corporis for 2 weeks and tinea pedis for 4 weeks. Do not use for diaper dermatitis.

MYCOLOG II **(nystatin + triamcinolone)** ▶L ♀C ▶? $

ADULT – Cutaneous candidiasis: Apply two times per day.

PEDS – Not approved in children.

UNAPPROVED PEDS – Sometimes used for diaper dermatitis, but not recommended due to risk of adrenal suppression.

FORMS – Generic only: Cream, Ointment 15, 30, 60, 120, 454 g.

NOTES – Avoid occlusive dressings.

DERMATOLOGY: Corticosteroids (Topical)

NOTE: After long-term use, do not discontinue abruptly; switch to a less potent agent or alternate use of corticosteroids and emollient products. Monitor for hyperglycemia/adrenal suppression if used for long period of time or over a large area of the body, especially in children. Chronic administration may cause skin atrophy and interfere with pediatric growth and development.

ALCLOMETASONE DIPROPIONATE (***Aclovate***) ▶L ♀C ▶? $$

ADULT – Inflammatory and pruritic manifestations of corticosteroid-responsive dermatoses: Apply sparingly two to three times per day.

PEDS – Inflammatory and pruritic manifestations of corticosteroid-responsive dermatoses: Apply sparingly two to three times per day for age 1 yo or older. Safety and efficacy for more than 3 weeks have not been established.

FORMS – Generic/Trade: Ointment, Cream 0.05% 15, 45, 60 g.

AMCINONIDE (***Cyclocort***) ▶L ♀C ▶? $$

ADULT – Inflammatory and pruritic manifestations of corticosteroid-responsive dermatoses: Apply sparingly two to three times per day.

PEDS – Inflammatory and pruritic manifestations of corticosteroid-responsive dermatoses: Apply sparingly two to three times per day.

FORMS – Generic only: Cream, Ointment 0.1% 15, 30, 60 g. Lotion 0.1% 60 mL.

CORTICOSTEROIDS—TOPICAL

*Potency**	*Generic*	*Trade Name*	*Forms*	*Frequency*
Low	alclometasone dipropionate	Aclovate	0.05% C/O	bid–tid
Low	clocortolone pivalate	Cloderm	0.1% C	tid
Low	desonide	DesOwen, Tridesilon	0.05% C/L/O	bid–tid
Low	hydrocortisone	Hytone, others	0.5% C/L/O; 1% C/L/O; 2.5% C/L/O	bid-qid
Low	hydrocortisone acetate	Cortaid, Corticaine	0.5% C/O; 1% C/O/Sp	bid–qid
Medium	betamethasone valerate	Luxiq	0.1% C/L/O; 0.12% F (Luxiq)	daily–bid
Medium	desoximetasone‡	Topicort	0.05% C	bid
Medium	fluocinolone	Synalar	0.01% C/S; 0.025% C/O	bid–qid
Medium	flurandrenolide	Cordran	0.025% C/O; 0.05% C/L/O/T	bid–qid
Medium	fluticasone propionate	Cutivate	0.005% O; 0.05% C/L	daily–bid
Medium	hydrocortisone butyrate	Locoid	0.1% C/O/S	bid–tid
Medium	hydrocortisone valerate	Westcort	0.2% C/O	bid–tid
Medium	mometasone furoate	Elocon	0.1% C/L/O	daily
Medium	triamcinolone‡	Aristocort, Kenalog	0.025% C/L/O; 0.1% C/L/O/S	bid–tid
High	amcinonide	Cyclocort	0.1% C/L/O	bid–tid
High	betamethasone dipropionate‡	Maxivate, others	0.05% C/L/O (non-Diprolene)	daily–bid
High	desoximetasone‡	Topicort	0.05% G; 0.25% C/O	bid
High	diflorasone diacetate‡	Maxiflor	0.05% C/O	bid
High	fluocinonide	Lidex	0.05% C/G/O/S	bid–qid
High	halcinonide	Halog	0.1% C/O/S	bid–tid
High	triamcinolone‡	Aristocort, Kenalog	0.5% C/O	bid–tid
Very high	betamethasone dipropionate‡	Diprolene, Diprolene AF	0.05% C/G/L/O	daily–bid
Very high	clobetasol	Temovate, Cormax, Olux	0.05% C/G/O/L/S/Sp/F (Olux)	bid
Very high	diflorasone diacetate‡	Psorcon	0.05% C/O	daily-tid
Very high	halobetasol propionate	Ultravate	0.05% C/O	daily-bid

bid=two times per day; tid=three times per day; qid=four times per day.
*Potency based on vasoconstrictive assays, which may not correlate with efficacy. Not all available products are listed, including those lacking potency ratings.
‡These drugs have formulations in more than once potency category.
C, cream; O, ointment; L, lotion; T, tape; F, foam; S, solution; G, gel; Sp, spray.

AUGMENTED BETAMETHASONE DIPROPIONATE (***Diprolene, Diprolene AF,*** ✤ ***Topilene Glycol***) ▶L ♀C ▶? $$$

ADULT – Inflammatory and pruritic manifestations of corticosteroid-responsive dermatoses: Apply sparingly one to two times per day.

PEDS – Not approved younger than 12 yo.

FORMS – Generic/Trade: Diprolene: Ointment 0.05% 15, 50 g. Lotion 0.05% 30, 60 mL. Diprolene AF: Cream 0.05% 15, 50 g. Generic only: Gel 0.05% 15, 50 g.

NOTES – Do not use occlusive dressings. Do not use for longer than 2 consecutive weeks and do not exceed a total dose of 45 to 50 g per weeks or 50 mL per week of the lotion.

BETAMETHASONE DIPROPIONATE (*Diprosone, Maxivate, ♣ Propaderm, TARO-sone*) ▶L ♀C ▶? $

ADULT – Inflammatory and pruritic manifestations of corticosteroid-responsive dermatoses: Apply sparingly one to two times per day.

PEDS – Inflammatory and pruritic manifestations of corticosteroid-responsive dermatoses: Apply sparingly one to two times per day.

FORMS – Generic only: Ointment, Cream 0.05% 15, 45 g. Lotion 0.05% 30, 60 mL.

NOTES – Do not use occlusive dressings.

BETAMETHASONE VALERATE (*Luxiq foam, Beta-Val, ♣ Betaderm*) ▶L ♀C ▶? $

ADULT – Inflammatory and pruritic manifestations of corticosteroid-responsive dermatoses: Apply sparingly one to two times per day. Dermatoses of scalp: Apply small amount of foam to scalp two times per day.

PEDS – Inflammatory and pruritic manifestations of corticosteroid-responsive dermatoses: Apply sparingly one to two times per day.

FORMS – Generic only: Ointment, Cream 0.1% 15, 45 g. Lotion 0.1% 60 mL. Trade only: Foam (Luxiq) 0.12% 50, 100, 150 g.

CLOBETASOL (*Temovate, Olux, Clobex, Cormax, ♣ Dermasone*) ▶L ♀C ▶? $$

ADULT – Inflammatory and pruritic manifestations of corticosteroid-responsive dermatoses: Apply sparingly two times per day. For scalp apply foam two times per day.

PEDS – Not approved in children.

FORMS – Generic/Trade: Cream, Ointment 0.05% 15, 30, 45, 60 g. Scalp application 0.05% 25, 50 mL. Gel 0.05% 15, 30, 60 g. Foam (Olux) 0.05% 50, 100 g. Lotion (Clobex) 0.05% 30, 60, 120 mL. Trade only (Clobex): Spray 0.05% 60, 125 mL. Shampoo 0.05% 118 mL.

NOTES – Adrenal suppression at doses as low as 2 g per day. Do not use occlusive dressings. Do not use for longer than 2 consecutive weeks and do not exceed a total dose of 50 g per week.

CLOCORTOLONE PIVALATE (*Cloderm*) ▶L ♀C ▶? $$$

ADULT – Inflammatory and pruritic manifestations of corticosteroid-responsive dermatoses: Apply sparingly three times per day.

PEDS – Inflammatory and pruritic manifestations of corticosteroid-responsive dermatoses: Apply sparingly three times per day.

FORMS – Trade only: Cream 0.1% 30, 45, 75, 90 g.

DESONIDE (*DesOwen, Desonate, Tridesilon, Verdeso*) ▶L ♀C ▶? $$

ADULT – Inflammatory and pruritic manifestations of corticosteroid-responsive dermatoses: Apply sparingly two to three times per day.

PEDS – Inflammatory and pruritic manifestations of corticosteroid-responsive dermatoses: Apply sparingly two to three times per day.

FORMS – Generic/Trade: Cream, Ointment 0.05%, 15, 60 g. Lotion 0.05%, 60, 120 mL. Trade only: Gel (Desonate) 0.05% 60 g, Foam (Verdeso) 0.05%, 50, 100 g.

NOTES – Do not use with occlusive dressings.

DESOXIMETASONE (*Topicort, Topicort LP, ♣ Desoxi*) ▶L ♀C ▶? $$$

ADULT – Inflammatory and pruritic manifestations of corticosteroid-responsive dermatoses: Apply sparingly two times per day.

PEDS – Safety and efficacy have not been established for Topicort 0.25% ointment. Inflammatory and pruritic manifestations of corticosteroid-responsive dermatoses (cream and gel): Apply sparingly two times per day.

FORMS – Generic/Trade: Cream, Gel 0.05% 15, 60 g. Cream, Ointment 0.25% 15, 60, 100 g.

DIFLORASONE (*Psorcon E, Maxiflor*) ▶L ♀C ▶? $$$

ADULT – Inflammatory and pruritic manifestations of corticosteroid-responsive dermatoses: Apply sparingly one to three times per day.

PEDS – Not approved in children.

FORMS – Generic/Trade: Cream, Ointment 0.05% 15, 30, 60 g.

NOTES – Doses of 30 g/day of diflorasone 0.05% cream for 1 week resulted in adrenal suppression in some psoriasis patients.

FLUOCINOLONE (*Synalar, Capex, Derma-Smoothe/FS, ♣ Caprex*) ▶L ♀C ▶? $

ADULT – Inflammatory and pruritic manifestations of corticosteroid-responsive dermatoses: Apply sparingly two to three times per day. Psoriasis of the scalp (Derma-Smoothe/FS): Massage into scalp, cover with shower cap and leave on 4 h or longer or overnight and then wash off.

PEDS – Inflammatory and pruritic manifestations of corticosteroid-responsive dermatoses: Apply sparingly two to four times per day. Atopic dermatitis: Moisten skin and apply to affected areas two times per day for up to 4 weeks (Derma-Smoothe/FS).

FORMS – Generic/Trade: Cream, Ointment 0.025% 15, 30, 60 g. Soln 0.01% 20, 60 mL. Generic only: Cream 0.01% 15, 60 g. Trade only (Derma-Smoothe/FS): Topical oil 0.01% 120 mL. (Capex) Shampoo 0.01% 120 mL.

FLUOCINONIDE (*Lidex, Lidex-E, Vanos, ♣ Lidemol, Topsyn, Tiamol*) ▶L ♀C ▶? $$

ADULT – Inflammatory and pruritic manifestations of corticosteroid-responsive dermatoses: Apply sparingly two to four times per day. Plaque-type psoriasis: Apply 0.1% cream

(cont.)

FLUOCINONIDE (*cont.*)

(Vanos) one to two times per day for 2 consecutive weeks only; no more than 60 g per week. Atopic dermatitis: Apply 0.1% cream (Vanos) once a day.

PEDS – Inflammatory and pruritic manifestations of corticosteroid-responsive dermatoses: Apply sparingly two to four times per day.

FORMS – Generic/Trade: Cream, Ointment, Gel 0.05% 15, 30, 60 g. Soln 0.05% 20, 60 mL. Trade only: Cream 0.1% 30, 60, 120 g (Vanos).

FLURANDRENOLIDE (***Cordran, Cordran SP***) ▶L ♀C ▶? $$$

ADULT – Inflammatory and pruritic manifestations of corticosteroid-responsive dermatoses: Apply sparingly two to three times per day.

PEDS – Inflammatory and pruritic manifestations of corticosteroid-responsive dermatoses: Apply sparingly two to three times per day.

FORMS – Trade only: Ointment, Cream 0.05% 15, 30, 60 g. Lotion 0.05% 15, 60 mL. Tape 4 mcg/cm^2.

FLUTICASONE—TOPICAL (***Cutivate, ✤ Flixonase, Flixotide***) ▶L ♀C ▶? $$

ADULT – Eczema: Apply sparingly one to two times per day. Other inflammatory and pruritic manifestations of corticosteroid-responsive dermatoses: Apply sparingly two times per day.

PEDS – Children older than 3 mo: Eczema: Apply sparingly one to two times per day. Other inflammatory and pruritic manifestations of corticosteroid-responsive dermatoses: Apply sparingly two times per day.

FORMS – Generic/Trade: Cream 0.05% 15, 30, 60 g. Ointment 0.005% 15, 30, 60 g. Trade only: Lotion 0.05% 120 mL.

NOTES – Do not use with an occlusive dressing.

HALCINONIDE (***Halog***) ▶L ♀C ▶? $$

ADULT – Inflammatory and pruritic manifestations of corticosteroid-responsive dermatoses: Apply sparingly two to three times per day.

PEDS – Inflammatory and pruritic manifestations of corticosteroid-responsive dermatoses: Apply sparingly two to three times per day.

FORMS – Trade only: Cream, Ointment 0.1% 15, 30, 60 g. Soln 0.1% 20, 60 mL.

HALOBETASOL PROPIONATE (***Ultravate***) ▶L ♀C ▶? $$

ADULT – Inflammatory and pruritic manifestations of corticosteroid-responsive dermatoses: Apply sparingly one to two times per day.

PEDS – Not approved in children.

FORMS – Generic/Trade: Cream, Ointment 0.05% 15, 50 g.

NOTES – Do not use occlusive dressings. Do not use for more than 2 consecutive weeks and do not exceed a total dose of 50 g/week.

HYDROCORTISONE ACETATE (***Cortaid, Corticaine, Cortifoam, Micort-HC Lipocream, ✤ Hyderm, Cortamed***) ▶L ♀C ▶? $

ADULT – Inflammatory and pruritic manifestations of corticosteroid-responsive dermatoses: Apply sparingly two to four times per day.

PEDS – Inflammatory and pruritic manifestations of corticosteroid-responsive dermatoses: Apply sparingly two to four times per day.

FORMS – OTC Generic/Trade: Ointment 0.5% 15 g. Ointment 1% 15, 30 g. Cream 0.5% 15 g. Cream 1% 15, 30, 60 g. Topical spray 1% 60 mL. Rx Trade only: Cream 2.5% 30 g (Micort-HC Lipocream). Rectal foam 15 g (Cortifoam).

HYDROCORTISONE BUTYRATE (***Locoid, Locoid Lipocream***) ▶L ♀C ▶? $$

ADULT – Inflammatory and pruritic manifestations of corticosteroid-responsive dermatoses: Apply sparingly two to three times per day. Seborrheic dermatitis (soln only): Apply two to three times per day.

PEDS – Inflammatory and pruritic manifestations of corticosteroid-responsive dermatoses: Apply sparingly two to three times per day. Seborrheic dermatitis (soln only): Apply two to three times per day.

FORMS – Generic/Trade: Cream, Ointment 0.1% 15, 45 g. Soln 0.1% 20, 60 mL. Trade only: Cream 0.1% (Lipocream) 15, 45, 60 g.

HYDROCORTISONE PROBUTATE (***Pandel***) ▶L ♀C ▶? $$

ADULT – Inflammatory and pruritic manifestations of corticosteroid-responsive dermatoses: Apply sparingly one to two times per day.

PEDS – Not approved in children.

FORMS – Trade only: Cream 0.1% 15, 45, 80 g.

HYDROCORTISONE VALERATE (***Westcort, ✤ Hydroval***) ▶L ♀C ▶? $$

ADULT – Inflammatory and pruritic manifestations of corticosteroid-responsive dermatoses: Apply sparingly two to three times per day.

PEDS – Safety and efficacy of Westcort ointment have not been established in children. Inflammatory and pruritic manifestations of corticosteroid-responsive dermatoses (cream only): Apply sparingly two to three times per day.

FORMS – Generic/Trade: Cream, Ointment 0.2% 15, 45, 60 g.

HYDROCORTISONE—TOPICAL (***Cortizone, Hycort, Hytone, Tegrin-HC, Dermolate, Synacort, Anusol-HC, Proctocream HC, ✤ Cortoderm, Prevex-HC, Cortate, Emo-Cort***) ▶L ♀C ▶? $

(cont.)

HYDROCORTISONE—TOPICAL (*cont.*)

ADULT – Inflammatory and pruritic manifestations of corticosteroid-responsive dermatoses: Apply sparingly two to four times per day. External anal itching: Apply cream three to four times per day prn or suppository two times per day or rectal foam one to two times per day.

PEDS – Inflammatory and pruritic manifestations of corticosteroid-responsive dermatoses: Apply sparingly two to four times per day.

FORMS – Products available OTC and Rx depending on labeling. 2.5% preparation available Rx only. Generic/Trade: Ointment 0.5% 30 g. Ointment 1% 15, 20, 30, 60, 454 g. Ointment 2.5% 5, 20, 30, 454 g. Cream 0.5% 30 g. Cream 1% 5, 15, 20, 30, 120 g. Cream 2.5% 5, 20, 30, 454 g. Lotion 1% 120 mL. Lotion 2.5% 60 mL. Anal preparations: Generic/Trade: Cream 2.5% 30 g (Anusol HC, Proctocream HC). Suppositories 25 mg (Anusol HC).

MOMETASONE—TOPICAL (***Elocon,*** ✤ ***Elocom***) ▸L ♀C ▸? $

ADULT – Inflammatory and pruritic manifestations of corticosteroid-responsive dermatoses: Apply sparingly once a day.

PEDS – Inflammatory and pruritic manifestations of corticosteroid-responsive dermatoses: Apply sparingly once a day for age 2 yo or older. Safety and efficacy for more than 3 weeks have not been established.

FORMS – Generic/Trade: Cream, Ointment 0.1% 15, 45 g. Lotion 0.1% 30, 60 mL.

NOTES – Do not use an occlusive dressing. Not for ophthalmic use.

PREDNICARBATE (***Dermatop***) ▸L ♀C ▸? $$

ADULT – Inflammatory and pruritic manifestations of corticosteroid-responsive dermatoses: Apply sparingly two times per day.

PEDS – Inflammatory and pruritic manifestations of corticosteroid-responsive dermatoses: Apply sparingly two times per day for age 1 yo or older. Safety and efficacy for more than 3 weeks have not been established.

FORMS – Generic/Trade: Cream, Ointment 0.1% 15, 60 g.

NOTES – Can damage latex (condoms, diaphragms, etc.). Avoid contact with latex.

TRIAMCINOLONE—TOPICAL (***Kenalog, Kenalog in Orabase,*** ✤ ***Oracort, Triaderm***) ▸L ♀C ▸? $

ADULT – Inflammatory and pruritic manifestations of corticosteroid-responsive dermatoses: Apply sparingly three to four times per day. Oral paste: Aphthous ulcers: Using finger, apply about 1 cm of paste to oral lesion and a thin film will develop. Apply paste two to three times per day, ideally after meals and at bedtime.

PEDS – Inflammatory and pruritic manifestations of corticosteroid-responsive dermatoses: Apply sparingly three to four times per day.

FORMS – Generic/Trade: Cream, Ointment 0.1% 15, 60, 80 g. Cream 0.5% 20 g. Lotion 0.025% and 0.1% 60 mL. Oral paste (in Orabase) 0.1% 5 g. Generic only: Cream, Ointment 0.025% 15, 80 g. Cream, Ointment 0.5% 15 g. Trade only: Aerosol topical spray 0.147 mg/g, 63 g.

DERMATOLOGY: Hemorrhoid Care

DIBUCAINE (***Nupercainal***) ▸L ♀? ▸? $

ADULT – Hemorrhoids or other anorectal disorders: Apply three to four times per day prn.

PEDS – Not approved in children.

UNAPPROVED PEDS – Hemorrhoids or other anorectal disorders: Apply three to four times per day prn for age older than 2 yo or wt greater than 35 lbs or 15.9 kg.

FORMS – OTC Trade only: Ointment 1% 30, 60 g.

NOTES – Do not use if younger than 2 yo or wt less than 35 pounds.

HYDROCORTISONE + PRAMOXINE—TOPICAL (***Analpram-HC, Epifoam, Proctofoam HC***) ▸L ♀C ▸? $$$

ADULT – Inflammatory and pruritic manifestations of corticosteroid-responsive dermatoses of the anal region: Apply two to four times per day.

PEDS – Use with caution. Inflammatory and pruritic manifestations of corticosteroid-responsive dermatoses of the anal region: Apply two to four times per day.

FORMS – Trade only: Topical aerosol foam (Proctofoam HC, Epifoam 1% hydrocortisone + 1% pramoxine) 10 g. Cream (Analpram-HC 1% hydrocortisone + 1% pramoxine, 2.5% hydrocortisone + 1% pramoxine) 4 g, 30 g. Lotion (Analpram-HC 2.5% hydrocortisone + 1% pramoxine) 60 mL.

PRAMOXINE (***Tucks Hemorrhoidal Ointment, Fleet Pain Relief, ProctoFoam NS***) ▸Not absorbed ♀+ ▸+ $

ADULT – Hemorrhoids: Apply ointment, pads, or foam up to 5 times per day prn.

PEDS – Not approved in children.

FORMS – OTC Trade only: Ointment (Tucks Hemorrhoidal Ointment) 30 g. Pads (Fleet Pain

(cont.)

PRAMOXINE (*cont.*)

Relief) 100 each. Aerosol foam (ProctoFoam NS) 15 g.

STARCH (*Tucks Suppositories*) ▶Not absorbed ♀+ ▶+ $

ADULT – Hemorrhoids: 1 suppository PR up to 6 times per day prn or after each bowel movement.

PEDS – Not approved in children.

FORMS – OTC Trade only: Suppository (51% topical starch; vegetable oil, tocopheryl acetate) 12, 24 each.

WITCH HAZEL (*Tucks*) ▶? ♀+ ▶+ $

ADULT – Hemorrhoids: Apply to anus/perineum up to 6 times per day prn.

PEDS – Not approved in children.

FORMS – OTC Generic/Trade: Pads 50% 12, 40, 100 ea, generically available in various quantities.

DERMATOLOGY: Other Dermatologic Agents

ALITRETINOIN (*Panretin,* ✦ *Toctino*) ▶Not absorbed ♀D ▶– $$$$$

WARNING – May cause fetal harm if significant absorption were to occur. Women of child-bearing age should be advised to avoid becoming pregnant during treatment.

ADULT – Cutaneous lesions of AIDS-related Kaposi's sarcoma: Apply two to four times per day.

PEDS – Not approved in children.

FORMS – Trade only: Gel 0.1% 60 g.

ALUMINUM CHLORIDE (*Drysol, Certain Dri*) ▶K ♀? ▶? $

ADULT – Hyperhidrosis: Apply at bedtime. For maximum effect, cover area with plastic wrap held in place with tight shirt and wash area following morning. Once excessive sweating stopped, use once a week or twice a week.

PEDS – Not approved in children.

FORMS – Rx Trade only: Soln 20% 37.5 mL bottle, 35, 60 mL bottle with applicator. OTC Trade only (Certain Dri): Soln 12.5% 36 mL bottle.

NOTES – To prevent irritation, apply to dry area.

BECAPLERMIN (*Regranex*) ▶Minimal absorption ♀C ▶? $$$$$

WARNING – Increased rate of mortality due to malignancy in patients who used 3 or more tubes. Use with caution in patients with known malignancy.

ADULT – Diabetic neuropathic ulcers: Apply daily and cover with saline-moistened gauze for 12 h. Rinse after 12 h and cover with saline gauze without medication.

PEDS – Not approved in children.

FORMS – Trade only: Gel 0.01%, 2, 15 g.

NOTES – Length of gel to be applied calculated by size of wound (length × width × 0.6 = amount of gel in inches). If ulcer does not decrease by 30% in size by 10 weeks or complete healing has not occurred by 20 weeks, continued therapy should be reassessed. Ineffective for stasis ulcers and pressure ulcers. Increased cancer mortality in patients who use 3 or more tubes of the product.

CALAMINE ▶? ♀? ▶? $

ADULT – Itching due to poison ivy/oak/sumac, insect bites, or minor irritation: Apply up to three to four times per day prn.

PEDS – Itching due to poison ivy/oak/sumac, insect bites, or minor irritation: Apply up to three to four times per day prn for age older than 2 yo.

FORMS – OTC Generic only: Lotion 120, 240, 480 mL.

CAPSAICIN (*Zostrix, Zostrix-HP*) ▶? ♀? ▶? $

ADULT – Pain due to RA, OA, and neuralgias such as zoster or diabetic neuropathies: Apply to affected area up to three to four times per day.

PEDS – Children older than 2 yo: Pain due to RA, OA, and neuralgias such as zoster or diabetic neuropathies: Apply to affected area up to three to four times per day.

UNAPPROVED ADULT – Psoriasis and intractable pruritus, postmastectomy/postamputation neuromas (phantom limb pain), vulvar vestibulitis, apocrine chromhidrosis, and reflex sympathetic dystrophy.

FORMS – OTC Generic/Trade: Cream 0.025% 60 g, 0.075% (HP) 60 g. OTC Generic only: Lotion 0.025% 59 mL, 0.075% 59 mL.

NOTES – Burning occurs in 30% or more of patients but diminishes with continued use. Pain more commonly occurs when applied less than three to four times per day. Wash hands immediately after application.

CARMOL HC **(hydrocortisone acetate + urea)** ▶L ♀C ▶? $$

ADULT – Inflammatory and pruritic manifestations of corticosteroid-responsive dermatoses: Apply sparingly two to four times per day.

PEDS – Inflammatory and pruritic manifestations of corticosteroid-responsive dermatoses: Apply sparingly two to four times per day.

(cont.)

CARMOL HC (cont.)

FORMS – Generic/Trade: Hydrocortisone acetate 1% + urea 10% cream 85 g (Trade), 30 g (U-cort).

COAL TAR (***Polytar, Tegrin, Cutar, Tarsum***) ▶? ♀? ▶? $

ADULT – Dandruff, seborrheic dermatitis: Apply shampoo at least twice a week. Psoriasis: Apply to affected areas one to four times per day or use shampoo on affected areas.

PEDS – Children older than 2 yo: Dandruff, seborrheic dermatitis: Apply shampoo at least twice a week. Psoriasis: Apply to affected areas one to four times per day or use shampoo on affected areas.

FORMS – OTC Generic/Trade: Shampoo, cream, ointment, gel, lotion, liquid, oil, soap.

NOTES – May cause photosensitivity for up to 24 h after application.

DEET (***Off, Cutter, Repel, Ultrathon,* n-n-diethyl-m-toluamide**) ▶L ♀+ ▶+ $

ADULT – Mosquito repellant: 10% to 50% q 2 to 6 h. Higher concentration products do not work better, but have a longer duration of action.

PEDS – Up to 30% spray/lotion q 2 to 6 h for age 2 mo or older.

FORMS – OTC Generic/Trade: Spray, lotion, towelette 4.75% to 100%.

NOTES – Duration of action varies by concentration. For example, 23.8% DEET provides approximately 5 h of protection from mosquito bites, 20% DEET provides approximately 4 h of protection, 6.65% DEET provides approximately 2 h of protection, and 4.75% DEET provides approximately 1.5 h of protection. Apply sunscreen prior to application of DEET-containing products.

DOXEPIN—TOPICAL (***Zonalon***) ▶L ♀B ▶– $$$$

ADULT – Pruritus associated with atopic dermatitis, lichen simplex chronicus, eczematous dermatitis: Apply four times per day for up to 8 days.

PEDS – Not approved in children.

FORMS – Trade only: Cream 5% 30, 45 g.

NOTES – Risk of systemic toxicity increased if applied to more than 10% of body. Can cause contact dermatitis.

EFLORNITHINE (***Vaniqa***) ▶K ♀C ▶? $$$

ADULT – Reduction of facial hair: Apply to face two times per day at least 8 h apart.

PEDS – Not approved in children.

FORMS – Trade only: Cream 13.9% 30 g.

NOTES – Takes 4 to 8 weeks or more to see an effect.

EMLA (**prilocaine + lidocaine—topical**) ▶LK ♀B ▶? $$

ADULT – Topical anesthesia for minor dermal procedures (eg, IV cannulation, venipuncture): Apply 2.5 g over 20 to 25 cm^2 area or 1 disc at least 1 h prior to procedure, for major dermal procedures (ie, skin grafting harvesting) apply 2 g/10 cm^2 area at least 2 h prior to procedure.

PEDS – Prior to circumcision in infants older than 37 weeks gestation: Apply a max 1 g dose over max of 10 cm^2. Topical anesthesia: Children age 1 to 3 mo or less than 5 kg: Apply a max 1 g dose over max of 10 cm^2; age 4 to 12 mo and more than 5 kg: Apply max 2 g dose over a max of 20 cm^2; age 1 to 6 yo and more than 10 kg: Apply max 10 g dose over max of 100 cm^2; age 7 to 12 yo and more than 20 kg: Apply max 20 g dose over max of 200 cm^2.

FORMS – Generic/Trade: Cream (2.5% lidocaine + 2.5% prilocaine) 5, 30 g.

NOTES – Cover cream with an occlusive dressing. Do not use in children younger than 12 mo if child is receiving treatment with methemoglobin-inducing agents. Do not use on open wounds. Patients with glucose-6-phosphate deficiencies are more susceptible to methemoglobinemia. Use caution with amiodarone, bretylium, sotalol, dofetilide; possible additive cardiac effects. Dermal analgesia increases for up to 3 h under occlusive dressings and persists for 1 to 2 h after removal.

HYALURONIC ACID (***Bionect, Restylane, Perlane***) ▶? ♀? ▶? $$$

ADULT – Moderate to severe facial wrinkles: Inject into wrinkle/fold (Restylane, Perlane). Protection of dermal ulcers: Apply gel/cream/spray to wound two or three times per day (Bionect).

PEDS – Not approved in children.

FORMS – OTC Trade only: Cream 2% 15, 30 g. Rx Generic/Trade: Soln 3% 30 mL. Gel 4% 30 g. Cream 4% 15, 30, 60 g. Injectable gel 2%.

NOTES – Do not use more than 1.5 mL of injectable form per treatment area. Injectable product contains trace amounts of Gram-positive bacterial proteins; contraindicated if history of anaphylaxis or severe allergy.

HYDROQUINONE (***Eldopaque, Eldoquin, Eldoquin Forte, EpiQuin Micro, Esoterica, Glyquin, Lustra, Melanex, Solaquin, Claripel, ♣ Ultraquin***) ▶? ♀C ▶? $

ADULT – Temporary bleaching of hyperpigmented skin conditions (ie, chloasma, melasma, freckles, senile lentigines, ultraviolet-induced discoloration from oral contraceptives, pregnancy, or hormone

(cont.)

HYDROQUINONE (*cont.*)

therapy): Apply two times per day to affected area.

PEDS – Not approved in children.

FORMS – OTC Trade only: Cream 2% 15, 30 g. Rx Generic/Trade: Soln 3% 30 mL. Gel 4% 30 g. Cream 4% 15, 30, 60 g.

NOTES – Responses may take 3 weeks to 6 months. Use a sunscreen on treated exposed areas.

LACTIC ACID (***Lac-Hydrin, AmLactin,*** ✤ ***Dermalac***) ▸? ♀? ▸? $$

ADULT – Ichthyosis vulgaris and xerosis (dry, scaly skin): Apply two times per day to affected area.

PEDS – Ichthyosis vulgaris and xerosis (dry, scaly skin) in children older than 2 yo: Apply two times per day to affected area.

FORMS – Trade only: Lotion 12% 150, 360 mL. Generic/OTC: Cream 12% 140, 385 g. AmLactin AP is lactic acid (12%) with pramoxine (1%).

NOTES – Frequently causes irritation in non-intact skin. Minimize exposure to sun, artificial sunlight.

LIDOCAINE—TOPICAL (***Xylocaine, Lidoderm, Numby Stuff, LMX, Zingo,*** ✤ ***Maxilene***) ▸LK ♀B ▸+ $$

WARNING – Contraindicated in allergy to amide-type anesthetics.

ADULT – Topical anesthesia: Apply to affected area prn. Dose varies with anesthetic procedure, degree of anesthesia required, and individual patient response. Postherpetic neuralgia (patch): Apply up to 3 patches to affected area at once for up to 12 h within a 24 h period.

PEDS – Topical anesthesia: Apply to affected area prn. Dose varies with anesthetic procedure, degree of anesthesia required, and individual patient response. Max 3 mg/kg/dose, do not repeat dose within 2 h. Intradermal powder injection for venipuncture/IV cannulation, for age 3 to 18 yo (Zingo): 0.5 mg to site 1 to 10 min prior.

UNAPPROVED PEDS – Topical anesthesia prior to venipuncture: Apply 30 min prior to procedure (ELA-Max 4%).

FORMS – For membranes of mouth and pharynx: Spray 10%, Ointment 5%, Liquid 5%, Soln 2%, 4%, Dental patch. For urethral use: Jelly 2%. Patch (Lidoderm) 5%. Intradermal powder injection system: 0.5 mg (Zingo). OTC Trade only: Liposomal lidocaine 4% (ELA-Max).

NOTES – Apply patches only to intact skin to cover the most painful area. Patches may be cut into smaller sizes with scissors prior to removal of the release liner. Store and dispose out of the reach of children and pets to avoid possible toxicity from ingestion.

MINOXIDIL—TOPICAL (***Rogaine, Women's Rogaine, Rogaine Extra Strength, Minoxidil for Men***) ▸K ♀C ▸– $

ADULT – Androgenetic alopecia in men or women: 1 mL to dry scalp two times per day.

PEDS – Not approved in children.

UNAPPROVED ADULT – Alopecia areata.

UNAPPROVED PEDS – Alopecia: Apply to dry scalp two times per day.

FORMS – OTC Generic/Trade: Soln 2% 60 mL (Rogaine, Women's Rogaine). Soln 5% 60 mL (Rogaine Extra Strength). Foam 5% 60 g (Rogaine Extra Strength).

NOTES – 5% strength for men only. Alcohol content may cause burning and stinging. Evidence of hair growth usually takes at least 4 months. If treatment is stopped, new hair will be shed in a few months.

MONOBENZONE (***Benoquin***) ▸Minimal absorption ♀C ▸? $$$

ADULT – Extensive vitiligo: Apply two to three times per day.

PEDS – Not approved for younger than 12 yo.

FORMS – Trade only: Cream 20% 35.4 g.

NOTES – Avoid prolonged exposure to sunlight. May take 1 to 4 months for depigmentation to occur. Depigmentation is permanent and can cause lifelong increase in photosensitivity.

OATMEAL (***Aveeno***) ▸Not absorbed ♀? ▸? $

ADULT – Pruritus from poison ivy/oak, varicella: Apply lotion four times per day prn. Also available in packets to be added to bath.

PEDS – Pruritus from poison ivy/oak, varicella: Apply lotion four times per day prn. Also available in bath packets for tub.

FORMS – OTC Generic/Trade: Lotion. Bath packets.

PANAFIL **(papain + urea + chlorophyllin copper complex)** ▸? ♀? ▸? $$$

ADULT – Debridement of acute or chronic lesions: Apply to clean wound and cover one to two times per day.

PEDS – Not approved in children.

FORMS – Trade only: Ointment 6, 30 g. Spray 33 mL.

NOTES – Longer redressings (2 to 3 days) are acceptable. May be applied under pressure dressings. Hydrogen peroxide inactivates papain; avoid concomitant use.

PLIAGIS **(tetracaine + lidocaine—topical)** ▸Minimal absorption ♀B ▸? $$

WARNING – Contraindicated in allergy to amide-type anesthetics.

(cont.)

PLIAGIS (*cont.*)

ADULT – Prior to venipuncture, intravenous cannulation, superficial dermatological procedure: Apply 20 to 30 min prior to procedure (60 min for tattoo removal).

PEDS – Not approved in children.

FORMS – Trade only: Cream lidocaine 7% + tetracaine 7%.

POLY-L-LACTIC ACID (***Sculptra***) ▶Not absorbed ♀? ▶? $$$$$

ADULT – Restoration of facial fat loss due to HIV lipoatrophy: Dose based on degree of correction needed.

PEDS – Not approved in children younger than 18 yo.

PRAMOSONE **(pramoxine + hydrocortisone,** ***✤ Pramox HC*****)** ▶Not absorbed ♀C ▶? $$$

ADULT – Apply three to four times per day.

PEDS – Apply two to three times per day.

FORMS – Trade only: 1% pramoxine/1% hydrocortisone: Cream 30, 60 g. Ointment 30 g. Lotion 60, 120, 240 mL. 1% pramoxine/2.5% hydrocortisone acetate: Cream 30, 60 g. Ointment 30 g. Lotion 60, 120 mL.

NOTES – Monitor for hyperglycemia/adrenal suppression if used for long period of time or over a large area of the body, especially in children. Chronic administration may interfere with pediatric growth and development.

SELENIUM SULFIDE (***Selsun, Exsel, Versel***) ▶? ♀C ▶? $

ADULT – Dandruff, seborrheic dermatitis: Massage 5 to 10 mL of shampoo into wet scalp, allow to remain 2 to 3 min, rinse. Apply twice a week for 2 weeks. For maintenance, less frequent administration needed. Tinea versicolor: Apply 2.5% shampoo/lotion to affected area, allow to remain on skin 10 min, rinse. Repeat daily for 7 days.

PEDS – Dandruff, seborrheic dermatitis: Massage 5 to 10 mL of shampoo into wet scalp, allow to remain 2 to 3 min, rinse. Apply twice a week for 2 weeks. For maintenance, less frequent administration needed. Tinea versicolor: Apply 2.5% lotion/shampoo to affected area, allow to remain on skin 10 min, rinse. Repeat daily for 7 days.

FORMS – OTC Generic/Trade: Lotion/Shampoo 1% 120, 210, 240, 325 mL, 2.5% 120 mL. Rx Generic/Trade: Lotion/Shampoo 2.5% 120 mL.

SOLAG **(mequinol + tretinoin)** ▶Not absorbed ♀X ▶? $$$$

ADULT – Solar lentigines: Apply two times per day separated by at least 8 h.

PEDS – Not approved in children.

FORMS – Trade only: Soln 30 mL (mequinol 2% + tretinoin 0.01%).

NOTES – Use in non-Caucasians has not been evaluated. Avoid in patients taking photosensitizers. Minimize exposure to sunlight.

SUNSCREEN ▶Not absorbed ♀? ▶+ $

ADULT – Apply at least 2 tablespoons for full body coverage 30 minutes before going outdoors. If in the sun between 10 am and 4 pm, reapply sunscreen q 2 h (more often if swimming or sweating).

PEDS – Avoid sun exposure if younger than 6 mo. For age 6 mo or older: Apply at least 2 tablespoons for full body coverage 30 minutes before going outdoors. If in the sun between 10 am and 4 pm, reapply sunscreen q 2 h (more often if swimming or sweating). Apply prior to sun exposure.

FORMS – Many formulations available.

NOTES – Sun protection factor (SPF) numbers equal the ratio of doses of ultraviolet radiation (predominantly UVB radiation) that result in sunburn with protection to the doses that result in erythema without protection. SPF 2 equals a 50% block, SPF 15 equals a 93% block, and SPF 45 equals a 98% block.

SYNERA **(tetracaine + lidocaine—topical)** ▶Minimal absorption ♀B ▶? $$

WARNING – Contraindicated in allergy to amide-type anesthetics.

ADULT – Prior to venipuncture, intravenous cannulation, superficial dermatological procedure: Apply 20 to 30 min prior to procedure.

PEDS – Children 3 yo or older: Prior to venipuncture, IV cannulation, superficial dermatological procedure: Apply 20 to 30 min prior to procedure.

FORMS – Trade only: Topical patch (lidocaine 70 mg + tetracaine 70 mg).

NOTES – Do not cut patch or remove top cover.

TRI-LUMA **(fluocinolone + hydroquinone + tretinoin)** ▶Minimal absorption ♀C ▶? $$$$

ADULT – Melasma of the face: Apply at bedtime for 4 to 8 weeks.

PEDS – Not approved in children.

FORMS – Trade only: Cream 30 g (fluocinolone 0.01% + hydroquinone 4% + tretinoin 0.05%).

NOTES – Minimize exposure to sunlight. Not intended for melasma maintenance therapy.

UREA (***Carmol 40***) ▶? ♀B ▶? $$$$

ADULT – Debridement of hyperkeratotic surface lesions: Apply two times per day.

PEDS – Debridement of hyperkeratotic surface lesions: Apply two times per day.

FORMS – Trade only: Urea 40% Cream 30, 85, 200 g. Lotion 240 mL. Gel 15 mL.

VUSION **(miconazole—topical + zinc oxide + white petrolatum)** ▶Minimal absorption ♀C ▶? $$$$$

ADULT – Not approved in adults.

PEDS – Apply to affected diaper area with each change for 7 days.

FORMS – Trade only: Ointment 50 g.

NOTES – Use only in documented cases of candidiasis.

ENDOCRINE AND METABOLIC: Androgens / Anabolic Steroids

NOTE: See OB/GYN section for other hormones.

FLUOXYMESTERONE (***Halotestin, Androxy***) ▶L ♀X ▶?©III $$$$

ADULT – Palliative treatment of androgen-responsive recurrent breast cancer in women who are 1 to 5 years postmenopausal: 5 to 10 mg PO two to four times per day for 1 to 3 months.

PEDS – Delayed puberty in males: 2.5 to 10 mg PO daily for 4 to 6 months.

FORMS – Generic only: Tabs 10 mg.

NOTES – Transdermal or injectable therapy preferred for hypogonadism. Pediatric use by specialists who monitor bone maturation q 6 months. Prolonged high-dose use may cause hepatic adenomas, hepatocellular carcinoma, and peliosis hepatitis. Monitor LFTs. Monitor Hb for polycythemia.

METHYLTESTOSTERONE (***Android, Methitest, Testred, Virilon***) ▶L ♀X ▶?©III $$$

ADULT – Advancing inoperable breast cancer in women who are 1 to 5 years postmenopausal: 50 to 200 mg/day PO in divided doses.

PEDS – Delayed puberty in males: 10 mg PO daily for 4 to 6 months.

FORMS – Trade/Generic: Caps 10 mg, Tabs 10, 25 mg.

NOTES – Transdermal or injectable therapy preferred to oral for hypogonadism. Pediatric use by specialists who monitor bone maturation q 6 months. Prolonged high-dose use may cause hepatic adenomas, hepatocellular carcinoma, and peliosis hepatitis. Monitor LFTs. Monitor Hb for polycythemia.

OXANDROLONE (***Oxandrin***) ▶L ♀X ▶?©III $$$$$

WARNING – Peliosis hepatitis, liver cell tumors, and lipid changes have occurred secondary to anabolic steroid use.

ADULT – Weight gain promotion following extensive surgery, chronic infection, or severe trauma; in some patients who fail to gain or maintain wt without a physiologic cause; to offset protein catabolism associated with long-term corticosteroid therapy: 2.5 mg/day to 20 mg/day PO divided two to four times per day for 2 to 4 weeks. May repeat therapy intermittently as indicated.

PEDS – Weight gain: Up to 0.1 mg/kg or up to 0.045 mg/pound PO divided two to four times per day for 2 to 4 weeks. May repeat therapy intermittently as indicated.

FORMS – Generic/Trade: Tabs 2.5, 10 mg.

NOTES – Contraindicated in known or suspected prostate/breast cancer. Not shown to enhance athletic ability. Associated with dyslipidemia; monitor lipids. Pediatric use by specialists who monitor bone maturation q 6 months. Long-term use may cause hepatic adenomas, hepatocellular carcinoma, and peliosis hepatitis; monitor LFTs. May increase anticoagulant effects of warfarin. Monitor Hb for polycythemia.

OXYMETHOLONE (***Anadrol-50***) ▶L ♀X ▶–©III $$$$$

WARNING – Peliosis hepatitis, liver cell tumors, and lipid changes have occurred secondary to anabolic steroid use.

ADULT – Anemia caused by deficient red cell production: 1 to 5 mg/kg/day PO. Usual effective dose is 1 to 2 mg/kg/day PO, but higher doses may be required, and the dose should be individualized. Max 100 mg/day.

PEDS – Anemia caused by deficient red cell production: 1 to 5 mg/kg/day PO. Usual effective dose is 1 to 2 mg/kg/day PO, but higher doses may be required, and the dose should be individualized.

FORMS – Trade only: Tabs 50 mg (scored)

NOTES – Not recommended by National Kidney Foundation. Response is not rapid and may require 3 to 6 months. Some patients may need to be maintained on a lower dose following remission. Continued use is usually necessary for congenital aplastic anemia. Contraindicated in known or suspected prostate/breast cancer. Avoid if nephrosis or nephritis. Not shown to enhance athletic ability. Associated with dyslipidemia, monitor lipids. Pediatric use by specialists who monitor bone maturation q 6 months. Long-term use may cause hepatic adenomas, hepatocellular carcinoma, and peliosis hepatitis; monitor LFTs. May increase anticoagulant effects of warfarin. May cause iron deficiency anemia; monitor serum iron and iron-binding capacity.

TESTOSTERONE (*Androderm, AndroGel, Axiron, Delatestryl, Depo-Testosterone, Striant, Testim, Testopel, Testro AQ,* ✦ *Andriol*) ▶L ♀X ▶?©III $ – varies by therapy

WARNING – Risk of transfer and secondary exposure with topical products. Virilization has been reported in children after secondary exposure to gel. Women and children should avoid contact with skin areas to which gel has been applied. Advise patient to wash hands with soap and water following application and cover area with clothing once gel has dried.

ADULT – Hypogonadism in men: Injectable enanthate or cypionate, 50 to 400 mg IM q 2 to 4 weeks. Androderm, Start 4 mg patch at bedtime to clean, dry area of skin on back, abdomen, upper arms, or thighs. Nonvirilized patients start with 2 mg patch at bedtime. Adjust based on serum testosterone concentrations; see prescribing information. AndroGel 1%: Apply 5 g from gel pack or 4 pumps (5 g gel; 50 mg testosterone) from dispenser daily to clean, dry, intact skin of the shoulders, upper arms, or abdomen. May increase dose to 7.5 to 10 g (100 mg testosterone) after 2 weeks. Androgel 1.62%: Apply 2 pumps (40.5 mg testosterone) from dispenser daily to shoulders or upper arms. Adjust based on serum testosterone concentration q 14 to 28 days. Dose range: 1 to 4 pumps daily. Axiron: 60 mg (1 pump of 30 mg to each axilla) once daily. Testim: 1 tube (5 g) daily to the clean, dry intact skin of the shoulders or upper arms. May increase dose to 2 tubes (10 g) after 2 weeks. Testopel: 2 to 6 pellets (150 to 450 mg testosterone) SC q 3 to 6 months. 2 pellets for each 25 mg testosterone propionate required weekly. Buccal (Striant): 30 mg q 12 h on upper gum above the incisor tooth; alternate sides for each application.

PEDS – Not approved in children.

FORMS – Trade only: Patch 2, 4 mg/24 h (Androderm). Gel 1% 2.5, 5 g packet, 75 g multidose pump (AndroGel 1% 1.25 g gel containing 12.5 mg testosterone per actuation). Gel 1.62%, 20.25 mg testosterone/actuation (AndroGel 1.62%). Gel 1%, 5 g tube (Testim). Gel 110 mL multidose pump (Axiron, 30 mg/actuation). Pellet 75 mg (Testopel). Buccal: Blister packs: 30 mg (Striant). Generic/Trade: Injection 100, 200 mg/mL (cypionate), 200 mg/mL (ethanate).

NOTES – Do not apply Androderm or AndroGel to scrotum. Apply Axiron only to axilla. Do not apply Testim to the scrotum or abdomen. Wash hands after topical product administration. Do not shower or swim for 5 h after applying AndroGel. Pellet implantation is less flexible for dosage adjustment, therefore, take great care when estimating the amount of testosterone. For testosterone gel form, obtain serum testosterone level 2 weeks after initiation, then increase dose if necessary. Inject IM formulations slowly into gluteal muscle; rare reports of cough or respiratory distress following injection. Prolonged high-dose use of oral forms of testosterone have caused hepatic adenomas, hepatocellular carcinoma, and peliosis hepatitis. May promote the development of prostatic hyperplasia or prostate cancer. Monitor prostate exam, PSA, and hemoglobin to detect polycythemia. Advise patient to regularly inspect the gum region where Striant is applied and report any abnormality; refer for dental consultation as appropriate. Injectable forms less expensive than gel or patch.

ENDOCRINE AND METABOLIC: Bisphosphonates

NOTE: Supplemental Vitamin D and calcium are recommended for osteoporosis prevention and treatment. Osteonecrosis of the jaw has been reported with bisphosphonates; generally associated with tooth extraction and/or local infection with delayed healing. Prior to treatment, consider dental exam and appropriate preventative dentistry, particularly with risk factors (eg, cancer, chemotherapy, corticosteroids, poor oral hygiene). While on bisphosphonate therapy, avoid invasive dental procedures when possible. Severe musculoskeletal pain has been reported; may occur at any time during therapy. Atypical, low trauma femoral shaft fractures have been reported; evaluate new thigh/groin pain for possible fracture. AACE guidelines recommend considering a drug holiday for 1 to 2 years in patients with stable bone mineral density after 4 to 5 years of treatment in patients with mild osteoporosis and after 10 years of treatment in patients with high fracture risk. Monitor bone density and resume treatment if it declines, if bone turnover markers increase, or if fracture.

ALENDRONATE (*Fosamax, Fosamax Plus D,* ✤ *Fosavance*) ▸K ♀C ◗– $$

ADULT – Prevention of postmenopausal osteoporosis: 5 mg PO daily or 35 mg PO weekly). Treatment of postmenopausal osteoporosis: 10 mg daily, 70 mg PO weekly, 70 mg/vitamin D3 2800 international units PO weekly, or 70 mg/vitamin D3 5600 international units PO weekly. Treatment of glucocorticoid-induced osteoporosis: 5 mg PO daily in men and women or 10 mg PO daily postmenopausal women not taking estrogen. Treatment of osteoporosis in men: 10 mg PO daily, 70 mg PO weekly, 70 mg/vitamin D3 2800 international units PO weekly, or 70 mg/vitamin D3 5600 international units PO weekly. Paget's disease: 40 mg PO daily for 6 months.

PEDS – Not approved in children.

UNAPPROVED ADULT – Prevention of glucocorticoid-induced osteoporosis men and women: 5 mg PO daily or 35 mg PO weekly; 10 mg PO daily or 70 mg PO weekly (postmenopausal women not taking estrogen). Treatment of glucocorticoid-induced osteoporosis in men and women: 35 mg weekly or 70 mg weekly (postmenopausal women not taking estrogen).

FORMS – Generic/Trade (Fosamax): Tabs 5, 10, 35, 40, 70 mg. Trade only: Oral soln 70 mg/75 mL (single-dose bottle). Fosamax Plus D: 70 mg + either 2800 or 5600 units of vitamin D3.

NOTES – May cause esophagitis, esophageal ulcers, and esophageal erosions, occasionally with bleeding and rarely followed by esophageal stricture or perforation. Monitor frequently for dysphagia, odynophagia, and retrosternal pain. Take 30 min before first food, beverage, and medication of the day with a full glass of water only. Remain in upright position for at least 30 min following dose. Caution if CrCl less than 35 mL/min. For patients requiring invasive dental procedures, discontinuation may reduce the risk for osteonecrosis of the jaw.

CLODRONATE (✤ *Clasteon, Bonefos*) ▸K ♀D ◗– $$$$$

ADULT – Canada only. Hypercalcemia of malignancy; management of osteolysis resulting from bone metastases of malignant tumors: IV single dose, 1500 mg slow infusion over at least 4 h. IV multiple dose, 300 mg slow infusion daily over 2 to 6 h up to 10 days. Oral, following IV therapy, maintenance 1600 to 2400 mg/day in single or divided doses. Max PO dose 3200 mg/day; duration of therapy is usually 6 months.

PEDS – Not approved in children.

FORMS – Generic/Trade: Caps 400 mg.

NOTES – Contraindicated if creatinine is more than 5 mg/dL or if severe GI tract inflammation. Avoid rapid bolus which may cause severe local reactions, thrombophlebitis, or renal failure. Do not mix with calcium-containing infusions. Ensure adequate hydration prior to infusion. Normocalcemia usually occurs within 2 to 5 days after initiation of therapy with multiple-dose infusion. Monitor serum calcium, renal function in those with renal insufficiency, LFTs, and hematological parameters.

ETIDRONATE (*Didronel*) ▸K ♀C ◗? $$$$$

ADULT – Paget's disease: 5 to 10 mg/kg PO daily for 6 months or 11 to 20 mg/kg daily for 3 months. Heterotopic ossification with hip replacement: 20 mg/kg/day PO for 1 month before and 3 months after surgery. Heterotopic ossification with spinal cord injury: 20 mg/kg/day PO for 2 weeks, then 10 mg/kg/day PO for 10 weeks.

PEDS – Not approved in children.

FORMS – Generic/Trade: Tabs 400 mg. Generic only: Tabs 200 mg.

NOTES – Divide dose if GI discomfort occurs. Avoid in abnormalities of the esophagus that may delay esophageal emptying (eg, stricture). Avoid food, vitamins with minerals, or antacids within 2 h of dose.

IBANDRONATE (*Boniva*) ▸K ♀C ◗? $$$$

ADULT – Prevention and treatment of postmenopausal osteoporosis. Oral: 2.5 mg PO daily or 150 mg PO q month. IV: 3 mg IV q 3 months.

PEDS – Not approved in children.

FORMS – Trade only: Tabs 2.5, 150 mg. IV: 3 mg.

NOTES – May cause esophagitis. Avoid in abnormalities of the esophagus that may delay esophageal emptying (eg, stricture). Avoid if CrCl less than 30 mL/min. Oral: Take 1 h before first food/beverage with a full glass of water only; remain in upright position 1 h after taking. IV: Administer over 15 to 30 sec.

PAMIDRONATE (*Aredia*) ▸K ♀D ◗? $$$$$

WARNING – Single dose should not exceed 90 mg due to risk of renal impairment/failure.

ADULT – Hypercalcemia of malignancy, moderate (corrected Ca in the range of 12 to 13.5 mg/dL): 60 to 90 mg IV single dose infused over 2 to 24 h. Hypercalcemia of malignancy, severe (Ca more than 13.5 mg/dL): 90 mg IV single dose infused over 2 to 24 h. Wait at least 7 days before considering retreatment. Paget's disease: 30 mg IV over 4 h daily for 3 days. Osteolytic bone lesions: 90 mg IV over 4

(cont.)

PAMIDRONATE (*cont.*)

h once a month. Osteolytic bone metastases: 90 mg IV over 2 h q 3 to 4 weeks.

PEDS – Not approved in children.

UNAPPROVED ADULT – Mild hypercalcemia: 30 mg IV single dose over 4 h. Treatment of osteoporosis: 30 mg IV q 3 months. Prevention of bone loss during androgen deprivation treatment for prostate cancer: 60 mg IV q 12 weeks.

NOTES – Fever occurs in more than 20% of patients. Monitor creatinine (prior to each dose), lytes, calcium, phosphate, magnesium, and CBC (regularly). Avoid in severe renal impairment and hold dosing if worsening renal function. Longer infusions (more than 2 h) may reduce renal toxicity. Not studied in patients with SCr above 3 mg/dL. Maintain adequate hydration.

RISEDRONATE (***Actonel, Atelvia***) ▶K ♀C ▶? $$$$

ADULT – Prevention and treatment of postmenopausal osteoporosis: 5 mg PO daily, 35 mg PO weekly or 150 mg once a month. Treatment of osteoporosis in men: 35 mg PO weekly. Prevention and treatment of glucocorticoid-induced osteoporosis: 5 mg PO daily. Paget's disease: 30 mg PO daily for 2 months.

PEDS – Not approved in children.

UNAPPROVED ADULT – Prevention and treatment of glucocorticoid-induced osteoporosis: 35 mg PO weekly.

FORMS – Trade only: Tabs 5, 30, 35, 150 mg, Delayed-release tab (Atelvia): 35 mg.

NOTES – May cause esophagitis, monitor frequently for dysphagia, odynophagia, and retrosternal pain. Remain in upright position for at least 30 min following dose. Take Actonel 30 min before first food, beverage, or medication of the day with a full glass of water only. Take delayed-release (Atelvia) in the morning immediately following breakfast with 4 oz or more of water only. Avoid in abnormalities of the esophagus that may delay esophageal emptying (eg, stricture).

TILUDRONATE (***Skelid***) ▶K ♀C ▶? $$$$$

ADULT – Paget's disease: 400 mg PO daily for 3 months.

PEDS – Not approved in children.

FORMS – Trade only: Tabs 200 mg.

NOTES – May cause esophagitis, esophageal ulcers, and esophageal erosions, occasionally with bleeding and rarely followed by esophageal stricture or perforation. Monitor frequently for dysphagia, odynophagia, and retrosternal pain. Take 30 min before first food, beverage, or medication of the day with a full glass of water only. Remain in upright position for at least 30 min following dose.

ZOLEDRONIC ACID (***Reclast, Zometa,*** ✤***Aclasta***) ▶K ♀D ▶? $$$$$

ADULT – Treatment of osteoporosis: 5 mg (Reclast) once yearly IV infusion over 15 min or longer. Prevention and treatment of glucocorticoid-induced osteoporosis in patients expected to receive glucocorticoids for at least 12 months: 5 mg (Reclast) once yearly IV infusion over 15 min or longer. Hypercalcemia of malignancy (corrected Ca at least 12 mg/dL, Zometa): 4 mg single-dose IV infusion over 15 min or longer. Wait at least 7 days before considering retreatment. Paget's disease (Reclast): 5 mg IV single dose. Multiple myeloma and metastatic bone lesions from solid tumors (Zometa): 4 mg (CrCl more than 60 mL/min), 3.5 mg (CrCl 50 to 60 mL/min), 3.3 mg (CrCl 40 to 49 mL/min) or 3 mg (CrCl 30 to 39 mL/min) IV infusion over 15 min or longer q 3 to 4 weeks.

PEDS – Not approved in children.

UNAPPROVED ADULT – Osteoporosis: 4 mg (Zometa) once yearly IV infusion over 15 min or longer. Paget's disease (Zometa; approved in Canada): 5 mg IV single dose. Treatment of hormone-refractory prostate cancer metastatic to bone (Zometa): 4 mg IV q 3 to 4 weeks. Prevention of bone loss during androgen-deprivation treatment for nonmetastatic prostate cancer (Zometa): 4 mg IV q 3 months for 1 year or 4 mg q 12 months. Prevention of bone loss during aromatase inhibitor use in breast cancer (Zometa): 4 mg IV q 6 months. Suppression of breast cancer in combination with adjuvant endocrine therapy (tamoxifen): 4 mg IV q 6 months for 3 years.

NOTES – Contraindicated in severe renal impairment (CrCl less than 35 mL/min) and hold dosing with worsening renal function. Monitor creatinine (before each dose), lytes, calcium, phosphate, magnesium, and Hb/HCT (regularly). Avoid single doses higher than 4 mg (Zometa) or higher than 5 mg (Reclast), infusions less than 15 min. Fever occurs in more than 15%. In treatment of Paget's disease, correct preexisting hypocalcemia with calcium and vitamin D before therapy. Maintain adequate hydration for those with hypercalcemia of malignancy, and give 500 mg calcium supplement and vitamin D 400 international units PO daily to those with multiple myeloma or metastatic bone lesions.

ENDOCRINE AND METABOLIC: Corticosteroids

NOTE: See also Dermatology, Ophthalmology.

BETAMETHASONE (*Celestone, Celestone Soluspan, ✤ Betaject*) ▸L ♀C ▸– $$$$$

ADULT – Anti-inflammatory/Immunosuppressive: 0.6 to 7.2 mg/day PO divided two to four times per day or up to 9 mg/day IM. 0.25 to 2 mL intra-articular depending on location and size of joint.

PEDS – Dosing guidelines not established.

UNAPPROVED ADULT – Fetal lung maturation, maternal antepartum between 24 and 34 weeks gestation: 12 mg IM q 24 h for 2 doses.

UNAPPROVED PEDS – Anti-inflammatory, immunosuppressive: 0.0175 to 0.25 mg/kg/day PO divided three to four times per day. Fetal lung maturation, maternal antepartum: 12 mg IM q 24 h for 2 doses.

FORMS – Trade only: Syrup 0.6 mg/5 mL.

NOTES – Avoid prolonged use in children due to possible bone growth retardation. If such therapy necessary monitor growth and development.

CORTISONE (*Cortone*) ▸L ♀D ▸– $

ADULT – Adrenocortical insufficiency: 25 to 300 mg PO daily.

PEDS – Dosing guidelines not established.

UNAPPROVED PEDS – Adrenocortical insufficiency: 0.5 to 0.75 mg/kg/day PO divided q 8 h.

FORMS – Generic only: Tabs 25 mg.

DEXAMETHASONE (*Decadron, Dexpak, ✤ Dexasone*) ▸L ♀C ▸– $

ADULT – Anti-inflammatory/immunosuppressive: 0.5 to 9 mg/day PO/IV/IM divided two to four times per day. Cerebral edema: 10 to 20 mg IV load, then 4 mg IM q 6 h (off-label IV use common) or 1 to 3 mg PO three times per day.

PEDS – Dosing varies by indication; start 0.02 to 0.3 mg/kg/day divided three to four times per day.

UNAPPROVED ADULT – Initial treatment of immune thrombocytopenic purpura: 40 mg PO daily for 4 days. Fetal lung maturation, maternal antepartum between 24 and 34 weeks gestation: 6 mg IM q 12 h for 4 doses. Bacterial meningitis (controversial): 0.15 mg/kg IV q 6 h for 2 to 4 days; start 10 to 15 min before the 1st dose of antibiotic. Antiemetic, prophylaxis: 8 mg IV or 12 mg PO prior to chemotherapy; 8 mg PO daily for 2 to 4 days. Antiemetic, treatment: 10 to 20 mg PO/IV q 4 to 6 h.

UNAPPROVED PEDS – Anti-inflammatory/immunosuppressive: 0.08 to 0.3 mg/kg/day PO/IV/IM divided q 6 to 12 h. Croup: 0.6 mg/kg PO/IV/IM for one dose. Bacterial meningitis (controversial): 0.15 mg/kg IV q 6 h for 2 to 4 days; start 10 to 15 min before the 1st dose of antibiotic. Bronchopulmonary dysplasia in preterm infants: 0.5 mg/kg PO/IV divided q 12 h for 3 days, then taper. Acute asthma: Older than 2 yo: 0.6 mg/kg to max 16 mg PO daily for 2 days.

FORMS – Generic/Trade: Tabs 0.5, 0.75. Generic only: Tabs 0.25, 1.0, 1.5, 2, 4, 6 mg; elixir 0.5 mg/5 mL; Soln 0.5 mg/5 mL, 1 mg/1 mL (concentrate). Trade only: Dexpak 13 day (51 total 1.5 mg tabs for a 13-day taper), Dexpak 10 day (35 total 1.5 mg tabs for 10-day taper), Dexpak 6 days (21 total 1.5 mg tabs for 6-day taper).

NOTES – Avoid prolonged use in children due to possible bone growth retardation. If such therapy necessary monitor growth and development.

FLUDROCORTISONE (*Florinef*) ▸L ♀C ▸? $

ADULT – Adrenocortical insufficiency/Addison's disease: 0.1 mg PO 3 times a week to 0.2 mg PO daily. Salt-losing adrenogenital syndrome: 0.1 to 0.2 mg PO daily.

PEDS – Not approved in children.

UNAPPROVED ADULT – Postural hypotension: 0.05 to 0.4 mg PO daily.

UNAPPROVED PEDS – Adrenocortical insufficiency: 0.05 to 0.2 mg PO daily.

FORMS – Generic only: Tabs 0.1 mg.

NOTES – For primary adrenocortical insufficiency usually given in conjunction with cortisone or hydrocortisone.

HYDROCORTISONE (*Cortef, Cortenema, Solu-Cortef*) ▸L ♀C ▸– $

ADULT – Adrenocortical insufficiency: 20 to 240 mg/day PO divided three to four times per day or 100 to 500 mg IV/IM q 2 to 10 h prn (sodium succinate). Ulcerative colitis: 100 mg retention enema at bedtime (laying on side for 1 h or longer) for 21 days. May use for 2 to 3 months for severe cases; when course extends more than 3 weeks then discontinue gradually by decreasing frequency to every other night for 2 to 3 weeks. Multiple sclerosis acute exacerbation: 800 mg daily then 320 mg every other day for 1 month.

PEDS – Dosing guidelines not established. Prescribing information suggests tailoring doses to the specific disease being treated with a range of initial doses of 0.56 to 8 mg/kg/day IV/PO divided three to four times per day.

(cont.)

HYDROCORTISONE (*cont.*)

UNAPPROVED PEDS – Chronic adrenocortical insufficiency: 0.5 to 0.75 mg/kg/day PO divided q 8 h or 0.25 to 0.35 mg/kg/day IM daily. Acute adrenocortical insufficiency: Infants and young children 1 to 2 mg/kg IV bolus, then 25 to 150 mg/day divided q 6 to 8 h. Older children 1 to 2 mg/kg IV bolus, then 150 to 250 mg/day IV q 6 to 8 h.

FORMS – Generic/Trade: Tabs 5, 10, 20 mg; Enema 100 mg/60 mL.

NOTES – Agent of choice for adrenocortical insufficiency because of mixed glucocorticoid and mineralocorticoid properties at doses more than 100 mg/day.

METHYLPREDNISOLONE (***Solu-Medrol, Medrol, Depo-Medrol***) ▶L ♀C ▶– $

ADULT – Anti-inflammatory, immunosuppressive: Parenteral (Solu-Medrol) 10 to 250 mg IV/IM q 4 h prn. Oral (Medrol) 4 to 48 mg PO daily. Medrol Dosepak tapers 24 to 0 mg PO over 7 days. IM/joints (Depo-Medrol) 4 to 120 mg IM q 1 to 2 weeks. Multiple sclerosis flare: 200 mg PO/IV daily for 1 week followed by 80 mg PO daily for 1 month.

PEDS – Dosing guidelines not established.

UNAPPROVED ADULT – Acute asthma exacerbation ("burst" therapy): 40 to 60 mg PO daily or divided two times per day for 3 to 10 days. Acute asthma exacerbation (vomiting or nonadherent): 240 mg IM once. Optic neuritis: 1 g IV daily (or in divided doses) for 3 days, then PO prednisone 1 mg/kg/day for 11 days (followed by a 3-day taper). Multiple sclerosis flare: 1 g IV daily (or in divided doses) for 3 to 5 days. May follow with PO prednisone 1 mg/kg/day for 14 days, then taper off. Spinal cord injury: 30 mg/kg IV over 15 min, followed in 45 min by 5.4 mg/kg/h IV infusion for 23 h (if initiated within 3 h of injury) or for 47 h (if initiated 3 to 8 h after injury). Due to insufficient evidence, routine use in spinal cord injury not recommended.

UNAPPROVED PEDS – Anti-inflammatory, immunosuppressive: 0.5 to 1.7 mg/kg/day PO/IV/IM divided q 6 to 12 h. Spinal cord injury: 30 mg/kg IV over 15 min, followed in 45 min by 5.4 mg/kg/h IV infusion for 23 h. Due to insufficient evidence, routine use in spinal cord injury not recommended. Acute asthma exacerbation ("burst" therapy): 1 to 2 mg/kg/day PO; max 60 mg daily for 3 to 10 days. Acute asthma exacerbation (vomiting or nonadherent): Age younger than 5 yo: 7.5 mg/kg IM once; age 5 to 11 yo: 240 mg IM once; age at least 12 yo: 240 mg IM once.

FORMS – Trade only: Tabs 2, 16, 32 mg. Generic/Trade: Tabs 4, 8 mg. Medrol Dosepak (4 mg, 21 tabs).

NOTES – Other dosing regimens have been used for MS and optic neuritis. Avoid initial treatment of optic neuritis with oral steroids, as it may increase the risk of new episodes. Contains benzyl alcohol, contraindicated in premature infants and for intrathecal administration. Do not use for traumatic brain injury.

PREDNISOLONE (***Flo-Pred, Prelone, Pediapred, Orapred, Orapred ODT***) ▶L ♀C ▶+ $$

ADULT – Anti-inflammatory/Immunosuppressive: 5 to 60 mg/day PO; individualize to severity of disease and response. Multiple sclerosis: 200 mg PO daily for 1 week, then 80 mg every other day for 1 month.

PEDS – Anti-inflammatory/Immunosuppressive: 0.14 to 2 mg/kg/day PO divided three to four times per day (4 to 60 mg/m^2/day); individualize to severity of disease and response. Acute asthma: 1 to 2 mg/kg/day daily or divided two

(cont.)

CORTICOSTEROIDS	Approximate Equivalent Dose (mg)	Relative Anti-inflammatory Potency	Relative Mineralocorticoid Potency	Biological Half-life (h)
betamethasone	0.6–0.75	20–30	0	36–54
cortisone	25	0.8	2	8–12
dexamethasone	0.75	20–30	0	36–54
fludrocortisone	n.a.	10	125	18–36
hydrocortisone	20	1	2	8–12
methylprednisolone	4	5	0	18–36
prednisolone	5	4	1	18–36
prednisone	5	4	1	18–36
triamcinolone	4	5	0	12–36

n.a.= not available.

PREDNISOLONE (*cont.*)

times per day for 3 to 10 days. Nephrotic syndrome: 60 mg/m²/day divided three times per day for 4 weeks; then 40 mg/m²/day every other day for 4 weeks.

UNAPPROVED ADULT – Acute asthma exacerbation ("burst" therapy): 40 to 60 mg PO daily or divided two times per day for 3 to 10 days.

UNAPPROVED PEDS – Acute asthma exacerbation ("burst" therapy): 1 to 2 mg/kg/day PO; max 60 mg daily for 3 to 10 days. Early active RA: 10 mg/day PO.

FORMS – Generic/Trade: Syrup 15 mg/5 mL (Prelone; wild cherry flavor). Soln 5 mg/5 mL (Pediapred, raspberry flavor), 15 mg/5 mL (Orapred; grape flavor). Trade only: Orally disintegrating tabs 10, 15, 30 mg (Orapred ODT); Susp 5 mg/5 mL, 15 mg/5 mL (Flo-Pred; cherry flavor). Generic only: Tabs 5 mg. Syrup 5 mg/5 mL.

PREDNISONE (***Deltasone, Sterapred,*** ✤ ***Winpred***) ▸L ♀C ▸+ $

ADULT – Anti-inflammatory, immunosuppressive: 5 to 60 mg/day PO daily or divided two to four times per day.

PEDS – Dosing guidelines not established.

UNAPPROVED ADULT – Acute asthma exacerbation ("burst" therapy): 40 to 60 mg PO daily or divided two times per day for 3 to 10 days.

UNAPPROVED PEDS – Anti-inflammatory, immunosuppressive: 0.05 to 2 mg/kg/day divided one to four times per day. Acute asthma exacerbation ("burst" therapy): 1 to 2 mg/kg/day PO; max 60 mg daily for 3 to 10 days.

FORMS – Trade only: Sterapred (5 mg tabs: Tapers 30 to 5 mg PO over 6 days or 30 to 10 mg over 12 days), Sterapred DS (10 mg tabs: Tapers 60 to 10 mg over 6 days, or 60 to 20 mg PO over 12 days) taper packs. Generic only: Tabs 1, 2.5, 5, 10, 20, 50 mg. Soln 5 mg/5 mL, 5 mg/mL (Prednisone Intensol).

NOTES – Conversion to prednisolone may be impaired in liver disease.

TRIAMCINOLONE (***Aristospan, Kenalog, Trivaris***) ▸L ♀C ▸– $

ADULT – Anti-inflammatory/Immunosuppressive: 4 to 48 mg/day PO divided one to four times per day. 2.5 to 60 mg IM daily (Kenalog, Trivaris). Intra-articular: Small joints 2.5 to 5 mg (Kenalog, Trivaris), 2 to 6 mg (Aristospan); large joints 5 to 15 mg (Kenalog, Trivaris); 10 to 20 mg (Aristospan). Intravitreal: 4 mg (Trivaris).

PEDS – Dosing guidelines not established.

UNAPPROVED PEDS – Anti-inflammatory, immunosuppressive: 0.117 to 1.66 mg/kg/day PO divided four times per day.

FORMS – Trade only: Injection 10 mg/mL, 40 mg/mL (Kenalog), 5 mg/mL, 20 mg/mL (Aristospan), 8 mg (80 mg/mL) syringe (Trivaris).

NOTES – Parenteral form not for IV use. Kenalog and Aristospan contain benzyl alcohol; do not use in neonates. Due to Trivaris availability in a syringe, multiple injections may be required for dose.

ENDOCRINE AND METABOLIC: Diabetes-Related—Alpha-Glucosidase Inhibitors

NOTE: No clinical studies have established conclusive evidence of decreased macrovascular outcomes with antidiabetic drugs. Alpha-glucosidase inhibitor administered alone should not cause hypoglycemia. If hypoglycemia occurs, treat with oral glucose rather than sucrose (table sugar). Adverse GI effects (ie, flatulence, diarrhea, abdominal pain) may occur with initial therapy.

ACARBOSE (***Precose,*** ✤ ***Glucobay***) ▸Gut/K ♀B ▸– $$$

ADULT – DM, Type 2: Initiate therapy with 25 mg PO three times per day with the first bite of each meal. May start with 25 mg PO daily to minimize GI adverse effects. May increase to 50 mg PO three times per day after 4 to 8 weeks. Usual range is 50 to 100 mg PO three times per day. Max dose for patients wt 60 kg or less is 50 mg three times per day, wt greater than 60 kg max is 100 mg three times per day.

PEDS – Not approved in children.

UNAPPROVED ADULT – DM prevention, Type 2: 100 mg PO three times per day or to maximum tolerated dose.

FORMS – Generic/Trade: Tabs 25, 50, 100 mg.

MIGLITOL (***Glyset***) ▸K ♀B ▸– $$$

ADULT – DM, Type 2: Initiate therapy with 25 mg PO three times per day with the first bite of each meal. Use 25 mg PO daily to start if GI adverse effects. May increase dose to 50 mg PO three times per day after 4 to 8 weeks, max 300 mg/day.

PEDS – Not approved in children.

FORMS – Trade only: Tabs 25, 50, 100 mg.

ENDOCRINE AND METABOLIC: Diabetes-Related—Combinations

NOTE: No clinical studies have established conclusive evidence of decreased macrovascular outcomes with antidiabetic drugs. Metformin-containing products may cause life-threatening lactic acidosis, usually in setting of decreased tissue perfusion, hypoxia, hepatic dysfunction, or impaired renal clearance. Hold prior to IV contrast agents and for 48 h after. Avoid if ethanol abuse, heart failure (requiring treatment), hepatic or renal insufficiency (creatinine 1.4 mg/dL or greater in women, 1.5 mg/dL or greater in men), or hypoxic states (cardiogenic shock, septicemia, acute MI). Initial GI upset may be minimized by starting with lower dose of metformin component. Glitazone-containing products may cause edema, wt gain, new heart failure, or exacerbate existing heart failure (avoid in NYHA Class III or IV). Monitor for signs of heart failure (rapid wt gain, dyspnea, edema) following initiation or dose increase. If occurs, manage fluid retention and consider discontinuation or dosage decrease. Rosiglitazone (Avandia) is not recommended with nitrates or insulin, and its labeling includes boxed warning regarding increased risk of myocardial ischemic events and notes that studies are currently inconclusive. Avoid if liver disease or ALT greater than 2.5 times normal. Monitor LFTs before therapy and periodically thereafter. Discontinue if ALT is greater than 3 times upper normal limit. Full effect may not be apparent for up to 12 weeks. May cause resumption of ovulation in premenopausal anovulatory women; recommend contraception use. Sulfonylureas can lead to hemolytic anemia in patients with G6PD deficiency; use caution or consider alternate agents. DPP-IV inhibitors: Report pancreatitis and discontinue drug if occurs.

ACTOPLUS MET **(pioglitazone + metformin)** ▶KL ♀C ▶? $$$$$

ADULT – DM, Type 2: 1 tab PO daily to two times per day. If inadequate control with metformin monotherapy, start 15/500 or 15/850 PO one to two times per day. If inadequate control with pioglitazone monotherapy, start 15/500 two times per day or 15/850 daily. Max 45/2550 mg/day. Extended release, start 1 tab (15/100 mg or 30/1000 mg) daily with evening meal. Max: 45/2000 mg/day.

PEDS – Not approved in children.

FORMS – Trade only: Tabs 15/500, 15/850 mg, Extended release, tabs: 15/1000 mg, 30/1000 mg.

NOTES – Urinary bladder tumors reported; advise patients to report macroscopic hematuria or dysuria.

AVANDAMET **(rosiglitazone + metformin)** ▶KL ♀C ▶? $$$$$

ADULT – DM, Type 2, initial therapy (drug-naive): Start 2/500 mg PO one or two times per day. If inadequate control with metformin alone, select tab strength based on adding 4 mg/day rosiglitazone to existing metformin dose. If inadequate control with rosiglitazone alone, select tab strength based on adding 1000 mg/day metformin to existing rosiglitazone dose. Max 8/2000 mg/day.

PEDS – Not approved in children.

FORMS – Trade only: Tabs 2/500, 4/500, 2/1000, 4/1000 mg.

NOTES – Due to potential for elevated cardiovascular risks, rosiglitazone products restricted by FDA to use in patients where other medications cannot control Type 2 diabetes. May be given concomitantly with sulfonylureas.

AVANDARYL **(rosiglitazone + glimepiride)** ▶LK ♀C ▶? $$$$

ADULT – DM, Type 2, initial therapy (drug-naive): Start 4/1 mg PO daily. If switching from monotherapy with a sulfonylurea or glitazone, consider 4/2 mg PO daily. Max 8/4 mg/day. Give with breakfast or the first main meal of the day. Use low starting dose of 4/1 mg and titrate more slowly in elderly, malnourished, and in renal and hepatic impairment.

PEDS – Not approved in children.

FORMS – Trade only (restricted access): Tabs 4/1, 4/2, 4/4, 8/2, 8/4 mg rosiglitazone/glimepiride.

NOTES – Due to potential for elevated cardiovascular risks, rosiglitazone products restricted by FDA to use in patients where other medications cannot control Type 2 diabetes.

DUETACT **(pioglitazone + glimepiride)** ▶LK ♀C ▶– $$$$

ADULT – DM, Type 2: Start 30/2 mg PO daily. Start up to 30/4 mg PO daily if prior glimepiride therapy, or 30/2 mg PO daily if prior pioglitazone therapy; max 30/4 mg/day. Give with breakfast or the first main meal of the day. In the elderly, the malnourished, or those with renal/hepatic impairment, precede therapy with trial of glimepiride 1 mg/day and then titrate Duetact more slowly.

PEDS – Not approved in children.

FORMS – Trade only: Tabs 30/2, 30/4 mg pioglitazone/glimepiride.

NOTES – Urinary bladder tumors reported; advise patients to report macroscopic hematuria or dysuria.

DIABETES NUMBERS*

Criteria for diagnosis	**Self-monitoring glucose goals**
Pre-diabetes: Fasting glucose 100–125 mg/dL or A1C 5.7–6.4% or 140–199 mg/dL 2 h after 75 g oral glucose load	Preprandial: 70–130 mg/dL Postprandial: < 180 mg/dL
Diabetes:[†] A1C ≥ 6.5% Fasting glucose ≥ 126 mg/dL. Random glucose with symptoms: ≥ 200 mg/dL, or ≥ 200 mg/dL 2 h after 75 g oral glucose load	A1C goal: < 7% for most non-pregnant adults, individualize based on comorbid conditions, hypoglycemia, and other patient specific factors.
Hospitalized patients: may consider more stringent goal if safely achievable without hypoglycemia Critically ill glucose goal: 140–180 mg/d Non-critically ill glucose goal (hospitalized patients): premeal blood glucose < 140 mg/dL, random < 180 mg/dL	
Estimated average glucose (eAG): eAG (mg/dL) = (28.7 × A1C) – 46.7	
Complications prevention & management: ASA[‡] (75–162 mg/day) in Type 1 & 2 adults for primary prevention if 10-year cardiovascular risk > 10% (includes most men older than 50 yo or women older than 60 yo with at least one other major risk factor) and secondary prevention (those with vascular disease); statin therapy to achieve goal LDL regardless of baseline LDL (for those with vascular disease, those older than 40 yo and additional risk factor, or those younger than 40 yo but LDL > 100 mg/dL); ACE inhibitor or ARB if hypertensive or micro-/macro-albuminuria; pneumococcal vaccine (revaccinate one time if age 65 yo or older and previously received vaccine at age younger than 65 or older and more than 5 years ago). Every visit: Measure wt & BP (goal < 130/80 mm Hg); visual foot exam; review self-monitoring glucose record; review/adjust meds; review self-mgmt skills, dietary needs, and physical activity; smoking cessation counseling. Twice a year: A1C in those meeting treatment goals with stable glycemia (quarterly if not); dental exam. Annually: Fasting lipid profile** [goal LDL < 100 mg/dL, cardiovascular disease consider LDL < 70 mg/dL; HDL > 40 mg/dL (> 50 mg/dL in women), TG < 150 mg/dL], q 2 years with low-risk lipid values; creatinine; albumin to creatinine ratio spot collection; dilated eye exam; flu vaccine.	

*See recommendations at: care.diabetesjournals.org. Reference: *Diabetes Care* 2012;35(Suppl 1):S11-63. Glucose values are plasma.

[†]In the absence of symptoms, confirm diagnosis with glucose testing on subsequent day.

[‡]Avoid ASA if younger than 21 yo due to Reye's Syndrome risk; use if younger than 30 yo has not been studied.

**LDL is primary target of therapy, consider 30 to 40% LDL reduction from baseline as alternate goal if unable to reach targets on maximal tolerated statin.

GLUCOVANCE **(glyburide + metformin)** ▶KL ♀B ▶? $$$

ADULT – DM, Type 2, initial therapy (drug-naive): Start 1.25/250 mg PO daily or two times per day with meals; max 10/2000 mg daily. Inadequate control with a sulfonylurea or metformin alone: Start 2.5/500 or 5/500 mg PO two times per day with meals; max 20/2000 mg daily.

PEDS – Not approved in children.

FORMS – Generic/Trade: Tabs 1.25/250, 2.5/500, 5/500 mg.

JANUMET, JANUMET XR **(sitagliptin + metformin)** ▶K ♀B ▶? $$$$

ADULT – DM, Type 2: Individualize based on patient's current therapy. Immediate-release: Start 1 tab PO two times per day. Extended-release: 1 tab PO daily. If inadequate control with metformin monotherapy, start 50/500 or 50/1000 two times per day based on current metformin dose. Extended-release: Start 100 mg sitagliptin daily plus current daily metformin If inadequate control on sitagliptin monotherapy: Immediate-release: Start 50/500

(cont.)

JANUMET, JANUMET XR ***(cont.)***

two times per day. Extended-release: Start 100/1000 mg daily. Max 100/2000 mg daily. Give with meals.

PEDS – Not approved in children.

FORMS – Trade only: Immediate-release tabs 50/500, 50/1000 mg, extended-release tabs 100/1000, 50/500, 50/1000 mg sitagliptin/metformin.

NOTES – Not for use in Type 1 DM or DKA. Assess renal function and hematologic parameters prior to initiating and at least annually thereafter. Assess renal function more often if risk factors for dysfunction and discontinue if renal dysfunction. Do not split, crush, or chew extended-release formulation. Discontinue if signs of hypersensitivity, including anaphylaxis, angioedema, and severe dermatologic reactions.

JENTADUETO **(linagliptin + metformin)** ▶KL – ♀B ▶? $$$$$

ADULT – DM, Type 2: If prior metformin, start 2.5 mg linagliptin and current metformin dose two times per day. If no prior metformin, start 2.5/5 mg PO two times per day. If current linagliptin/metformin, start at current doses. Max 2.5/1000 mg.

PEDS – Not approved in children.

FORMS – Trade only: 2.5/500, 2.5/850, 2.5/1000 mg.

NOTES – Not for use in Type 1 DM or DKA. May cause hypoglycemia when adding to sulfonylurea therapy, consider reducing dose of sulfonylurea to decrease risk of hypoglycemia. Metformin may lower B12 levels, monitor hematologic parameters anually.

JUVISYNC **(sitagliptin + simvastatin)** ▶KL – ♀X ▶? $$$$$

ADULT – DM, Type 2 with hyperlipidemia: 100/40 (sitagliptin/simvatatin) mg PO once daily in evening. Or, may start on current dose of sitagliptin/simvastatin.

PEDS – Not approved in pediatrics.

FORMS – Trade only: Tabs 100/10, 100/20, 100/40 mg sitagliptin/simvastain.

NOTES – Not for use in Type 1 DM or DKA. Not recommended in moderate or severe renal impairment. Assess renal function periodically and dose adjust for renal function. Not studied in combination with insulin. When adding to sulfonylurea therapy, consider reducing dose of sulfonylurea to decrease risk of hypoglycemia. Discontinue if signs of hypersensitivity, including anaphylaxis, angioedema, and severe dermatologic reactions. Monitor for myopathy. Check LFTs at baseline and when clinically indicated; discontinue if persistent elevations. See simvastatin notes/warnings for additional considerations and dosing with drug interactions.

KOMBIGLYZE XR **(saxagliptin + metformin)** ♀B ▶? $$$$$

ADULT – DM, Type 2: If inadequately controlled on metformin alone, start 2.5 to 5 mg of saxagliptin plus current dose of metformin; give once daily with evening meal. If inadequately controlled on saxagliptin, start 5/500 mg once daily with evening meal. Max: 5/2000 mg/day.

PEDS – Not approved in children.

FORMS – Trade only: Tabs 5/500, 2.5/1000, 5/1000 mg.

NOTES – Reduce saxagliptin dose to 2.5 mg when administered with strong CYP3A4/5 inhibitors such as ketoconazole; use individual products instead of combination product if needed to achieve appropriate dose. Not for use in Type 1 DM or DKA. Assess renal function periodically. To minimize risk of hypoglycemia if used with insulin or a sulfonylurea, consider lower dose of insulin or sulfonylurea. Do not split, crush, or chew. Hypersensitivity, including angioedema, reported; caution if history of angioedema to other DPP4 inhibitors.

METAGLIP **(glipizide + metformin)** ▶KL ♀C ▶? $$$

ADULT – DM, Type 2, initial therapy (drug-naive): Start 2.5/250 mg PO daily to 2.5/500 mg PO twice per day with meals; max 10/2000 mg daily. Inadequate control with a sulfonylurea or metformin alone: Start 2.5/500 or 5/500 mg PO twice per day with meals; max 20/2000 mg daily.

PEDS – Not approved in children.

FORMS – Generic/Trade: Tabs 2.5/250, 2.5/500, 5/500 mg.

NOTES – May add thiazolidinedione if glycemic control is not obtained.

PRANDIMET **(repaglinide + metformin)** ▶KL ♀C ▶? $$$

ADULT – DM, Type 2, initial therapy (drug-naive): Start 1/500 mg PO daily before meals; max 10/2500 mg daily or 4/1000 mg/meal. Inadequate control with metformin alone: Start 1/500 mg PO two times per day before meals. Inadequate control with repaglinide alone: Start 500 mg metformin component PO two times per day before meals. In patients taking repaglinide and metformin concomitantly: Start at current dose and titrate to achieve adequate response.

PEDS – Not approved in children.

FORMS – Trade: Tabs 1/500, 2/500 mg.

NOTES – May take dose immediately preceding meal to as long as 30 min before the meal.

(cont.)

PRANDIMET *(cont.)*

Patients should be advised to skip dose if skipping meal. Gemfibrozil and itraconazole increase blood repaglinide levels and may result in an increased risk of hypoglycemia. Do not use with NPH insulin.

ENDOCRINE AND METABOLIC: Diabetes-Related—"Gliptins" (DPP-4 inhibitors)

NOTE: No clinical studies have established conclusive evidence of decreased macrovascular outcomes with antidiabetic drugs. Not for use in Type 1 DM or DKA. Not studied in combination with insulin. When adding to sulfonylurea therapy, consider reducing dose of sulfonylurea to decrease risk of hypoglycemia. Monitor for pancreatitis at initiation of therapy and dosage increases; discontinue drug if occurs.

LINAGLIPTIN (*Tradjenta*, ✤ *Trajenta*) ▶L - ♀B ◗? $$$$$

ADULT – DM, Type 2: 5 mg PO once daily.

FORMS – Trade only: Tabs 5 mg.

SAXAGLIPTIN (*Onglyza*) ▶LK ♀B ◗? $$$$$

ADULT – DM, Type 2: 2.5 or 5 mg PO daily. If CrCl is 50 mL/min or less reduce dose to 2.5 mg daily.

PEDS – Not approved in children.

FORMS – Trade only: Tabs 2.5, 5 mg.

NOTES – Not for use in Type 1 DM or DKA. Assess renal function periodically. Not studied in combination with insulin. When adding to sulfonylurea or insulin therapy, consider reducing dose of sulfonylurea or insulin to decrease risk of hypoglycemia. Reduce dose when administered with strong CYP3A4/5 inhibitors such as ketoconazole. No clinical studies have established conclusive evidence of decreased macrovascular outcomes with antidiabetic drugs. Observe for signs/symptoms of pancreatitis and discontinue if occurs. Hypersensitivity, including angioedema, reported; caution if history of angioedema to other DPP4 inhibitors.

SITAGLIPTIN (*Januvia*) ▶K ♀B ◗? $$$$$

ADULT – DM, Type 2: 100 mg PO daily. If CrCl 30 to 49 mL/min reduce dose to 50 mg daily; if CrCl less than 30 mL/min then 25 mg daily.

PEDS – Not approved in children.

FORMS – Trade only: Tabs 25, 50, 100 mg.

NOTES – Discontinue if signs of hypersensitivity, including anaphylaxis, angioedema, and severe dermatologic reactions.

ENDOCRINE AND METABOLIC: Diabetes-Related — GLP-1 agonists

NOTE: No clinical studies have established conclusive evidence of decreased macrovascular outcomes with antidiabetic drugs. Start with low dose to increase GI tolerance. May promote slight wt loss. May give SC in upper arm, abdomen, or thigh. Take medications that require rapid GI absorption at least 1 h prior to exenatide immediate-release or liraglutide. Risk of hypoglycemia is higher when used with insulin or insulin secretagogue (sulfonylurea, meglitinides), therefore, consider reduction in sulfonylurea or insulin dose. Pancreatitis reported, monitor for signs and symptoms including abdominal pain and vomiting upon initiation and dose increases. Discontinue if pancreatitis occurs. Extended-release exenatide and liraglutide: Thyroid C-cell tumors reported in animal studies. Contraindicated if history or family history of medullary thyroid cancer or in patients with multiple endocrine neoplasia syndrome type 2. Counsel patients on risk of thyroid tumors.

EXENATIDE (*Byetta, Bydureon*) ▶K ♀C ◗? $$$$$

ADULT – DM, Type 2, adjunctive therapy: Immediate-release: 5 mcg SC two times per day (within 1 h before the morning and evening meals, or 1 h before the two main meals of the day at least 6 h apart). May increase to 10 mcg SC two times per day after 1 month. Extended-release: 2 mg SC once weekly.

PEDS – Not approved in children.

FORMS – Trade only: Byetta, prefilled pen (60 doses each) 5 mcg/dose, 1.2 mL; 10 mcg/dose, 2.4 mL. Bydureon (extended-release): 2 mg/vial.

NOTES – Protect from light. Prior to initial use, keep refrigerated. After initial use, store at temperature below 78°F; do not freeze. Discard pen 30 days after first use. Avoid use if renal insufficiency (CrCl less than 30 mL/min). Caution recommended if increasing dose from 5 to 10 mcg in patients with CrCl 30 to 50 mL/min (immediate release). Monitor for kidney dysfunction. Not recommended in severe GI disease, including gastroparesis. Do not substitute for insulin in the insulin-dependent; concurrent use with prandial insulin has not been studied. Use with short- or rapid-acting insulins not recommended. May potentiate warfarin.

LIRAGLUTIDE (*Victoza*) ♀C ▸? $$$$$

ADULT – DM, Type 2: Start 0.6 mg SC daily for 1 week, then increase to 1.2 mg SC daily. May increase to 1.8 mg SC daily.

PEDS – Not approved in children.

FORMS – Trade only: Multidose pen (18 mg/3 mL) delivers doses of 0.6 mg, 1.2 mg or 1.8 mg.

NOTES – May be given any time of day, independent of meals. Use caution in patients with renal or hepatic impairment or history of pancreatitis. Concurrent use with insulin has not been studied. Not recommended as first-line therapy or for use in DM, Type 1 or DKA.

ENDOCRINE AND METABOLIC: Diabetes-Related—Insulins

NOTE: Adjust insulin dosing to achieve glycemic control. See table Diabetes Numbers for goals. Administer rapid-acting insulin (Humalog, NovoLog, Apidra) within 15 min before or immediately after a meal. Administer regular insulin 30 min before meals. May mix NPH with aspart, lispro, glulisine or regular. Draw up rapid/short-acting insulin first. Do not mix Lantus (glargine) or Levemir (detemir) with other insulins. Pens for use by one person only.

INSULIN—INJECTABLE COMBINATIONS (***Humalog Mix 75/25, Humalog Mix 50/50, Humulin 70/30, Novolin 70/30, Novolog Mix 70/30***) ▸LK ♀B/C ▸+ $$$$

ADULT – Doses vary, but typically total insulin 0.3 to 1 unit/kg/day SC in divided doses (Type 1), and 0.5 to 1.5 unit/kg/day SC in divided doses (Type 2).

PEDS – Not approved in children.

UNAPPROVED PEDS – Diabetes: Maintenance: Total insulin 0.5 to 1 unit/kg/day SC, but doses vary.

FORMS – Trade only: Insulin lispro protamine susp/insulin lispro (Humalog Mix 75/25, Humalog Mix 50/50). Insulin aspart protamine/insulin aspart (Novolog Mix 70/30). NPH and regular mixtures (Humulin 70/30, Novolin 70/30). Insulin available in pen form: Novolin 70/30 InnoLet, Novolog Mix 70/30 FlexPen, Humulin 70/30, Humalog Mix 75/25 KwikPen, Humalog Mix 50/50 KwikPen.

INSULIN—INJECTABLE INTERMEDIATE/LONG ACTING (***Novolin N, Humulin N, Lantus, Levemir***) ▸LK ♀B/C ▸+ $$$$

ADULT – Doses vary, but typically total insulin 0.3 to 0.5 unit/kg/day SC in divided doses (Type 1), and 1 to 1.5 unit/kg/day SC in divided doses (Type 2). Generally, 50 to 70% of

(cont.)

INJECTABLE INSULINS*

		Onset (h)	Peak (h)	Duration (h)
Rapid-/short acting	Insulin aspart (NovoLog)	<0.2	1–3	3–5
	Insulin glulisine (Apidra)	0.30–0.4	1	4–5
	Insulin lispro (Humalog)	0.25–0.5	0.5–2.5	≤5
	Regular (Novolin R, Humulin R)	0.5–1	2–3	3–6
Intermediate-/long acting	NPH (Novolin N, Humulin N)	2–4	4–10	10–16
	Insulin detemir (Levemir)	n.a.	flat action profile	up to 23†
	Insulin glargine (Lantus)	2–4	peakless	24
Mixtures	Insulin aspart protamine susp/aspart (NovoLog Mix 70/30)	0.25	1–4 (biphasic)	up to 24
	Insulin lispro protamine susp/insulin lispro (Humalog Mix 75/25, Humalog Mix 50/50)	<0.25	1–3 (biphasic)	10–20
	NPH/Reg (Humulin 70/30, Novolin 70/30)	0.5–1	2–10 (biphasic)	10–20

*These are general guidelines, as onset, peak, and duration of activity are affected by the site of injection, physical activity, body temperature, and blood supply.

†Dose-dependent duration of action, range from 6 to 23 h.

n.a.= not available.

INSULIN—INJECTABLE INTERMEDIATE/LONG ACTING (*cont.*)

insulin requirements are provided by rapid- or short-acting insulin and the remainder from intermediate- or long-acting insulin. Lantus: Start 10 units SC daily (same time everyday) in insulin-naive patients, adjust to usual dose of 2 to 100 units/day. When transferring from twice a day NPH human insulin, the initial Lantus dose should be reduced by about 20% from the previous total daily NPH dose, then adjust dose based on patient response. Levemir: Type 2 DM (inadequately controlled on oral meds): Start 0.1 to 0.2 units/kg once a day; or 10 units SC one or two times per day. When transferring from basal insulin (Lantus, NPH) in type 1 or 2 DM, change on a unit-to-unit basis; more Levemir may be required than NPH insulin.

PEDS – Diabetes: Maintenance: Total insulin 0.5 to 1 unit/kg/day SC, but doses vary. Generally, 50 to 70% of insulin requirements are provided by rapid-acting insulin and the remainder from intermediate- or long-acting insulin. Age 6 to 15 yo (Lantus): Start 10 units SC daily (same time everyday) in insulin-naive patients, adjust to usual dose of 2 to 100 units/day. When transferring from twice a day NPH human insulin, the initial Lantus dose should be reduced by about 20% from the previous total daily NPH dose, then adjust dose based on patient response. Levemir (Type 1 DM): When transferring from NPH, change on a unit-to-unit basis; more Levemir may be required than NPH.

FORMS – Trade only: Injection NPH (Novolin N, Humulin N). Insulin glargine (Lantus). Insulin detemir (Levemir). Insulin available in pen form: Novolin N InnoLet, Humulin N Pen, Lantus OptiClik (reusable), Lantus SoloStar (prefilled-disposable), Levemir InnoLet, Levemir FlexPen. Premixed preparations of NPH and regular insulin also available.

INSULIN—INJECTABLE SHORT/RAPID ACTING (***Apidra, Novolin R, NovoLog, Humulin R, Humalog, ✦ NovoRapid***) ▶LK ♀B/C ▶+ $$$

ADULT – Doses vary, but typically total insulin 0.3 to 0.5 unit/kg/day SC in divided doses (Type 1), and 1 to 1.5 unit/kg/day SC in divided doses (Type 2). Generally, 50 to 70% of insulin requirements are provided by rapid- or short-acting insulin and the remainder from intermediate- or long-acting insulin.

PEDS – Diabetes age older than 4 yo (Apidra), older than 3 yo (Humalog) or older than 2 yo (NovoLog): Doses vary, but typically total insulin maintenance dose 0.5 to 1 unit/kg/day SC in divided doses. Generally, 50 to 70% of insulin requirements are provided by rapid-acting insulin and the remainder from intermediate- or long-acting insulin.

UNAPPROVED ADULT – Severe hyperkalemia: 5 to 10 units regular insulin plus concurrent dextrose IV. Profound hyperglycemia (eg, DKA): 0.1 unit/kg regular insulin IV bolus, then begin IV infusion 100 units in 100 mL NS (1 unit/mL) at 0.1 units/kg/h. 70 kg: 7 units/h (7 mL/h). Titrate to clinical effect.

UNAPPROVED PEDS – Profound hyperglycemia (eg, DKA): 0.1 unit/kg regular insulin IV bolus, then IV infusion 100 units in 100 mL NS (1 unit/mL) at 0.1 unit/kg/h. Titrate to clinical effect. Severe hyperkalemia: 0.1 unit/kg regular insulin IV with glucose over 30 min. May repeat in 30 to 60 min or start 0.1 unit/kg/h.

FORMS – Trade only: Injection regular 100 units/mL (Novolin R, Humulin R) Injection regular 500 units/mL (Humulin U-500, concentrated). Insulin glulisine (Apidra). Insulin lispro (Humalog). Insulin aspart (NovoLog). Insulin available in pen form: Novolin R InnoLet, Humulin R, Apidra OptiClik, Humalog KwikPen, Novolog FlexPen.

NOTES – Apidra, Humalog, and NovoLog approved for use by continuous SC infusion in insulin pump. Do not mix insulins in pump. Consult manufacturer instructions for frequency of reservoir change when used in pump. Caution: Med errors have occurred when using concentrated Humulin R U-500, note strength 500 units/mL.

ENDOCRINE AND METABOLIC: Diabetes-Related—Meglitinides

NOTE: No clinical studies have established conclusive evidence of decreased macrovascular outcomes with antidiabetic drugs.

NATEGLINIDE (***Starlix***) ▶L ♀C ▶? $$$

ADULT – DM, Type 2, monotherapy or in combination with metformin or thiazolidinedione: 120 mg PO three times per day within 30 min before meals; use 60 mg PO three times per day in patients who are near goal A1C.

PEDS – Not approved in children.

FORMS – Generic/Trade: Tabs 60, 120 mg.

NOTES – Not to be used as monotherapy in patients inadequately controlled with glyburide or other antidiabetic agents previously. Patients with severe renal impairment are at risk for hypoglycemic episodes.

REPAGLINIDE (*Prandin,* ✤ *Gluconorm*) ▶L ♀C ▶? $$$$$

ADULT – DM, Type 2: 0.5 to 2 mg PO three times per day within 30 min before a meal. Allow 1 week between dosage adjustments. Usual range is 0.5 to 4 mg PO three to four times per day, max 16 mg/day.

PEDS – Not approved in children.

FORMS – Trade only: Tabs 0.5, 1, 2 mg.

NOTES – May take dose immediately preceding meal to as long as 30 min before the meal. Gemfibrozil and itraconazole increase blood repaglinide levels and may result in an increased risk of hypoglycemia. Do not use with NPH insulin.

ENDOCRINE AND METABOLIC: Diabetes-Related—Sulfonylureas—1st Generation

NOTE: No clinical studies have established conclusive evidence of decreased macrovascular outcomes with antidiabetic drugs. Sulfonylureas can lead to hemolytic anemia in patients with G6PD deficiency; use caution or consider alternate agents.

CHLORPROPAMIDE (*Diabinese*) ▶LK ♀C ▶– $$

ADULT – DM, Type 2: Initiate therapy with 100 to 250 mg PO daily. Titrate after 5 to 7 days by increments of 50 to 125 mg at intervals of 3 to 5 days to obtain optimal control. Max 750 mg/day.

PEDS – Not approved in children.

FORMS – Generic/Trade: Tabs 100, 250 mg.

NOTES – Clinical use in the elderly has not been properly evaluated. Elderly are more prone to hypoglycemia and/or hyponatremia possibly from renal impairment or drug interactions. May cause disulfiram-like reaction with alcohol.

TOLAZAMIDE (*Tolinase*) ▶LK ♀C ▶? $

ADULT – DM, Type 2: Initiate therapy with 100 mg PO daily in patients with fasting blood glucose less than 200 mg/dL, and in patients who are malnourished, underweight, or elderly. Initiate therapy with 250 mg PO daily in patients with fasting blood glucose more than 200 mg/dL. Give with breakfast or the first main meal of the day. If daily doses exceed 500 mg, divide the dose two times per day. Max 1000 mg/day.

PEDS – Not approved in children.

FORMS – Generic only: Tabs 100, 250, 500 mg.

TOLBUTAMIDE ▶LK ♀C ▶+ $

ADULT – DM, Type 2: Start 1 g PO daily. Maintenance dose is usually 250 mg to 2 g PO daily. Total daily dose may be taken in the morning; divide doses if GI intolerance occurs. Max 3 g/day.

PEDS – Not approved in children.

FORMS – Generic only: Tabs 500 mg.

ENDOCRINE AND METABOLIC: Diabetes-Related—Sulfonylureas—2nd Generation

NOTE: No clinical studies have established conclusive evidence of decreased macrovascular outcomes with antidiabetic drugs. Sulfonylureas can lead to hemolytic anemia in patients with G6PD deficiency; use caution or consider alternate agents.

GLICLAZIDE (✤ *Diamicron, Diamicron MR*) ▶KL ♀C ▶? $

ADULT – Canada only, DM, Type 2: Immediate-release: Start 80 to 160 mg PO daily, max 320 mg PO daily (160 mg or more per day should be in divided doses). Modified-release: Start 30 mg PO daily, max 120 mg PO daily.

PEDS – Not approved in children.

FORMS – Generic/Trade: Tabs 80 mg (Diamicron). Trade only: Tabs, modified-release 30 mg (Diamicron MR).

NOTES – Immediate, and modified-release not equipotent; 80 mg of immediate-release can be changed to 30 mg of modified-release.

GLIMEPIRIDE (*Amaryl*) ▶LK ♀C ▶– $$

ADULT – DM, Type 2: Initiate therapy with 1 to 2 mg PO daily. Start with 1 mg PO daily in elderly, malnourished patients or those with renal or hepatic insufficiency. Give with breakfast or the first main meal of the day. Titrate in increments of 1 to 2 mg at 1- to 2-week intervals based on response. Usual maintenance dose is 1 to 4 mg PO daily, max 8 mg/day.

PEDS – Not approved in children.

FORMS – Generic/Trade: Tabs 1, 2, 4 mg. Generic only: Tabs 3, 6, 8 mg.

NOTES – Allergy may develop if allergic to other sulfonamide derivatives.

GLIPIZIDE (*Glucotrol, Glucotrol XL*) ▶LK ♀C ▶? $

ADULT – DM, Type 2: Initiate therapy with 5 mg PO daily. Give 2.5 mg PO daily to geriatric patients or those with liver disease. Adjust dose in increments of 2.5 to 5 mg to a usual maintenance dose of 10 to 20 mg/day, max 40 mg/day. Doses more than 15 mg should be

(cont.)

GLIPIZIDE (*cont.*)

divided two times per day. Extended-release (Glucotrol XL): Initiate therapy with 5 mg PO daily. Usual dose is 5 to 10 mg PO daily, max 20 mg/day.

PEDS – Not approved in children.

FORMS – Generic/Trade: Tabs 5, 10 mg; Extended-release tabs 2.5, 5, 10 mg.

NOTES – Maximum effective dose is generally 20 mg/day.

GLYBURIDE (***DiaBeta, Glynase PresTab***) ▶LK ♀B ▶? $

ADULT – DM, Type 2: Initiate therapy with 2.5 to 5 mg PO daily. Start with 1.25 mg PO daily in elderly or malnourished patients or those with renal or hepatic insufficiency. Give with breakfast or the first main meal of the day. Titrate in increments of no more than 2.5 mg at weekly intervals based on response. Usual maintenance dose is 1.25 to 20 mg PO daily or divided two times per day, max 20 mg/day. Micronized tabs: Initiate therapy with 1.5 to 3 mg PO daily. Start with 0.75 mg PO daily in elderly, malnourished patients, or those with renal or hepatic insufficiency. Give with breakfast or the first main meal of the day. Titrate in increments of no more than 1.5 mg at weekly intervals based on response. Usual maintenance dose is 0.75 to 12 mg PO daily, max 12 mg/day. May divide dose two times per day if more than 6 mg/day.

PEDS – Not approved in children.

FORMS – Generic/Trade: Tabs (scored) 1.25, 2.5, 5 mg. Micronized Tabs (scored) 1.5, 3, 4.5, 6 mg.

NOTES – Maximum effective dose is generally 10 mg/day.

ENDOCRINE AND METABOLIC: Diabetes-Related—Thiazolidinediones

NOTE: No clinical studies have established conclusive evidence of decreased macrovascular outcomes with antidiabetic drugs. May cause edema, wt gain, new heart failure, or exacerbate existing heart failure (contraindicated in NYHA Class III or IV). Monitor for signs of heart failure (rapid wt gain, dyspnea, edema) following initiation or dose increase. If signs occur, manage fluid retention and consider discontinuation or dosage decrease. Avoid if liver disease or ALT more than 2.5 times normal. Monitor LFTs before therapy and periodically thereafter. Discontinue if ALT more than 3 times upper normal limit. Full effect may not be apparent for up to 12 weeks. May cause resumption of ovulation in premenopausal anovulatory women; recommend contraception use.

PIOGLITAZONE (***Actos***) ▶L ♀C ▶– $$$$$

ADULT – DM, Type 2: Start 15 to 30 mg PO daily, may adjust dose after 3 months to max 45 mg/day.

PEDS – Not approved in children.

FORMS – Trade only: Tabs 15, 30, 45 mg.

NOTES – Reports of fracture risk. Do not use in Type 1 DM or diabetic ketoacidosis. Urinary bladder tumors reported; advise patients to report macroscopic hematuria or dysuria.

ROSIGLITAZONE (***Avandia***) ▶L ♀C ▶– $$$$

ADULT – Type 2 DM monotherapy or in combination with metformin or sulfonylurea: Start 4 mg PO daily or divided two times per day, may increase after 8 to 12 weeks to max 8 mg/day.

PEDS – Not approved in children younger than 18 yo.

FORMS – Trade only (restricted access): Tabs 2, 4, 8 mg.

NOTES – Due to potential for elevated cardiovascular risks, restricted by FDA to use in patients where other medications cannot control Type 2 diabetes. In order to prescribe, providers must enroll in the Avandia-Rosiglitazone Medicines Access Program. Not recommended with nitrates or insulin, and its labeling includes boxed warning regarding increased risk of myocardial ischemic events and notes that studies are currently inconclusive. Reports of fracture risk.

ENDOCRINE AND METABOLIC: Diabetes-Related—Other

DEXTROSE (***Glutose, B-D Glucose, Insta-Glucose, Dex-4***) ▶L ♀C ▶? $

ADULT – Hypoglycemia: 0.5 to 1 g/kg (1 to 2 mL/kg) up to 25 g (50 mL) of 50% soln by slow IV injection. Hypoglycemia in conscious diabetics: 10 to 20 g PO q 10 to 20 min prn.

PEDS – Hypoglycemia in neonates: 0.25 to 0.5 g/kg/dose (5 to 10 mL of 25% dextrose in a 5 kg infant). Severe hypoglycemia or older infants may require larger doses up to 3 g (12 mL of 25% dextrose) followed by a continuous IV infusion of 10% dextrose. Non-neonates may require 0.5 to 1 g/kg.

FORMS – OTC Generic/Trade: Chewable tabs 4 g (Dex-4), 5 g (Glutose). Trade only: Oral gel 40%.

NOTES – Do not exceed an infusion rate of 0.5 g/kg/h.

GLUCAGON (*GlucaGen*) ▶LK ♀B ▶? $$$

ADULT – Hypoglycemia: 1 mg IV/IM/SC. If no response within 15 min, may repeat dose 1 to 2 times (preferred via IV for repeat). Diagnostic aid for GI tract radiography: 1 mg IV/IM/SC.

PEDS – Hypoglycemia in children wt greater than 20 kg: Same as adults. Hypoglycemia in children wt less than 20 kg: 0.5 mg IV/IM/SC or 20 to 30 mcg/kg. If no response in 5 to 20 min, may repeat dose 1 to 2 times.

UNAPPROVED ADULT – The following indications are based upon limited data. Esophageal obstruction caused by food: 1 mg IV over 1 to 3 min. Symptomatic bradycardia/hypotension, especially with beta-blocker therapy: 3 to 10 mg IV bolus (0.05 mg/kg general recommendation) may repeat in 10 min; may be followed by continuous infusion of 1 to 5 mg/h or 0.07 mg/kg/h. Infusion rate should be titrated to the desired response.

FORMS – Trade only: Injection 1 mg.

NOTES – Should be reserved for refractory/severe cases or when IV dextrose cannot be administered. Advise patients to educate family members and co-workers how to administer a dose. Give supplemental carbohydrates when patient responds.

METFORMIN (*Glucophage, Glucophage XR, Glumetza, Fortamet, Riomet*) ▶K ♀B ▶? $

ADULT – DM, type 2: Immediate-release: Start 500 mg PO one to two times per day or 850 mg PO daily with meals. Increase by 500 mg q week or 850 mg q 2 weeks to max 2550 mg/day. Higher doses may be divided three times per day with meals. Extended-release: Glucophage XR: 500 mg PO daily with evening meal; increase by 500 mg q week to max 2000 mg/day (may divide two times per day). Glumetza: 1000 mg PO daily with evening meal; increase by 500 mg q week to max 2000 mg/day (may divide two times per day). Fortamet: 500 to 1000 mg daily with evening meal; increase by 500 mg q week to max 2500 mg/day. All products started at low doses to improve GI tolerability, gradually increase as tolerated.

PEDS – DM, Type 2, 10 yo or older: Start 500 mg PO one to two times per day (Glucophage) with meals, increase by 500 mg q week to max 2000 mg/day in divided doses (10 to 16 yo). Glucophage XR and Fortamet are indicated for age 17 yo or older.

UNAPPROVED ADULT – Polycystic ovary syndrome: 500 mg PO three times per day or 850 mg PO two times per day. Prevention/delay DM Type 2 (with lifestyle modifications): 850 mg PO daily for 1 month, then increase to 850 mg PO two times per day.

FORMS – Generic/Trade: Tabs 500, 850, 1000 mg, extended-release 500, 750 mg. Trade only, extended-release: Fortamet 500, 1000 mg; Glumetza 500, 1000 mg. Trade only: Oral soln 500 mg/5 mL (Riomet).

NOTES – May reduce the risk of progression to Type 2 diabetes in those with impaired glucose tolerance, but less effectively than intensive lifestyle modification. Metformin-containing products may cause life-threatening lactic acidosis, usually in setting of decreased tissue perfusion, hypoxia, hepatic dysfunction, unstable congestive heart failure or impaired renal clearance. Hold prior to IV contrast agents and for 48 h after. Avoid if ethanol abuse, hepatic or renal insufficiency (creatinine 1.4 mg/dL or greater in women, 1.5 mg/dL or greater in men), or hypoxic states (cardiogenic shock, septicemia, acute MI). No clinical studies have established conclusive evidence of decreased macrovascular outcomes with antidiabetic drugs.

MIFEPRISTONE (*Korlym*) ♀X ▶– $$$$$

ADULT – DM, Type 2 in Cushing's syndrome (failed surgery or not surgical candidate): 300 mg PO once daily with meal. Titrate to max of 1200 mg daily. Max 20 mg/kg/day. In renal impairment or mild to moderate hepatic impairment, max 600 mg/day.

PEDS – Not approved in peds.

FORMS – Trade only: Tabs 300 mg.

NOTES – Contraindicated in pregnancy; antiprogestational effects result in termination. Confirm no pregnancy prior to initiation and if treatement is interrupted for more than 14 days in women of reproductive age. Do not use in women with endometrial hyperplasia or carcinoma or unexplained vaginal bleeding. Not for use in Type 2 diabetes unrelated to Cushing's syndrome.

PRAMLINTIDE (*Symlin, Symlinpen*) ▶K ♀C ▶? $$$$

WARNING – May cause severe insulin-induced hypoglycemia, especially in Type 1 DM, usually within 3 h. Avoid if hypoglycemic unawareness, gastroparesis, GI motility medications, alpha-glucosidase inhibitors, A1C more than 9%, poor compliance, or hypersensitivity to the metacresol preservative. Appropriate patient selection, careful patient instruction, and insulin dose adjustments (reduction in premeal short-acting insulin of 50%) are critical for reducing the hypoglycemia risk.

ADULT – DM, Type 1 with mealtime insulin therapy: Initiate 15 mcg SC immediately before major meals and titrate by 15-mcg increments (if significant nausea has not

(cont.)

PRAMLINTIDE *(cont.)*

occurred for at least 3 days) to maintenance 30 to 60 mcg as tolerated. If significant nausea, decrease to 30 mcg. DM, Type 2 with mealtime insulin therapy: Initiate 60 mcg SC immediately before major meals and increase to 120 mcg as tolerated (if significant nausea has not occurred for 3 to 7 days). If significant nausea, decrease dose to 60 mcg.

PEDS – Not approved in children.

FORMS – Trade only: 600 mcg/mL in 5 mL vials, 1000 mcg/mL pen injector (Symlinpen) 1.5, 2.7 mL.

NOTES – Keep unopened vials refrigerated. Opened vials can be kept at room temperature or refrigerated up to 28 days. May give SC in abdomen or thigh. Take medications that require rapid onset 1 h prior or 2 h after. Careful patient selection and skilled health care supervision are critical for safe and effective use. Monitor pre-/postmeal and bedtime glucose. Decrease initial premeal short-acting insulin doses by 50% including fixed-mix insulin (ie, 70/30). Do not mix with insulin. Use new needle and syringe for each dose.

ENDOCRINE AND METABOLIC: Diagnostic Agents

CORTICOTROPIN (*H.P. Acthar Gel*) ▸K ♀C ▸– $$$$$

ADULT – Diagnostic testing of adrenocortical function: 80 units IM or SC. Acute exacerbation of multiple sclerosis: 80 to 120 units IM daily for 2 to 3 weeks.

UNAPPROVED PEDS – Various dosing regimens have been used for infantile spasms.

NOTES – Limited therapeutic value in conditions responsive to corticosteroid therapy; corticosteroids should be the treatment of choice if responsive. Prolonged use in children may inhibit skeletal growth. Cosyntropin preferred for diagnostic testing as it is less allergenic and more potent.

COSYNTROPIN (*Cortrosyn*, ✤*Synacthen*) ▸L ♀C ▸? $

ADULT – Rapid screen for adrenocortical insufficiency: 0.25 mg IM/IV over 2 min; measure serum cortisol before and 30 to 60 min after.

PEDS – Rapid screen for adrenocortical insufficiency: 0.25 mg (0.125 mg if age younger than 2 yo) IM/IV over 2 min; measure serum cortisol before and 30 to 60 min after.

METYRAPONE (*Metopirone*) ▸KL ♀C ▸? $

WARNING – May cause acute adrenal insufficiency.

ADULT – Diagnostic aid for testing hypothalamic-pituitary adrenocorticotropic hormone (ACTH) function: Specialized single- and multiple-test dose available.

PEDS – Diagnostic aid for testing hypothalamic-pituitary adrenocorticotropic hormone (ACTH) function: Specialized single- and multiple-test dose available.

UNAPPROVED ADULT – Cushing's syndrome: Dosing varies.

FORMS – Trade only: Caps 250 mg. Only available from manufacturer due to limited supply: 1-800-988-7768.

NOTES – Ability of adrenals to respond to exogenous ACTH should be demonstrated before metyrapone is employed as a test. In the presence of hypo- or hyperthyroidism, response to the test may be subnormal. May suppress aldosterone synthesis. May cause dizziness and sedation.

ENDOCRINE AND METABOLIC: Gout-Related

ALLOPURINOL (*Aloprim, Zyloprim*) ▸K ♀C ▸+ $

ADULT – Mild gout or recurrent calcium oxalate stones: 200 to 300 mg PO daily (start with 100 mg PO daily). Moderately severe gout: 400 to 600 mg PO daily. Secondary hyperuricemia: 600 to 800 mg PO daily. Doses in excess of 300 mg should be divided. Max 800 mg/day. Reduce dose in renal insufficiency (CrCl 10 to 20 mL/min: 200 mg/day, CrCl 3 to 10 mL/min: 100 mg/day, CrCl less than 3 mL/min: 100 mg/day at extended intervals). Prevention of hyperuricemia secondary to chemotherapy and unable to tolerate PO: 200 to 400 mg/m^2/day as a single IV infusion or in equally divided infusions q 6 to 12 h. Max 600 mg/day. Reduce dose in renal insufficiency (CrCl 10 to 20 mL/min: 200 mg/day, CrCl 3 to 10 mL/min: 100 mg/day, CrCl less than 3 mL/min: 100 mg/day at extended intervals). Initiate 24 to 48 h before chemotherapy.

PEDS – Secondary hyperuricemia: Age younger than 6 yo give 150 mg PO daily; age 6 to 10 yo give 300 mg PO daily or 1 mg/kg/day divided q 6 h to max 600 mg/day. Prevention

(cont.)

ALLOPURINOL (*cont.*)

of hyperuricemia secondary to chemotherapy and unable to tolerate PO: Initiate with 200 mg/m²/day as a single IV infusion or in equally divided infusions q 6 to 12 h.

FORMS – Generic/Trade: Tabs 100, 300 mg.

NOTES – May precipitate acute gout; consider using NSAIDs or colchicine prophylactically. Start with 100 mg PO daily and increase weekly to target serum uric acid of less than 6 mg/dL. Incidence of rash and allopurinol hypersensitivity syndrome is increased in renal impairment. Discontinue if rash or allergic symptoms, do not restart after severe rash. Drug interaction with warfarin and azathioprine. Normal serum uric acid levels are usually achieved after 1 to 3 weeks of therapy. Ensure hydration before IV administration.

COLBENEMID **(colchicine + probenecid)** ▶KL ♀C ◗? $

ADULT – Chronic gouty arthritis: Start 1 tab PO daily for 1 week, then 1 tab PO two times per day.

PEDS – Not approved in children.

FORMS – Generic only: Tabs 0.5 mg colchicine + 500 mg probenecid.

NOTES – Maintain alkaline urine. Probenecid ineffective if CrCl is less than 30 ml/min.

COLCHICINE (***Colcrys***) ▶L ♀C ◗? $$$$

ADULT – Acute gout: 1.2 mg (2 tabs) PO at signs of attack then 0.6 mg (1 tab) 1 h later. CrCl less than 30 mL/min: Do not repeat more than q 2 weeks. CrCl less than 15 mL/min: 0.6 mg PO for 1 dose; do not repeat more than q 2 weeks. Familial Mediterranean fever: 1.2 to 2.4 mg PO daily or divided two times per day. See prescribing information in renal insufficiency.

PEDS – Familial Mediterranean fever: Age 4 to 6 yo: 0.3 to 1.8 mg PO daily or divided two times per day; age 6 to 12 yo: 0.9 to 1.8 mg daily or divided two times per day; age 12 yo or older: See adult dosing.

UNAPPROVED ADULT – Gout prophylaxis: 0.6 mg PO two times per day if CrCl is 50 mL/min or greater, 0.6 mg PO daily if CrCl is 35 to 49 mL/min, 0.6 mg PO q 2 to 3 days if CrCl is 10 to 34 mL/min. Primary biliary cirrhosis: 0.6 mg PO two times per day.

FORMS – Trade: Tabs 0.6 mg.

NOTES – Contraindicated with P-glycoprotein or strong CYP3A4 inhibitors. Lower max doses with specific concomitant drugs. For familial Mediterranean fever, increase or decrease by 0.3 mg/day to effect/tolerability up to max. Most effective when initiated on the 1st day of gouty arthritis.

FEBUXOSTAT (***Uloric***) ▶LK ♀C ◗? $$$$

ADULT – Hyperuricemia with gout: Start 40 mg daily. After 2 weeks, if uric acid is greater than 6 mg/dL may increase to 80 mg daily.

PEDS – Not approved in children.

FORMS – Trade only: Tabs 40, 80 mg.

NOTES – May precipitate acute gout; consider using NSAIDs or colchicine prophylactically for up to 6 months. Monitor LFTs periodically. Do not use with azathioprine, mercaptopurine, or theophylline. May increase risk of thromboembolic events, monitor for cardiovascular events (MI, CVA). Caution in severe renal or hepatic impairment.

PEGLOTICASE (***Krystexxa***) ▶NA ♀C ◗? $$$$$

WARNING – Anaphylaxis and infusion reactions reported. Premedicate with antihistamines and corticosteroids and administer in a healthcare setting. Anaphylaxis and infusion reactions more common if loss of therapeutic response. Monitor uric acid levels before infusion and discontinue if greater than 6 mg/dL, especially if two consecutive levels greater than 6.

ADULT – Chronic gout (refractory): 8 mg IV infusion q 2 weeks. Administer over 120 minutes or longer.

FORMS – Trade only: single-use vial (8 mg/mL).

NOTES – Gout flares frequent upon initiation. Recommend gout flare prophylaxis with NSAID or colchicine to start 1 week prior to therapy and continuing for first 6 months. Discontinue urate-lowering therapy. Contraindicated in G6PD deficiency due to risk of hemolysis and methemoglobinemia; screen those at high risk including those of African and Mediterranean ancestry.

PROBENECID ▶KL ♀B ◗? $

ADULT – Gout: 250 mg PO two times per day for 7 days, then 500 mg PO two times per day. May increase by 500 mg/day q 4 weeks not to exceed 2 g/day. Adjunct to penicillin: 2 g/day PO in divided doses.

PEDS – Adjunct to penicillin: In children 2 to 14 yo use 25 mg/kg PO initially, then 40 mg/kg/day divided four times per day. For children greater than 50 kg, use adult dose. Contraindicated in children age younger than 2 yo.

FORMS – Generic only: Tabs 500 mg.

NOTES – Decrease dose if GI intolerance occurs. Maintain alkaline urine. Begin therapy 2 to 3 weeks after acute gouty attack subsides. Ineffective if CrCl is less than 30 ml/min. Not recommended in combination with penicillin if renal impairment.

ENDOCRINE AND METABOLIC: Minerals

CALCIUM ACETATE (*PhosLo, Eliphos*) ▶K ♀C ◗? $$$$

ADULT – Phosphate binder to reduce serum phosphorous in end-stage renal disease: Initially 2 tabs/caps PO three times per day with each meal. Titrate dose gradually based on serum phosphorus. Usual dose 3 to 4 tabs/caps per meal.

PEDS – Not approved in children.

UNAPPROVED PEDS – Titrate to response.

FORMS – Generic/Trade: Gelcaps 667 mg (169 mg elem Ca). Trade: Tab 667 mg (169 mg elem Ca).

NOTES – Avoid calcium supplements and antacids with calcium. Monitor serum calcium twice weekly initially and during dosage adjustment. Monitor for signs of hypercalcemia and discontinue if occurs. Consider decreasing or discontinuing vitamin D supplementation if mild hypercalcemia occurs. Maintain serum calcium-phosphorous product (Ca × P) less than 55. Hypercalcemia may aggrevate digoxin toxicity.

CALCIUM CARBONATE (*Caltrate, Mylanta Children's, Os-Cal, Oyst-Cal, Tums, Surpass, Viactiv,* ✤ *Calsan*) ▶K ♀+ (? 1st trimester) ◗? $

ADULT – Supplement: 1 to 2 g elem Ca/day or more PO with meals divided two to four times per day. Prevention of osteoporosis: 1000 to 1500 mg elem Ca/day PO divided two to three times per day with meals. Adequate intake in most adults is 1000 to 1200 mg elem Ca/day. Antacid: 1000 to 3000 mg (2 to 4 tab) PO q 2 h prn or 1 to 2 pieces gum chewed prn, max 7000 mg/day.

PEDS – Hypocalcemia: Neonates: 50 to 150 mg elem Ca/kg/day PO in 4 to 6 divided doses; Children: 45 to 65 mg elem Ca/kg/day PO divided four times per day. Adequate intake for children (in elem calcium): Age younger than 6 mo: 210 mg/day when fed human milk and 315 mg/day when fed cow's milk; 6 to 12 mo: 270 mg/day when fed human milk plus solid food and 335 mg/day when fed cow's milk plus solid food; 1 to 3 yo: 500 mg/day; 4 to 8 yo: 800 mg/day; 9 to 18 yo 1300 mg/day.

UNAPPROVED ADULT – May lower BP in patients with HTN. May reduce PMS symptoms such as fluid retention, pain, and negative affect.

FORMS – OTC Generic/Trade: Tabs 500, 650, 750, 1000, 1250, 1500 mg, Chewable tabs 400, 500, 750, 850, 1000, 1177, 1250 mg, Caps 1250 mg, Gum 300, 450 mg, Susp 1250 mg/5 mL. Calcium carbonate is 40% elem Ca and contains 20 mEq of elem Ca/g calcium carbonate. Not more than 500 to 600 mg elem Ca/dose. Available in combination with sodium fluoride, vitamin D, and/or vitamin K. Trade examples: Caltrate 600 + D = 600 mg elemental Ca/200 units vitamin D, Os-Cal 500 + D = 500 mg elemental Ca/200 units vitamin D, Os-Cal Extra D = 500 mg elemental Ca/400 units vitamin D, Tums (regular strength) = 200 mg elemental Ca, Tums (ultra) = 400 mg elemental Ca, Viactiv (chewable) 500 mg elemental Ca+ 100 units vitamin D + 40 mcg vitamin K.

NOTES – Decreases absorption of levothyroxine, tetracycline, and fluoroquinolones.

CALCIUM CHLORIDE ▶K ♀+ ◗+ $

ADULT – Hypocalcemia: 500 to 1000 mg slow IV q 1 to 3 days. Magnesium intoxication: 500 mg IV. Hyperkalemic ECG changes: Dose based on ECG.

PEDS – Hypocalcemia: 0.2 mL/kg IV up to 10 mL/day. Cardiac resuscitation: 0.2 mL/kg IV.

UNAPPROVED ADULT – Has been used in calcium channel blocker toxicity and to treat or prevent calcium channel blocker–induced hypotension.

UNAPPROVED PEDS – Has been used in calcium channel blocker toxicity.

FORMS – Generic only: Injectable 10% (1000 mg/10 mL) 10 mL ampules, vials, syringes.

NOTES – Calcium chloride contains 14.4 mEq Ca/g versus calcium gluconate 4.7 mEq Ca/g. For IV use only; do not administer IM or SC. Avoid extravasation. Administer no faster than 0.5 to 1 mL/min. Use cautiously in patients receiving digoxin; inotropic and toxic effects are synergistic and may cause arrhythmias. Usually not recommended for hypocalcemia associated with renal insufficiency because calcium chloride is an acidifying salt.

CALCIUM CITRATE (*Citracal*) ▶K ♀+ ◗+ $

ADULT – 1 to 2 g elem Ca/day or more PO with meals divided two to four times per day. Prevention of osteoporosis: 1000 to 1500 mg elem Ca/day PO divided two to three times per day with meals. The adequate intake in most adults is 1000 to 1200 mg elem Ca/day.

PEDS – Not approved in children.

FORMS – OTC Trade/generic (mg elem Ca/units vitamin D): 200/250, 250/200, 315/250, 600/500 (slow release); some products available with magnesium and/or phosphorous.

(cont.)

CALCIUM CITRATE (*cont.*)

Chewable gummies: 250 mg with 250 units vitamin D.

NOTES – Calcium citrate is 21% elem Ca. Not more than 500 to 600 mg elem Ca/dose. Decreases absorption of levothyroxine, tetracycline, and fluoroquinolones. Acidic environment not needed for absorption; preferred calcium salt in patients on PPI or H2RA.

CALCIUM GLUCONATE ▶K ♀+ ▶+ $

ADULT – Emergency correction of hypocalcemia: 7 to 14 mEq slow IV prn. Hypocalcemic tetany: 4.5 to 16 mEq IM prn. Hyperkalemia with cardiac toxicity: 2.25 to 14 mEq IV while monitoring ECG. May repeat after 1 to 2 min. Magnesium intoxication: 4.5 to 9 mEq IV, adjust dose based on patient response. If IV not possible, give 2 to 5 mEq IM. Exchange transfusions: 1.35 mEq calcium gluconate IV concurrent with each 100 mL of citrated blood. Oral calcium gluconate: 1 to 2 g elem Ca/day or more PO with meals divided two to four times per day. Prevention of osteoporosis: 1000 to 1500 mg elem Ca/day PO with meals in divided doses.

PEDS – Emergency correction of hypocalcemia: Children: 1 to 7 mEq IV prn. Infants: 1 mEq IV prn. Hypocalcemic tetany: Children: 0.5 to 0.7 mEq/kg IV three to four times per day. Neonates: 2.4 mEq/kg/day IV in divided doses. Exchange transfusions: Neonates: 0.45 mEq IV/100 mL of exchange transfusions. Oral calcium gluconate: Hypocalcemia: Neonates: 50 to 150 mg elem Ca/kg/day PO in 4 to 6 divided doses; children: 45 to 65 mg elem Ca/kg/day PO divided four times per day.

UNAPPROVED ADULT – Has been used in calcium channel blocker toxicity and to treat or prevent calcium channel blocker-induced hypotension.

UNAPPROVED PEDS – Has been used in calcium channel blocker toxicity.

FORMS – Generic only: Injectable 10% (1000 mg/10 mL, 4.65 mEq/10 mL) 1, 10, 50, 100, 200 mL. OTC Generic only: Tabs 50, 500, 650, 975, 1000 mg. Chewable tabs 650 mg.

NOTES – Calcium gluconate is 9.3% elem Ca and contains 4.6 mEq elem Ca/g calcium gluconate. Administer IV calcium gluconate not faster than 0.5 to 2 mL/min. Use cautiously in patients receiving digoxin; inotropic and toxic effects are synergistic and may cause arrhythmias.

COPPER GLUCONATE ▶L – ♀A ▶? $

ADULT – Supplementation: 2 to 5 mg PO daily. RDA: Adults: 900 mcg PO daily; pregnancy: 1000 mcg PO daily; breastfeeding: 1300 mcg PO daily.

PEDS – RDA: 14 to 18 yo: 890 mcg PO daily; 9 to 13 yo: 700 mcg PO daily; 4 to 8 yo: 440 mcg PO daily; 1 to 3 yo: 340 mcg PO daily; 7 to 12 mo: 220 mcg PO daily; 0 to 6 mo: 200 mcg PO daily.

FORMS – OTC Generic: 2, 5 mg.

FERRIC GLUCONATE COMPLEX (***Ferrlecit***) ▶KL ♀B ▶? $$$$$

WARNING – Potentially fatal hypersensitivity reactions rarely reported with sodium ferric gluconate complex. Facilities for CPR must be available during dosing.

ADULT – Iron deficiency in chronic hemodialysis patients: 125 mg elem iron IV over 10 min or diluted in 100 mL NS IV over 1 h. Most hemodialysis patients require 1 g of elem iron over 8 consecutive hemodialysis sessions.

PEDS – Iron deficiency in chronic hemodialysis, age 6 yo or older: 1.5 mg/kg elem iron diluted in 25 mL NS and administered IV over 1 h at 8 sequential dialysis sessions. Max 125 mg/dose.

UNAPPROVED ADULT – Iron deficiency in cancer and chemotherapy-induced anemia: 125 mg elem iron IV over 60 min, repeat weekly for 8 doses, or 200 mg IV over 3 to 4 h repeated q 3 weeks for 5 doses.

NOTES – Potentially fatal hypersensitivity reactions, including serious hypotension, reported with sodium ferric gluconate complex. Facilities for CPR must be available during dosing.

FERROUS GLUCONATE (***Fergon***) ▶K ♀+ ▶+ $

WARNING – Severe iron toxicity possible in overdose, especially in children. Store out of reach of children and in child-resistant containers. Iron overdose is a leading cause of poisoning in children younger than 6 yo.

ADULT – Iron deficiency: 800 to 1600 mg ferrous gluconate (100 to 200 mg elem iron) PO divided three times per day. RDA (elem iron): 8 mg for adult males age 19 yo or older, 18 mg for adult premenopausal females age 19 to 50 yo, 8 mg for females age 51 yo or older, 27 mg during pregnancy, 10 mg during lactation if age 14 to 18 yo and 9 mg if age 19 to 50 yo. Upper limit: 45 mg/day.

PEDS – Mild to moderate iron deficiency: 3 mg/kg/day of elem iron PO in 1 to 2 divided doses. Severe iron deficiency: 4 to 6 mg/kg/day PO in 3 divided doses. RDA (elem iron): 0.27 mg for age younger than 6 mo, 11 mg for age 7 to 12 mo, 7 mg for age 1 to 3 yo, 10 mg for age 4 to 8 yo, 8 mg for age 9 to 13 yo, 11 mg for males age 14 to 18 yo, 15 mg for females age 14 to 18 yo.

(cont.)

FERROUS GLUCONATE (*cont.*)

UNAPPROVED ADULT – Adjunct to epoetin to maximize hematologic response: 200 mg elem iron/day PO.

UNAPPROVED PEDS – Adjunct to epoetin to maximize hematologic response: 2 to 3 mg/kg elem iron/day PO.

FORMS – OTC Generic/Trade: Tabs (ferrous gluconate) 240 mg (27 mg elemental iron). Generic only: Tabs 324, 325 mg.

NOTES – Ferrous gluconate is 12% elem iron. For iron deficiency, 4 to 6 months of therapy generally necessary to replete stores even after hemoglobin has returned to normal. Do not take within 2 h of antacids, tetracyclines, levothyroxine, or fluoroquinolones. May cause black stools, constipation, or diarrhea.

FERROUS SULFATE (***Fer-in-Sol, Feosol, Slow FE, ♣ Ferodan, Slow-Fe***) ▶K ♀+ ▶+ $

WARNING – Severe iron toxicity possible in overdose, especially in children. Store out of reach of children and in child-resistant containers. Iron overdose is the leading cause of poisoning in children younger than 6 yo.

ADULT – Iron deficiency: 500 to 1000 mg ferrous sulfate (100 to 200 mg elem iron) PO divided three times per day. For iron supplementation RDA see ferrous gluconate.

PEDS – Mild to moderate iron deficiency: 3 mg/kg/day of elem iron PO in 1 to 2 divided doses; Severe iron deficiency: 4 to 6 mg/kg/day PO in 3 divided doses. For iron supplementation RDA see ferrous gluconate.

UNAPPROVED ADULT – Adjunct to epoetin to maximize hematologic response: 200 mg elem iron/day PO.

FORMS – OTC Generic/Trade (mg ferrous sulfate): Tabs extended-release 160 mg. Tabs 200, 324, 325 mg. OTC Generic only (mg ferrous sulfate): Soln 75 mg/0.6 mL, Elixir 220 mg/5 mL.

NOTES – Iron sulfate is 20% elem iron. For iron deficiency, 4 to 6 months of therapy generally necessary. Do not take within 2 h of antacids, tetracyclines, levothyroxine, or fluoroquinolones. May cause black stools, constipation or diarrhea.

FERUMOXYTOL (***Feraheme***) ▶KL ♀C ▶? $$$$$

ADULT – Iron deficiency in chronic kidney disease: Give 510 mg IV push, followed by 510 mg IV push for 1 dose given 3 to 8 days after initial injection. May readminister if persistent/recurrent iron deficiency anemia.

PEDS – Not studied in pediatrics.

NOTES – Administer IV push undiluted up to 30 mg/sec. Monitor hemoglobin and iron studies at least 1 month following second injection. Observe for hypersensitivity for at least 30 min following injection, life-threatening hypersensitivity reported. May alter MRI imaging studies. Contraindicated in anemias not due to iron deficiency.

FLUORIDE (***Luride, ♣ Fluor-A-Day***) ▶K ♀? ▶? $

ADULT – Prevention of dental cavities: 10 mL of topical rinse swish and spit daily.

PEDS – Prevention of dental caries: Dose based on age and fluoride concentrations in water. See table.

FORMS – Generic only: Chewable tabs 0.5, 1 mg; Tabs 1 mg, gtts 0.125 mg, 0.25 mg, and 0.5 mg/dropperful, Lozenges 1 mg, Soln 0.2 mg/mL, Gel 0.1%, 0.5%, 1.23%, Rinse (sodium fluoride) 0.05, 0.1, 0.2%.

NOTES – In communities without fluoridated water, fluoride supplementation should be used until 13 to 16 yo. Chronic overdosage of fluorides may result in dental fluorosis (mottling of tooth enamel) and osseous changes. Use rinses and gels after brushing and flossing and before bedtime.

IRON DEXTRAN (***InFed, DexFerrum, ♣ Dexiron, Infufer***) ▶KL ♀C ▶? $$$$

WARNING – Administer a test dose prior to 1st dose. Parenteral iron therapy has resulted in anaphylactic reactions, even with test dose and after uneventful test doses. Potentially

(cont.)

IV SOLUTIONS

Solution	Dextrose	Calories/ Liter	Na*	Ca*	Lactate*	Osm*
0.9 NS	0 g/L	0	154	0	0	310
LR	0 g/L	9	130	3	28	273
D5 W	50 g/L	170	0	0	0	253
D5 0.2 NS	50 g/L	170	34	0	0	320
D5 0.45 NS	50 g/L	170	77	0	0	405
D5 0.9 NS	50 g/L	170	154	0	0	560
D5 LR	50 g/L	179	130	2.7	28	527

* All given in mEq/L

FLUORIDE SUPPLEMENTATION

Age	<0.3 ppm in drinking water	0.3–0.6 ppm in drinking water	>0.6 ppm in drinking water
0–6 mo	none	none	none
6 mo–3 yo	0.25 mg PO daily	none	none
3–6 yo	0.5 mg PO daily	0.25 mg PO daily	none
6–16 yo	1 mg PO daily	0.5 mg PO daily	none

JADA 2010;141:1480-1489

IRON DEXTRAN (*cont.*)

fatal hypersensitivity reactions have been reported with iron dextran injection. Facilities for CPR must be available during dosing. Use only when clearly warranted.

ADULT – Iron deficiency: Dose based on patient wt and hemoglobin. Total dose (mL) = 0.0442 × (desired Hgb – observed Hgb) × wt (kg) + [0.26 × wt (kg)]. For wt, use lesser of lean body wt or actual body wt. Iron replacement for blood loss: Replacement iron (mg) = blood loss (mL) × hematocrit. Max daily IM dose 100 mg.

PEDS – Not recommended for infants younger than 4 mo. Iron deficiency in children greater than 5 kg: Dose based on patient wt and hemoglobin. Dose (mL) = 0.0442 × (desired Hgb – observed Hgb) × wt (kg) + [0.26 × wt (kg)]. For wt, use lesser of lean body wt or actual body wt. Iron replacement for blood loss: Replacement iron (mg) = blood loss (mL) × hematocrit. Max daily IM dose: Infant wt less than 5 kg give 25 mg; children 5 to 10 kg give 50 mg; children wt greater than 10 kg give 100 mg.

UNAPPROVED ADULT – Adjunct to epoetin to maximize hematologic response. Total dose (325 to 1500 mg) as a single, slow (6 mg/min) IV infusion has been used.

UNAPPROVED PEDS – Adjunct to epoetin to maximize hematologic response.

NOTES – A 0.5 mL IV test dose (0.25 mL in infants) over 30 sec or longer should be given at least 1 h before therapy. Infuse no faster than 50 mg/min. For IM administration, use Z-track technique.

IRON POLYSACCHARIDE (***Niferex, Niferex-150, Nu-Iron 150, Ferrex 150***) ▶K ♀+ ▶+ $$

WARNING – Severe iron toxicity possible in overdose, especially in children. Store out of reach of children and in child-resistant containers. Iron overdose is the leading cause of poisoning in children younger than 6 yo.

ADULT – Iron deficiency: 50 to 200 mg PO divided one to three times per day. For iron supplementation RDA see ferrous gluconate.

PEDS – Mild to moderate iron deficiency: 3 mg/kg/day of elem iron PO in 1 to 2 divided doses. Severe iron deficiency: 4 to 6 mg/kg/day PO in 3 divided doses. For iron supplementation RDA see ferrous gluconate.

UNAPPROVED ADULT – Adjunct to epoetin to maximize hematologic response: 200 mg elem iron/day PO.

UNAPPROVED PEDS – Adjunct to epoetin to maximize hematologic response: 2 to 3 mg/kg elem iron/day PO.

FORMS – OTC Trade only: Caps 60 mg (Niferex). OTC Generic/Trade: Caps 150 mg (Niferex-150, Nu-Iron 150, Ferrex-150), Elixir 100 mg/5 mL (Niferex). 1 mg iron polysaccharide = 1 mg elemental iron.

NOTES – For iron deficiency, 4 to 6 months of therapy generally necessary. Do not take within 2 h of antacids, tetracyclines, levothyroxine, or fluoroquinolones. May cause black stools, constipation, or diarrhea.

IRON SUCROSE (***Venofer***) ▶KL ♀B ▶? $$$$$

WARNING – Potentially fatal hypersensitivity reactions have been rarely reported with iron sucrose injection. Facilities for CPR must be available during dosing.

ADULT – Iron deficiency in chronic hemodialysis patients: 5 mL (100 mg elem iron) IV over 5 min or diluted in 100 mL NS IV over 15 min or longer. Iron deficiency in nondialysis chronic kidney disease patients: 10 mL (200 mg elem iron) IV over 5 min or 500 mg diluted in 250 mL NS IV over 4 h.

PEDS – Not approved in children.

UNAPPROVED ADULT – Iron deficiency: 5 mL (100 mg elem iron) IV over 5 min or diluted in 100 mL NS IV over 15 min or longer.

NOTES – Most hemodialysis patients require 1 g of elem iron over 10 consecutive hemodialysis sessions. Nondialysis patients require 1 g of elemental iron divided and given over 14 days. Observe patients for at least 30 minutes following administration; anaphylaxis reported.

MAGNESIUM CHLORIDE (*Slow-Mag*) ▶K ♀A ▶+ $

ADULT – Dietary supplement: 2 tabs PO daily. RDA (elem Mg): Adult males: 400 mg if 19 to 30 yo, 420 mg if older than 30 yo. Adult females: 310 mg if 19 to 30 yo, 320 mg if older than 30 yo.

PEDS – Not approved in children.

UNAPPROVED ADULT – Hypomagnesemia: 300 mg elem magnesium PO divided four times per day.

FORMS – OTC Trade only: Enteric-coated tab 64 mg. 64 mg tab Slow-Mag = 64 mg elemental magnesium.

NOTES – May cause diarrhea. May accumulate in renal insufficiency.

MAGNESIUM GLUCONATE (*Almora, Magtrate, Maganate,* ✤ *Maglucate*) ▶K ♀A ▶+ $

ADULT – Dietary supplement: 500 to 1000 mg/day PO divided three times per day. RDA (elem Mg): Adult males: 19 to 30 yo: 400 mg; older than 30 yo: 420 mg. Adult females: 19 to 30 yo: 310 mg; older than 30 yo: 320 mg.

PEDS – Not approved in children.

UNAPPROVED ADULT – Hypomagnesemia: 300 mg elem magnesium PO divided four times per day. Unproven efficacy for oral tocolysis following IV magnesium sulfate.

UNAPPROVED PEDS – Hypomagnesemia: 10 to 20 mg elem magnesium/kg/dose PO four times per day. RDA (elem Mg): Age 0 to 6 mo: 30 mg/day; age 7 to 12 mo: 75 mg/day; age 1 to 3 yo: 80 mg; age 4 to 8 yo: 130 mg; age 9 to 13 yo: 240 mg; age 14 to 18 yo (males): 410 mg; age 14 to 18 yo (females): 360 mg.

FORMS – OTC Generic only: Tabs 500 mg (27 mg elemental Mg), liquid 54 mg elemental Mg/5 mL.

NOTES – May cause diarrhea. Use caution in renal failure; may accumulate.

MAGNESIUM OXIDE (*Mag-200, Mag-Ox 400*) ▶K ♀A ▶+ $

ADULT – Dietary supplement: 400 to 800 mg PO daily. RDA (elem Mg): Adult males: 19 to 30 yo: 400 mg; older than 30 yo: 420 mg. Adult females: 19 to 30 yo: 310 mg; older than 30 yo: 320 mg.

PEDS – Not approved in children.

UNAPPROVED ADULT – Hypomagnesemia: 300 mg elem magnesium PO four times per day. Has also been used as oral tocolysis following IV magnesium sulfate (unproven efficacy) and in the prevention of calcium-oxalate kidney stones.

FORMS – OTC Generic/Trade: Caps: 140 (84.5 mg elemental Mg), 250 (elemental), 400 (240 mg elemental Mg), 420 (253 mg elemental Mg), 500 mg (elemental).

NOTES – Take with food. Magnesium oxide is approximately 60% elemental magnesium. May accumulate in renal insufficiency.

MAGNESIUM SULFATE ▶K ♀A ▶+ $

ADULT – Hypomagnesemia: Mild deficiency: 1 g IM q 6 h for 4 doses; severe deficiency: 2 g IV over 1 h (monitor for hypotension). Hyperalimentation: Maintenance requirements not precisely known; adults generally require 8 to 24 mEq/day. Seizure prevention in preeclampsia or eclampsia: 4 to 6 g IV over 30 min, then 1 to 2 g IV per h. 5 g in 250 mL D5W

(cont.)

PEDIATRIC REHYDRATION SOLUTIONS

Brand	Glucose	Calories/ Liter	Na*	K*	Cl*	Citrate*	Phos*	Ca*	Mg*
CeraLyte 50†	0 g/L	160	50	20	40	30	0	0	0
CeraLyte 70†	0 g/L	160	70	20	60	30	0	0	0
CeraLyte 90†	0 g/L	160	90	20	80	30	0	0	0
Infalyte	30 g/L	140	50	25	45	34	0	0	0
Kao Lectrolyte†	20 g/L	90	50	20	40	30	0	0	0
Lytren (Canada)	20 g/L	80	50	25	45	30	0	0	0
Naturalyte	25 g/L	100	45	20	35	48	0	0	0
Pedialyte and Pedialyte Freezer Pops	25 g/L	100	45	20	35	30	0	0	0
Rehydralyte	25 g/L	100	75	20	65	30	0	0	0
Resol	20 g/L	80	50	20	50	34	5	4	4

* All given in mEq/L

† Premeasured powder packet

MAGNESIUM SULFATE (*cont.*)

(20 mg/mL), 2 g/h = 100 mL/h. 4 to 5 g of a 50% soln IM q 4 h prn.

PEDS – Not approved in children.

UNAPPROVED ADULT – Preterm labor: 6 g IV over 20 min, then 1 to 3 g/h titrated to decrease contractions. Has been used as an adjunctive bronchodilator in very severe acute asthma (2 g IV over 10 to 20 min), and in chronic fatigue syndrome. Torsades de pointes: 1 to 2 g IV in D5W over 5 to 60 min.

UNAPPROVED PEDS – Hypomagnesemia: 25 to 50 mg/kg IV/IM q 4 to 6 h for 3 to 4 doses, max single dose 2 g. Hyperalimentation: Maintenance requirements not precisely known; infants require 2 to 10 mEq/day. Acute nephritis: 20 to 40 mg/kg (in 20% soln) IM prn. Adjunctive bronchodilator in very severe acute asthma: 25 to 100 mg/kg IV over 10 to 20 min.

NOTES – 1000 mg magnesium sulfate contains 8 mEq elem magnesium. Do not give faster than 1.5 mL/min (of 10% soln) except in eclampsia or seizures. Use caution in renal insufficiency; may accumulate. Monitor urine output, patellar reflex, respiratory rate and serum magnesium level. Concomitant use with terbutaline may lead to fatal pulmonary edema. IM administration must be diluted to a 20% soln. If needed, may reverse toxicity with calcium gluconate 1 g IV.

PHOSPHORUS (***Neutra-Phos, K-Phos***) ▶K ♀C ◗? $

ADULT – Dietary supplement: 1 cap/packet (Neutra-Phos) PO four times per day or 1 to 2 tabs (K-Phos) PO four times per day after meals and at bedtime. Severe hypophosphatemia (less than 1 mg/dL): 0.08 to 0.16 mmol/kg IV over 6 h. In TPN, 310 to 465 mg/day (10 to 15 mmol/1000 kcal.) IV is usually adequate, although higher amounts may be necessary in hypermetabolic states. RDA for adults is 800 mg.

PEDS – RDA(elem phosphorus): 0 to 6 mo: 100 mg; 6 to 12 mo: 275 mg; 1 to 3 yo: 460 mg; 4 to 8 yo: 500 mg; 9 to 18: 1250 mg. Severe hypophosphatemia (less than 1 mg/dL): 0.25 to 0.5 mmol/kg IV over 4 to 6 h. Infant TPN: 1.5 to 2 mmol/kg/day in TPN.

FORMS – OTC Trade only: (Neutra-Phos, Neutra-Phos K) tab/cap/packet 250 mg (8 mmol) phosphorus. Rx: Trade only: (K-Phos) tab 250 mg (8 mmol) phosphorus.

NOTES – Dissolve caps/tabs/powder in 75 mL water prior to ingestion.

POTASSIUM (oral forms)*

Effervescent Granules	
20 mEq	Klorvess Effervescent, K-vescent
Effervescent Tabs	
10 mEq	Effer-K
20 mEq	Effer-K
25 mEq	Effer-K, K+Care ET, K-Lyte, K-Lyte/Cl, Klor-Con/EF
50 mEq	K-Lyte DS, K-Lyte/Cl 50
Liquids	
20 mEq/15 mL	Cena-K, Kaochlor S-F, K-G Elixir, Kaochlor 10%, Kay Ciel, Kaon, Kaylixir, Kolyum, Potasalan, Twin-K
30 mEq/15 mL	Rum-K
40 mEq/15 mL	Cena-K, Kaon-Cl 20%
45 mEq/15 mL	Tri-K
Powders	
15 mEq/pack	K+Care
20 mEq/pack	Gen-K, K+Care, Kay Ciel, K-Lor, Klor-Con
25 mEq/pack	K+Care, Klor-Con 25
Tabs/Caps	
8 mEq	K+8, Klor-Con 8, Slow-K, Micro-K
10 mEq	K+10, K-Norm, Kaon-Cl 10, Klor-Con M10 Klotrix, K-Tab, K-Dur 10, Micro-K 10
20 mEq	Klor-Con M20, K-Dur 20

*Table provides examples and is not intended to be all inclusive.

POTASSIUM (***Cena-K, Effer-K, K+8, K+10, Kaochlor, Kaon, Kaon Cl, Kay Ciel, Kaylixir, K+Care, K+Care ET, K-Dur, K-G Elixir, K-Lease, K-Lor, Klor-con, Klorvess Effervescent, Klotrix, K-Lyte, K-Lyte Cl, K-Norm, Kolyum, K-Tab, K-vescent, Micro-K, Micro-K LS, Sl***) ▶K ♀C ▶? $

ADULT – Hypokalemia: 20 to 40 mEq/day or more IV or immediate-release PO. Intermittent infusion: 10 to 20 mEq/dose IV over 1 to 2 h prn. Consider monitoring for infusions greater than 10 mEq/h. Prevention of hypokalemia: 20 to 40 mEq/day PO one to two times per day.

PEDS – Not approved in children.

UNAPPROVED ADULT – Diuretic-induced hypokalemia: 20 to 60 mEq/day PO.

UNAPPROVED PEDS – Hypokalemia: 2.5 mEq/kg/day given IV/PO one to two times per day. Intermittent infusion: 0.5 to 1 mEq/kg/dose IV at 0.3 to 0.5 mEq/kg/h prn. Infusions faster than 0.5 mEq/kg/h require continuous monitoring.

FORMS – Injectable, many different products in a variety of salt forms (ie, chloride, bicarbonate, citrate, acetate, gluconate), available in tabs, caps, liquids, effervescent tabs, packets. Potassium gluconate is available OTC. See table.

NOTES – Use potassium chloride for hypokalemia associated with alkalosis; use potassium bicarbonate, citrate, acetate, or gluconate when associated with acidosis.

ZINC ACETATE (***Galzin***) ▶Minimal absorption ♀A ▶– $$$

ADULT – RDA (elemental Zn): Adult males: 11 mg daily. Adult females: 8 to 12 mg daily. Zinc deficiency: 25 to 50 mg (elemental) daily. Wilson's disease, previously treated with chelating agent: 25 to 50 mg (elemental) PO three times per day.

PEDS – RDA (elem Zn): Age 7 mo to 3 yo: 3 mg; 4 to 8 yo: 5 mg; 9 to 13 yo: 8 mg; 14 to 18 yo (males): 8 mg; 14 to 18 yo (females): 9 to 14 mg. Zinc deficiency: 0.5 to 1 mg elemental zinc mg/kg/day divided two to three times per day. Wilson's disease (age 10 yo or older): 25 to 50 mg (elemental) three times per day.

FORMS – Trade only: Caps 25, 50 mg elemental zinc.

NOTES – Poorly absorbed; take 1 h before or 2 to 3 h after meals. Decreases absorption of tetracycline and fluoroquinolones.

ZINC SULFATE (***Orazinc, Zincate***) ▶Minimal absorption ♀A ▶– $

ADULT – RDA (elemental Zn): Adult males: 11 mg daily. Adult females: 8 to 12 mg daily. Zinc deficiency: 25 to 50 mg (elemental) PO daily.

PEDS – RDA (elemental Zn): Age 7 mo to 3 yo: 3 mg; 4 to 8 yo: 5 mg; 9 to 13 yo: 8 mg; 14 to 18 yo (males): 8 mg; 14 to 18 yo (females): 9 to 14 mg. Zinc deficiency: 0.5 to 1 mg elemental zinc mg/kg/day PO divided two to three times per day.

UNAPPROVED ADULT – Wound healing in zinc deficiency: 200 mg PO three times per day.

FORMS – OTC Generic/Trade: Tabs 66, 110, 200 mg. Rx Generic/Trade: Caps 220 mg.

NOTES – Zinc sulfate is 23% elemental Zn. Decreases absorption of tetracycline and fluoroquinolones. Poorly absorbed; increased absorption on empty stomach; however, administration with food decreases GI upset.

ENDOCRINE AND METABOLIC: Nutritionals

BANANA BAG ▶KL ♀+ ▶+ $

UNAPPROVED ADULT – Alcoholic malnutrition (one formula): Add thiamine 100 mg + folic acid 1 mg + IV multivitamins to 1 liter NS and infuse over 4 h. Magnesium sulfate 2 g may be added. "Banana bag" is jargon and not a valid drug order; also known as "rally pack"; specify individual components.

FAT EMULSION (***Intralipid, Liposyn***) ▶L ♀C ▶? $$$$$

WARNING – Deaths have occurred in preterm infants after infusion of IV fat emulsions. Autopsy results showed intravascular fat accumulation in the lungs. Strict adherence to total daily dose and administration rate is mandatory. Premature and small for gestational age infants have poor clearance of IV fat emulsion. Monitor infant's ability to eliminate fat (ie, triglycerides or plasma-free fatty acid levels).

ADULT – Calorie and essential fatty acids source: As part of TPN, fat emulsion should be no more than 60% of total calories; when correcting essential fatty acid deficiency, 8 to 10% of caloric intake should be supplied by lipids. Initial infusion rate 1 mL/min IV (10% fat emulsion) or 0.5 mL/min (20% fat emulsion) IV for first 15 to 30 min. If tolerated, increase rate. If using 10% fat emulsion, infuse no more than 500 mL 1st day and increase the next day. Max daily dose 2.5 g/kg. If using 20% fat emulsion, infuse up to

(cont.)

FAT EMULSION (*cont.*)

250 mL (Liposyn II) or up to 500 mL (Intralipid) first day and increase the next day. Max daily dose 2.5 g/kg.

PEDS – Calorie and essential fatty acids source: As part of TPN, fat emulsion should be no more than 60% of total calories; when correcting essential fatty acid deficiency, 8 to 10% of caloric intake should be supplied by lipids. Initial infusion rate 0.1 mL/min IV (10% fat emulsion) or 0.05 mL/min (20% fat emulsion) for first 10 to 15 min. If tolerated increase rate up to 1 mL/kg/h (10% fat emulsion) or 0.5 mL/kg/h (20% fat emulsion). Max daily dose 3 g/kg. For premature infants, start at 0.5 g/kg/day and increase based on infant's ability to eliminate fat. Max infusion rate 1 g fat/kg in 4 h.

NOTES – Do not use in patients with severe egg allergy; contains egg yolk phospholipids. Use caution in severe liver disease, pulmonary disease, anemia, blood coagulation disorders, when there is danger of fat embolism or in jaundiced or premature infants. Monitor CBC, blood coagulation, LFTs, plasma lipid profile, and platelet count.

LEVOCARNITINE (***Carnitor***) ▶KL ♀B ◗? $$$$$

ADULT – Prevention of levocarnitine deficiency in dialysis patients: 10 to 20 mg/kg IV at each dialysis session. Titrate dose based on serum concentration.

PEDS – Prevention of deficiency in dialysis patients: 10 to 20 mg/kg IV at each dialysis session. Titrate dose based on serum concentration.

FORMS – Generic/Trade: Tabs 330 mg, Oral soln 1 g/10 mL.

NOTES – Adverse neurophysiologic effects may occur with long-term, high doses of oral levocarnitine in patients with renal dysfunction. Only the IV formulation is indicated in patients receiving hemodialysis.

OMEGA-3-ACID ETHYL ESTERS (***Lovaza,* fish oil, omega 3 fatty acids**) ▶L ♀C ◗? $

ADULT – Adjunct to diet to reduce high triglycerides (500 mg/dL or above): 4 caps PO daily or divided two times per day.

PEDS – Not approved in children.

UNAPPROVED ADULT – Hypertriglyceridemia: 2 to 4 g EPA plus DHA content daily under physician's care. Secondary prevention of CHD: 1 to 2 g EPA plus DHA content daily. Adjunctive treatment in RA: 20 g/day PO. Psoriasis: 10 to 15 g/day PO. Prevention of early restenosis after coronary angioplasty in combination with dipyridamole and aspirin: 18 g/day PO.

FORMS – Trade only: (Lovaza) 1 g cap (total 840 mg EPA + DHA).

NOTES – Lovaza is only FDA-approved fish oil, previously known as Omacor. Other products available with varying EPA and DHA content. May increase LDL-cholesterol, monitor periodically. Effect on cardiovascular morbidity and mortality has not been determined. Treatment doses lower triglycerides by 30 to 50%. Prolongs bleeding time, may potentiate warfarin. Caution in seafood allergy; derived from fish oil. Monitor AST/ALT if hepatic impairment.

RALLY PACK ▶KL ♀C ◗– $

UNAPPROVED ADULT – See "Banana Bag". "Rally pack" is jargon and not a valid drug order; specify individual components.

ENDOCRINE AND METABOLIC: Phosphate Binders

LANTHANUM CARBONATE (***Fosrenol***) ▶Not absorbed ♀C ◗? $$$$$

ADULT – Treatment of hyperphosphatemia in end-stage renal disease: Start 1500 mg/day PO in divided doses with meals. Titrate dose q 2 to 3 weeks in increments of 750 mg/day until acceptable serum phosphate is reached. Most will require 1500 to 3000 mg/day to reduce serum phosphate less than 6.0 mg/dL. Chew or crush tabs completely before swallowing; not to be swallowed whole.

PEDS – Not approved in children.

FORMS – Trade only: Chewable tabs 500, 750, 1000 mg.

NOTES – Divided doses up to 3750 mg/day have been used. Caution if acute peptic ulcer, ulcerative colitis, or Crohn's disease. Serious GI obstructions reported; contraindicated if preexisting bowel obstruction, ileus, and fecal impaction. Avoid medications known to interact with antacids within 2 h. May be radio-opaque enough to appear on abdominal x-ray.

SEVELAMER (***Renagel, Renvela***) ▶Not absorbed ♀C ◗? $$$$$

ADULT – Hyperphosphatemia in kidney disease on dialysis: Start 800 to 1600 mg PO three times per day with meals, adjust according to serum phosphorus concentration.

PEDS – Not approved in children.

FORMS – Trade only (Renagel—sevelamer hydrochloride): Tabs 400, 800 mg.

(cont.)

SEVELAMER (*cont.*)

(Renvela—sevelamer carbonate): Tabs 800 mg; Powder: 800, 2400 mg packets.

NOTES – Titrate by 800 mg/meal at 2-week intervals to keep phosphorus less than 5.5 mg/dL; highest daily dose in studies: Renagel, 13 g; Renvela, 14 g. Decreases absorption of ciprofloxacin; may decrease absorption of antiarrhythmic and antiseizure medications; administer these meds 1 h before or 3 h after. Caution in GI motility disorders, including severe constipation. Contraindicated if bowel obstruction. Dysphagia and esophageal tablet retention reported; consider susp form if history of swallowing difficulties.

ENDOCRINE AND METABOLIC: Thyroid Agents

LEVOTHYROXINE (***L-Thyroxine, Levolet, Levo-T, Levothroid, Levoxyl, Novothyrox, Synthroid, Thyro-Tabs, Tirosint, Unithroid, T4 ✤ Eltroxin, Euthyrox***) ▶L ♀A ▶+ $

WARNING – Do not use for obesity/wt loss; possible serious or life-threatening toxic effects when used in euthyroid patients.

ADULT – Hypothyroidism: Start 100 to 200 mcg PO daily (healthy adults) or 12.5 to 50 mcg PO daily (elderly or CV disease), increase by 12.5 to 25 mcg/day at 3- to 8-week intervals. Usual maintenance dose 100 to 200 mcg PO daily, max 300 mcg/day.

PEDS – Hypothyroidism: 0 to 6 mo: 8 to 10 mcg/kg/day PO; 6 to 12 mo: 6 to 8 mcg/kg/day PO; 1 to 5 yo: 5 to 6 mcg/kg/day PO; 6 to 12 yo: 4 to 5 mcg/kg/day PO; older than 12 yo: 2 to 3 mcg/kg/day PO, max 300 mcg/day.

UNAPPROVED ADULT – Hypothyroidism: 1.6 mcg/kg/day PO; start with lower doses (25 mcg PO daily) in elderly and patients with cardiac disease.

FORMS – Generic/Trade: Tabs 25, 50, 75, 88, 100, 112, 125, 137, 150, 175, 200, 300 mcg. Trade only: Caps: 25, 50, 75, 100, 125, 150 mcg in 7-day blister packs, Tabs: 13 mcg (Tirosint).

NOTES – May crush tabs for infants and children. May give IV or IM at ½ oral dose in adults and ½ to ¾ oral dose in children; then adjust based on tolerance and therapeutic response. Generics are not necessarily bioequivalent to brand products; reevaluate thyroid function when switching.

LIOTHYRONINE (***T3, Cytomel, Triostat***) ▶L ♀A ▶? $$

WARNING – Do not use for obesity/wt loss; possible serious or life-threatening toxic effects when used in euthyroid patients.

ADULT – Mild hypothyroidism: 25 mcg PO daily, increase by 12.5 to 25 mcg/day at 1- to 2-week intervals to desired response. Usual maintenance dose 25 to 75 mcg PO daily. Goiter: 5 mcg PO daily, increase by 5 to 10 mcg/day at 1- to 2-week intervals. Usual maintenance dose 75 mcg PO daily. Myxedema: 5 mcg PO daily, increase by 5 to 10 mcg/day at 1- to 2-week intervals. Usual maintenance dose 50 to 100 mcg/day.

PEDS – Congenital hypothyroidism: 5 mcg PO daily, increase by 5 mcg/day at 3- to 4-day intervals to desired response.

FORMS – Generic/Trade: Tabs 5, 25, 50 mcg.

NOTES – Levothyroxine is preferred maintenance treatment for hypothyroidism. Start therapy at 5 mcg/day in children and elderly and increase by 5-mcg increments only. Rapidly absorbed from the GI tract. Monitor T3 and TSH. Elderly may need lower doses due to potential decreased renal function.

METHIMAZOLE (***Tapazole***) ▶L ♀D ▶+ $$$

ADULT – Hyperthyroidism. Mild: 5 mg PO three times per day. Moderate: 10 mg PO three times per day. Severe: 20 mg PO three times per day (q 8 h intervals). Maintenance dose is 5 to 30 mg/day.

PEDS – Hyperthyroidism: 0.4 mg/kg/day PO divided q 8 h. Maintenance dose is ½ initial dose, max 30 mg/day.

UNAPPROVED ADULT – Start 10 to 30 mg PO daily, then adjust.

FORMS – Generic/Trade: Tabs 5, 10. Generic only: Tabs 15, 20 mg.

NOTES – Check CBC for evidence of marrow suppression if fever, sore throat, or other signs of infection. Propylthiouracil preferred over methimazole in first trimester of pregnancy.

POTASSIUM IODIDE (***Iosat, SSKI, Thyrosafe, Thyroshield***) ▶L ♀D ▶– $

WARNING – Do not use for obesity.

ADULT – Thyroidectomy preparation: 50 to 250 mg PO three times per day for 10 to 14 days prior to surgery. Thyroid storm: 1 mL (Lugol's) PO three times per day at least 1 h after initial propylthiouracil or methimazole dose. Thyroid blocking in radiation emergency: 130 mg PO daily for 10 days or as directed by state health officials.

PEDS – Thyroid blocking in radiation emergency age 3 to 18 yo: 65 mg (½ of a 130 mg tab) PO

(cont.)

POTASSIUM IODIDE (*cont.*)

daily, or 130 mg PO daily in adolescents greater than 70 kg. 1 mo to 3 yo: 32 mg (¼ of a 130 mg tab) PO daily. Birth to 1 mo: 16 mg (⅛ of a 130-mg tab) PO daily. Duration is until risk of exposure to radioiodines no longer exists.

FORMS – OTC Trade only: Tabs 130 mg (Iosat). Trade only Rx: Soln 1 g/mL (30, 240 mL, SSKI). OTC Generic only: Tabs 65 mg (Thyrosafe), Soln 65 mg/mL (30 mL, Thyroshield).

PROPYLTHIOURACIL (***PTU,*** ***✤ Propyl Thyracil***) ▶L ♀D (but preferred over methimazole in first trimester) ▶+ $

WARNING – Acute liver failure and severe liver injury reported, including fatal injury and need for liver transplantation. Use only if patient cannot tolerate methimazole or if not a candidate for radioactive iodine therapy or surgery.

ADULT – Hyperthyroidism: 100 to 150 mg PO three times per day. Severe hyperthyroidism and/or large goiters: 200 to 400 mg PO three times per day. Continue initial dose for approximately 2 months. Adjust dose to desired response. Usual maintenance dose 100 to 150 mg/day. Thyroid storm: 200 mg PO q 4 to 6 h once daily, decrease dose gradually to usual maintenance dose.

PEDS – Hyperthyroidism in children age 6 to 10 yo: 50 mg PO daily to three times per day. Children 10 yo or older: 50 to 100 mg PO three times per day. Continue initial dose for 2 months, then maintenance dose is ⅓ to ⅔ initial dose.

UNAPPROVED PEDS – Hyperthyroidism in neonates: 5 to 10 mg/kg/day PO divided q 8 h. Children: 5 to 7 mg/kg/day PO divided q 8 h.

FORMS – Generic only: Tabs 50 mg.

NOTES – Monitor CBC for marrow suppression if fever, sore throat, or other signs of infection. Vasculitic syndrome with positive antineutrophilic icytoplasmic antibodies (ANCAs) reported requiring discontinuation. Propylthiouracil preferred over methimazole in first trimester of pregnancy.

SODIUM IODIDE I-131 (***Hicon, Iodotope, Sodium Iodide I-131 Therapeutic***) ▶K ♀X ▶– $$$$$

ADULT – Specialized dosing for hyperthyroidism and thyroid carcinoma.

PEDS – Not approved in children.

FORMS – Generic/Trade: Caps Oral soln: Radioactivity range varies at the time of calibration. Hicon is a kit containing caps and a concentrated oral soln for dilution and cap preparation.

NOTES – Hazardous substance, handle with necessary precautions and use proper disposal. Avoid if preexisting vomiting or diarrhea. Discontinue antithyroid therapy at least 3 days before starting. Low serum chloride or nephrosis may increase uptake; renal insufficiency may decrease excretion and thus increase radiation exposure. Ensure adequate hydration before and after administration. Follow low-iodine diet for 1 to 2 weeks before treatment. Women should have negative pregnancy test prior to treatment; advise not to conceive for at least 6 months.

THYROID—DESICCATED (***Thyroid USP, Armour Thyroid***) ▶L ♀A ▶? $

WARNING – Do not use for wt loss; possible serious or life-threatening toxic effects when used in euthyroid patients.

ADULT – Obsolete; use levothyroxine instead. Hypothyroidism: Start 30 mg PO daily, increase by 15 mg/day at 2- to 3-week intervals to max 180 mg/day.

PEDS – Congenital hypothyroidism: 15 mg PO daily. Increase at 2-week intervals.

FORMS – Generic/Trade: Tabs 15, 30, 60, 90, 120, 180, 300 mg. Trade only: Tabs 240 mg.

NOTES – 60 mg thyroid desiccated is roughly equivalent to 100 mcg levothyroxine. Combination of levothyroxine (T4) and liothyronine (T3); content varies (range 2:1 to 5:1).

THYROLAR, LIOTRIX **(levothyroxine + liothyronine)** ▶L ♀A ▶? $

WARNING – Do not use for wt loss; possible serious or life-threatening toxic effects when used in euthyroid patients.

ADULT – Hypothyroidism: 1 tab PO daily, starting with small doses initially (¼ to ½ strength), then increase at 2-week intervals.

PEDS – Not approved in children.

FORMS – Trade only: Tabs T4/T3 12.5 mcg/3.1 mcg (¼ strength), 25 mcg/6.25 mcg (half-strength), 50 mcg/12.5 mcg (#1), 100 mcg/25 mcg (#2), 150 mcg/37.5 mcg (#3).

NOTES – Combination of levothyroxine (T4) and liothyronine (T3).

ENDOCRINE AND METABOLIC: Vitamins

ASCORBIC ACID **(vitamin C,** ***✤ Redoxon***) ▶K ♀C ▶? $

ADULT – Prevention of scurvy: 70 to 150 mg/day PO. Treatment of scurvy: 300 to 1000 mg/day PO. RDA females: 75 mg/day; males: 90 mg/day. Smokers: Add 35 mg/day more than nonsmokers.

PEDS – Prevention of scurvy: Infants: 30 mg/day PO. Treatment of scurvy: Infants: 100 to 300 mg/day PO. Adequate daily intake for

(cont.)

ASCORBIC ACID (*cont.*)

infants 0 to 6 mo: 40 mg; 7 to 12 mo: 50 mg. RDA for children: 1 to 3 yo: 15 mg; 4 to 8 yo: 25 mg; 9 to 13 yo: 45 mg; 14 to 18 yo: 75 mg (males), 65 mg (females).

UNAPPROVED ADULT – Urinary acidification with methenamine: More than 2 g/day PO. Idiopathic methemoglobinemia: 150 mg/day or more PO. Wound healing: 300 to 500 mg/day or more PO for 7 to 10 days. Severe burns: 1 to 2 g/day PO.

FORMS – OTC Generic only: Tabs 25, 50, 100, 250, 500, 1000 mg, Chewable tabs 100, 250, 500 mg, Timed-release tabs 500, 1000, 1500 mg, Timed-release caps 500 mg, Lozenges 60 mg, Liquid 35 mg/0.6 mL, Oral soln 100 mg/mL, Syrup 500 mg/5 mL.

NOTES – Use IV/IM/SC ascorbic acid for acute deficiency or when oral absorption is uncertain. Avoid excessive doses in diabetics, patients prone to renal calculi, those undergoing stool occult blood tests (may cause false-negative), those on sodium-restricted diets and those taking anticoagulants (may decrease INR). Doses in adults more than 2 g/day may cause osmotic diarrhea.

CALCITRIOL (***Rocaltrol, Calcijex***) ▶L ♀C ▶? $$

ADULT – Hypocalcemia in chronic renal dialysis: Oral: 0.25 mcg PO daily, increase by 0.25 mcg q 4 to 8 weeks until normocalcemia achieved. Most hemodialysis patients require 0.5 to 1 mcg/day PO. Hypocalcemia and/or secondary hyperparathyroidism in chronic renal dialysis IV: 1 to 2 mcg, 3 times a week; increase dose by 0.5 to 1 mcg q 2 to 4 weeks. If PTH decreased less than 30% then increase dose; if PTH decreased 30 to 60% then maintain current dose; if PTH decreased more than 60% then decrease dose; if PTH 1.5 to 3 times the upper normal limit then maintain current dose. Hypoparathyroidism: 0.25 mcg PO q am; increase dose q 2 to 4 weeks if inadequate response. Most adults respond to 0.5 to 2 mcg/day PO. Secondary hyperparathyroidism in predialysis patients: 0.25 mcg PO q am; may increase dose to 0.5 mcg q am.

PEDS – Hypoparathyroidism 1 to 5 yo: 0.25 to 0.75 mcg PO q am. If age 6 yo or older then 0.25 mcg PO q am; increase dose in 2 to 4 weeks; usually respond to 0.5 to 2 mcg/day PO. Secondary hyperparathyroidism in predialysis patients age 3 yo or older: 0.25 mcg q am; may increase dose to 0.5 mcg q am. If younger than 3 yo: 0.01 to 0.015 mcg/kg/day PO.

UNAPPROVED ADULT – Psoriasis vulgaris: 0.5 mcg/day PO or 0.5 mcg/g petrolatum topically daily.

FORMS – Generic/Trade: Caps 0.25, 0.5 mcg. Oral soln 1 mcg/mL. Injection 1, 2 mcg/mL.

NOTES – Calcitriol is the activated form of vitamin D. During titration period, monitor serum calcium at least twice a week. Successful therapy requires an adequate daily calcium intake. Topical preparation must be compounded (not commercially available).

CYANOCOBALAMIN (**vitamin B12,** ***CaloMist, Nascobal***) ▶K ♀C ▶+ $

ADULT – See also UNAPPROVED ADULT dosing. Maintenance of nutritional deficiency following IM correction: 500 mcg intranasal weekly (Nascobal: 1 spray 1 nostril once a week) or 50 to 100 mcg intranasal daily (CaloMist: 1 to 2 sprays each nostril daily). Pernicious anemia: 100 mcg IM/SC daily, for 6 to 7 days, then every other day for 7 doses, then q 3 to 4 days for 2 to 3 weeks, then q month. Other patients with vitamin B12 deficiency: 30 mcg IM daily for 5 to 10 days, then 100 to 200 mcg IM q month. RDA for adults is 2.4 mcg.

PEDS – Nutritional deficiency: 100 mcg/24 h deep IM/SC for 10 to 15 days then at least 60 mcg/month IM/deep SC. Pernicious anemia: 30 to 50 mcg/24 h for 14 days or more to total dose of 1000 to 5000 mcg deep IM/SC then 100 mcg/month deep IM/SC. Adequate daily intake for infants: 0 to 6 mo: 0.4 mcg; 7 to 11 mo: 0.5 mcg. RDA for children: 1 to 3 yo: 0.9 mcg; 4 to 8 yo: 1.2 mcg; 9 to 13 yo: 1.8 mcg; 14 to 18 yo: 2.4 mcg.

UNAPPROVED ADULT – Pernicious anemia and nutritional deficiency states: 1000 to 2000 mcg PO daily for 1 to 2 weeks, then 1000 mcg PO daily. Prevention and treatment of cyanide toxicity associated with nitroprusside.

UNAPPROVED PEDS – Prevention/treatment of nitroprusside-associated cyanide toxicity.

FORMS – OTC Generic only: Tabs 100, 500, 1000, 5000 mcg; Lozenges 100, 250, 500 mcg. Rx Trade only: Nasal spray 500 mcg/spray (Nascobal 2.3 mL), 25 mcg/spray (CaloMist, 18 mL).

NOTES – Prime nasal pump before use per package insert directions. Although official dose for deficiency states is 100 to 200 mcg IM q month, some give 1000 mcg IM periodically. Oral supplementation is safe and effective for B12 deficiency even when intrinsic factor is not present. Monitor B12, folate, iron, and CBC.

DOXERCALCIFEROL (*Hectorol*) ▶L ♀B ▶? $$$$$

ADULT – Secondary hyperparathyroidism on dialysis: Oral: If PTH is greater than 400 pg/mL then start 10 mcg PO 3 times a week; if PTH is greater than 300 pg/mL then increase by 2.5 mcg/dose q 8 weeks prn; if PTH is 150 to 300 pg/mL then maintain current dose; if PTH is less than 100 pg/mL then stop for 1 week, then resume at a dose at least 2.5 mcg lower. Max 60 mcg/week. IV: If PTH is greater than 400 pg/mL then 4 mcg IV 3 times a week; if PTH decreased by less than 50% and greater than 300 pg/mL then increase by 1 to 2 mcg q 8 weeks as necessary; if PTH decreased by greater than 50% and greater than 300 pg/mL then maintain current dose; if PTH is 150 to 300 pg/mL then maintain current dose; if PTH is less than 100 pg/mL then stop for 1 week, then resume at a dose that is at least 1 mcg lower. Max 18 mcg/week. Secondary hyperparathyroidism not on dialysis: If PTH is greater than 70 pg/mL (Stage 3) or greater than 110 pg/mL (Stage 4) then start 1 mcg PO daily; if PTH is greater than 70 pg/mL (Stage 3) or greater than 110 pg/mL (Stage 4) then increase by 0.5 mcg/dose q 2 weeks; if PTH is 35 to 70 pg/mL (Stage 3) or 70 to 110 pg/mL (Stage 4) then maintain current dose; if less than 35 pg/mL (Stage 3) or less than 70 pg/mL (Stage 4) then stop for 1 week, then resume at a dose that is at least 0.5 mcg lower. Max 3.5 mcg/day.

PEDS – Not approved in children.

FORMS – Generic/Trade: Caps 0.5 mcg. Trade only: Caps 2.5 mcg.

NOTES – Monitor PTH, serum calcium, and phosphorus weekly during dose titration; may need to monitor patients with hepatic insufficiency more closely.

ERGOCALCIFEROL (**vitamin D2,** ***Calciferol, Drisdol,*** ✦ ***Osteoforte***) ▶L ♀A (C if exceed RDA) ▶+ $

ADULT – Familial hypophosphatemia (Vitamin D-resistant Rickets): 12,000 to 500,000 units PO daily. Hypoparathyroidism: 50,000 to 200,000 units PO daily. Adequate daily intake: 18 to 70 yo: 600 units (15 mcg); older than 70 yo: 800 units (20 mcg).

PEDS – Adequate daily intake: 1 to 18 yo 600 units (15 mcg). Hypoparathyroidism: 1.25 to 5 mg PO daily.

UNAPPROVED ADULT – Osteoporosis prevention and treatment (age 50 or older): 800 to 1000 units PO daily with calcium supplements. Fanconi syndrome: 50,000 to 200,000 units PO daily. Osteomalacia: 1000 to 5000 units PO daily. Anticonvulsant-induced osteomalacia: 2000 to 50,000 units PO daily. Vitamin D deficiency: 50,000 units PO weekly or biweekly for 8 to 12 weeks.

UNAPPROVED PEDS – Familial hypophosphatemia: 400,000 to 800,000 units PO daily, increased by 10,000 to 20,000 units/day q 3 to 4 months as needed. Hypoparathyroidism: 50,000 to 200,000 units PO daily. Fanconi syndrome: 250 to 50,000 units PO daily.

FORMS – OTC Generic only: Caps 400, 1000, 5000 units, Soln 8000 units/mL (Calciferol). Rx Generic/Trade: Caps 50,000 units. Rx Generic only: Caps 25,000 units.

NOTES – 1 mcg ergocalciferol = 40 units vitamin D. Sufficient level of 25-OH vitamin D is greater than 20 ng/mL, optimal is greater than 30 ng/mL. Vitamin D2 (ergocalciferol) is less effective than vitamin D3 (cholecalciferol) in maintaining 25-OH vitamin D levels; higher doses may be needed. IM or high-dose oral therapy may be necessary if malabsorption exists. Familial hypophosphatemia also requires phosphate supplementation; hypoparathyroidism also requires calcium supplementation.

FOLGARD (**folic acid + cyanocobalamin + pyridoxine**) ▶K ♀? ▶? $

ADULT – Nutritional supplement: 1 tab PO daily.

PEDS – Not approved in children.

FORMS – OTC Trade only: Folic acid 0.8 mg + cyanocobalamin 0.115 mg + pyridoxine 10 mg tab.

NOTES – Folic acid doses greater than 0.1 mg may obscure pernicious anemia, preventable with the concurrent cyanocobalamin.

FOLGARD RX (**folic acid + cyanocobalamin + pyridoxine**) ▶K – ▶? $

ADULT – Nutritional supplement: 1 tab PO daily.

PEDS – Not approved in children.

FORMS – Trade only: Folic acid 2.2 mg + cyanocobalamin 1000 mcg + pyridoxine 25 mg tab.

NOTES – Folic acid doses greater than 0.1 mg may obscure pernicious anemia, preventable with the concurrent cyanocobalamin.

FOLIC ACID (**folate,** ***Folvite***) ▶K ♀A ▶+ $

ADULT – Megaloblastic anemia: 1 mg PO/IM/IV/SC daily. When symptoms subside and CBC normalizes, give maintenance dose of 0.4 mg PO daily and 0.8 mg PO daily in pregnant and lactating females. RDA for adults 0.4 mg, 0.6 mg for pregnant females, and 0.5 mg for lactating women. Max recommended daily dose 1 mg.

(cont.)

FOLIC ACID (*cont.*)

PEDS – Megaloblastic anemia: Infants: 0.05 mg PO daily, maintenance of 0.04 mg PO daily. Children: 0.5 to 1 mg PO daily, maintenance of 0.4 mg PO daily. Adequate daily intake for infants: 0 to 6 mo: 65 mcg; 7 to 12 mo: 80 mcg. RDA for children: 1 to 3 yo: 150 mcg; 4 to 8 yo: 200 mcg; 9 to 13 yo: 300 mcg, 14 to 18 yo: 400 mcg.

UNAPPROVED ADULT – Hyperhomocysteinemia: 0.5 to 1 mg PO daily.

FORMS – OTC Generic only: Tabs 0.4, 0.8 mg. Rx Generic 1 mg.

NOTES – Folic acid doses greater than 0.1 mg/day may obscure pernicious anemia. Prior to conception all women should receive 0.4 mg/day to reduce the risk of neural tube defects in infants. Consider high dose (up to 4 mg) in women with prior history of infant with neural tube defect. Use oral route except in cases of severe intestinal absorption.

FOLTX **(folic acid + cyanocobalamin + pyridoxine)** ▶K ♀A ▶+ $$

ADULT – Nutritional supplement for end-stage renal failure, dialysis, hyperhomocysteinemia, homocystinuria, nutrient malabsorption, or inadequate dietary intake: 1 tab PO daily.

PEDS – Not approved in children.

FORMS – Trade only: Folic acid 2.5 mg/cyanocobalamin 2 mg/pyridoxine 25 mg tab.

NOTES – Folic acid doses greater than 0.1 mg may obscure pernicious anemia, preventable with the concurrent cyanocobalamin.

MULTIVITAMINS (***MVI***) ▶LK ♀+ ▶+ $

WARNING – Severe iron toxicity possible in overdose, especially in children. Store out of reach of children and in child-resistant containers. Iron overdose is a leading cause of poisoning in children younger than 6 yo.

ADULT – Dietary supplement: Dose varies by product.

PEDS – Dietary supplement: Dose varies by product.

FORMS – OTC and Rx: Many different brands and forms available with and without iron (tabs, caps, chewable tabs, gtts, liquid).

NOTES – Do not take within 2 h of antacids, tetracyclines, levothyroxine, or fluoroquinolones.

NEPHROCAP **(ascorbic acid + folic acid + niacin + thiamine + riboflavin + pyridoxine + pantothenic acid + biotin + cyanocobalamin)** ▶K ♀? ▶? $

ADULT – Nutritional supplement for chronic renal failure, uremia, impaired metabolic functions of the kidney and to maintain levels when the dietary intake of vitamins is inadequate or excretion and loss are excessive: 1 cap PO daily. If on dialysis, take after treatment.

PEDS – Not approved in children.

FORMS – Generic/Trade: Vitamin C 100 mg/folic acid 1 mg/niacin 20 mg/thiamine 1.5 mg/riboflavin 1.7 mg/pyridoxine 10 mg/pantothenic acid 5 mg/biotin 150 mcg/cyanocobalamin 6 mcg.

NOTES – Folic acid doses greater than 0.1 mg/day may obscure pernicious anemia (preventable with the concurrent cyanocobalamin).

NEPHROVITE **(ascorbic acid + folic acid + niacin + thiamine + riboflavin + pyridoxine + pantothenic acid + biotin + cyanocobalamin)** ▶K ♀? ▶? $

ADULT – Nutritional supplement for chronic renal failure, dialysis, hyperhomocysteinemia, or inadequate dietary vitamin intake: 1 tab PO daily. If on dialysis, take after treatment.

PEDS – Not approved in children.

FORMS – Generic/Trade: Vitamin C 60 mg/folic acid 1 mg/niacin 20 mg/thiamine 1.5 mg/riboflavin 1.7 mg/pyridoxine 10 mg/pantothenic acid 10 mg/biotin 300 mcg/cyanocobalamin 6 mcg.

NOTES – Folic acid doses greater than 0.1 mg/day may obscure pernicious anemia (preventable with the concurrent cyanocobalamin).

NIACIN (vitamin B3, nicotinic acid, *Niacor, Nicolar, Slo-Niacin, Niaspan*) ▶K ♀C ▶? $

ADULT – Niacin deficiency: 100 mg PO daily. RDA: 16 mg for males, 14 mg for females. Hyperlipidemia: Start 50 to 100 mg PO two to three times per day with meals, increase slowly, usual maintenance range 1.5 to 3 g/day, max 6 g/day. Extended-release (Niaspan): Start 500 mg at bedtime with a low-fat snack for 4 weeks, increase prn q 4 weeks to max 2000 mg.

PEDS – Safety and efficacy not established for doses which exceed nutritional requirements. Adequate daily intake for infants: 0 to 6 mo: 2 mg; 7 to 12 mo: 3 mg. RDA for children: 1 to 3 yo: 6 mg; 48 yo: 8 mg; 9 to 13 yo: 12 mg; 14 to 18 yo: 16 mg (males) and 14 mg (females).

UNAPPROVED ADULT – Pellagra: 50 to 100 mg three to four times per day, up to 500 mg PO daily.

FORMS – OTC Generic only: Tabs 50, 100, 250, 500 mg; Timed-release cap 125, 250, 400 mg; Timed-release tab 250, 500 mg; Liquid 50 mg/5 mL. Trade only: 250, 500, 750 mg (Slo-Niacin). Rx: Trade only: Tabs 500 mg (Niacor), Timed-release caps 500 mg, Timed-release tabs 500, 750, 1000 mg (Niaspan, $$$$).

NOTES – Start with low doses and increase slowly to minimize flushing; 325 mg aspirin

(cont.)

NIACIN (*cont.*)

(non-EC) 30 to 60 min prior to niacin ingestion will minimize flushing. Use caution in diabetics, patients with gout, peptic ulcer, liver, or gallbladder disease. Extended-release formulations may have greater hepatotoxicity.

PARICALCITOL (***Zemplar***) ▶L ♀C ▶? $$$$$

ADULT – Prevention/treatment of secondary hyperparathyroidism with renal insufficiency: If PTH is less than 500 pg/mL then start 1 mcg PO daily or 2 mcg PO three times per week. If PTH is greater than 500 pg/mL then start 2 mcg PO daily or 4 mcg PO three times per week. Can increase PO dose by 1 mcg daily or 2 mcg three times per week based on PTH in 2- to 4-week intervals. Prevention/treatment of secondary hyperparathyroidism with renal failure (CrCl less than 15 mL/min): PO: To calculate initial dose divide baseline iPTH by 80 and then administer this dose in mcg three times per week. To titrate dose based on response, divide recent iPTH by 80 and then administer this dose in mcg three times per week. IV: Initially 0.04 to 0.1 mcg/kg (2.8 to 7 mcg) IV three times per week during dialysis. Can increase IV dose 2 to 4 mcg based on PTH in 2- to 4-week intervals. PO/IV: If PTH level decreased less than 30% then increase dose; if PTH level decreased 30 to 60% then maintain current dose; if PTH level decreased greater than 60% then decrease dose.

PEDS – Prevention/treatment of secondary hyperparathyroidism with renal failure (CrCl less than 15 mL/min): 0.04 to 0.1 mcg/kg (2.8 to 7 mcg) IV three times per week at dialysis; increase dose by 2 to 4 mcg or 0.04 mcg/kg q 2 to 4 weeks until desired PTH level is achieved. Max dose 0.24 mcg/kg (16.8 mcg).

FORMS – Trade only: Caps 1, 2, 4 mcg.

NOTES – Monitor serum PTH, calcium, and phosphorous. IV doses up to 0.24 mcg/kg (16.8 mcg) have been administered. Do not initiate PO therapy in renal failure until calcium is 9.6 mg/dL or lower. Avoid prescription-based doses of vitamin D and derivatives to minimize the risk of hypercalemia. Monitor closely (eg, twice weekly) during dosage adjustment for acute hypercalcemia. Chronic hypercalemia may lead to vascular and soft-tissue calcification. Do not administer with aluminum-containing medications; risk of aluminum toxicity. Risk of digoxin toxicity if hypercalcemia.

PHYTONADIONE (**vitamin K**, ***Mephyton, AquaMephyton***) ▶L ♀C ▶+ $

WARNING – Severe reactions, including fatalities, have occurred during and immediately after IV injection, even with diluted injection and slow administration. Restrict IV use to situations where other routes of administration are not feasible.

ADULT – Excessive oral anticoagulation: Dose varies based on INR. INR 4.5 to 10: 2012 CHEST guidelines recommend AGAINST routine vitamin K administration; INR greater than 10 with no bleeding: 2012 CHEST guidelines recommend giving vitamin K, but do not specify a dose, 2008 guidelines previously recommended 5 to 10 mg PO; serious bleeding and elevated INR: 5 to 10 mg slow IV infusion. Hypoprothrombinemia due to other causes: 2.5 to 25 mg PO/IM/SC. Adequate daily intake: 120 mcg (males) and 90 mcg (females).

PEDS – Hemorrhagic disease of the newborn: Prophylaxis: 0.5 to 1 mg IM 1 h after birth; Treatment: 1 mg SC/IM.

UNAPPROVED PEDS – Nutritional deficiency: Children: 2.5 to 5 mg PO daily or 1 to 2 mg IM/SC/IV. Excessive oral anticoagulation: Infants: 1 to 2 mg IM/SC/IV q 4 to 8 h. Children: 2.5 to 10 mg PO/IM/SC/IV, may be repeated 12 to 48 h after PO dose or 6 to 8 h after IM/SC/IV dose.

FORMS – Trade only: Tabs 5 mg.

NOTES – Excessive doses of vitamin K in a patient receiving warfarin may cause warfarin resistance for up to a week. Avoid IM administration in patients with a high INR.

PYRIDOXINE (**vitamin B6**) ▶K ♀A ▶+ $

ADULT – Dietary deficiency: 10 to 20 mg PO daily for 3 weeks. Prevention of deficiency due to isoniazid in high-risk patients: 10 to 25 mg PO daily. Treatment of neuropathies due to isoniazid: 50 to 200 mg PO daily. Isoniazid overdose (greater than 10 g): 4 g IV followed by 1 g IM over 30 min, repeat until total dose of 1 g for each g of isoniazid ingested. RDA for adults: 19 to 50 yo: 1.3 mg; older than 50 yo: 1.7 mg (males), 1.5 mg (females). Max recommended: 100 mg/day.

PEDS – Adequate daily intake for infants: 0 to 6 mo: 0.1 mg; 7 to 12 mo: 0.3 mg. RDA for children: 1 to 3 yo: 0.5 mg; 4 to 8 yo: 0.6 mg; 9 to 13 yo: 1 mg; 14 to 18 yo: 1.3 (boys) and 1.2 mg (girls).

UNAPPROVED ADULT – Premenstrual syndrome: 50 to 500 mg/day PO. Hyperoxaluria type I and oxalate kidney stones: 25 to 300 mg/day PO. Prevention of oral contraceptive–induced deficiency: 25 to 40 mg PO daily. Hyperemesis of pregnancy: 10 to 50 mg PO q 8 h. Has been used in hydrazine poisoning.

UNAPPROVED PEDS – Dietary deficiency: 5 to 10 mg PO daily for 3 weeks. Prevention

(cont.)

PYRIDOXINE (*cont.*)

of deficiency due to isoniazid: 1 to 2 mg/kg PO daily. Treatment of neuropathies due to isoniazid: 10 to 50 mg PO daily. Pyridoxine-dependent epilepsy: Neonatal: 25 to 50 mg/dose IV; older infants and children: 100 mg/dose IV for 1 dose then 100 mg PO daily.

FORMS – OTC Generic only: Tabs 25, 50, 100 mg; Timed-release tab 100 mg.

RIBOFLAVIN (**vitamin B2**) ▶K ♀A ▶+ $

ADULT – Deficiency: 5 to 25 mg/day PO. RDA for adults: 1.3 mg (males) and 1.1 mg (females), 1.4 mg for pregnant women, 1.6 mg for lactating women.

PEDS – Deficiency: 5 to 10 mg/day PO. Adequate daily intake for infants: 0 to 6 mo: 0.3 mg; 7 to 12 mo: 0.4 mg. RDA for children: 1 to 3 yo: 0.5 mg; 4 to 8 yo: 0.6 mg; 9 to 13 yo: 0.9 mg; 14 to 18 yo: 1.3 mg (males) and 1 mg (females).

UNAPPROVED ADULT – Prevention of migraine headaches: 400 mg PO daily.

FORMS – OTC Generic only: Tabs 25, 50, 100 mg.

NOTES – May cause yellow/orange discoloration of urine.

THIAMINE (**vitamin B1**) ▶K ♀A ▶+ $

ADULT – Beriberi: 10 to 20 mg IM 3 times per week for 2 weeks. Wet beriberi with MI: 10 to 30 mg IV three times per day. Wernicke encephalopathy: 50 to 100 mg IV and 50 to 100 mg IM for 1 dose then 50 to 100 mg IM daily until patient resumes normal diet. Give before starting glucose. RDA for adults: 1.2 mg (males) and 1.1 mg (females).

PEDS – Beriberi: 10 to 25 mg IM daily or 10 to 50 mg PO daily for 2 weeks then 5 to 10 mg PO daily for 1 month. Adequate daily intake, infants: 0 to 6 mo: 0.2 mg; 7 to 12 mo: 0.3 mg. RDA for children: 1 to 3 yo: 0.5 mg; 4 to 8 yo: 0.6 mg; 9 to 13 yo: 0.9 mg; 14 to 18 yo: 1.2 mg (males), 1.0 mg (females).

FORMS – OTC Generic only: Tabs 50, 100, 250, 500 mg; Enteric-coated tab 20 mg.

TOCOPHEROL (**vitamin E,** ✤ ***Aquasol E***) ▶L ♀A ▶? $

ADULT – RDA is 22 units (natural, d-alpha-tocopherol) or 33 units (synthetic, d,l-alpha-tocopherol) or 15 mg (alpha-tocopherol). Max recommended 1000 mg (alpha-tocopherol).

PEDS – Adequate daily intake (alpha-tocopherol): Infants 0 to 6 mo: 4 mg; 7 to 12 mo: 6 mg. RDA for children (alpha-tocopherol): 1 to 3 yo: 6 mg; 4 to 8 yo: 7 mg; 9 to 13 yo: 11 mg; 14 to 18 yo: 15 mg.

UNAPPROVED PEDS – Nutritional deficiency: Neonates: 25 to 50 units PO daily. Children: 1 unit/kg PO daily. Cystic fibrosis: 5 to 10 units/kg PO daily (use water soluble form), max 400 units/day.

FORMS – OTC Generic only: Tabs 200, 400 units; Caps 73.5, 100, 147, 165, 200, 330, 400, 500, 600, 1000 units; Gtts 50 mg/mL.

NOTES – 1 mg alpha-tocopherol equivalents equals ~1.5 units. Natural vitamin E (d-alpha-tocopherol) recommended over synthetic (d,l-alpha-tocopherol). Higher doses may increase risk of bleeding. Large randomized trials have failed to demonstrate cardioprotective effects.

VITAMIN A ▶L ♀A (C if exceed RDA, X in high doses) ▶+ $

ADULT – Treatment of deficiency states: 100,000 units IM daily for 3 days, then 50,000 units IM daily for 2 weeks. RDA: 1000 mcg RE (males), 800 mcg RE (females). Max recommended daily dose in nondeficiency 3000 mcg (see NOTES).

PEDS – Treatment of deficiency states: Infants: 7500 to 15,000 units IM daily for 10 days; children 1 to 8 yo: 17,500 to 35,000 units IM daily for 10 days. Kwashiorkor: 30 mg IM of water-soluble palmitate followed by 5000 to 10,000 units PO daily for 2 months. Xerophthalmia: Older than 1 yo: 110 mg retinyl palmitate PO or 55 mg IM plus 110 mg PO next day. Administer another 110 mg PO prior to discharge. Vitamin E (40 units) should be coadministered to increase efficacy of retinol. RDA for children: 0 to 6 mo: 400 mcg (adequate intake); 7 to 12 mo: 500 mcg; 1 to 3 yo: 300 mcg; 4 to 8 yo: 400 mcg; 9 to 13 yo: 600 mcg; 14 to 18 yo: 900 mcg (males), 700 mcg (females).

UNAPPROVED ADULT – Test for fat absorption: 7000 units/kg (2100 RE/kg) PO for 1 dose. Measure serum vitamin A concentrations at baseline and 4 h after ingestion. Dermatologic disorders such as follicularis keratosis: 50,000 to 500,000 units PO daily for several weeks.

UNAPPROVED PEDS – Has been tried in reduction of malaria episodes in children older than 12 mo and to reduce the mortality in HIV-infected children.

FORMS – OTC Generic only: Caps 10,000, 15,000 units. Trade only: Tabs 5000 units. Rx: Generic: 25,000 units. Trade only: Soln 50,000 units/mL.

NOTES – 1 RE (retinol equivalent) = 1 mcg retinol or 6 mcg beta-carotene. Continued vitamin A/retinol intake of 2000 mcg/day or more may increase risk of hip fracture in postmenopausal women.

VITAMIN D3 (**cholecalciferol,** ***DDrops***) ▶L –◗+ $

ADULT – Familial hypophosphatemia (vitamin D–resistant Rickets): 12,000 to 500,000 units PO daily. Hypoparathyroidism: 50,000 to 200,000 units PO daily. Adequate daily intake adults: 1 to 70 yo: 600 units; older than 70 yo: 800 units. Max recommended daily dose in nondeficiency 4000 units.

PEDS – Adequate daily intake: 1 to 18 yo 600 units. Hypoparathyroidism: 1.25 to 5 mg PO daily.

UNAPPROVED ADULT – Osteoporosis prevention and treatment (age 50 or older): 800 to 1000 units PO daily with calcium supplements.

UNAPPROVED PEDS – Familial hypophosphatemia: 400,000 to 800,000 units PO daily, increased by 10,000 to 20,000 units/day q 3 to 4 months as needed. Hypoparathyroidism: 50,000 to 200,000 units PO daily. Fanconi syndrome: 250 to 50,000 units PO daily.

FORMS – OTC Generic: 200 units, 400 units, 800 units, 1000 units, 2000 units (caps/tabs).Trade only: Soln 400 units/drop, 1000 units/drop, 2000 units/drop.

NOTES – Sufficient level of 25(OH) vitamin D is greater than 20 ng/mL, optimal is greater than 30 ng/mL.

ENDOCRINE AND METABOLIC: Other

AMMONUL (**sodium phenylacetate + sodium benzoate**) ▶KL ♀C ◗? $$$$$

ADULT – Acute hyperammonemia with encephalopathy in urea cycle enzyme deficiency: 55 mL/m^2 IV over 90 to 120 min, followed by maintenance 55 mL/m^2 over 24 h. Stop when hyperammonemia resolved or oral nutrition and medications are tolerated.

PEDS – Acute hyperammonemia with encephalopathy in urea cycle enzyme deficiency: If wt 20 kg or less, then 2.5 mL/kg IV over 90 to 120 min, followed by maintenance 2.5 mL/kg over 24 h. If greater than 20 kg, then 55 mL/m^2 IV over 90 to 120 min, followed by maintenance 55 mL/m^2 over 24 h. Consider coadministration of arginine in hyperammonemic infants. Stop when hyperammonemia resolved or oral nutrition and medications are tolerated.

FORMS – Single-use vial 50 mL (10% sodium phenylacetate/10% sodium benzoate).

NOTES – Administer through a central line. Closely monitor if renal insufficiency. Monitor plasma ammonia level, neurological status, electrolytes, blood pH, blood pCO_2, and clinical response. May cause hypokalemia. Consider coadministration of antiemetic. Penicillin and probenecid may affect renal secretion.

BELIMUMAB (***Benlysta***) ▶? – ♀C ◗? $$$$$

ADULT – Systemic lupus erythematosus (SLE): 10 mg/kg IV infusion q 2 weeks for first 3 doses. Then, 10 mg/kg IV infusion q 4 weeks. Infuse over 1 h.

PEDS – Not approved in children.

FORMS – Trade: 120 mg, 400 mg vials.

NOTES – Use for autoantibody-positive SLE in patients on standard therapy. Do not give live immunizations during therapy. More deaths reported with belimumab than placebo during clinical trials. Use with caution in patients with chronic infections and consider stopping therapy if new serious infection develops; reports of serious or fatal infections. Suicide and depression reported.

BROMOCRIPTINE (***Cycloset, Parlodel***) ▶L ♀B ◗– $$$$$

ADULT – Type 2 DM: Start 0.8 mg PO q am, may increase by 0.8 mg weekly to max 4.8 mg. Hyperprolactinemia: Start 1.25 to 2.5 mg PO at bedtime, then increase q 3 to 7 days to usual effective dose of 2.5 to 15 mg/day, max 40 mg/day. Acromegaly: Usual effective dose is 20 to 30 mg/day, max 100 mg/day. Doses greater than 20 mg/day can be divided two times per day. Also approved for Parkinson's disease, but rarely used. Take with food to minimize dizziness and nausea.

PEDS – Not approved in children.

UNAPPROVED ADULT – Neuroleptic malignant syndrome: 2.5 to 5 mg PO 2 to 6 times per day. Hyperprolactinemia: 2.5 to 7.5 mg/day vaginally if GI intolerance occurs with PO dosing.

FORMS – Generic/Trade: Tabs 2.5 mg. Caps 5 mg. Trade only: Tabs 0.8 mg (Cycloset).

NOTES – Take with food to minimize dizziness and nausea. Ergots have been associated with potentially life-threatening fibrotic complications. Seizures, CVA, HTN, arrhythmias, and MI have been reported. Should not be used for postpartum lactation suppression. Contraindicated in Raynaud's syndrome. Avoid concomitant use of other ergot medications.

CABERGOLINE (***Dostinex***) ▶L ♀B ◗– $$$$$

ADULT – Hyperprolactinemia: Initiate therapy with 0.25 mg PO twice a week. Increase by 0.25 mg twice a week at 4-week intervals up to max 1 mg twice a week.

(cont.)

CABERGOLINE (*cont.*)

PEDS – Not approved in children.
UNAPPROVED ADULT – Acromegaly: 0.5 mg PO twice a week. Increase as needed up to 3.5 mg/week based on plasma IGF-1 levels.
FORMS – Generic/Trade: Tabs 0.5 mg.
NOTES – Monitor serum prolactin levels. Hepatically metabolized; use with caution in hepatic insufficiency. Contraindicated if cardiac vascular disease; perform pretreament cardiovascular evaluation for valvular disease. Associated with vavlular disease, especially during use for Parkinson's with higher doses and longer durations of use, but also reported with lower doses in hyperprolactinemia. Monitor for valvular disease via echocardiogram q 6 to 12 months or as clinically indicated. Discontinue if signs of valvular thickening, regurgitation, or restriction. Postmarketing reports of pathological gambling, increased libido, and hypersexuality. Reports of fibrosis. Monitor for signs of pleural fibrosis (dyspnea, shortness of breath, cough), retroperitoneal fibrosis (renal insufficiency, flank pain, abdominal mass) and cardiac fibrosis (cardiac failure).

CALCITONIN (***Miacalcin, Fortical,*** ✤ ***Calcimar, Caltine***) ▶Plasma ♀C ▶? $$$$

ADULT – Osteoporosis: 100 units SC/IM every other day or 200 units (1 spray) intranasal daily (alternate nostrils). Paget's disease: 50 to 100 units SC/IM daily or 3 times per week. Hypercalcemia: 4 units/kg SC/IM q 12 h. May increase after 2 days to max 8 units/kg q 6 h.
PEDS – Not approved in children.
UNAPPROVED ADULT – Acute osteoporotic vertebral fracture pain: 100 units SC/IM daily or 200 units intranasal daily (alternate nostrils).
UNAPPROVED PEDS – Osteogenesis imperfecta, age 6 mo to 15 yo: 2 units/kg SC/IM 3 times per week with oral calcium supplements.
FORMS – Generic/Trade: Nasal spray 200 units/activation in 3.7 mL bottle (minimum of 30 doses/bottle).
NOTES – Skin test before using injectable product: 1 unit intradermally and observe for local reaction. Hypocalcemic effect diminishes in 2 to 7 days, therefore, only useful during acute short-term management of hypercalcemia.

CINACALCET (***Sensipar***) ▶LK ♀C ▶? $$$$$

ADULT – Treatment of secondary hyperparathyroidism in dialysis patients: 30 mg PO daily. May titrate q 2 to 4 weeks through sequential doses of 60, 90, 120, and 180 mg daily to target intact parathyroid hormone level of 150 to 300 pg/mL. Treatment of hypercalcemia in parathyroid carcinoma or primary hyperparathyroidism unable to undergo parathyroidectomy: 30 mg PO two times per day. May titrate q 2 to 4 weeks through sequential doses of 60 mg two times per day, 90 mg two times per day, and 90 mg three to four times per day as necessary to normalize serum calcium levels.
PEDS – Not approved in children.
FORMS – Trade only: Tabs 30, 60, 90 mg.
NOTES – Monitor serum calcium and phosphorus 1 week after initiation or dose adjustment, then monthly after a maintenance dose has been established. Intact parathyroid hormone should be checked 1 to 4 weeks after initiation or dose adjustment, and then 1 to 3 months after a maintenance dose has been established. For parathyroid carcinoma, monitor serum calcium within 1 week after initiation or dose adjustment, then q 2 months after a maintenance dose has been established. Withhold if serum calcium falls below 7.5 mg/dL or if signs and symptoms of hypocalcemia. May restart when calcium level reaches 8.0 mg/dL or when signs and symptoms of hypocalcemia resolve. Reinitiate using the next lowest dose. Use calcium-containing phosphate binder and/or vitamin D to raise calcium if it falls between 7.5 and 8.4 mg/dL. Seizure threshold reduced if hypocalcemia. Reduce dose or discontinue if intact parathyroid hormone level is less than 150 to 300 pg/mL to prevent adynamic bone disease. Do not check parathyroid hormone levels within 12 h after administration of a dose. Inhibits metabolism by CYP2D6; may increase levels of flecainide, vinblastine, thioridazine, TCAs. Dose adjustment may be needed when initiating/discontinuing a strong CYP3A4 inhibitor (ie, ketoconazole, erythromycin, and itraconazole). Closely monitor parathyroid hormone and serum calcium if moderate to severe hepatic impairment.

CONIVAPTAN (***Vaprisol***) ▶LK ♀C ▶? $$$$$

ADULT – Euvolemic or hypervolemic hyponatremia: Loading dose of 20 mg IV over 30 min, then continuous infusion 20 mg over 24 h for 1 to 4 days. Titrate to desired serum sodium. Max dose 40 mg daily as continuous infusion.
PEDS – Not approved in children.
NOTES – No benefit exepected in anuric patients. Avoid concurrent use of CYP3A4 inhibitors (ketoconazole, itraconazole, clarithromycin, ritonavir, indinavir). May increase digoxin levels. Discontinue if hypovolemia, hypotension, or rapid rise in serum sodium

(cont.)

CONIVAPTAN (*cont.*)

(greater than 12 mEq/L/24 h) occurs. Rapid correction of serum sodium may cause osmotic demyelination syndrome. Requires frequent monitoring of serum sodium, volume, and neurologic status. Administer through large veins and change infusion site daily to minimize irritation. Not approved for hyponatremia in heart failure. Increased exposure to conivaptan in renal or hepatic impairment. Not recommended if CrCl less than 30 mL/min.

DENOSUMAB (*Prolia*) ▶? ♀X ▶? $$$$

ADULT — Postmenopausal osteoporosis, androgen deprivation-induced bone loss in men with prostate cancer, aromatase inhibitor-induced bone loss in women with breast cancer: 60 mg SC q 6 months.

PEDS — Not approved in children

FORMS — Trade only: 60 mg/1 mL vial, prefilled syringe.

NOTES — Must correct hypocalcemia before administration, monitor calcium especially in renal insufficiency. Administered by a healthcare professional SC in upper arm, upper thigh, or abdomen. Give calcium 1000 mg and at least 400 International units vitamin D daily. Prolia contains same active ingredient (denosumab) as Xgeva; see Oncology section for Xgeva indications.

DESMOPRESSIN (*DDAVP, Stimate,* ✤ *Minirin, Octostim*) ▶LK ♀B ▶? $$$$

WARNING — Adjust fluid intake downward to decrease potential water intoxication and hyponatremia; use cautiously in those at risk.

ADULT — Diabetes insipidus: 10 to 40 mcg (0.1 to 0.4 mL) intranasally daily or divided two to three times per day or 0.05 to 1.2 mg PO daily or divided two to three times per day or 0.5 to 1 mL (2 to 4 mcg) SC/IV daily in 2 divided doses. Hemophilia A, von Willebrand's disease: 0.3 mcg/kg IV over 15 to 30 min; 300 mcg intranasally if wt 50 kg or more (1 spray in each nostril), 150 mcg intranasally if wt less than 50 kg (single spray in 1 nostril). Primary nocturnal enuresis: 0.2 to 0.6 mg PO at bedtime.

PEDS — Diabetes insipidus 3 mo to 12 yo: 5 to 30 mcg (0.05 to 0.3 mL) intranasally once or twice daily or 0.05 mg PO daily. Hemophilia A, von Willebrand's disease (age 3 mo or older for IV, age 11 mo 12 yo for nasal spray): 0.3 mcg/kg IV over 15 to 30 min; 300 mcg intranasally if wt 50 kg or greater (1 spray in each nostril), 150 mcg intranasally if wt less than 50 kg (single spray in 1 nostril). Primary nocturnal enuresis, age 6 yo or older: 0.2 to 0.6 mg PO at bedtime.

UNAPPROVED ADULT — Uremic bleeding: 0.3 mcg/kg IV single dose or q 12 h (onset 1 to 2 h; duration 6 to 8 h after single dose). Intranasal is 20 mcg/day (onset 24 to 72 h; duration 14 days during 14-day course).

UNAPPROVED PEDS — Hemophilia A and type 1 von Willebrand's disease: 2 to 4 mcg/kg intranasally or 0.2 to 0.4 mcg/kg IV over 15 to 30 min.

FORMS — Trade only: Stimate nasal spray 150 mcg/0.1 mL (1 spray), 2.5 mL bottle (25 sprays). Generic/Trade (DDAVP nasal spray): 10 mcg/0.1 mL (1 spray), 5 mL bottle (50 sprays). Note difference in concentration of nasal soln. Rhinal tube: 2.5 mL bottle with 2 flexible plastic tube applicators with graduation marks for dosing. Generic only: Tabs 0.1, 0.2 mg.

NOTES — Monitor serum sodium and for signs/symptoms of hyponatremia, including headache, wt gain, altered mental status, muscle weakness/cramps, seizure, coma, or respiratory arrest. Restrict fluid intake 1 h before to 8 h after PO administration. Hold PO treatment for enuresis during acute illnesses that may cause fluid/electrolyte imbalances. Start at lowest dose with diabetes insipidus. IV/SC doses are approximately $\frac{1}{10}$ the intranasal dose. Anaphylaxis reported with both IV and intranasal forms. Do not give if type IIB von Willebrand's disease. Changes in nasal mucosa may impair absorption of nasal spray. Refrigerate nasal spray; stable for 3 weeks at room temperature. 10 mcg = 40 units desmopressin.

DIAZOXIDE (*Hyperstat, Proglycem*) ▶L ♀C ▶– $$$$$

ADULT — Hypoglycemia from hyperinsulinism: Initially 3 mg/kg/day PO divided equally q 8 h, usual maintenance dose 3 to 8 mg/kg/day divided equally q 8 to 12 h, max 10 to 15 mg/kg/day.

PEDS — Hypoglycemia from hyperinsulinism: Neonates and infants, initially 10 mg/kg/day divided equally q 8 h, usual maintenance dose 8 to 15 mg/kg/day divided equally q 8 to 12 h; children, same as adult.

FORMS — Trade only: Susp 50 mg/mL (30 mL).

NOTES — Close monitoring of blood glucose required. Consider reduced dose in renal impairment. Used for hyperinsulinism associated with islet cell adenoma, carcinoma, or hyperplasia; extrapancreatic malignancy, leucine sensitivty in children, nesidioblastosis. Avoid if hypersensitivity to thiazides

(cont.)

DIAZOXIDE (*cont.*)

or sulfonamide derivatives. Caution in gout; may increase uric acid. Monitor for edema and heart failure exacerbation during administration; diuretic therapy may be needed.

GALLIUM (***Ganite***) ▶K ♀C ▶? $$$$$

WARNING – Monitor creatinine (contraindicated if greater than 2.5 mg/dL), urine output, calcium, and phosphorous. Avoid concurrent nephrotoxic drugs (eg, aminoglycosides, amphotericin B). Establish urinary output of at least 2 L/day prior to treatment and maintain adequate hydration during therapy.

ADULT – Hypercalcemia of malignancy: 200 mg/m²/day for 5 days. Shorten course if hypercalcemia is corrected. If mild hypercalcemia with few symptoms, consider 100 mg/m²/day for 5 days. Administer as slow IV infusion over 24 h.

PEDS – Not approved in children.

NOTES – Monitor creatinine (contraindicated if greater than 2.5 mg/dL), urine output, calcium and phosphorous. Avoid concurrent nephrotoxic drugs (eg, aminoglycosides, amphotericin B). Ensure adequate hydration prior to infusion.

SODIUM POLYSTYRENE SULFONATE (***Kayexalate***) ▶Fecal excretion ♀C ▶? $$$$

ADULT – Hyperkalemia: 15 g PO one to four times per day or 30 to 50 g retention enema (in sorbitol) q 6 h prn. Retain for 30 min to several h. Irrigate with tap water after enema to prevent necrosis.

PEDS – Hyperkalemia: 1 g/kg PO q 6 h.

UNAPPROVED PEDS – Hyperkalemia: 1 g/kg PR q 2 to 6 h.

FORMS – Generic only: Susp 15 g/60 mL. Powdered resin.

NOTES – 1 g binds approximately 1 mEq of potassium. Avoid in bowel obstruction, constipation, or abnormal bowel function, including patients without a bowel movement post-surgery. Avoid administration with sorbitol as intestinal necrosis has been reported. Discontinue use if constipation develops. Follow aspiration cautions during oral administration.

SOMATROPIN (**human growth hormone, *Genotropin, Humatrope, Norditropin, Norditropin NordiFlex, Nutropin, Nutropin AQ, Nutropin Depot, Omnitrope, Protropin, Serostim, Serostim LQ, Saizen, Tev-Tropin, Valtropin, Zorbtive***) ▶LK ♀B/C ▶? $$$$$

WARNING – Avoid in patients with Prader-Willi syndrome who are severely obese, have severe respiratory impairment or sleep apnea, or unidentified respiratory infection; fatalities have been reported.

ADULT – Growth hormone deficiency (Genotropin, Humatrope, Nutropin, Nutropin AQ, Norditropin, Nutropin, Nutropin AQ, Omnitrope, Saizen, Valtropin): Doses vary according to product. AIDS wasting or cachexia (Serostim, Serostim LQ): 0.1 mg/kg SC daily, max 6 mg daily. Short bowel syndrome (Zorbtive): 0.1 mg/kg SC daily, max 8 mg daily.

PEDS – Growth hormone deficiency (Genotropin, Humatrope, Norditropin, Nutropin, Nutropin AQ, Nutropin Depot, Omnitrope, Tev-Tropin, Saizen): Doses vary according to product used. Turner syndrome (Genotropin, Humatrope, Norditropin, Nutropin, Nutropin AQ, Valtropin): Doses vary according to product used. Growth failure in Prader-Willi syndrome (Genotropin, Omnitrope): Individualized dosing. Idiopathic short stature (Genotropin, Humatrope): Individualized dosing. SHOX deficiency (Humatrope): Individualized dosing. Short stature in Noonan syndrome (Norditropin): Individualized dosing. Growth failure in chronic renal insufficiency (Nutropin, Nutropin AQ): Individualized dosing. Short stature in small for gestational age children (Humatrope, Norditropin, Omnitrope): Individualized dosing.

FORMS – Single-dose vials (powder for injection with diluent). Tev-Tropin: 5 mg vial (powder for injection with diluent, stable for 14 days when refrigerated). Genotropin: 1.5, 5.8, 13.8 mg cartridges. Humatrope: 6, 12, 24 mg pen cartridges; 5 mg vial (powder for injection with diluent, stable for 14 days when refrigerated). Nutropin AQ: 10 mg multidose vial, 5, 10, 20 mg/pen cartridges. Norditropin: 5, 10, 15 mg pen cartridges. Norditropin NordiFlex: 5, 10, 15 mg prefilled pens. Omnitrope: 1.5, 5.8 mg vial (powder for injection with diluent). Saizen: Preassembled reconstitution device with autoinjector pen. Serostim: 4, 5, 6 mg single-dose vials; 4, 8.8 mg multidose vials; and 8.8 mg cartridges for autoinjector. Valtropin: 5 mg single-dose vials, 5 mg prefilled syringe. Zorbtive: 8.8 mg vial (powder for injection with diluent, stable for 14 days when refrigerated).

NOTES – Do not use in children with closed epiphyses. Contraindicated in active malignancy or acute critical illness. Monitor glucose for insulin resistance; use with caution if diabetes or risk for diabetes. Transient and dose-dependent fluid retention may occur in adults. May cause hypothyroidism. Monitor thyroid function periodically. Evaluate patients with Prader-Willi syndrome for upper airway obstruction and sleep apnea

(cont.)

SOMATROPIN (*cont.*)

prior to treatment; control wt and monitor for signs and symptoms of respiratory infection. Avoid if pre-proliferative or proliferative diabetic retinopathy. Perform funduscopic exam initially and then periodically. Monitor other hormonal replacement treatments closely in patients with hypopituitarism. Risk of pancreatitis may be greater in children, especially girls with Turner syndrome; consider pancreatitis if perisistent abdominial pain.

TERIPARATIDE (*Forteo*) ▶LK ♀C ▶– $$$$$

WARNING – Osteosarcoma in animal studies; avoid in those at risk (eg, Paget's disease, prior skeletal radiation).

ADULT – Treatment of postmenopausal osteoporosis, treatment of men and women with glucocorticoid-induced osteoporosis, or to increase bone mass in men with primary or hypogonadal osteoporosis and high risk for fracture: 20 mcg SC daily in thigh or abdomen for no longer than 2 years.

PEDS – Not approved in children.

FORMS – Trade only: 28-dose pen injector (20 mcg/dose).

NOTES – Take with calcium and vitamin D. Pen-like delivery device requires education, and should be discarded 28 days after 1st injection even if not empty.

TOLVAPTAN (*Samsca*) ▶K ♀C ▶? $$$$$

WARNING – Start and restart therapy in the hospital setting to closely monitor serum sodium. Avoid rapid correction of serum sodium (greater than 12 mEq/L/24 h); rapid correction may cause osmotic demyelination causing death or symptoms including dysarthria, dysphagia, lethargy, seizures, or coma. Slower correction advised in higher risk patients including malnutrition, alcoholism, or advanced liver disease.

ADULT – Euvolemic or hypervolemic hyponatremia (sodium less than 125 mEq/L): Start 15 mg PO daily. Titrate to desired serum sodium. If needed, increase q 24 h or more slowly to 30 mg PO daily; max dose 60 mg daily.

PEDS – Not approved in children.

FORMS – Trade only: Tabs 15, 30 mg.

NOTES – Avoid fluid restriction for first 24 h. May use for hyponatremia secondary to heart failure, cirrhosis, or SIADH. May use in hyponatremia with sodium greater than 125 mEq/L if resistant to fluid restriction and symptomatic. Do not use if urgent rise in serum sodium needed or serious neurologic symptoms. Requires frequent monitoring of serum sodium, volume, and neurologic status; monitor potassium if baseline K greater than 5 mEq/L. Administer through large veins and change infusion site daily to minimize irritation. Avoid concurrent use of strong or moderate CYP3A4 inhibitors or inducers.

VASOPRESSIN (*Pitressin, ADH,* ✤ *Pressyn AR*) ▶LK ♀C ▶? $$$$$

ADULT – Diabetes insipidus: 5 to 10 units IM/SC two to four times per day prn.

PEDS – Not approved in children.

UNAPPROVED ADULT – Cardiac arrest: 40 units IV; may repeat if no response after 3 min. Septic shock: 0.01 to 0.1 units/min IV infusion, usual dose less than 0.04 units/min. Bleeding esophageal varices: 0.2 to 0.4 units/min initially (max 0.8 units/min).

UNAPPROVED PEDS – Diabetes insipidus: 2.5 to 10 units IM/SC two to four times per day prn. Bleeding esophageal varices: Start 0.002 to 0.005 units/kg/min IV, increase prn to 0.01 units/kg/min. Growth hormone and corticotropin provocative test: 0.3 units/kg IM, max 10 units.

NOTES – Monitor serum sodium. Injectable form may be given intranasally. May cause tissue necrosis with extravasation.

ENT: Antihistamines—Non-Sedating

NOTE: Antihistamines ineffective when treating the common cold.

DESLORATADINE (*Clarinex,* ✤ *Aerius*) ▶LK ♀C ▶+ $$$

ADULT – Allergic rhinitis, urticaria: 5 mg PO daily.

PEDS – Allergic rhinitis, urticaria: 2 mL (1 mg) PO daily for age 6 to 11 mo, ½ teaspoonful (1.25 mg) PO daily for age 12 mo to 5 yo, 1 teaspoonful (2.5 mg) PO daily for age 6 to 11 yo, 5 mg PO daily for age older than 12 yo.

FORMS – Trade only: Tabs 5 mg. Fast-dissolve RediTabs 2.5, 5 mg. Syrup 0.5 mg/mL.

NOTES – Increase dosing interval in liver or renal insufficiency to every other day. Use a measured dropper for syrup.

FEXOFENADINE (*Allegra*) ▶LK ♀C ▶+ $$$

ADULT – Allergic rhinitis, urticaria: 60 mg PO two times per day or 180 mg PO daily. 60 mg PO daily if decreased renal function.

(cont.)

FEXOFENADINE (*cont.*)

PEDS – Allergic rhinitis, urticaria: 30 mg PO two times per day or orally disintegrating tab two times per day for age 2 to 11 yo. Use adult dose for age older than 12 yo. 30 mg PO daily if decreased renal function. Urticaria: 15 mg (2.5 mL) twice daily for age 6 mo to younger than 2 yo. 15 mg PO daily if decreased renal function.

FORMS – OTC Generic/Trade: Tabs 30, 60, 180 mg, Caps 60 mg. Trade only: Susp 30 mg/5 mL, orally disintegrating tab 30 mg.

NOTES – Avoid taking with fruit juice due to a large decrease in bioavailability. Do not remove orally disintegrating tab from its blister package until time of administration.

LORATADINE (*Claritin, Claritin Hives Relief, Claritin RediTabs, Alavert, Tavist ND*) ▶LK ♀B ▶+ $

ADULT – Allergic rhinitis, urticaria: 10 mg PO daily.

PEDS – Allergic rhinitis, urticaria: 10 mg PO daily for age older than 6 yo, 5 mg PO daily (syrup) for age 2 to 5 yo.

FORMS – OTC Generic/Trade: Tabs 10 mg. Fast-dissolve tabs (Alavert, Claritin RediTabs) 5, 10 mg. Syrup 1 mg/mL. Rx Trade only (Claritin): Chewable tabs 5 mg, Liqui-gel caps 10 mg.

NOTES – Decrease dose in liver failure or renal insufficiency. Fast-dissolve tabs dissolve on tongue without water. ND indicates nondrowsy (Tavist).

ENT: Antihistamines—Other

NOTE: Antihistamines ineffective when treating the common cold. Contraindicated in narrow-angle glaucoma, BPH, stenosing peptic ulcer disease, and bladder obstruction. Use half the normal dose in the elderly. May cause drowsiness and/or sedation, which may be enhanced with alcohol, sedatives, and other CNS depressants. Deaths have occurred in children younger than 2 yo attributed to toxicity from cough and cold medications; the FDA does not recommend their use in this age group.

CARBINOXAMINE (*Palgic*) ▶L ♀C ▶– $$$

ADULT – Allergic/vasomotor rhinitis, urticaria: 4 to 8 mg PO three to four times per day.

PEDS – Allergic/vasomotor rhinitis, urticaria: Give 2 mg PO three to four times per day for age 2 to 3 yo, give 2 to 4 mg PO three to four times per day for age 3 to 6 yo, give 4 to 6 mg PO three to four times per day for age 6 yo or older.

FORMS – Generic/Trade: Oral soln 4 mg/5 mL. Tab 4 mg.

NOTES – Decrease dose in hepatic impairment.

CETIRIZINE (*Zyrtec, ✤ Reactine, Aller-Relief*) ▶LK ♀B ▶– $$$

ADULT – Allergic rhinitis, urticaria: 5 to 10 mg PO daily.

PEDS – Allergic rhinitis, urticaria: 5 to 10 mg PO daily for age older than 6 yo. Give 2.5 mg PO daily for age 6 to 23 mo, give 2.5 mg PO daily to two times per day or 5 mg PO daily for age 2 to 5 yo. If age older than 12 mo, may increase to 2.5 mg PO two times per day.

FORMS – OTC Generic/Trade: Tabs 5, 10 mg. Syrup 5 mg/5 mL. Chewable tabs, grape flavored 5, 10 mg.

NOTES – Decrease dose in renal or hepatic impairment.

CHLORPHENIRAMINE (*Chlor-Trimeton, Aller-Chlor*) ▶LK ♀B ▶– $

ADULT – Allergic rhinitis: 4 mg PO q 4 to 6 h. 8 mg PO q 8 to 12 h (timed-release) or 12 mg PO q 12 h (timed-release). Max 24 mg/day.

PEDS – Allergic rhinitis: 2 mg PO q 4 to 6 h (up to 12 mg/day) for age 6 to 11 yo, give adult dose for age 12 yo or older.

UNAPPROVED PEDS – Allergic rhinitis age 2 to 5 yo: 1 mg PO q 4 to 6 h (up to 6 mg/day). Timed release age 6 to 11 yo: 8 mg PO q 12 h prn.

FORMS – OTC Trade only: Tabs extended-release 12 mg. Generic/Trade: Tabs 4 mg. Syrup 2 mg/5 mL. Tabs extended-release 8 mg.

CLEMASTINE (*Tavist-1*) ▶LK ♀B ▶– $

ADULT – Allergic rhinitis: 1.34 mg PO two times per day. Max 8.04 mg/day. Urticaria, angioedema: 2.68 mg PO one to three times per day. Max 8.04 mg/day.

PEDS – Allergic rhinitis: Give 0.67 mg PO two times per day. Max 4.02 mg/day for age 6 to 12 yo, give adult dose for age 12 yo or older. Urticaria, angioedema: Give 1.34 mg PO two times per day (up to 4.02 mg/day) for age 6 to 12 yo, give adult dose for age 6 to 12 yo.

UNAPPROVED PEDS – Allergic rhinitis for age younger than 6 yo: 0.05 mg/kg/day (as clemastine base) PO divided two to three times per day. Max dose 1 mg/day.

FORMS – OTC Generic/Trade: Tabs 1.34 mg. Rx: Generic/Trade: Tabs 2.68 mg, Syrup 0.67 mg/5 mL. Rx: Generic only: Syrup 0.5 mg/5 mL.

NOTES – 1.34 mg is equivalent to 1 mg clemastine base.

CYPROHEPTADINE (*Periactin*) ▶LK ♀B ▶– $

ADULT – Allergic rhinitis, urticaria: Start 4 mg PO three times per day, usual effective dose is 12 to 16 mg/day. Max 32 mg/day.

PEDS – Allergic rhinitis, urticaria: Start 2 mg PO two to three times per day (up to 12 mg/day) for age 2 to 6 yo, Start 4 mg PO two to three times per day (up to 16 mg/day) for age 7 to 14 yo.

UNAPPROVED ADULT – Appetite stimulant: 2 to 4 mg PO three times per day 1 h before meals. Prevention of cluster headaches: 4 mg PO four times per day. Treatment of acute serotonin syndrome: 12 mg PO/NG followed by 2 mg q 2 h until symptoms clear, then 8 mg q 6 h maintenance while syndrome remains active.

FORMS – Generic only: Tabs 4 mg. Syrup 2 mg/5 mL.

DEXCHLORPHENIRAMINE (*Polaramine*) ▶LK ♀? ▶– $$

ADULT – Allergic rhinitis, urticaria: 2 mg PO q 4 to 6 h. Timed-release tabs: 4 or 6 mg PO at bedtime or q 8 to 10 h.

PEDS – Allergic rhinitis, urticaria: Immediate-release tabs and syrup: Give 0.5 mg PO q 4 to 6 h for age 2 to 5 yo, give 1 mg PO q 4 to 6 h for age 6 to 11 yo, give adult dose for age 12 yo or older. Timed-release tabs age 6 to 12 yo: 4 mg PO daily, preferably at at bedtime.

FORMS – Generic only: Tabs immediate-release 2 mg, timed-release 4, 6 mg. Syrup 2 mg/5 mL.

DIPHENHYDRAMINE (*Benadryl, Banophen, Allermax, Diphen, Diphenhist, Dytan, Siladryl, Sominex, ✤Allerdryl, Nytol*) ▶LK ♀B ▶– $

ADULT – Allergic rhinitis, urticaria, hypersensitivity reactions: 25 to 50 mg PO/IM/IV q 4 to 6 h. Max 300 to 400 mg/day. Motion sickness: 25 to 50 mg PO preexposure and q 4 to 6 h prn. Drug-induced parkinsonism: 10 to 50 mg IV/IM. Antitussive: 25 mg PO q 4 h. Max 100 mg/day. EPS: 25 to 50 mg PO three to four times per day or 10 to 50 mg IV/IM three to four times per day. Insomnia: 25 to 50 mg PO at bedtime.

PEDS – Hypersensitivity reactions: Give 12.5 to 25 mg PO q 4 to 6 h or 5 mg/kg/day PO/IV/IM divided four times per day for age 6 to 11 yo, give adult dose for age 12 yo or older. Max 150 mg/day. Antitussive (syrup): Give 6.25 mg PO q 4 h (up to 25 mg/day) for age 2 to 5 yo, give 12.5 mg PO q 4 h (up to 50 mg/day) for age 6 to 12 yo. EPS: 12.5 to 25 mg PO three to four times per day or 5 mg/kg/day IV/IM divided four times per day, max 300 mg/day. Insomnia age 12 yo or older: 25 to 50 mg PO at bedtime.

FORMS – OTC Trade only: Tabs 25, 50 mg, Chewable tabs 12.5 mg. OTC and Rx: Generic only: Caps 25, 50 mg, softgel cap 25 mg. OTC Generic/Trade: Soln 6.25 or 12.5 mg per 5 mL. Rx: Trade only: (Dytan) Susp 25 mg/mL, Chewable tabs 25 mg.

NOTES – Anticholinergic side effects are enhanced in the elderly and may worsen dementia or delirium. Avoid use with donepezil, rivastigmine, galantamine, or tacrine.

HYDROXYZINE (*Atarax, Vistaril*) ▶L ♀C ▶– $$

ADULT – Pruritus: 25 to 100 mg IM/PO one to four times per day or prn.

PEDS – Pruritus: Give 50 mg/day PO divided four times per day for age younger than 6 yo, give 50 to 100 mg/day PO divided four times per day for age 6 or older.

FORMS – Generic only: Tabs 10, 25, 50, 100 mg; Caps 100 mg; Syrup 10 mg/5 mL. Generic/Trade: Caps 25, 50 mg, Susp 25 mg/5 mL (Vistaril). (Caps = Vistaril, Tabs = Atarax).

NOTES – Atarax (hydrochloride salt), Vistaril (pamoate salt).

LEVOCETIRIZINE (*Xyzal*) ▶K ♀B ▶– $$$

ADULT – Allergic rhinitis, urticaria: 5 mg PO daily.

PEDS – Allergic rhinitis, urticaria: Give 2.5 mg PO daily for age 6 to 11 yo, give 5 mg PO daily for age 12 yo or older.

FORMS – Trade only: Tabs scored 5 mg; Oral soln 2.5 mg/5 mL (148 mL).

NOTES – Decrease dose in renal impairment.

MECLIZINE (*Antivert, Bonine, Medivert, Meclicot, Meni-D, ✤Bonamine*) ▶L ♀B ▶? $

ADULT – Motion sickness: 25 to 50 mg PO 1 h prior to travel, then 25 to 50 mg PO daily.

PEDS – Not approved in children.

UNAPPROVED ADULT – Vertigo: 25 mg PO one to four times per day prn.

FORMS – Rx/OTC/Generic/Trade: Tabs 12.5, 25 mg; Chewable tabs 25 mg. Rx/Trade only: Tabs 50 mg.

NOTES – FDA classifies meclizine as "possibly effective" for vertigo. May cause dizziness and drowsiness.

ENT: Antitussives / Expectorants

BENZONATATE (*Tessalon, Tessalon Perles*) ▶L ♀C ▶? $$

ADULT – Cough: 100 to 200 mg PO three times per day. Max 600 mg/day.

PEDS – Cough: give adult dose for age older than 10 yo.

FORMS – Generic/Trade: Softgel caps: 100, 200 mg.

NOTES – Swallow whole. Do not chew. Numbs mouth; possible choking hazard.

DEXTROMETHORPHAN (*Benylin, Delsym, DexAlone, Robitussin Cough, Vick's 44 Cough*) ▶L ♀+ ▶+ $

ADULT – Cough: 10 to 20 mg PO q 4 h or 30 mg PO q 6 to 8 h. 60 mg PO q 12 h (Delsym).

PEDS – Cough: Give either 2.5 to 5 mg PO q 4 h or 7.5 mg PO q 6 to 8 h of regular susp or 15 mg PO q 12 h of sustained action liquid for age 2 to 5 yo, give either 5 to 10 mg PO q 4 h or 15 mg PO q 6 to 8 h of regular susp, or 30 mg PO q 12 h of sustained-action liquid for age 6 to 12 yo, give adult dose for age older than 12 yo.

FORMS – OTC Trade only: Caps 15 mg (Robitussin), 30 mg (DexAlone), Susp, extended-release 30 mg/5 mL (Delsym). Generic/Trade: Syrup 5, 7.5, 10, 15 mg/5 mL. Generic only: Lozenges 5, 10 mg.

NOTES – Contraindicated with MAOIs due to potential for serotonin syndrome.

GUAIFENESIN (*Robitussin, Hytuss, Guiatuss, Mucinex*) ▶L ♀C ▶+ $

ADULT – Expectorant: 100 to 400 mg PO q 4 h. 600 to 1200 mg PO q 12 h (extended-release). Max 2.4 g/day.

PEDS – Expectorant: 50 to 100 mg/dose for age 2 to 5 yo, give 100 to 200 mg/dose for age 6 to 11 yo, give adult dose for age 12 yo or older.

UNAPPROVED PEDS – Expectorant: Give 25 mg PO q 4 h (up to 150 mg/day) for age 6 to 11 mo, give 50 mg po q 4 h (up to 300 mg/day) for age 12 to 23 mo.

FORMS – Rx Generic/Trade: Extended-release tabs 600, 1200 mg. OTC Generic/Trade: Liquid, Syrup 100 mg/5 mL. OTC Trade only: Caps 200 mg (Hytuss), Extended-release tabs 600 mg (Mucinex). OTC Generic only: Tabs 100, 200, 400 mg.

NOTES – Lack of convincing studies to document efficacy.

ENT: Combination Products—OTC

NOTE: Decongestants in some ENT combination products can increase BP, aggravate anxiety, or cause insomnia (use caution). Some contain sedating antihistamines. Sedation can be enhanced by alcohol and other CNS depressants. Some states have restricted or ended OTC sale of pseudoephedrine and pseudoephedrine combination products or reclassified it as a scheduled drug due to the potential for diversion to methamphetamine labs. Deaths have occurred in children younger than 2 yo attributed to toxicity from cough and cold medications; the FDA does not recommend their use in this age group.

ACTIFED COLD AND ALLERGY **(phenylephrine + chlorpheniramine)** ▶L ♀C ▶+ $

ADULT – Allergic rhinitis, nasal congestion: 1 tab PO q 4 to 6 h. Max 4 tabs/day.

PEDS – Allergic rhinitis, nasal congestion: Give ½ tab PO q 4 to 6 h (up to 2 tabs/day) for age 6 to 12 yo, give adult dose for age older than 12 yo.

FORMS – OTC Trade only: Tabs 10 mg phenylephrine/4 mg chlorpheniramine.

ACTIFED COLD AND SINUS **(pseudoephedrine + chlorpheniramine + acetaminophen)** ▶L ♀C ▶+ $$

ADULT – Allergic rhinitis, nasal congestion, headache: 2 caps PO q 6 h. Max 8 caps/day.

PEDS – Allergic rhinitis, nasal congestion/headache: Age older than 12 yo: Use adult dose.

FORMS – OTC Trade only: Tabs 30 mg pseudoephedrine/2 mg chlorpheniramine/500 mg acetaminophen.

ALAVERT D-12 **(pseudoephedrine + loratadine)** ▶LK ♀B ▶– $

ADULT – Allergic rhinitis, nasal congestion: 1 tab PO two times per day.

PEDS – Not approved in children.

FORMS – OTC Generic/Trade: Tabs, 12 h extended-release, 120 mg pseudoephedrine/5 mg loratadine.

NOTES – Decrease dose to 1 tab PO daily with CrCl less than 30 mL/min. Avoid in hepatic insufficiency.

ALEVE COLD AND SINUS **(naproxen + pseudoephedrine)** ▶L ♀C (D in 3rd trimester) ▶+ $

ADULT – Nasal/sinus congestion, fever, and pain: 1 cap PO q 12 h.

PEDS – Nasal/sinus congestion, fever, and pain: Age older than 12 yo: Use adult dose.

FORMS – OTC Generic/Trade: Extended-release caps: 220 mg naproxen sodium/120 mg pseudoephedrine.

ALLERFRIM **(pseudoephedrine + triprolidine)** ▶L ♀C ▶+ $

ADULT – Allergic rhinitis, nasal congestion: 1 tab or 10 mL PO q 4 to 6 h. Max 4 tabs/day or 40 mL/day.

PEDS – Allergic rhinitis, nasal congestion: Give ½ tab or 5 mL PO q 4 to 6 h (up to 2 tabs/day or 20 mL/day) for age 6 to 12 yo, give adult dose for age older than 12 yo.

FORMS – OTC Trade only: Tabs 60 mg pseudoephedrine/2.5 mg triprolidine. Syrup 30 mg pseudoephedrine/1.25 mg triprolidine/5 mL.

APRODINE **(pseudoephedrine + triprolidine)** ▶L ♀C ▶+ $

ADULT – Allergic rhinitis, nasal congestion: 1 tab or 10 mL PO q 4 to 6 h. Max 4 tabs/day or 40 mL/day.

PEDS – Allergic rhinitis, nasal congestion: Age older than 12 yo: Use adult dose. 6 to 12 yo: ½ tab or 5 mL PO q 4 to 6 h. Max 2 tabs/day or 20 mL/day.

FORMS – OTC Trade only: Tabs 60 mg pseudoephedrine/2.5 mg triprolidine. Syrup 30 mg pseudoephedrine/1.25 mg triprolidine/5 mL.

BENADRYL ALLERGY AND COLD **(phenylephrine + diphenhydramine + acetaminophen)** ▶L ♀C ▶– $

ADULT – Allergic rhinitis, nasal congestion, headache: 2 tabs PO q 4 h. Max 12 tabs/day.

PEDS – Allergic rhinitis, nasal congestion, headache: Give 1 tab PO q 4 h (up to 5 tabs/day) for age 6 to 12 yo, give adult dose for age older than 12 yo.

FORMS – OTC Trade only: Tabs 5/12.5/325 mg of phenylephrine/diphenhydramine/acetaminophen.

BENADRYL-D ALLERGY AND SINUS **(phenylephrine + diphenhydramine)** ▶L ♀C ▶– $

ADULT – Allergic rhinitis, nasal congestion: 1 tab PO q 4 h. Max 6 tabs/day.

PEDS – Allergic rhinitis, nasal congestion: Age older than 12 yo: Use adult dose.

FORMS – OTC Trade only: Tabs 10/25 mg phenylephrine/diphenhydramine.

CHERACOL D COUGH **(guaifenesin + dextromethorphan)** ▶L ♀C ▶? $

ADULT – Cough: 10 mL PO q 4 h.

PEDS – Cough: Give 2.5 mL PO q 4 h (up to 15 mL/day) for age 2 to 5 yo, give 5 mL PO q 4 h for age 6 to 11 yo, give adult dose for age 12 yo or older.

FORMS – OTC Generic/Trade: Syrup 100 mg guaifenesin/10 mg dextromethorphan/5 mL.

CHILDREN'S ADVIL COLD **(ibuprofen + pseudoephedrine)** ▶L ♀C (D in 3rd trimester) ▶+ $

ADULT – Not approved for use in adults.

PEDS – Nasal congestion, sore throat, fever: Give 5 mL PO q 6 h for age 2 to 5 yo, give 10 mL PO q 6 h for age 6 to 11 yo.

FORMS – OTC Trade only: Susp: 100 mg ibuprofen/15 mg pseudoephedrine/5 mL. Grape flavor, alcohol-free.

NOTES – Shake well before using. Do not use for more than 7 days for cold, sinus, and flu symptoms.

CLARITIN-D 12 HR **(pseudoephedrine + loratadine)** ▶LK ♀B ▶+ $

ADULT – Allergic rhinitis, nasal congestion: 1 tab PO two times per day.

PEDS – Not approved in children.

FORMS – OTC Generic/Trade: Tabs, 12 h extended-release: 120 mg pseudoephedrine/5 mg loratadine.

NOTES – Decrease dose to 1 tab PO daily with CrCl less than 30 mL/min. Avoid in hepatic insufficiency.

CLARITIN-D 24 HR **(pseudoephedrine + loratadine)** ▶LK ♀B ▶+ $

ADULT – Allergic rhinitis, nasal congestion: 1 tab PO daily.

PEDS – Not approved in children.

FORMS – OTC Generic/Trade: Tabs, 24 h extended-release: 240 mg pseudoephedrine/10 mg loratadine.

NOTES – Decrease dose to 1 tab PO every other day with CrCl less than 30 mL/min. Avoid in hepatic insufficiency.

CORICIDIN HBP CONGESTION AND COUGH **(guaifenesin + dextromethorphan)** ▶LK ♀B ▶+ $$

ADULT – Productive cough: 1 to 2 softgels PO q 4 h. Max 12 softgels/day.

PEDS – Productive cough: Give adult dose for 12 yo or older.

FORMS – OTC Trade only: Softgels 200 mg guaifenesin/10 mg dextromethorphan.

CORICIDIN HBP COUGH AND COLD **(chlorpheniramine + dextromethorphan)** ▶LK ♀B ▶+ $

ADULT – Rhinitis, cough: 1 tab q 6 h. Max 4 doses/day.

PEDS – Rhinitis, cough: Give adult dose for 12 yo or older.

FORMS – OTC Trade only: Tabs 4 mg chlorpheniramine/30 mg dextromethorphan.

DIMETAPP COLD AND ALLERGY **(phenylephrine + brompheniramine)** ▶LK ♀C ▶– $

ADULT – Allergic rhinitis, nasal congestion: 20 mL PO q 4 h. Max 4 doses/day.

PEDS – Allergic rhinitis, nasal congestion: 10 mL PO q 4 h for age 6 to 11 yo, give adult dose for 12 yo or older.

FORMS – OTC Trade only: Liquid, Tabs 2.5 mg phenylephrine/1 mg brompheniramine per tab or 5 mL.

NOTES – Grape flavor, alcohol-free.

DIMETAPP COLD AND COUGH **(phenylephrine + brompheniramine + dextromethorphan)** ▶LK ♀C ▶– $
ADULT – Nasal congestion, cough: 20 mL PO q 4 h. Max 6 doses/day.
PEDS – Nasal congestion, cough: Give 10 mL PO q 4 h (up to 6 doses/day) for age 6 to 11 yo, give adult dose for 12 yo or older.
FORMS – OTC Trade only: Liquid 2.5 mg phenylephrine/1 mg brompheniramine/5 mg dextromethorphan/5 mL.
NOTES – Red grape flavor, alcohol-free.

DIMETAPP NIGHTTIME COLD AND CONGESTION **(phenylephrine + diphenydramine)** ▶LK ♀C ▶– $
ADULT – Nasal congestion, runny nose, fever, cough, sore throat: 20 mL PO q 4 h. Max 5 doses/day.
PEDS – Nasal congestion, runny nose, fever, cough, sore throat: Give 10 mL PO q 4 h (up to 5 doses/day) for age 6 to 11 yo, give adult dose for 12 yo or older.
FORMS – OTC Trade only: Syrup 2.5 mg phenylephrine and 6.25 mg diphenhydramine.
NOTES – Bubble gum flavor, alcohol-free.

DRIXORAL COLD AND ALLERGY **(pseudoephedrine + dexbrompheniramine)** ▶LK ♀C ▶– $
ADULT – Allergic rhinitis, nasal congestion: 1 tab PO q 12 h.
PEDS – Allergic rhinitis, nasal congestion: Give adult dose for 12 yo or older.
FORMS – OTC Trade only: Tabs, sustained-action 120 mg pseudoephedrine/6 mg dexbrompheniramine.

GUIATUSS PE **(pseudoephedrine + guaifenesin)** ▶L ♀C ▶– $
ADULT – Nasal congestion, cough: 10 mL PO q 4 h. Max 40 mL/day.
PEDS – Nasal congestion, cough: Give 2.5 mL PO q 4 h for age 2 to 5 yo, give 5 mL PO q 4 h for age 6 to 11 yo, give adult dose for 12 yo or older. Max 4 doses/day.
FORMS – OTC Trade only: Syrup 30 mg pseudoephedrine/100 mg guaifenesin/5 mL.
NOTES – PE indicates pseudoephedrine.

MUCINEX D **(guaifenesin + pseudoephedrine)** ▶L ♀C ▶? $
WARNING – Multiple strengths; write specific product on Rx.
ADULT – Cough, congestion: 2 tabs (600/60) PO q 12 h; max 4 tabs/24 h. 1 tab (1200/120) PO q 12 h; max 2 tabs/24 h.
PEDS – Cough: Give adult dose for 12 yo or older.
FORMS – OTC Trade only: Tabs, extended-release: 600/60, 1200/120 mg guaifenesin/pseudoephedrine.
NOTES – Do not crush, chew, or break the tab. Take with a full glass of water.

MUCINEX DM **(guaifenesin + dextromethorphan)** ▶L ♀C ▶? $
WARNING – Multiple strengths; write specific product on Rx.
ADULT – Cough: 1 to 2 tabs (600/30) PO q 12 h; max 4 tabs/24 h. 1 tab (1200/60) PO q 12 h; max 2 tabs/24 h.
PEDS – Cough: Give adult dose for 12 yo or older.
FORMS – OTC Trade only: Tabs, extended-release: 600/30, 1200/60 mg guaifenesin/dextromethorphan.
NOTES – DM indicates dextromethorphan. Do not crush, chew, or break the tab. Take with a full glass of water.

ROBITUSSIN CF **(phenylephrine + guaifenesin + dextromethorphan)** ▶L ♀C ▶– $
ADULT – Nasal congestion, cough: 10 mL PO q 4 h.
PEDS – Nasal congestion, cough: Give 2.5 mL PO q 4 h for age 2 to 5 yo, give 5 mL PO q 4 h for age 6 to 11 yo, give adult dose for 12 yo or older.
FORMS – OTC Generic/Trade: Syrup 5 mg phenylephrine/100 mg guaifenesin/10 mg dextromethorphan/5 mL.
NOTES – CF indicates cough formula.

ROBITUSSIN DM **(guaifenesin + dextromethorphan)** ▶L ♀C ▶+ $
ADULT – Cough: 10 mL PO q 4 h. Max 60 mL/day.
PEDS – Cough: Give 2.5 mL PO q 4 h (up to 15 mL/day) for age 2 to 5 yo, give 5 mL PO q 4 h (up to 30 mL/day) for age 6 to 11 yo, give adult dose for 12 yo or older.
FORMS – OTC Generic/Trade: Syrup 100 mg guaifenesin/10 mg dextromethorphan/5 mL.
NOTES – Alcohol-free. DM indicates dextromethorphan.

TRIAMINIC CHEST AND NASAL CONGESTION **(phenylephrine + guaifenesin)** ▶LK ♀C ▶– $
ADULT – Child-only preparation.
PEDS – Chest, nasal congestion: Give 5 mL PO q 4 h (up to 6 doses/day) for age 2 to 6 yo, give 10 mL PO q 4 h (up to 6 doses/day) for age 6 to 12 yo.
FORMS – OTC Trade only, yellow label: Syrup 2.5 mg phenylephrine/50 mg guaifenesin/5 mL, tropical flavor.

TRIAMINIC COLD AND ALLERGY **(phenylephrine + chlorpheniramine)** ▶LK ♀C ▶– $
ADULT – Child-only preparation.
PEDS – Allergic rhinitis, nasal congestion: 10 mL PO q 4 h to max 6 doses/day for age 6 to 12 yo.
FORMS – OTC Trade only, orange label: Syrup 2.5 mg phenylephrine/1 mg chlorpheniramine/5 mL, orange flavor.

TRIAMINIC COUGH AND SORE THROAT **(dextromethorphan + acetaminophen)** ▶LK ♀C ▶– $
ADULT – Child-only preparation.
PEDS – Cough, sore throat: Give PO q 4 h to max 5 doses/day: 5 mL or 1 softchew tab per dose for age 2 to 6 yo, give 10 mL or 2 softchew tabs per dose for age 7 to 12 yo.
FORMS – OTC Trade only, purple label: Syrup, softchew tabs 5 mg dextromethorphan/160 mg acetaminophen/5 mL or tab, grape flavor.

TRIAMINIC DAY TIME COLD AND COUGH **(phenylephrine + dextromethorphan)** ▶LK ♀C ▶– $
ADULT – Child-only preparation.
PEDS – Nasal congestion, cough: Give PO q 4 h to max 6 doses/day: 5 mL or 1 strip per dose for age 2 to 6 yo, give 10 mL or 2 strips per dose for age 7 to 12 yo.
FORMS – OTC Trade only, red label: Syrup, thin strips 2.5 mg phenylephrine/5 mg dextromethorphan/5 mL, cherry flavor.
NOTES – Allow strips to dissolve on the tongue.

TRIAMINIC FLU COUGH AND FEVER **(acetaminophen + chlorpheniramine + dextromethorphan)** ▶LK ♀C ▶– $
ADULT – Child-only preparation.
PEDS – Fever, cough: 10 mL PO q 6 h to max 4 doses/day for age 6 to 12 yo.
FORMS – OTC Trade only, pink label: Syrup 160 mg acetaminophen/1 mg chlorpheniramine/7.5 mg dextromethorphan/5 mL, bubble gum flavor.

TRIAMINIC NIGHT TIME COLD AND COUGH **(phenylephrine + diphenhydramine)** ▶LK ♀C ▶– $
ADULT – Child-only preparation.
PEDS – Nasal congestion, cough: 10 mL PO q 4 h to max 6 doses/day for age 6 to 12 yo.
FORMS – OTC Trade only, blue label: Syrup 2.5 mg phenylephrine/6.25 mg diphenhydramine/5 mL, grape flavor.

ENT: Combination Products—Rx Only

NOTE: Decongestants in some ENT combination products can increase BP, aggravate anxiety, or cause insomnia (use caution). Some contain sedating antihistamines. Sedation can be enhanced by alcohol and other CNS depressants. Deaths have occurred in children younger than 2 yo attributed to toxicity from cough and cold medications; the FDA does not recommend their use in this age group.

ALLEGRA-D 12-HOUR **(fexofenadine + pseudoephedrine)** ▶LK ♀C ▶+ $$$$
ADULT – Allergic rhinitis, nasal congestion: 1 tab PO q 12 h.
PEDS – Not approved in children.
FORMS – Trade only: Tabs, extended-release 60/120 mg fexofenadine/pseudoephedrine.
NOTES – Decrease dose to 1 tab PO daily with decreased renal function. Take on an empty stomach. Avoid taking with fruit juice due to a large decrease in bioavailability.

ALLEGRA-D 24-HOUR **(fexofenadine + pseudoephedrine)** ▶LK ♀C ▶+ $$$$
ADULT – Allergic rhinitis, nasal congestion: 1 tab PO daily.
PEDS – Not approved in children.
FORMS – Trade only: Tabs, extended-release 180/240 mg fexofenadine/pseudoephedrine.
NOTES – Decrease dose to 1 tab PO every other day with decreased renal function. Take on an empty stomach. Avoid taking with fruit juice due to a large decrease in bioavailability.

ALLERX **(pseudoephedrine + methscopolamine + chlorpheniramine)** ▶LK ♀C ▶– $$$
ADULT – Allergic rhinitis, vasomotor rhinitis, nasal congestion: 1 yellow am tab q am and 1 blue pm tab q pm.
PEDS – Allergic rhinitis, vasomotor rhinitis, nasal congestion: Use adult dose for age older than 12 yo.
FORMS – Trade only: Tabs, am (yellow): 120 mg pseudoephedrine/2.5 mg methscopolamine. Tabs, pm (blue): 8 mg chlorpheniramine/2.5 mg methscopolamine.
NOTES – Contraindicated in severe HTN, CAD, MAOI therapy, narrow-angle glaucoma, urinary retention, and peptic ulcer. Caution in elderly, hepatic, and renal disease.

BROMFENEX **(pseudoephedrine + brompheniramine)** ▶LK ♀C ▶– $
ADULT – Allergic rhinitis, nasal congestion: 1 cap PO q 12 h. Max 2 caps/day.
PEDS – Allergic rhinitis, nasal congestion: Age older than 12 yo: Use adult dose. 6 to 11 yo: 1 cap PO daily.
FORMS – Generic/Trade: Caps, sustained-release 120 mg pseudoephedrine/12 mg brompheniramine.

BROMFENEX PD **(pseudoephedrine + brompheniramine)** ▶LK ♀C ▶– $
ADULT – Allergic rhinitis, nasal congestion: 1 to 2 caps PO q 12 h. Max 4 caps/day.
PEDS – Allergic rhinitis, nasal congestion: Age older than 12 yo: 1 cap PO q 12 h. Max 2 caps/day.

(cont.)

BROMFENEX PD *(cont.)*

FORMS – Generic/Trade: Caps, sustained-release 60 mg pseudoephedrine/6 mg brompheniramine.

NOTES – PD indicates pediatric.

CARBODEC DM **(pseudoephedrine + carbinoxamine + dextromethorphan)** ▶L ♀C ▶– $

ADULT – Allergic rhinitis, nasal congestion, cough: 5 mL PO four times per day.

PEDS – Allergic rhinitis, nasal congestion, cough: Syrup: Give 2.5 mL PO four times per day for age 18 mo to 5 yo, give 5 mL PO four times per day for age older than 6 yo. Infant gtts: Give 0.25 mL PO four times per day for age 1 to 3 mo, give 0.5 mL PO four times per day for age 4 to 6 mo, give 0.75 mL PO four times per day for age 7 to 9 mo, give 1 mL PO four times per day for age 10 mo to 17 mo.

FORMS – Generic only: Syrup, 60/4/15 mg pseudoephedrine/carbinoxamine/dextromethorphan/ 5 mL. Gtts, 25/2/4 mg/mL, grape flavor 30 mL with dropper, sugar-free.

NOTES – Carbinoxamine has potential for sedation similar to diphenhydramine. DM indicates dextromethorphan.

CHERATUSSIN AC **(guaifenesin + codeine)** ▶L ♀C ▶?©V $

ADULT – Cough: 10 mL PO q 4 h. Max 60 mL/day.

PEDS – Cough: Give 1.25 to 2.5 mL PO q 4 h (up to 15 mL/day) for age 6 to 23 mo, give 2.5 to 5 mL PO q 4 h (up to 30 mL/day) for age 2 to 5 yo, give 5 mL PO q 4 h (up to 30 mL/day) for age 6 to 11 yo, give adult dose for age 12 or older.

FORMS – Generic/Trade: Syrup 100 mg guaifenesin/10 mg codeine/5 mL. Sugar-free.

CHERATUSSIN DAC **(pseudoephedrine + guaifenesin + codeine)** ▶L ♀C ▶?©V $

ADULT – Nasal congestion, cough: 10 mL PO q 4 h. Max 40 mL/day.

PEDS – Nasal congestion, cough: Give 5 mL PO q 4 h (up to 20 mL/day) for age 6 to 11 yo, give adult dose for 12 yo or older.

FORMS – Generic/Trade: Syrup 30 mg pseudoephedrine/100 mg guaifenesin/10 mg codeine/5 mL. Sugar-free.

NOTES – DAC indicates decongestant and codeine.

CHLORDRINE SR **(pseudoephedrine + chlorpheniramine)** ▶LK ♀C ▶– $

ADULT – Allergic rhinitis, nasal congestion: 1 cap PO q 12 h. Max 2 caps/day.

PEDS – Allergic rhinitis, nasal congestion: 1 cap PO daily for age 6 to 11 yo, use adult dose for age 12 yo or older.

FORMS – Generic only: Caps, sustained-release 120 mg pseudoephedrine/8 mg chlorpheniramine.

CLARINEX-D 12 HOUR **(pseudoephedrine + desloratadine)** ▶LK ♀C ▶+ $$$$

ADULT – Allergic rhinitis: 1 tab PO q 12 h.

PEDS – Allergic rhinitis, age 12 yo or older: Use adult dose.

FORMS – Trade only: Tabs, extended-release 120 mg pseudoephedrine/2.5 mg desloratadine.

NOTES – Swallow tabs whole. Avoid with hepatic or renal insufficiency.

CLARINEX-D 24 HOUR **(pseudoephedrine + desloratadine)** ▶LK ♀C ▶+ $$$$

ADULT – Allergic rhinitis: 1 tab PO daily.

PEDS – Allergic rhinitis age 12 yo or older: Use adult dose.

FORMS – Trade only: Tabs, extended-release pseudoephedrine + desloratadine, 120/2.5, 240/5 mg.

NOTES – Instruct patients to swallow the tab whole. Increase dosing interval in renal insufficiency to every other day. Avoid with hepatic insufficiency.

DECONAMINE **(pseudoephedrine + chlorpheniramine)** ▶LK ♀C ▶– $$

WARNING – Multiple strengths; write specific product on Rx.

ADULT – Allergic rhinitis, nasal congestion: 1 tab or 10 mL PO three to four times per day. Max 6 tabs or 60 mL/day. Sustained-release: 1 cap PO q 12 h. Max 2 caps/day.

PEDS – Allergic rhinitis, nasal congestion: Age older than 12 yo: Use adult dose. 6 to 11 yo: ½ tab or 5 mL PO three to four times per day. Max 3 tabs or 30 mL/day.

FORMS – Trade only: Tabs 60/4 mg pseudoephedrine/chlorpheniramine, scored. Syrup 30/2 mg per 5 mL. Chewable tabs 15/1 mg. Generic/Trade: Caps, sustained-release 120/8 mg (Deconamine SR).

DECONSAL II **(phenylephrine + guaifenesin)** ▶L ♀C ▶– $$

ADULT – Nasal congestion, cough: 1 to 2 tabs PO q 12 h. Max 4 tabs/day.

PEDS – Nasal congestion, cough: Give ½ tab PO q 12 h (up to 1 tab/day) for age 2 to 5 yo, give 1 tab PO q 12 h up to 2 tabs/day for 6 to 12 yo, give adult dose for age older than 12 yo.

FORMS – Trade only: Caps, sustained-release 20 mg phenylephrine/375 mg guaifenesin.

DICEL **(pseudoephedrine + chlorpheniramine)** ▶L ♀C ▶– $$

ADULT – Allergic rhinitis, nasal congestion: 10 to 20 mL PO q 12 h. Max 40 mL/day.

(cont.)

DICEL *(cont.)*

PEDS – Allergic rhinitis, nasal congestion: Give 2.5 to 5 mL (up to 10 mL/day) PO q 12 h for age 2 to 5 yo, give 5 to 10 mL PO q 12 h (up to 20 mL/day) for age 6 to 11 yo, give adult dose for age 12 yo or older.

FORMS – Generic/Trade: Susp 75 mg pseudoephedrine/4.5 mg chlorpheniramine/5 mL, strawberry-banana flavor.

DIMETANE-DX COUGH SYRUP **(pseudoephedrine + brompheniramine + dextromethorphan)** ▶L ♀C ▶– $$$

ADULT – Nasal congestion, rhinitis, cough: 10 mL PO q 4 h prn.

PEDS – Nasal congestion, rhinitis, cough: Dose by wt: Give 1.25 mL PO four times per day prn for wt 12 to 22 kg, give 2.5 mL PO four times per day prn for wt 23 to 40 kg. Dose by age: Give 2.5 mL PO q 4 h for age 2 to 5 yo, give 5 mL PO q 4 h for age 6 to 11 yo, give adult dosing for age older than 12 yo.

FORMS – Trade only: Liquid 30 mg pseudoephedrine/2 mg brompheniramine/10 mg dextromethorphan/5 mL, butterscotch flavor. Sugar-free.

DURATUSS **(phenylephrine + guaifenesin)** ▶L ♀C ▶– $

ADULT – Nasal congestion, cough: 1 tab PO q 12 h.

PEDS – Nasal congestion, cough: Give ½ tab PO q 12 h for age 6 to 12, use adult dosing for age older than 12 yo.

FORMS – Generic/Trade: Tabs, long-acting 25 mg phenylephrine/900 mg guaifenesin.

DURATUSS GP **(phenylephrine + guaifenesin)** ▶L ♀C ▶– $

ADULT – Nasal congestion, cough: 1 tab PO q 12 h.

PEDS – Not approved in children.

FORMS – Generic/Trade: Tabs, long-acting 25 mg phenylephrine/1200 mg guaifenesin.

DURATUSS HD **(hydrocodone + phenylephrine + guaifenesin)** ▶L ♀C ▶–©III $$$

ADULT – Cough, nasal congestion: 10 mL PO q 4 to 6 h.

PEDS – Cough, nasal congestion: Give 5 mL PO q 4 to 6 h for age 6 to 12, use adult dosing for age older than 12 yo.

FORMS – Generic/Trade: Elixir 2.5 mg hydrocodone/10 mg phenylephrine/225 mg guaifenesin/5 mL. 5% alcohol.

ENTEX LA **(phenylephrine + guaifenesin)** ▶L ♀C ▶– $$

ADULT – Nasal congestion, cough: 1 tab PO q 12 h.

PEDS – Nasal congestion, cough: Give ½ tab PO q 12 h for age 6 to 11 yo, give adult dose for 12 yo or older.

FORMS – Generic/Trade: Tabs, long-acting 30/600 mg phenylephrine/guaifenesin. Caps, long-acting 30/400 mg.

NOTES – Do not crush or chew.

ENTEX LIQUID **(phenylephrine + guaifenesin)** ▶L ♀C ▶– $$$

ADULT – Nasal congestion, cough: 5 to 10 mL PO q 4 to 6 h. Max 40 mL/day.

PEDS – Nasal congestion, cough: Give 2.5 mL PO q 4 to 6 h (up 10 mL/day) for age 2 to 5 yo, give 5 mL PO q 4 to 6 h (up to 20 mL/day) for age 6 to 11 yo, give adult dose for age 12 yo or older.

FORMS – Generic/Trade: Liquid 7.5 mg phenylephrine/100 mg guaifenesin/5 mL. Punch flavor, alcohol-free.

ENTEX PSE **(pseudoephedrine + guaifenesin)** ▶L ♀C ▶– $

ADULT – Nasal congestion, cough: 1 tab PO q 12 h.

PEDS – Nasal congestion, cough: Give ½ tab PO q 12 h for age 6 to 12 yo, use adult dosing for age older than 12 yo.

FORMS – Generic/Trade: Tabs, long-acting 120 mg pseudoephedrine/600 mg guaifenesin, scored.

NOTES – PSE indicates pseudoephedrine.

GANI-TUSS NR **(guaifenesin + codeine)** ▶L ♀C ▶?©V $

ADULT – Cough: 10 mL PO q 4 h. Max 60 mL/day.

PEDS – Cough: Give 1.25 to 2.5 mL PO q 4 h (up to 15 mL/day) for age 6 to 23 mo, give 2.5 to 5 mL PO q 4 h (up to 30 mL/day) for age 2 to 5 yo, give 5 mL PO q 4 h (up to 30 mL/day) for age 6 to 11 yo, give adult dosing for age 12 yo or older.

FORMS – Generic/Trade: Syrup 100 mg guaifenesin/10 mg codeine/5 mL. Sugar-free.

GUAIFENEX DM **(guaifenesin + dextromethorphan)** ▶L ♀C ▶? $

ADULT – Cough: 1 to 2 tabs PO q 12 h. Max 4 tabs/day.

PEDS – Cough: Give ½ tab PO q 12 h (up to 1 tab/day) for age 2 to 6 yo, give 1 tab PO q 12 h (up to 2 tabs/day) for age 6 to 12 yo, give adult dose for age 12 yo or older.

FORMS – Generic/Trade: Tabs, sustained-release 600 mg guaifenesin/30 mg dextromethorphan, scored.

NOTES – DM indicates dextromethorphan.

GUAIFENEX PSE **(pseudoephedrine + guaifenesin)** ▶L ♀C ▶– $

WARNING – Multiple strengths; write specific product on Rx.

ADULT – Nasal congestion, cough: PSE 60: 1 to 2 tabs PO q 12 h. Max 4 tabs/day. PSE 120: 1 tab PO q 12 h.

PEDS – Nasal congestion, cough: PSE 60: Give ½ tab PO q 12 h (up to 1 tab/day) for age 2

(cont.)

***GUAIFENEX PSE** (cont.)*
to 6 yo, give 1 tab PO q 12 h (up to 2 tabs/day) for age 6 to 12 yo, give adult dose for age 12 yo or older. PSE 120: ½ tab PO q 12 h for age 6 to 12 yo, give adult dose for age older than 12 yo.
FORMS – Generic/Trade: Tabs, extended-release 60/600 mg pseudoephedrine/guaifenesin, scored (Guaifenex PSE 60). Trade only: Tabs, extended-release 120/600 mg (Guaifenex PSE 120).
NOTES – PSE indicates pseudoephedrine.

GUAITEX II SR/PSE **(pseudoephedrine + guaifenesin)** ▶L ♀C ▶– $
WARNING – Multiple strengths; write specific product on Rx.
ADULT – Nasal congestion, cough: 1 to 2 tabs PO q 12 h. Max 4 tabs/day (Guaitex II SR). 1 tab PO q 12 h. Max 2 tabs/day (Guaitex PSE).
PEDS – Nasal congestion, cough: Guaitex II SR: Give ½ tab PO q 12 h (up to 1 tab/day) for age 2 to 6 yo, give 1 tab PO q 12 h (up to 2 tabs/day) for age 6 to 12 yo, give adult dose for age 12 yo or older. Guaitex PSE: Give ½ tab PO q 12 h for age 6 to 12 yo, give adult dose for age older than 12 yo.
FORMS – Generic/Trade: Tabs, sustained-release 60 mg pseudoephedrine/600 mg guaifenesin (Guaitex II SR). Trade only: Tabs, long-acting 120 mg pseudoephedrine/600 mg guaifenesin (Guaitex PSE).
NOTES – PSE indicates pseudoephedrine.

GUIATUSS AC **(guaifenesin + codeine)** ▶L ♀C ▶? ©V $
ADULT – Cough: 10 mL PO q 4 h. Max 60 mL/day.
PEDS – Cough: Give 5 mL PO q 4 h (up to 30 mL/day) for age 6 to 11 yo, give adult dose for 12 yo or older.
FORMS – Generic/Trade: Syrup 100 mg guaifenesin/10 mg codeine/5 mL. Sugar-free.
NOTES – AC indicates before meals and codeine.

GUIATUSSIN DAC **(pseudoephedrine + guaifenesin + codeine)** ▶L ♀C ▶– ©V $
ADULT – Nasal congestion, cough: 10 mL PO q 4 h. Max 40 mL/day.
PEDS – Nasal congestion, cough: Give 5 mL PO q 4 h (up to 20 mL/day) for age 6 to 11 yo, give adult dose for 12 yo or older.
FORMS – Generic/Trade: Syrup 30 mg pseudoephedrine/100 mg guaifenesin/10 mg codeine/5 mL. Sugar-free.
NOTES – DAC indicates decongestant and codeine.

HALOTUSSIN AC **(guaifenesin + codeine)** ▶L ♀C ▶? ©V $
ADULT – Cough: 10 mL PO q 4 h. Max 60 mL/day.
PEDS – Cough: Give 5 mL PO q 4 h (up to 30 mL/day) for age 6 to 11 yo, give adult dose for 12 yo or older.
FORMS – Generic/Trade: Syrup 100 mg guaifenesin/10 mg codeine/5 mL. Sugar-free.
NOTES – AC indicates before meals and codeine.

HALOTUSSIN DAC **(pseudoephedrine + guaifenesin + codeine)** ▶L ♀C ▶– ©V $
ADULT – Nasal congestion, cough: 10 mL PO q 4 h. Max 40 mL/day.
PEDS – Nasal congestion, cough: Give 5 mL PO q 4 h (up to 20 mL/day) for age 6 to 11 yo, give adult dose for 12 yo or older.
FORMS – Generic/Trade: Syrup 30 mg pseudoephedrine/100 mg guaifenesin/10 mg codeine/5 mL. Sugar-free.
NOTES – DAC indicates decongestant and codeine.

HISTINEX HC **(phenylephrine + chlorpheniramine + hydrocodone)** ▶L ♀C ▶– ©III $
ADULT – Allergic rhinitis, congestion, cough: 10 mL PO q 4 h. Max 40 mL/day.
PEDS – Allergic rhinitis, congestion, cough: Give 5 mL PO q 4 h (up to 20 mL/day) for age 6 to 11 yo, give adult dose for 12 yo or older.
FORMS – Generic/Trade: Syrup 5 mg phenylephrine/2 mg chlorpheniramine/2.5 mg hydrocodone/5 mL. Alcohol- and sugar-free.

HISTUSSIN D **(pseudoephedrine + hydrocodone)** ▶L ♀C ▶– ©III $$
ADULT – Nasal congestion, cough: 5 mL PO four times per day prn.
PEDS – Nasal congestion, cough: Give 1.25 mL PO four times per day prn for wt 12 to 22 kg, give 2.5 mL PO four times per day prn for wt 22 to 40 kg.
FORMS – Generic/Trade: Liquid 60 mg pseudoephedrine/5 mg hydrocodone/5 mL, cherry/black raspberry flavor.

HISTUSSIN HC **(phenylephrine + dexbrompheniramine + hydrocodone)** ▶L ♀C ▶– ©III $$
ADULT – Allergic rhinitis, congestion, cough: 10 mL PO q 4 h. Max 40 mL/day.
PEDS – Allergic rhinitis, congestion, cough: Give 5 mL PO q 4 h (up to 20 mL/day) for age 6 to 11 yo, give adult dose for 12 yo or older.
FORMS – Generic/Trade: Syrup 5 mg phenylephrine/ 1 mg dexbrompheniramine/2.5 mg hydrocodone/ 5 mL.

HUMIBID DM **(guaifenesin + guaiacolsulfonate + dextromethorphan)** ▶L ♀C ▶? $

ADULT – Cough: 1 cap PO q 12 h. Max 2 caps/day.

PEDS – Cough: Give 1 cap PO daily for age 6 to 12 yo, give adult dose for 12 yo or older.

FORMS – Trade only: Caps, sustained-release 400 mg guaifenesin/200 mg guaiacolsulfonate/50 mg dextromethorphan.

NOTES – DM indicates dextromethorphan.

HUMIBID LA **(guaifenesin + guaiacolsulfonate)** ▶L ♀C ▶+ $

ADULT – Expectorant: 1 tab PO q 12 h (extended-release). Max 2 tabs/day.

PEDS – Expectorant age older than 12 yo: Use adult dose.

FORMS – Trade only: Tabs, extended-release 600 mg guaifenesin/300 mg guaiacolsulfonate.

HYCOCLEAR TUSS **(hydrocodone + guaifenesin)** ▶L ♀C ▶– ©III $

ADULT – Cough: 5 mL PO after meals and at bedtime. Max 6 doses/day.

PEDS – Cough: Give 2.5 mL PO after meals and at bedtime (up to 6 doses/day) for age 6 to 12 yo, give adult dose for age older than 12 yo.

FORMS – Generic/Trade: Syrup 5 mg hydrocodone/ 100 mg guaifenesin/5 mL. Generic is alcohol- and sugar-free.

HYCODAN **(hydrocodone + homatropine)** ▶L ♀C ▶– ©III $

ADULT – Cough: 1 tab or 5 mL PO q 4 to 6 h. Max 6 doses/day.

PEDS – Cough: Give 2.5 mg (based on hydrocodone) PO q 4 to 6 h prn (up to 15 mg/day) for age 6 to 12 yo, give adult dose for age older than 12 yo.

FORMS – Generic/Trade: Syrup 5 mg hydrocodone/ 1.5 mg homatropine methylbromide/5 mL. Tabs 5/1.5 mg.

NOTES – May cause drowsiness/sedation. Dosing based on hydrocodone content.

HYCOTUSS **(hydrocodone + guaifenesin)** ▶L ♀C ▶– ©III $

ADULT – Cough: 5 mL PO after meals and at bedtime. Max 6 doses/day.

PEDS – Cough: Give 2.5 mL PO after meals and at bedtime (up to 6 doses/day) for age 6 to 12 yo, give adult dose for age older than 12 yo.

FORMS – Generic/Trade: Syrup 5 mg hydrocodone/ 100 mg guaifenesin/5 mL. Generic is alcohol- and sugar-free.

NOVAFED A **(pseudoephedrine + chlorpheniramine)** ▶LK ♀C ▶– $

ADULT – Allergic rhinitis, nasal congestion: 1 cap PO q 12 h. Max 2 caps/day.

PEDS – Allergic rhinitis, nasal congestion: 1 cap PO daily for age 6 to 12 yo, use adult dose for age older than 12 yo.

FORMS – Generic/Trade: Caps, sustained-release 120 mg pseudoephedrine/8 mg chlorpheniramine.

PALGIC DS **(pseudoephedrine + carbinoxamine)** ▶L ♀C ▶– $$

ADULT – Allergic rhinitis, nasal congestion: 10 mL PO four times per day.

PEDS – Allergic rhinitis, nasal congestion: Give up to the following PO four times per day: 1.25 mL for age 1 to 3 mo, 2.5 mL for age 3 to 6 mo, 3.75 mL for age 6 to 9 mo, 3.75 to 5 mL for age 9 to 18 mo, 5 mL for age 18 mo to 6 yo, use adult dose for age older than 6 yo.

FORMS – Generic/Trade: Syrup, 25 mg pseudoephedrine/2 mg carbinoxamine/5 mL. Alcohol- and sugar-free.

NOTES – Carbinoxamine has potential for sedation similar to diphenhydramine.

PHENERGAN VC **(phenylephrine + promethazine)** ▶LK ♀C ▶? $

WARNING – Promethazine contraindicated if age younger than 2 yo due to risk of fatal respiratory depression; caution in older children.

ADULT – Allergic rhinitis, congestion: 5 mL PO q 4 to 6 h. Max 30 mL/day.

PEDS – Allergic rhinitis, congestion: Give 1.25 to 2.5 mL PO q 4 to 6 h (up to 15 mL/day) for age 2 to 5 yo, give 2.5 to 5 mL PO q 4 to 6 h for age 6 to 12 yo (up to 20 mL/day), give adult dose for age 12 yo or older.

FORMS – Trade unavailable. Generic only: Syrup 6.25 mg promethazine/5 mg phenylephrine/ 5 mL.

NOTES – VC indicates vasoconstrictor.

PHENERGAN VC W/CODEINE **(phenylephrine + promethazine + codeine)** ▶LK ♀C ▶? ©V $

WARNING – Promethazine contraindicated if younger than 2 yo due to risk of fatal respiratory depression; caution in older children.

ADULT – Allergic rhinitis, congestion, cough: 5 mL PO q 4 to 6 h. Max 30 mL/day.

PEDS – Allergic rhinitis, congestion, cough: Give 1.25 to 2.5 mL PO q 4 to 6 h (up to 10 mL/day) for age 2 to 5 yo, give 2.5 to 5 mL PO q 4 to 6 h for age 6 to 12 yo (up to 20 mL/day), give adult dose for age 12 yo or older.

FORMS – Trade unavailable. Generic only: Syrup 5 mg phenylephrine/6.25 mg promethazine/10 mg codeine/5 mL.

PHENERGAN WITH CODEINE **(promethazine + codeine)** ▶LK ♀C ▶? ©V $

WARNING – Promethazine contraindicated if younger than 2 yo due to risk of fatal respiratory depression; caution in older children.

(cont.)

PHENERGAN WITH CODEINE *(cont.)*

ADULT – Allergic rhinitis/cough: 5 mL PO q 4 to 6 h. Max 30 mL/day.

PEDS – Allergic rhinitis/cough: Give 1.25 to 2.5 mL PO q 4 to 6 h (up to 10 mL/day) for age 2 to 5 yo, give 2.5 to 5 mL PO q 4 to 6 h (up to 20 mL/day) for age 6 to 12 yo, give adult dose for age 12 yo or older.

FORMS – Trade unavailable. Generic only: Syrup 6.25 mg promethazine/10 mg codeine/5 mL.

PHENERGAN/DEXTROMETHORPHAN **(promethazine + dextromethorphan)** ▶LK ♀C ▶? $

WARNING – Promethazine contraindicated if younger than 2 yo due to risk of fatal respiratory depression; caution in older children.

ADULT – Allergic rhinitis, cough: 5 mL PO q 4 to 6 h. Max 30 mL/day.

PEDS – Allergic rhinitis, cough: Give 1.25 to 2.5 mL PO q 4 to 6 h (up to 10 mL/day) for age 2 to 5 yo, give 2.5 to 5 mL PO q 4 to 6 h (up to 20 mL/day) for age 6 to 12 yo, give adult dose for age 12 yo or older.

FORMS – Trade unavailable. Generic only: Syrup 6.25 mg promethazine/15 mg dextromethorphan/5 mL.

PSEUDO-CHLOR **(pseudoephedrine + chlorpheniramine)** ▶LK ♀C ▶– $

ADULT – Allergic rhinitis, nasal congestion: 1 cap PO q 12 h. Max 2 caps/day.

PEDS – Allergic rhinitis, nasal congestion: Age older than 12 yo: Use adult dose.

FORMS – Generic/Trade: Caps, sustained-release 120 mg pseudoephedrine/8 mg chlorpheniramine.

REZIRA **(hydrocodone + pseudoephedrine)** ▶LK – ♀C ▶–©III

ADULT – Nasal congestion, cough: 5 mL q 4 to 6 h. Max 20 mL/day.

PEDS – Not approved in children.

FORMS – Trade: Syrup 5 mg hydrocodone/ 60 mg pseudoephedrine/ 5 mL.

ROBITUSSIN AC **(guaifenesin + codeine)** ▶L ♀C ▶?©V $

ADULT – The "Robitussin AC" brand is no longer produced; corresponding generics include Cheratussin AC, Gani-Tuss NR, Guiatuss AC, and Halotussin AC.

ROBITUSSIN DAC **(pseudoephedrine + guaifenesin + codeine)** ▶L ♀C ▶–©V $

ADULT – The "Robitussin DAC" brand is no longer produced; corresponding generics include Cheratussin DAC, Guiatuss DAC, and Halotussin DAC.

RONDEC **(phenylephrine + chlorpheniramine)** ▶L ♀C ▶– $$

ADULT – Allergic rhinitis, nasal congestion: 5 mL syrup PO four times per day.

PEDS – Allergic rhinitis, nasal congestion: Give 1.25 mL PO four times per day for age 2 to 5 yo, give 2.5 mL PO four times per day for age 6 to 12 yo, give adult dose for age older than 12 yo.

FORMS – Trade only: Syrup 12.5 mg phenylephrine/4 mg chlorpheniramine/5 mL, bubblegum flavor. Alcohol- and sugar-free.

RONDEC DM **(phenylephrine + chlorpheniramine + dextromethorphan)** ▶L ♀C ▶– $$

ADULT – Allergic rhinitis, nasal congestion, cough: 5 mL syrup PO four times per day.

PEDS – Allergic rhinitis, nasal congestion, cough: Give 1.25 mL PO four times per day for age 2 to 5 yo, give 2.5 mL PO four times per day for age 6 to 12 yo, give adult dose for age older than 12 yo.

FORMS – Trade only: Syrup 12.5 mg phenylephrine/4 mg chlorpheniramine/15 mg dextromethorphan/5 mL, grape flavor. Alcohol- and sugar-free.

NOTES – DM indicates dextromethorphan.

RONDEC INFANT DROPS **(phenylephrine + chlorpheniramine)** ▶L ♀C ▶– $$

PEDS – Allergic rhinitis, nasal congestion: Give the following dose PO four times per day: 0.75 mL for age 6 to 12 mo, 1 mL for age 13 to 24 mo.

FORMS – Trade only: Gtts 3.5 mg phenylephrine/1 mg chlorpheniramine/mL, bubble-gum flavor, 30 mL. Alcohol- and sugar-free.

RYNA-12 S **(phenylephrine + pyrilamine)** ▶L ♀C ▶– $$

PEDS – Nasal congestion, allergic rhinitis, sinusitis: Give 2.5 to 5 ML PO q 12 h for age 2 to 6 yo, give 5 to 10 mL PO q 12 h for age older than 6 yo.

FORMS – Generic/Trade: Susp 5 mg phenylephrine/30 mg pyrilamine/5 mL strawberry-currant flavor with graduated oral syringe.

RYNATAN **(phenylephrine + chlorpheniramine)** ▶LK ♀C ▶– $$

ADULT – Allergic rhinitis, nasal congestion: 1 to 2 tabs PO q 12 h.

PEDS – Allergic rhinitis, nasal congestion age 12 yo or older: 1 tab PO q 12 h.

FORMS – Trade only: Tabs, extended-release: 25/9 mg phenylephrine/chlorpheniramine. Chewable tabs 5/4.5 mg.

RYNATAN PEDIATRIC SUSPENSION **(phenylephrine + chlorpheniramine)** ▶L ♀C ▶– $$$

PEDS – Nasal congestion, allergic rhinitis, sinusitis: Give 2.5 to 5 mL PO q 12 h for age 2 to 6 yo, give 5 to 10 mL PO q 12 h for age older than 6 yo.

FORMS – Trade only: Susp 5 mg phenylephrine/4.5 mg chlorpheniramine/5 mL strawberry-currant flavor.

SEMPREX-D **(pseudoephedrine + acrivastine)** ▶LK ♀C ▶– $$

ADULT – Allergic rhinitis, nasal congestion: 1 cap PO q 4 to 6 h. Max 4 caps/day.

PEDS – Not approved in children.

FORMS – Trade only: Caps 60 mg pseudoephedrine/8 mg acrivastine.

TANAFED DMX **(pseudoephedrine + dexchlorpheniramine + dextromethorphan)** ▶L ♀C ▶– $$

ADULT – Allergic rhinitis, nasal congestion: 10 to 20 mL PO q 12 h. Max 40 mL/day.

PEDS – Allergic rhinitis, nasal congestion: Give 2.5 to 5 mL PO q 12 h (up to 10 mL/day) for 2 to 5 yo, give 5 to 10 mL PO q 12 h (up to 20 mL/day) for age 6 to 11 yo, give adult dose for age 12 yo or older.

FORMS – Generic/Trade: Susp 75 mg pseudoephedrine/2.5 mg dexchlorpheniramine/25 mg dextromethorphan/5 mL, strawberry-banana flavor.

TUSS-HC **(phenylephrine + chlorpheniramine + hydrocodone)** ▶L ♀C ▶–©III $

ADULT – Allergic rhinitis, congestion, cough: 10 mL PO q 4 h. Max 40 mL/day.

PEDS – Allergic rhinitis, congestion, cough: Give 5 mL PO q 4 h (up to 20 mL/day) for age 6 to 12 yo, give adult dose for age older than 12 yo.

FORMS – Generic/Trade: Syrup 5 mg phenylephrine/2 mg chlorpheniramine/2.5 mg hydrocodone/5 mL.

TUSSICAPS **(chlorpheniramine + hydrocodone)** ▶L ♀C ▶–©III $$

ADULT – Allergic rhinitis, cough: 1 full-strength cap PO q 12 h. Max 2 caps/day.

PEDS – Allergic rhinitis, congestion, cough: Give half-strength cap PO q 12 h (up to 2 caps/day) for age 6 to 12 yo, give adult dose for age older than 12 yo.

FORMS – Trade only: Caps, extended-release 4/5 mg (half-strength), 8/10 mg (full strength) chlorpheniramine/hydrocodone.

TUSSIONEX **(chlorpheniramine + hydrocodone)** ▶L ♀C ▶–©III $$$

ADULT – Allergic rhinitis, cough: 5 mL PO q 12 h. Max 10 mL/day.

PEDS – Allergic rhinitis, cough: 2.5 mL PO q 12 h (up to 5 mL/day) for age 6 to 12 yo, give adult dose for age older than 12 yo.

FORMS – Generic/Trade: Extended-release susp 8 mg chlorpheniramine/10 mg hydrocodone/5 mL.

ZEPHREX-LA **(pseudoephedrine + guaifenesin)** ▶L ♀C ▶– $

ADULT – Nasal congestion, cough: 1 tab PO q 12 h.

PEDS – Nasal congestion, cough: Give ½ tab PO q 12 h for age 6 to 12 yo, give adult dosing for age older than 12 yo.

FORMS – Trade only: Tabs, extended-release 120 mg pseudoephedrine/600 mg guaifenesin.

ZUTRIPRO **(hydrocodone + chlorpheniramine + pseudoephedrine)** ▶LK – ♀C ▶–© III

ADULT – Cough, nasal congestion, allergic rhinitis: 5 mL PO q 4 to 6 h. Max 20 mL/day.

PEDS – Not approved in children.

FORMS – Trade: Syrup 5 mg hydrocodone/4 mg chlorpheniramine/60 mg pseudoephedrine/5 mL.

ZYRTEC-D **(cetirizine + pseudoephedrine)** ▶LK ♀C ▶– $$

ADULT – Allergic rhinitis, nasal congestion: 1 tab PO q 12 h.

PEDS – Not approved in children.

FORMS – OTC Generic/Trade: Tabs, extended-release 5 mg cetirizine/120 mg pseudoephedrine.

NOTES – Decrease dose to 1 tab PO daily with decreased renal or hepatic function. Take on an empty stomach.

ENT: Decongestants

NOTE: See ENT: Nasal Preparations for nasal spray decongestants (oxymetazoline, phenylephrine). Systemic decongestants are sympathomimetic and may aggravate HTN, anxiety, BPH, and insomnia. Use cautiously in such patients. Some states have restricted or ended OTC sale of pseudoephedrine or reclassified it as a schedule III or V drug due to the potential for diversion to methamphetamine labs. Deaths have occurred in children younger than 2 yo attributed to toxicity from cough and cold medications; the FDA does not recommend their use in this age group.

PHENYLEPHRINE (***Sudafed PE***) ▶L ♀C ▶+ $

ADULT – Nasal congestion: 10 mg PO q 4 h prn. Max 6 doses/day.

PEDS – Nasal congestion, age older than 12 yo: Use adult dose.

FORMS – OTC Trade only: Tabs 10 mg.

NOTES – Avoid with MAOIs.

PSEUDOEPHEDRINE (***Sudafed, Sudafed 12 Hour, Efidac/24, Dimetapp Decongestant Infant Drops, PediaCare Infants' Decongestant Drops, Triaminic Oral Infant Drops,*** ✤ ***Pseudofrin***) ▶L ♀C ▶+ $

ADULT – Nasal congestion: 60 mg PO q 4 to 6 h. 120 mg PO q 12 h (extended-release). 240 mg PO daily (extended-release). Max 240 mg/day.

(cont.)

PSEUDOEPHEDRINE (*cont.*)

PEDS – Nasal congestion: Give 15 mg PO q 4 to 6 h for age 2 to 5 yo, give 30 mg PO q 4 to 6 h for age 6 to 12 yo, use adult dose for age older than 12 yo.

FORMS – OTC Generic/Trade: Tabs 30, 60 mg, Tabs, extended-release 120 mg (12 h), Soln 15, 30 mg/5 mL. Trade only: Chewable tabs 15 mg, Tabs, extended-release 240 mg (24 h). Rx only in some states.

NOTES – 12 to 24 h extended-release dosage forms may cause insomnia; use a shorter acting form if this occurs.

ENT: Ear Preparations

AURALGAN **(benzocaine + antipyrine)** ▶Not absorbed ♀C ▶? $

ADULT – Otitis media, adjunct: Instill 2 to 4 gtts (or enough to fill the ear canal) three to four times per day or q 1 to 2 h prn. Cerumen removal: Instill 2 to 4 gtts (or enough to fill the ear canal) three times per day for 2 to 3 days to detach cerumen, then prn for discomfort. Insert cotton plug moistened with soln after instillation.

PEDS – Otitis media, adjunct: Use adult dose. Cerumen removal: Use adult dose.

FORMS – Generic/Trade: Otic soln 10, 15 mL.

CARBAMIDE PEROXIDE (***Debrox, Murine Ear***) ▶Not absorbed ♀? ▶? $

ADULT – Cerumen impaction: Instill 5 to 10 gtts into ear two times per day for 4 days.

PEDS – Not approved in children.

FORMS – OTC Generic/Trade: Otic soln 6.5%, 15, 30 mL.

NOTES – Drops should remain in ear more than 15 min. Do not use for more than 4 days. Remove excess wax by flushing with warm water using a rubber bulb ear syringe.

CIPRO HC OTIC **(ciprofloxacin + hydrocortisone)** ▶Not absorbed ♀C ▶– $$$$

ADULT – Otitis externa: Instill 3 gtts into affected ear(s) two times per day for 7 days.

PEDS – Otitis externa age 1 yo or older: Use adult dose.

FORMS – Trade only: Otic susp 10 mL.

NOTES – Shake well. Contains benzyl alcohol.

CIPRODEX OTIC **(ciprofloxacin + dexamethasone)** ▶Not absorbed ♀C ▶– $$$$

ADULT – Otitis externa: Instill 4 gtts into affected ear(s) two times per day for 7 days.

PEDS – Otitis externa and otitis media with tympanostomy tubes, age 6 mo or older: Instill 4 gtts into affected ear(s) two times per day for 7 days.

FORMS – Trade only: Otic susp 5, 7.5 mL.

NOTES – Shake well. Warm susp by holding bottle in hands for 1 to 2 min before instilling.

CIPROFLOXACIN (***Cetraxal***) ▶Not absorbed ♀C ▶– $$$$

ADULT – Otitis externa: Instill 1 single-use container into affected ear(s) twice per day for 7 days.

PEDS – Otitis externa age 1 yo or older: Use adult dose.

FORMS – Trade only: 0.25 mL single-use containers with 0.2% ciprofloxacin soln, #14.

NOTES – Protect from light.

CORTISPORIN OTIC (hydrocortisone + polymyxin + neomycin, Pediotic) ▶Not absorbed ♀? ▶? $

ADULT – Otitis externa: Instill 4 gtts in affected ear(s) three to four times per day up to 10 days.

PEDS – Otitis externa: Instill 3 gtts in affected ear(s) three to four times per day up to 10 days.

FORMS – Generic only: Otic soln or susp 7.5, 10 mL.

NOTES – Caveats with perforated TMs or tympanostomy tubes: 1) Risk of neomycin ototoxicity, especially if use prolonged or repeated; 2) use susp rather than acidic soln.

CORTISPORIN TC OTIC **(hydrocortisone + neomycin + thonzonium + colistin)** ▶Not absorbed ♀? ▶? $$$

ADULT – Otitis externa: Instill 5 gtts in affected ear(s) three to four times per day up to 10 days.

PEDS – Otitis externa: Instill 4 gtts in affected ear(s) three to four times per day up to 10 days.

FORMS – Trade only: Otic susp, 10 mL.

DOMEBORO OTIC **(acetic acid + aluminum acetate)** ▶Not absorbed ♀? ▶? $

ADULT – Otitis externa: Instill 4 to 6 gtts in affected ear(s) q 2 to 3 h.

PEDS – Otitis externa: Instill 2 to 3 gtts in affected ear(s) q 3 to 4 h.

FORMS – Generic only: Otic soln 60 mL.

NOTES – Insert a saturated wick. Keep moist for 24 h.

FLUNICOLONE—OTIC (***DermOtic***) ▶L ♀C ▶? $$

ADULT – Chronic eczematous external otitis: Instill 5 gtts in affected ear(s) two times per day for 7 to 14 days.

PEDS – Chronic eczematous external otitis: Age 2 yo or older: Use adult dose.

FORMS – Trade only: Otic oil 0.01% 20 mL.

NOTES – Contains peanut oil.

OFLOXACIN—OTIC (*Floxin Otic*) ▶Not absorbed ♀C ▶– $$$

ADULT – Otitis externa: Instill 10 gtts in affected ear(s) daily for 7 days. Chronic suppurative otitis media: Instill 10 gtts in affected ear(s) two times per day for 14 days.

PEDS – Otitis externa: Instill 5 gtts in affected ear(s) daily for 7 days for age 1 to 12 yo, use adult dose for age 12 yo or older. Chronic suppurative otitis media for age older than 12 yo: Use adult dose. Acute otitis media with tympanostomy tubes age 1 to 12 yo: Instill 5 gtts in affected ear(s) two times per day for 10 days.

FORMS – Generic/Trade: Otic soln 0.3% 5, 10 mL. Trade only: "Singles": Single-dispensing containers 0.25 mL (5 gtts), 2 per foil pouch.

SWIM-EAR **(isopropyl alcohol + anhydrous glycerins)** ▶Not absorbed ♀? ▶? $

ADULT – Otitis externa, prophylaxis: Instill 4 to 5 gtts in ears after swimming, showering, or bathing.

PEDS – Otitis externa, prophylaxis: Use adult dose.

FORMS – OTC Trade only: Otic soln 30 mL.

VOSOL HC **(acetic acid + propylene glycol + hydrocortisone)** ▶Not absorbed ♀? ▶? $

ADULT – Otitis externa: Instill 5 gtts in affected ear(s) three to four times per day. Insert cotton plug moistened with 3 to 5 gtts q 4 to 6 h for the 1st 24 h.

PEDS – Otitis externa age older than 3 yo: Instill 3 to 4 gtts in affected ear(s) three to four times per day. Insert cotton plug moistened with 3 to 4 gtts q 4 to 6 h for the 1st 24 h.

FORMS – Generic/Trade: Otic soln 2%/3%/1% 10 mL.

ENT: Mouth and Lip Preparations

AMLEXANOX (*Aphthasol, OraDisc A*) ▶LK ♀B ▶? $

ADULT – Aphthous ulcers: Apply ¼ inch paste or mucoadhesive patch to ulcer in mouth four times per day after oral hygiene for up to 10 days.

PEDS – Aphthous ulcers, age older than 12 yo: Use adult dose.

FORMS – Trade only: Oral paste 5% (Apthasol), 3, 5 g tube. Mucoadhesive patch (OraDisc) 2 mg, #20.

NOTES – Mucoadhesive patch should be applied at least 80 min before bedtime to ensure its erosion before sleep. Up to 3 patches may be applied at one time. Avoid food or liquid for 1 h after application.

CEVIMELINE (*Evoxac*) ▶L ♀C ▶– $$$$$

WARNING – May alter cardiac conduction/heart rate; caution in heart disease. May worsen bronchospasm in asthma/COPD.

ADULT – Dry mouth due to Sjögren's syndrome: 30 mg PO three times per day.

PEDS – Not approved in children.

FORMS – Trade only: Caps 30 mg.

NOTES – Contraindicated in narrow-angle glaucoma, acute iritis, and severe asthma. May potentiate beta-blockers.

CHLORHEXIDINE GLUCONATE (*Peridex, Periogard,* ✦ *Denticare*) ▶Fecal excretion ♀B ▶? $

ADULT – Gingivitis: Twice per day as an oral rinse, morning and evening after brushing teeth. Rinse with 15 mL of undiluted soln for 30 sec. Do not swallow. Spit after rinsing.

PEDS – Not approved in children.

FORMS – Generic/Trade: Oral rinse 0.12% 473 to 480 mL bottles.

DEBACTEROL **(sulfuric acid + sulfonated phenolics)** ▶Not absorbed ♀C ▶+ $$

ADULT – Aphthous stomatitis, mucositis: Apply to dry ulcer. Rinse with water.

PEDS – Not approved in children younger than 12 yo.

FORMS – Trade only: 1 mL prefilled, single-use applicator.

NOTES – 1 application per ulcer treatment. Dry ulcer area with cotton swab. Apply to ulcer and ring of normal mucosa around it for 5 to 10 sec. Rinse and spit. Return of ulcer pain right after rinsing indicates incomplete application; can be reapplied immediately once. Avoid eye contact. If excess irritation, rinse with diluted bicarbonate soln.

GELCLAIR **(maltodextrin + propylene glycol)** ▶Not absorbed ♀+ ▶+ $$$

ADULT – Aphthous ulcers, mucositis, stomatitis: Rinse mouth with 1 packet three times per day or prn.

PEDS – Not approved in children.

FORMS – Trade only: 21 packets/box.

NOTES – Mix packet with 3 tablespoons of water. Swish for 1 min, then spit. Do not eat or drink for 1 h after treatment.

LIDOCAINE—VISCOUS (*Xylocaine*) ▶LK ♀B ▶+ $

WARNING – Avoid swallowing during oral or labial use due to GI absorption and toxicity. Measure dose exactly. May apply to small areas in mouth with a cotton-tipped applicator.

(cont.)

LIDOCAINE—VISCOUS (*cont.*)

ADULT – Mouth or lip pain: 15 to 20 mL topically or swish and spit q 3 h. Max 8 doses/day.

PEDS – Use with extreme caution, as therapeutic doses approach potentially toxic levels. Use the lowest effective dose. Mouth or lip pain age older than 3 yo: 3.75 to 5 mL topically or swish and spit up to q 3 h.

FORMS – Generic/Trade: Soln 2%, 20 mL unit dose, 100 mL bottle.

NOTES – High risk of adverse effects and overdose in children. Consider benzocaine as a safer alternative. Clearly communicate the amount, frequency, max daily dose, and mode of administration (eg, cotton pledget to individual lesions, ½ dropper to each cheek q 4 h, or 20 min before meals). Do not prescribe on a prn basis without specified dosing intervals.

MAGIC MOUTHWASH **(diphenhydramine + *Mylanta* + sucralfate)** ▶LK ◗– $$$

ADULT – See components.

PEDS – Not approved in children.

UNAPPROVED ADULT – Stomatitis: 5 mL PO swish and spit or swish and swallow three times per day before meals and prn.

UNAPPROVED PEDS – Stomatitis: Apply small amounts to lesions prn.

FORMS – Compounded susp. A standard mixture is 30 mL diphenhydramine liquid (12.5 mg/5 mL)/60 mL Mylanta or Maalox/4 g Carafate.

NOTES – Variations of this formulation are available. The dose and decision to swish and spit or swallow may vary with the indication and/or ingredient. Some preparations may contain: Kaopectate, nystatin, tetracycline, hydrocortisone, 2% lidocaine, cherry syrup (for children). Check local pharmacies for customized formulations. Avoid diphenhydramine formulations that contain alcohol: May cause stinging of mouth sores.

PILOCARPINE (***Salagen***) ▶L ♀C ◗– $$$$

ADULT – Dry mouth due to radiation of head and neck: 5 mg PO three times per day. May increase to 10 mg PO three times per day. Dry mouth due to Sjögren's syndrome: 5 mg PO four times per day. Hepatic dysfunction: 5 mg PO two times per day.

PEDS – Not approved in children.

UNAPPROVED ADULT – Dry mouth due to Sjögren's syndrome: 2% pilocarpine eye gtts: Swish and swallow 4 gtts diluted in water three times per day ($).

FORMS – Generic/Trade: Tabs 5, 7.5 mg.

NOTES – Contraindicated in narrow-angle glaucoma, acute iritis, and severe asthma. May potentiate beta-blockers.

ENT: Nasal Preparations—Corticosteroids

NOTE: Decrease to the lowest effective dose for maintenance therapy. Tell patients to prime pump before first use and shake well before each subsequent use.

BECLOMETHASONE (***Vancenase, Vancenase AQ Double Strength, Beconase AQ, Qnasl***) ▶L ♀C ◗? $$$$

ADULT – Allergic rhinitis, nasal polyp prophylaxis: Vancenase: 1 spray in each nostril two to four times per day. Beconase AQ: 1 to 2 spray(s) in each nostril two times per day. Vancenase AQ Double Strength: 1 to 2 spray(s) in each nostril daily. Allergic rhinitis: Qnasl 1 to 2 spray(s) in each nostril daily.

PEDS – Allergic rhinitis, nasal polyp prophylaxis: 1 spray in each nostril three times per day for age 6 to 12 yo, give adult dose for age older than 12 yo. Beconase AQ: 1 to 2 spray(s) in each nostril two times per day for age older than 6 yo. Vancenase AQ Double Strength: 1 to 2 spray(s) in each nostril daily for age older than 6 yo. Allergic rhinitis: Qnasl 1 to 2 spray(s) in each nostril once daily for age 12 and over.

FORMS – Trade only: Vancenase 42 mcg/spray, 80 or 200 sprays/bottle. Beconase AQ 42 mcg/spray, 200 sprays/bottle. Vancenase AQ Double Strength 84 mcg/spray, 120 sprays/bottle. Qnasl: 80 mcg/spray, 120 sprays/bottle.

NOTES – AQ (aqueous) formulation may cause less stinging.

BUDESONIDE—NASAL (***Rhinocort Aqua***) ▶L ♀B ◗? $$$$

ADULT – Allergic rhinitis: 1 to 4 sprays per nostril daily.

PEDS – Allergic rhinitis age 6 yo or older: 1 to 2 sprays per nostril daily.

FORMS – Trade only: Nasal inhaler 120 sprays/bottle.

NOTES – CYP3A4 inhibitors, such as ketoconazole, erythromycin, and ritonavir, significantly increase systemic concentrations, possibly causing adrenal suppression.

CICLESONIDE (***Omnaris, Zetonna***) ▶L ♀C ◗? $$$

ADULT – Allergic rhinitis: Omnaris: 2 sprays per nostril daily. Zetonna: 1 actuation per nostril daily.

(cont.)

CICLESONIDE (*cont.*)

PEDS – Allergic rhinitis, seasonal: Omnaris: give adult dose for age 6 yo or older. Zetonna: give adult dose for age 12 yo or older. Allergic rhinitis, perennial: Omnaris and Zetonna: Give adult dose for age 12 yo or older.

FORMS – Trade only: Nasal spray, 50 mcg/spray, 120 sprays/bottle (Omnaris). Nasal aerosol, 37 mcg/actuation, 60 actuations/cannister (Zetonna).

FLUNISOLIDE (***Nasalide, Nasarel,*** ♣ ***Rhinalar***) ▶L ♀C ▶? $$$

ADULT – Allergic rhinitis: 2 sprays per nostril two times per day, may increase to three times per day. Max 8 sprays/nostril/day.

PEDS – Allergic rhinitis age 6 to 14 yo: 1 spray per nostril three times per day or 2 sprays per nostril two times per day. Max 4 sprays/nostril/day.

FORMS – Generic/Trade: Nasal soln 0.025%, 200 sprays/bottle. Nasalide with pump unit. Nasarel with meter pump and nasal adapter.

FLUTICASONE—NASAL (***Flonase, Veramyst***) ▶L ♀C ▶? $$$

ADULT – Allergic rhinitis: 2 sprays per nostril daily or 1 spray per nostril two times per day, decrease to 1 spray per nostril daily when appropriate. Seasonal allergic rhinitis alternative: 2 sprays per nostril daily prn.

PEDS – Allergic rhinitis for age older than 4 yo: 1 to 2 sprays per nostril daily. Max 2 sprays/nostril/day. Seasonal allergic rhinitis alternative for age older than 12 yo: 2 sprays per nostril daily prn.

FORMS – Generic/Trade: Flonase: Nasal spray 0.05%, 120 sprays/bottle. Trade only: (Veramyst): Nasal spray susp: 27.5 mcg/spray, 120 sprays/bottle.

NOTES – CYP3A4 inhibitors, such as ketoconazole, erythromycin, and ritonavir, significantly increase systemic concentrations, possibly causing adrenal suppression.

MOMETASONE—NASAL (***Nasonex***) ▶L ♀C ▶? $$$$

ADULT – Prevention or treatment of symptoms of allergic rhinitis: 2 sprays per nostril daily. Treatment of nasal polyps: 2 sprays per nostril two times per day (once daily may also be effective).

PEDS – Prevention or treatment of symptoms of allergic rhinitis age 12 yo or older: Use adult dose. 2 to 11 yo: 1 spray per nostril daily.

FORMS – Trade only: Nasal spray, 120 sprays/bottle.

TRIAMCINOLONE—NASAL (***Nasacort AQ, Nasacort HFA, Tri-Nasal, AllerNaze***) ▶L ♀C ▶– $$$$

ADULT – Allergic rhinitis: Nasacort HFA, Tri-Nasal, AllerNaze: Start 2 sprays per nostril daily, may increase to 2 sprays/nostril two times per day. Max 4 sprays/nostril/day. Nasacort AQ: 2 sprays per nostril daily.

PEDS – Allergic rhinitis: Nasacort and Nasacort AQ: 1 to 2 sprays per nostril daily for age 6 to 12 yo, give adult dose for age older than 12 yo. Nasacort AQ: 1 spray in each nostril once daily for age 2 to 5 yo.

FORMS – Trade only: Nasal inhaler 55 mcg/spray, 100 sprays/bottle (Nasacort HFA). Nasal spray, 55 mcg/spray, 120 sprays/bottle (Nasacort AQ). Nasal spray 50 mcg/spray, 120 sprays/bottle (Tri-Nasal, AllerNaze).

NOTES – AQ (aqueous) formulation may cause less stinging. Decrease to lowest effective dose after allergy symptom improvement.

ENT: Nasal Preparations—Other

NOTE: For *all* nasal sprays except saline, oxymetazoline, and phenylephrine, tell patients to prime pump before first use and shake well before each subsequent use.

AZELASTINE—NASAL (***Astelin, Astepro***) ▶L ♀C ▶? $$$$

ADULT – Allergic/vasomotor rhinitis: 1 to 2 sprays/nostril two times per day.

PEDS – Allergic rhinitis: 1 spray/nostril two times per day for age 5 to 11 yo, give adult dose for 12 yo or older. Vasomotor rhinitis: Give adult dose for 12 yo or older.

FORMS – Generic: Nasal spray, 200 sprays/bottle.

CETACAINE (**benzocaine + tetracaine + butamben**) ▶LK ♀C ▶? $$

WARNING – Do not use on the eyes. Hypersensitivity (rare). Methemoglobinemia (rare).

ADULT – Topical anesthesia of mucous membranes: Spray: Apply for 1 sec or less. Liquid or gel: Apply with cotton applicator directly to site.

PEDS – Use adult dose.

FORMS – Trade only: (14%/2%/2%) Spray 56 mL. Topical liquid 56 mL. Topical gel 5, 29 g.

NOTES – Do not hold cotton applicator in position for extended time due to increased risk of local reactions. Do not use multiple applications. Maximum anesthesia occurs 1 min after application; duration 30 min. May result in potentially dangerous methemoglobinemia; use minimum amount needed.

CROMOLYN—NASAL (***NasalCrom***) ▶LK ♀B ▶+ $

ADULT – Allergic rhinitis: 1 spray per nostril three to four times per day up to 6 times per day.

PEDS – Allergic rhinitis, age 2 yo or older: Use adult dose.

FORMS – OTC Generic/Trade: Nasal inhaler 200 sprays/bottle 13, 26 mL.

NOTES – Therapeutic effects may not be seen for 1 to 2 weeks.

DYMISTA **(azelastine + fluticasone)** ▶L – ♀C ▶? $$$$

ADULT – Seasonal allergic rhinitis: 1 spray per nostril 2 times per day.

PEDS – Seasonal allergic rhinitis: Give adult dose for 12 yo or older.

FORMS – Trade only: Nasal spray: 137 mcg astelazine/50 mcg fluticasone/spray, 120 sprays/bottle.

NOTES – CYP3A4 inhibitors, such as ketoconazole, erythromycin, and ritonavir, significantly increase systemic concentrations of fluticasone, possibly causing adrenal suppression.

IPRATROPIUM—NASAL (***Atrovent Nasal Spray***) ▶L ♀B ▶? $$

ADULT – Rhinorrhea due to allergic/nonallergic rhinitis: 2 sprays (0.03%) per nostril two to three times per day or 2 sprays (0.06%) per nostril four times per day. Rhinorrhea due to common cold: 2 sprays (0.06%) per nostril three to four times per day.

PEDS – Rhinorrhea due to allergic/nonallergic rhinitis: Give adult dose (0.03% strength) for age 6 yo or older, give adult dose (0.06% strength) for age 5 yo or older. Rhinorrhea due to common cold: 2 sprays (0.06% strength) per nostril three times per day for age 5 yo or older.

UNAPPROVED ADULT – Vasomotor rhinitis: 2 sprays (0.06%) in each nostril three to four times per day.

FORMS – Generic/Trade: Nasal spray 0.03%, 345 sprays/bottle, 0.06%, 165 sprays/bottle.

✤ **LEVOCABASTINE—NASAL** (***Livostin***) ▶L (but minimal absorption) ♀C ▶– $$

ADULT – Canada only. Allergic rhinitis: 2 sprays per nostril two times per day; increase prn to 2 sprays per nostril three to four times per day.

PEDS – Not approved in children younger than 12 yo.

FORMS – Trade only: Nasal spray 0.5 mg/mL, plastic bottles of 15 mL. 50 mcg/spray.

NOTES – Nasal spray is devoid of CNS effects. Safety/efficacy in patients older than 65 yo has not been established.

OLOPATADINE—NASAL (***Patanase***) ▶L ♀C ▶? $$$

ADULT – Allergic rhinitis: 2 sprays/nostril two times per day.

PEDS – Allergic rhinitis age 12 yo or older: Use adult dose. For age 6 to 11 yo: 1 spray/nostril two times per day.

FORMS – Trade only: Nasal spray, 240 sprays/bottle.

OXYMETAZOLINE (***Afrin, Dristan 12 Hr Nasal, Nostrilla, Vicks Sinex 12 Hr***) ▶L ♀C ▶? $

ADULT – Nasal congestion: 2 to 3 sprays or gtts (0.05%) per nostril two times per day for no more than 3 days.

PEDS – Nasal congestion: Give 2 to 3 gtts (0.025%) per nostril two times per day no more than 3 days for age 2 to 5 yo, give 2 to 3 sprays or gtts (0.05%) per nostril two times per day not more than 3 days.

FORMS – OTC Generic/Trade: Nasal spray 0.05% 15, 30 mL; Nose gtts 0.025%, 0.05% 20 mL with dropper.

NOTES – Overuse (more than 3 to 5 days) may lead to rebound congestion. If this occurs, taper to use in 1 nostril only, alternating sides, then discontinue. Substituting an oral decongestant or nasal steroid may also be useful.

PHENYLEPHRINE—NASAL (***Neo-Synephrine, Vicks Sinex***) ▶L ♀C ▶? $

ADULT – Nasal congestion: 2 to 3 sprays or gtts (0.25 or 0.5%) per nostril q 4 h prn for 3 days. Use 1% soln for severe congestion.

PEDS – Nasal congestion: Give 1 to 2 gtts (0.125% or 0.16%) per nostril q 4 h prn for 3 days for age 6 to 11 mo, give 2 to 3 gtts (0.125% or 0.16%) per nostril q 4 h prn for 3 days for age 1 to 5 yo, give 2 to 3 gtts or sprays (0.25%) per nostril q 4 h prn for 3 days for age 6 to 12 yo, give adult dose for age older than 12 yo.

FORMS – OTC Generic/Trade: Nasal gtts/spray 0.25, 0.5, 1% (15 mL).

NOTES – Overuse (more 3 to 5 days) may lead to rebound congestion. If this occurs, taper to use in 1 nostril only, alternating sides, then discontinue. Substituting an oral decongestant or nasal steroid may also be useful.

SALINE NASAL SPRAY (***SeaMist, Entsol, Pretz, NaSal, Ocean,*** ✤ ***HydraSense***) ▶Not metabolized ♀A ▶+ $

ADULT – Nasal dryness: 1 to 3 sprays per nostril prn.

PEDS – Nasal dryness: 1 to 3 gtts per nostril prn.

FORMS – Generic/Trade: Nasal spray 0.4, 0.5, 0.65, 0.75%, Nasal gtts 0.4, 0.65%.

(cont.)

SALINE NASAL SPRAY (*cont.*)

Trade only: Preservative-free nasal spray 3% (Entsol).

NOTES – May be prepared at home by combining: ¼ teaspoon salt with 8 ounces (1 cup) warm water. Add ¼ teaspoon baking soda (optional) and put in spray bottle, ear syringe, neti pot, or any container with a small spout. Discard after 1 week.

GASTROENTEROLOGY: Antidiarrheals

BISMUTH SUBSALICYLATE (*Pepto-Bismol, Kaopectate*) ▶K ♀D ▶? $

WARNING – Avoid in children and teenagers with chickenpox or flu due to possible association with Reye's syndrome.

ADULT – Diarrhea: 2 tabs or 30 mL (262 mg/15 mL) PO q 30 to 60 min up to 8 doses/day for up to 2 days.

PEDS – Diarrhea: 100 mg/kg/day divided into 5 doses or ⅓ tab or 5 mL (262 mg/15 mL) q 30 to 60 min prn up to 8 doses/day for age 3 to 6 yo, ⅔ tab or 10 mL (262 mg/15 mL) q 30 to 60 min prn up to 8 doses/day for age 7 to 9 yo, 1 tab or 15 mL (262 mg/15 mL) q 30 to 60 min prn up to 8 doses/day for age 10 to 12 yo. Do not take for more than 2 days.

UNAPPROVED ADULT – Prevention of traveler's diarrhea: 2.1 g/day or 2 tabs four times per day before meals and at bedtime. Has been used as part of a multidrug regimen for *Helicobacter pylori*.

UNAPPROVED PEDS – Chronic infantile diarrhea: 2.5 mL (262 mg/15 mL) PO q 4 h for age 2 to 24 mo, 5 mL (262 mg/15 mL) PO q 4 h for age 25 to 48 mo, 10 mL (262 mg/15 mL) PO q 4 h for age 49 to 70 mo.

FORMS – OTC Generic/Trade: Chewable tabs 262 mg. Susp 262, 525, 750 mg/15 mL. OTC Trade only: Caplets 262 mg (Pepto-Bismol). Susp 87 mg/5 mL (Kaopectate Children's Liquid).

NOTES – Use with caution in patients already taking salicylates or warfarin, children recovering from chickenpox or flu. Decreases absorption of tetracycline. May darken stools or tongue.

IMODIUM MULTI-SYMPTOM RELIEF **(loperamide + simethicone)** ▶L ♀C ▶– $

ADULT – Diarrhea: 2 tabs/caps PO initially, then 1 tab/cap PO after each unformed stool to a max of 4 tabs/caps/day.

PEDS – Diarrhea: 1 cap PO initially, then ½ tab/cap PO after each unformed stool (up to 2 tabs/caps/day for age 6 to 8 yo or wt 48 to 59 lbs, up to 3 tabs/caps/day for age 9 to 11 yo or wt 60 to 95 lbs).

FORMS – OTC Generic/Trade: Caplets, Chewable tabs 2 mg loperamide/125 mg simethicone.

NOTES – Not for *C. difficile*–associated diarrhea, toxigenic bacterial diarrhea, or most childhood diarrhea (difficult to exclude toxigenic).

LOMOTIL **(diphenoxylate + atropine)** ▶L ♀C ▶– ©V $

ADULT – Diarrhea: 2 tabs or 10 mL PO four times per day.

PEDS – Diarrhea: 0.3 to 0.4 mg diphenoxylate/kg/24 h in 4 divided doses. Max daily dose 20 mg. Not recommended for younger than 2 yo, 1.5 to 3 mL PO four times per day for age 2 yo or wt 11 to 14 kg; 2 to 3 mL PO four times per day for age 3 yo or wt 12 to 16 kg; 2 to 4 mL PO four times per day for age 4 yo or wt 14 to 20 kg; 2.5 to 4.5 mL PO four times per day for age 5 yo or wt 16 to 23 kg; 2.5 to 5 mL PO four times per day for age 6 to 8 yo or wt 17 to 32 kg; 3.5 to 5 mL PO four times per day for 9 to 12 yo or wt 23 to 55 kg.

FORMS – Generic/Trade: Oral soln or tab 2.5 mg/0.025 mg diphenoxylate/atropine per 5 mL or tab.

NOTES – Give with food to decrease GI upset. May cause atropinism in children, especially with Down syndrome, even at recommended doses. Can cause delayed toxicity. Has been reported to cause severe respiratory depression, coma, brain damage, death after overdose in children. Naloxone reverses toxicity. Do not use for *C. difficile*–associated diarrhea, toxigenic bacterial diarrhea, or most childhood diarrhea (difficult to exclude toxigenic).

LOPERAMIDE (***Imodium, Imodium AD,*** ✤ ***Loperacap, Diarr-eze***) ▶L ♀C ▶+ $

WARNING – Discontinue if abdominal distention or ileus. Caution in children due to variable response.

ADULT – Diarrhea: 4 mg PO initially, then 2 mg after each unformed stool to max 16 mg/day.

PEDS – Diarrhea: First dose: 1 mg PO three times per day for age 2 to 5 yo or wt 13 to 20 kg, 2 mg PO two times per day for age 6 to 8 yo or wt 21 to 30 kg, 2 mg PO three times per day for age 9 to 12 yo or wt greater than 30 kg. After 1st day: Give 0.1 mg/kg PO after each loose stool; daily dose not to exceed daily dose of 1st day.

(cont.)

LOPERAMIDE (*cont.*)

UNAPPROVED ADULT – Chronic diarrhea or ileostomy drainage: 4 mg initially then 2 mg after each stool until symptoms are controlled, then reduce dose for maintenance treatment, average adult maintenance dose 4 to 8 mg daily as a single dose or in divided doses.

UNAPPROVED PEDS – Chronic diarrhea: Limited information. Average doses of 0.08 to 0.24 mg/kg/day PO in 2 to 3 divided doses. Max 2 mg/dose. Max 16 mg/day.

FORMS – OTC Generic/Trade: Tabs 2 mg. Oral soln 1 mg/5 mL. OTC Oral soln 1 mg/7.5 mL.

NOTES – Not for *C. difficile*–associated diarrhea, toxigenic bacterial diarrhea, or most childhood diarrhea (difficult to exclude toxigenic). Doses greater than 16 mg/day have been used.

MOTOFEN **(difenoxin + atropine)** ▶L ♀C ▶– ©IV $$

ADULT – Diarrhea: 2 tabs PO initially, then 1 after each loose stool q 3 to 4 h prn (up to 8 tabs/day).

PEDS – Not approved in children. Contraindicated younger than 2 yo.

FORMS – Trade only: Tabs difenoxin 1 mg + atropine 0.025 mg.

NOTES – Do not use for *C. difficile*–associated diarrhea, toxigenic bacterial diarrhea, or most childhood diarrhea (difficult to exclude toxigenic). May cause atropinism in children, especially with Down syndrome, even at recommended doses. Can cause delayed toxicity. Has been reported to cause severe respiratory depression, coma, brain damage, death after overdose in children. Difenoxin is the primary metabolite of diphenoxylate.

OPIUM (opium tincture, paregoric) ▶L ♀B (D with long-term use) ▶? ©II (opium tincture), III (paregoric) $$

ADULT – Diarrhea: 5 to 10 mL paregoric PO daily (up to four times per day) or 0.3 to 0.6 mL PO opium tincture four times per day.

PEDS – Diarrhea: 0.25 to 0.5 mL/kg paregoric PO daily (up to four times per day) or 0.005 to 0.01 mL/kg PO opium tincture q 3 to 4 h (up to 6 doses/day).

FORMS – Trade only: Opium tincture 10% (deodorized opium tincture, 10 mg morphine equivalent/mL). Generic only: Paregoric (camphorated opium tincture, 2 mg morphine equivalent/5 mL).

NOTES – Opium tincture contains 25 times more morphine than paregoric. Do not use for *C. difficile*–associated diarrhea, toxigenic bacterial diarrhea, or most childhood diarrhea.

GASTROENTEROLOGY: Antiemetics—5-HT3 Receptor Antagonists

DOLASETRON (*Anzemet*) ▶LK ♀B ▶? $$$

ADULT – Prevention of N/V with chemo: 1.8 mg/kg (up to 100 mg) PO single dose 60 min before chemo. Prevention/treatment of postop N/V: 12.5 mg IV as a single dose 15 min before end of anesthesia or as soon as N/V starts. Alternative for prevention 100 mg PO 2 h before surgery.

PEDS – Prevention of N/V with chemo: 1.8 mg/kg up to 100 mg PO single dose 60 min before chemo for age 2 to 16 yo. Prevention/treatment of postop N/V: 0.35 mg/kg IV as single dose 15 minutes before end of anesthesia or as soon as N/V starts for age 2 to 16 yo. Max 12.5 mg. Prevention alternative 1.2 mg/kg PO to max of 100 mg 2 h before surgery. Contraindicated in Canada in children younger than 18 yo.

UNAPPROVED ADULT – N/V due to radiotherapy: 0.3 mg/kg IV as a single dose.

FORMS – Trade only: Tabs 50, 100 mg. Injectable no longer available in Canada.

NOTES – Use caution in patients of any age who have or may develop prolongation of QT interval (ie, hypokalemia, hypomagnesemia, concomitant antiarrhythmic therapy, cumulative high-dose anthracycline therapy). Cimetidine may increase serum concentrations, rifampin may reduce serum concentrations.

GRANISETRON (*Sancuso*) ▶L ♀B ▶? $$$$

ADULT – Prevention of N/V with chemo: 1 patch to upper outer arm at least 24 h (but up to 48 h) before chemotherapy. Remove 24 h after completion of chemotherapy. Can be worn up to 7 days depending on the duration of chemo.

PEDS – Not approved in children.

FORMS – Transdermal patch 34.3 mg of granisetron delivering 3.1 mg/24 h.

ONDANSETRON (*Zofran*) ▶L ♀B ▶? $$$$$

ADULT – Prevention of N/V with chemo: 8 mg PO 30 min before moderately emetogenic chemo and 8 h later. Can be given q 12 h for 1 to 2 days after completion of chemo. For single-day highly emetogenic chemo, 24 mg PO 30 min before chemo. Prevention of postop nausea: 4 mg IV over 2 to 5 min or 4 mg IM or 16 mg PO 1 h before anesthesia. Prevention of N/V associated with radiotherapy: 8 mg PO three times per day.

PEDS – Prevention of N/V with chemo: IV: 0.15 mg/kg 30 min prior to chemo and repeated at

(cont.)

ONDANSETRON (*cont.*)

4 and 8 h after 1st dose for age older than 6 mo. PO: Give 4 mg 30 min prior to chemo and repeat at 4 and 8 h after 1st dose for age 4 to 11 yo. Can be given q 8 h PO for 1 to 2 days after completion of chemo. Give 8 mg PO 30 min before chemo and 8 h later for age 12 yo or older. Prevention of postop N/V: 0.1 mg/kg IV over 2 to 5 min for age 1 mo to 12 yo if wt 40 kg or less; give 4 mg IV over 2 to 5 min if wt greater than 40 kg.

UNAPPROVED ADULT – Has been used in hyperemesis associated with pregnancy.

UNAPPROVED PEDS – Use with caution if younger than 4 yo. Dosing based on BSA: Give 1 mg PO three times per day for BSA less than 0.3 m^2, give 2 mg PO three times per day for BSA 0.3 to 0.6 m^2, give 3 mg PO three times per day for BSA 0.6 to 1 m^2, give 4 mg PO three times per day for BSA greater than 1 m^2. Use caution in infants younger than 6 mo.

FORMS – Generic/Trade: Tabs 4, 8, 24 mg. Orally disintegrating tab 4, 8 mg. Oral soln 4 mg/5 mL. Generic only: Tabs 16 mg.

NOTES – Maximum oral dose if severe liver disease is 8 mg/day. Use following abdominal surgery or in those receiving chemotherapy may mask a progressive ileus or gastric distension. Contraindicated with apomorphine; concomitant use can lead to hypotension and loss of consiousness.

PALONOSETRON (*Aloxi*) ▶L ♀B ▶? $$$$$

ADULT – Prevention of N/V with chemo: 0.25 mg IV over 30 sec, 30 min prior to chemo. Prevention of postop N/V: 0.075 mg IV over 10 sec just prior to anesthesia.

PEDS – Not approved in children.

UNAPPROVED PEDS – Limited information suggests 3 mcg/kg (maximum 0.25 mg) IV is effective and safe in children older than 2 yo.

FORMS – Trade only: injectable.

GASTROENTEROLOGY: Antiemetics—Other

APREPITANT (*Emend,* **fosaprepitant**) ▶L ♀B ▶? $$$$$

ADULT – Prevention of N/V with moderately to highly emetogenic chemo, in combination with a corticosteroid and a 5-HT3 antagonist: 125 mg PO on day 1 (1 h prior to chemo), then 80 mg PO q am on days 2 and 3. Alternative for 1st dose only is 115 mg IV (fosaprepitant form) over 15 min given 30 min prior to chemo. Prevention of postop N/V: 40 mg PO within 3 h prior to anesthesia.

PEDS – Not approved in children.

FORMS – Trade only (aprepitant): Caps 40, 80, 125 mg. IV prodrug form is fosaprepitant.

NOTES – Use caution with other medications metabolized by CYP3A4 hepatic enzyme system and an inducer of the CYP2C9 hepatic enzyme system. Contraindicated with pimozide. May decrease efficacy of oral contraceptives; women should use alternate/back-up method. Monitor INR in patients receiving warfarin. Fosaprepitant is a prodrug of aprepitant.

✤ ***DICLECTIN*** (**doxylamine + pyridoxine**) ▶LK ♀A ▶? $

ADULT – Canada only. N/V in pregnancy: 2 tabs PO at bedtime. May add 1 tab in am and 1 tab in afternoon, if needed.

PEDS – Not approved in children.

FORMS – Canada Trade only: Delayed-release tabs doxylamine 10 mg + pyridoxine 10 mg.

DIMENHYDRINATE (*Dramamine,* ✤ *Gravol*) ▶LK ♀B ▶– $

ADULT – Nausea: 50 to 100 mg/dose PO/IM/IV q 4 to 6 h prn. Maximum PO dose 400 mg/24 h, maximum IV/IM dose 600 mg/24 h.

PEDS – Nausea: Not recommended for age younger than 2 yo. Give 12.5 to 25 mg PO q 6 to 8 h or 5 mg/kg/day (up to 75 mg/day) PO divided q 6 h for age 2 to 5 yo, give 25 to 50 mg (up to 150 mg/day) PO q 6 to 8 h or for age 6 to 12 yo.

FORMS – OTC Generic/Trade: Tabs 50 mg. Trade only: Chewable tabs 50 mg. Generic only: Oral soln 12.5 mg/5 mL. Canada only: Suppository 25, 50, 100 mg.

NOTES – May cause drowsiness. Use with caution in conditions that may be aggravated by anticholinergic effects (ie, prostatic hypertrophy, asthma, narrow-angle glaucoma). Available as suppositories in Canada.

DOMPERIDONE ▶L ♀? ▶– $$

ADULT – Canada only. Postprandial dyspepsia: 10 to 20 mg PO three to four times per day, 30 min before a meal. N/V: 20 mg PO three to four times per day.

PEDS – Not approved in children.

UNAPPROVED ADULT – Has been used for diabetic gastroparesis, chemotherapy/radiation-induced N/V. Has also been used to increase milk production in lactating mothers although this is not currently recommended due to safety concerns.

(cont.)

DOMPERIDONE (*cont.*)

UNAPPROVED PEDS – Use in children generally not recommended except for chemotherapy- or radiation-induced N/V: 200 to 400 mcg/kg PO q 4 to 8 h.

FORMS – Canada only. Trade/generic: Tabs 10, 20 mg.

NOTES – Similar in efficacy to metoclopramide but less likely to cause EPS.

DOXYLAMINE (***Unisom Nighttime Sleep Aid,*** **others**) ▶L ♀A ▶? $

PEDS – Not approved in children.

UNAPPROVED ADULT – N/V associated with pregnancy: 12.5 mg PO two to four times per day; often used in combination with pyridoxine.

FORMS – Generic/Trade: Tabs 25 mg.

DRONABINOL (***Marinol***) ▶L ♀C ▶– ©III $$$$$

ADULT – Nausea with chemo: 5 mg/m² PO 1 to 3 h before chemo then 5 mg/m²/dose q 2 to 4 h after chemo for 4 to 6 doses/day. Dose can be increased to max 15 mg/m². Anorexia associated with AIDS: Initially 2.5 mg PO two times per day before lunch and dinner. Maximum 20 mg/day.

PEDS – Nausea with chemo: 5 mg/m² PO 1 to 3 h before chemo then 5 mg/m²/dose PO q 2 to 4 h after chemo (up to 4 to 6 doses/day). Dose can be increased to max 15 mg/m². Not approved for anorexia associated with AIDS in children.

UNAPPROVED ADULT – Appetitie stimulant: 2.5 mg PO twice daily.

UNAPPROVED PEDS – Nausea with chemo: 5 mg/m² PO 1 to 3 h before chemo then 5 mg/m²/dose PO q 2 to 4 h after chemo (up to 4 to 6 doses/day). Dose can be increased to max 15 mg/m².

FORMS – Generic/Trade: Caps 2.5, 5, 10 mg.

NOTES – Patient response varies; individualize dosing (start with low doses in elderly). Additive CNS effects with alcohol, sedatives, hypnotics, psychomimetics. Caution if history of seizures.

DROPERIDOL (***Inapsine***) ▶L ♀C ▶? $

WARNING – Cases of fatal QT prolongation and/or torsades de pointes have occurred in patients receiving droperidol at or below recommended doses (some without risk factors for QT prolongation). Reserve for nonresponse to other treatments, and perform 12-lead ECG prior to administration and continue ECG monitoring 2 to 3 h after treatment. Avoid if prolonged baseline QT.

ADULT – Antiemetic premedication: 0.625 to 2.5 mg IV or 2.5 mg IM then 1.25 mg prn.

PEDS – Preop: 0.088 to 0.165 mg/kg IV for age 2 to 12 yo. Children older than 12 yo: 2.5 mg IM/IV, additional doses of 1.25 mg can be given with caution. Postop antiemetic: 0.01 to 0.03 mg/kg/dose IV q 6 to 8 h prn. Usual dose 0.05 to 0.06 mg/kg/dose (up to 0.1 mg/kg/dose).

UNAPPROVED ADULT – Chemo-induced nausea: 2.5 to 5 mg IV/IM q 3 to 4 h prn.

UNAPPROVED PEDS – Chemo-induced nausea: 0.05 to 0.06 mg/kg/dose IV/IM q 4 to 6 h prn.

NOTES – Has no analgesic or amnestic effects. Consider lower doses in geriatric, debilitated, or high-risk patients such as those receiving other CNS depressants. May cause hypotension or tachycardia, extrapyramidal reactions, drowsiness.

METOCLOPRAMIDE (***Reglan, Metozolv ODT, ✤Maxeran***) ▶K ♀B ▶? $

WARNING – Irreversible tardive dyskinesia with high dose or long-term (more than 3 months) use.

ADULT – GERD: 10 to 15 mg PO four times per day 30 min before meals and at bedtime. Diabetic gastroparesis: 10 mg PO/IV/IM 30 min before meals and at bedtime. Prevention of chemo-induced emesis: 1 to 2 mg/kg PO/IV/IM 30 min before chemo and then q 2 h for 2 doses then q 3 h for 3 doses prn. Prevention of postop nausea: 10 to 20 mg IM/IV near end of surgical procedure, may repeat q 3 to 4 h prn. Intubation of small intestine: 10 mg IV. Radiographic exam of upper GI tract: 10 mg IV.

PEDS – Intubation of small intestine: 0.1 mg/kg IV for age younger than 6 yo; 2.5 to 5 mg IV for age 6 to 14 yo. Radiographic exam of upper GI tract: 0.1 mg/kg IV for age younger than 6 yo; 2.5 to 5 mg IV for age 6 to 14 yo.

UNAPPROVED ADULT – Prevention/treatment of chemo-induced emesis: 3 mg/kg IV over 1 h followed by continuous IV infusion of 0.5 mg/kg/h for 12 h. Migraine treatment: 10 mg IV. Migraine adjunct: 10 mg PO 5 to 10 min before ergotamine/analgesic/sedative.

UNAPPROVED PEDS – GERD: 0.4 to 0.8 mg/kg/day in 4 divided doses. Prevention of chemo-induced emesis: 1 to 2 mg/kg 30 min before chemo and then q 3 h prn (up to 5 doses/day or 5 to 10 mg/kg/day).

FORMS – Generic/Trade: Tabs 5, 10 mg. Trade: Orally disintegrating tabs 5, 10 mg (Metozolv). Generic only: Oral soln 5 mg/5 mL.

NOTES – To reduce incidence and severity of akathisia, consider giving IV doses over 15 min. If extrapyramidal reactions occur (especially with high IV doses) give diphenhydramine IM/IV. Adjust dose in renal dysfunction. Irreversible tardive dyskinesia with high

(cont.)

METOCLOPRAMIDE (*cont.*)

dose or long-term (more than 12 weeks) use. Avoid use for more than 12 weeks except in rare cases where benefit outweighs risk of tardive dyskinesia. May cause drowsiness, agitation, seizures, hallucinations, galactorrhea, hyperprolactinemia, constipation, diarrhea. Increases cyclosporine and ethanol absorption. Do not use if bowel perforation or mechanical obstruction present. Levodopa decreases metoclopramide effects.

NABILONE (*Cesamet*) ▶L ♀C ▶–©II $$$$$

ADULT – N/V in cancer chemotherapy patients with poor response to other agents: 1 to 2 mg PO two times per day, 1 to 3 h before chemotherapy. Max dose 6 mg/day in 3 divided doses.

PEDS – Not approved in children.

UNAPPROVED PEDS – Children 4 yo or older: wt less than 18 kg: 0.5 mg PO two times per day, wt 18 to 30 kg: 1 mg PO two times per day, wt 30 kg or greater: 1 mg PO three times per day.

FORMS – Trade only: Caps 1 mg.

NOTES – Contraindicated in known sensitivity to marijuana or other cannabinoids. Use with caution with current or past psychiatric reactions. Additive CNS effects with alcohol, sedatives, hypnotics, psychomimetics. Additive cardiac effects with amphetamines, antihistamines, anticholinergic medications.

PHOSPHORATED CARBOHYDRATES (*Emetrol*) ▶L ♀A ▶+ $

ADULT – Nausea: 15 to 30 mL PO q 15 min until nausea subsides or up to 5 doses.

PEDS – Nausea: 2 to 12 yo: 5 to 10 mL q 15 min until nausea subsides or up to 5 doses.

UNAPPROVED ADULT – Morning sickness: 15 to 30 mL PO upon rising, repeat q 3 h prn. Motion sickness or nausea due to drug therapy or anesthesia: 15 mL/dose.

UNAPPROVED PEDS – Regurgitation in infants: 5 to 10 mL PO 10 to 15 min prior to each feeding. Motion sickness or nausea due to drug therapy or anesthesia: 5 mL/dose.

FORMS – OTC Generic/Trade: Soln containing dextrose, fructose, and phosphoric acid.

NOTES – Do not dilute. Do not ingest fluids before or for 15 min after dose. Monitor blood glucose in diabetic patients.

PROCHLORPERAZINE (*Compazine*, ✤ *Stemetil*) ▶LK ♀C ▶? $

ADULT – N/V: 5 to 10 mg PO/IM three to four times per day (up to 40 mg/day); Sustained release: 10 mg PO q 12 h or 15 mg PO q am; Suppository: 25 mg PR q 12 h; IV/IM: 5 to 10 mg IV over at least 2 min q 3 to 4 h prn (up to 40 mg/day); 5 to 10 mg IM q 3 to 4 h prn (up to 40 mg/day).

PEDS – N/V: Not recommended in age younger than 2 yo or wt less than 10 kg, 0.4 mg/kg/day PO/PR in 3 to 4 divided doses for age older than 2 yo; 0.1 to 0.15 mg/kg/dose IM; IV not recommended in children.

UNAPPROVED ADULT – Migraine: 10 mg IV/IM or 25 mg PR single dose for acute headache.

UNAPPROVED PEDS – N/V during surgery: 5 to 10 mg IM 1 to 2 h before anesthesia induction, may repeat in 30 min; 5 to 10 mg IV 15 to 30 min before anesthesia induction, may repeat once.

FORMS – Generic only: Tabs 5, 10, 25 mg. Supp 25 mg.

NOTES – May cause extrapyramidal reactions (especially in elderly), hypotension (with IV), arrhythmias, sedation, seizures, hyperprolactinemia, gynecomastia, dry mouth, constipation, urinary retention, leukopenia, thrombocytopenia. Elderly more prone to adverse effects.

PROMETHAZINE (*Phenergan*) ▶LK ♀C ▶– $

WARNING – Contraindicated if age younger than 2 yo due to risk of fatal respiratory depression; caution in older children. Risks of severe tissue injury associated with IV administration including gangrene. Preferred route of administration is deep IM injection, subcutaneous injection is contraindicated.

ADULT – N/V: 12.5 to 25 mg q 4 to 6 h PO/IM/PR prn. Motion sickness: 25 mg PO/PR 30 to 60 min prior to departure and q 12 h prn. Hypersensitivity reactions: 25 mg IM/IV, may repeat in 2 h. Allergic conditions: 12.5 mg PO/PR/IM/IV four times per day or 25 mg PO/PR at bedtime.

PEDS – N/V: 0.25 to 1 mg/kg/dose PO/IM/PR (up to 25 mg/dose) q 4 to 6 h prn for age 2 yo or older. Motion sickness: 0.5 mg/kg (up to 25 mg/dose) PO 30 to 60 min prior to departure and q 12 h prn. Hypersensitivity reactions: 6.25 to 12.5 mg PO/PR/IM/IV q 6 h prn for age older than 2 yo.

UNAPPROVED ADULT – N/V: 12.5 to 25 mg IV q 4 h prn.

UNAPPROVED PEDS – N/V: 0.25 mg/kg/dose IV q 4 h prn for age 2 yo or older.

FORMS – Generic only: Tabs/Supp 12.5, 25, 50 mg. Syrup 6.25 mg/5 mL.

NOTES – May cause sedation, extrapyramidal reactions (especially with high IV doses), hypotension with rapid IV administration, anticholinergic side effects (eg, dry mouth, blurred vision).

SCOPOLAMINE (*Transderm-Scop, Scopace,* ✤ *Transderm-V*) ▶L ♀C ▶+ $$

ADULT – Motion sickness: 1 disc behind ear at least 4 h before travel and q 3 days prn or 0.4 to 0.8 mg PO 1 h before travel and q 8 h prn. Prevention of postop N/V: Apply patch behind ear 4 h before surgery, remove 24 h after surgery. Spastic states, postencephalitic parkinsonism: 0.4 to 0.8 mg PO q 8 h prn.

PEDS – Not approved for age younger than 12 yo.

UNAPPROVED PEDS – Preop and antiemetic: 6 mcg/kg/dose IM/IV/SC (max dose 0.3 mg/dose). May repeat q 6 to 8 h. Has also been used in severe drooling.

FORMS – Trade only: Topical disc 1.5 mg/72 h, box of 4. Oral tab 0.4 mg.

NOTES – Dry mouth common. Also causes drowsiness, blurred vision.

TRIMETHOBENZAMIDE (*Tigan*) ▶LK ♀C ▶? $

ADULT – N/V: 300 mg PO q 6 to 8 h, 200 mg IM q 6 to 8 h.

PEDS – Not approved for use in children.

UNAPPROVED PEDS – 100 to 200 mg PO q 6 to 8 h if wt 13.6 to 40.9 kg.

FORMS – Generic/Trade: Cap 300 mg.

NOTES – Not for IV use. May cause sedation. Reduce starting dose in the elderly or if reduced renal function to minimize risk of adverse effects.

GASTROENTEROLOGY: Antiulcer—Antacids

ALKA-SELTZER **(acetylsalicylic acid + citrate + bicarbonate)** ▶LK ♀? (– 3rd trimester) ▶? $

ADULT – Relief of upset stomach: 2 regular-strength tabs in 4 oz water q 4 h PO prn (up to 8 tabs daily for age younger than 60 yo, up to 4 tabs daily for age 60 yo or older) or 2 extra-strength tabs in 4 oz water q 6 h PO prn (up to 7 tabs daily for age younger than 60 yo, up to 3 tabs daily for age 60 yo or older).

PEDS – Not approved in children.

FORMS – OTC Trade only: Regular-strength, original: aspirin 325 mg + citric acid 1000 mg + sodium bicarbonate 1916 mg. Regular-strength lemon-lime and cherry: 325 mg + 1000 mg + 1700 mg. Extra-strength: 500 mg + 1000 mg + 1985 mg. Not all forms of Alka-Seltzer contain aspirin (eg, Alka-Seltzer Heartburn Relief).

NOTES – Avoid aspirin-containing forms in children and teenagers due to risk of Reye's syndrome.

ALUMINUM HYDROXIDE (*Alternagel, Amphojel, Alu-Tab, Alu-Cap*) ▶K ♀C ▶? $

ADULT – Hyperphosphatemia in chronic renal failure (short-term treatment only to avoid aluminum accumulation): 300 to 600 mg PO with meals. Titrate prn. Upset stomach, indigestion: 5 to 10 mL or 300 to 600 mg PO 6 times per day, between meals and at bedtime and prn.

PEDS – Not approved in children.

UNAPPROVED ADULT – Symptomatic reflux: 15 to 30 mL PO q 30 to 60 min. Long-term management of GERD: 15 to 30 mL PO 1 and 3 h after meals and at bedtime prn. Peptic ulcer disease: 15 to 45 mL or 1 to 3 tabs PO 1 and 3 h after meals and at bedtime. Prophylaxis against GI bleeding (titrate dose to maintain gastric pH greater than 3.5): 30 to 60 mL or 2 to 4 tabs PO q 1 to 2 h.

UNAPPROVED PEDS – Peptic ulcer disease: 5 to 15 mL PO 1 and 3 h after meals and at bedtime. Prophylaxis against GI bleeding (titrate dose to maintain gastric pH greater than 3.5): Neonates 0.5 to 1 mL/kg/dose PO q 4 h. Infants 2 to 5 mL PO q 1 to 2 h. Child: 5 to 15 mL PO q 1 to 2 h.

FORMS – OTC Generic/Trade: Susp 320, 600 mg/ 5 mL.

NOTES – For concentrated suspensions, use ½ the recommended dose. May cause constipation. Avoid administration with tetracyclines, digoxin, iron, isoniazid, buffered/enteric aspirin, diazepam, fluoroquinolones.

CITROCARBONATE **(bicarbonate + citrate)** ▶K ♀? ▶? $

ADULT – 1 to 2 teaspoons in cold water PO 15 min to 2 h after meals prn.

PEDS – ¼ to ½ teaspoon in cold water PO after meals prn for age 6 to 12 yo.

FORMS – OTC Trade only: Sodium bicarbonate 0.78 g + sodium citrate anhydrous 1.82 g per 1 teaspoonful 150, 300 g.

NOTES – Chronic use may cause metabolic alkalosis. Contains sodium.

GAVISCON **(aluminum hydroxide + magnesium carbonate)** ▶K ♀? ▶? $

ADULT – 2 to 4 tabs or 15 to 30 mL (regular-strength) or 10 mL (extra-strength) PO four times per day prn.

PEDS – Not approved in children.

(cont.)

GAVISCON *(cont.)*

UNAPPROVED PEDS – Peptic ulcer disease: 5 to 15 mL PO after meals and at bedtime.

FORMS – OTC Trade only: Tabs: Regular-strength (Al hydroxide 80 mg + Mg carbonate 20 mg), Extra-strength (Al hydroxide 160 mg + Mg carbonate 105 mg). Liquid: Regular-strength (Al hydroxide 95 mg + Mg carbonate 358 mg per 15 mL), Extra-strength (Al hydroxide 254 mg + Mg carbonate 237.5 mg per 5 mL).

NOTES – Contains alginic acid or sodium alginate, which is considered an "inactive" ingredient. Alginic acid forms foam barrier which floats in stomach to minimize esophageal contact with acid. Chronic use may cause metabolic alkalosis. Contains sodium.

MAALOX **(aluminum hydroxide + magnesium hydroxide)** ▶K ♀C ▶? $

ADULT – Heartburn/indigestion: 10 to 20 mL or 1 to 2 tabs PO four times per day, after meals and at bedtime and prn.

PEDS – Not approved in children.

UNAPPROVED ADULT – Peptic ulcer disease: 15 to 45 mL PO 1 and 3 h after meals and at bedtime. Symptomatic reflux: 15 to 30 mL PO q 30 to 60 min prn. Long-term management of GERD: 15 to 30 mL PO 1 and 3 h after meals and at bedtime prn. Prophylaxis against GI bleeding (titrate dose to maintain gastric pH greater than 3.5): 30 to 60 mL PO q 1 to 2 h.

UNAPPROVED PEDS – Peptic ulcer disease: 5 to 15 mL PO 1 and 3 h after meals and at bedtime. Prophylaxis against GI bleeding (titrate dose to maintain gastric pH greater than 3.5): Neonates 1 mL/kg/dose PO q 4 h. Infants 2 to 5 mL PO q 1 to 2 h. Child: 5 to 15 mL PO q 1 to 2 h.

FORMS – OTC Generic/Trade: Regular-strength chewable tabs (Al hydroxide + Mg hydroxide 200/200 mg), susp (225/200 mg per 5 mL). Other strengths available.

NOTES – Maalox Extra Strength and Maalox TC are more concentrated than Maalox. Maalox Plus has added simethicone. May cause constipation or diarrhea. Avoid concomitant administration with tetracyclines, digoxin, iron, isoniazid, buffered/enteric aspirin, diazepam, fluoroquinolones. Avoid chronic use in patients with renal dysfunction due to potential for magnesium accumulation.

MAGALDRATE *(**Riopan Plus**)* ▶K ♀C ▶? $

ADULT – Heartburn/indigestion: 5 to 10 mL between meals and at bedtime and prn.

PEDS – Younger than 12 yo: not approved. 12 yo or older: 5 to 10 mL between meals and at bedtime and prn.

UNAPPROVED PEDS – Peptic ulcer disease: 5 to 10 mL PO 1 and 3 h after meals and at bedtime.

FORMS – OTC Trade only: Riopan Plus (with simethicone) susp 540/20 mg/5 mL.

NOTES – Riopan Plus has added simethicone. Avoid concomitant administration with tetracyclines, fluoroquinolones, digoxin, iron, isoniazid, buffered/enteric aspirin, diazepam. Avoid chronic use in patients with renal failure.

MYLANTA **(aluminum hydroxide + magnesium hydroxide + simethicone)** ▶K ♀C ▶? $

ADULT – Heartburn/indigestion: 10 to 20 mL between meals and at bedtime.

PEDS – Safe dosing has not been established.

UNAPPROVED ADULT – Peptic ulcer disease: 15 to 45 mL PO 1 and 3 h after meals and at bedtime. Symptomatic reflux: 15 to 30 mL PO q 30 to 60 min. Long-term management of GERD: 15 to 30 mL PO 1 and 3 h postprandially and at bedtime prn.

UNAPPROVED PEDS – Peptic ulcer disease: 5 to 15 mL PO or 0.5 to 2 mL/kg/dose (max 15 mL/dose) after meals and and at bedtime.

FORMS – OTC Generic/Trade: Liquid (various concentrations, eg, regular-strength, maximum-strength, supreme).

NOTES – May cause constipation or diarrhea. Avoid concomitant administration with tetracyclines, fluoroquinolones, digoxin, iron, isoniazid, buffered/enteric aspirin, diazepam. Avoid chronic use in renal dysfunction.

ROLAIDS **(calcium carbonate + magnesium hydroxide)** ▶K ♀? ▶? $

ADULT – 2 to 4 tabs PO q 1 h prn, max 12 tabs/day (regular-strength) or 10 tabs/day (extra-strength).

PEDS – Not approved in children.

FORMS – OTC Trade only: Tabs regular-strength (Ca carbonate 550 mg, Mg hydroxide 110 mg), extra-strength (Ca carbonate 675 mg, Mg hydroxide 135 mg).

NOTES – Chronic use may cause metabolic alkalosis.

GASTROENTEROLOGY: Antiulcer—H2 Antagonists

CIMETIDINE (*Tagamet, Tagamet HB*) ▶LK ♀B ◗+ $

ADULT – Treatment of duodenal or gastric ulcer: 800 mg PO at bedtime or 300 mg PO four times per day with meals and at bedtime or 400 mg PO two times per day. Prevention of duodenal ulcer: 400 mg PO at bedtime. Erosive esophagitis: 800 mg PO two times per day or 400 mg PO four times per day. Prevention or treatment of heartburn (OTC product only approved for this indication): 200 mg PO prn max 400 mg/day for up to 14 days. Hypersecretory conditions: 300 mg PO four times per day with meals and at bedtime. Patients unable to take oral medications: 300 mg IV/IM q 6 to 8 h or 37.5 mg/h continuous IV infusion. Prevention of upper GI bleeding in critically ill patients: 50 mg/h continuous infusion.

PEDS – 16 yo and older: Duodenal ulcer/benign gastric ulcer: 300 mg IV/IM q 6 to 8 h. GI bleed: 50 mg/h IV. Pathological hypersecretory: 300 mg IV/IM q 6 to 8 h.

UNAPPROVED ADULT – Prevention of aspiration pneumonitis during surgery: 300 to 600 mg PO or 200 to 400 mg IV 60 to 90 min prior to anesthesia. Has been used as adjunctive therapy with H1 antagonist for severe allergic reactions.

UNAPPROVED PEDS – Treatment of duodenal or gastric ulcers, erosive esophagitis, hypersecretory conditions: Neonates: 5 to 10 mg/kg/day PO/IV/IM divided q 8 to 12 h. Infants: 10 to 20 mg/kg/day PO/IV/IM divided q 6 h. Children: 20 to 40 mg/kg/day PO/IV/IM divided q 6 h. Chronic viral warts in children: 25 to 40 mg/kg/day PO in divided doses.

FORMS – Tabs 200, 300, 400, 800 mg. Rx Generic only: Oral soln 300 mg/5 mL. OTC Generic/Trade: Tabs 200 mg.

NOTES – May cause dizziness, drowsiness, headache, diarrhea, nausea. Decreased absorption of ketoconazole, itraconazole. Increased levels of carbamazepine, cyclosporine, diazepam, labetalol, lidocaine, theophylline, phenytoin, procainamide, quinidine, propranolol, TCAs, valproic acid, warfarin. Stagger doses of cimetidine and antacids. Decrease dose with CrCl less than 30 mL/min.

FAMOTIDINE (***Pepcid, Pepcid AC, Maximum Strength Pepcid AC***) ▶LK ♀B ◗? $

ADULT – Treatment of duodenal ulcer: 40 mg PO at bedtime or 20 mg PO two times per day. Maintenance of duodenal ulcer: 20 mg PO at bedtime. Treatment of gastric ulcer: 40 mg PO at bedtime. GERD: 20 mg PO two times per day. Treatment or prevention of heartburn: (OTC product only approved for this indication) 10 to 20 mg PO prn, up to 2 tabs per day. Hypersecretory conditions: 20 mg PO q 6 h. Patients unable to take oral medications: 20 mg IV q 12 h.

PEDS – GERD: 0.5 mg/kg/day PO daily for up to 8 weeks for age younger than 3 mo; 0.5 mg/kg PO two times per day for age 3 to 12 mo; 1 mg/kg/day PO divided two times per day or 2 mg/kg/day PO daily, max 40 mg PO two times per day for age 1 to 16 yo. Peptic ulcer: 0.5 mg/kg/day PO at bedtime or divided two times per day up to 40 mg/day.

UNAPPROVED ADULT – Prevention of aspiration pneumonitis during surgery: 40 mg PO prior to anesthesia. Upper GI bleeding: 20 mg IV q 12 h. Has been used as adjunctive therapy with H1 antagonist for severe allergic reactions.

UNAPPROVED PEDS – Treatment of hypersecretory conditions: 0.25 mg/kg IV q 12 h (max 40 mg daily) or 1 to 1.2 mg/kg/day PO in 2 to 3 divided doses, max 40 mg/day.

FORMS – Generic/Trade: Tabs 10 mg (OTC, Pepcid AC Acid Controller), 20 mg (Rx and OTC, Maximum Strength Pepcid AC), 40 mg. Rx Generic/Trade: Susp 40 mg/5 mL.

NOTES – May cause dizziness, headache, constipation, diarrhea. Decreased absorption of ketoconazole, itraconazole. Adjust dose in patients with CrCl less than 50 mL/min.

NIZATIDINE (*Axid, Axid AR*) ▶K ♀B ◗? $$$$

ADULT – Treatment of duodenal or gastric ulcer: 300 mg PO at bedtime or 150 mg PO two times per day. Maintenance of duodenal ulcer: 150 mg PO at bedtime. GERD: 150 mg PO two times per day. Treatment or prevention of heartburn: (OTC product only approved for this indication) 75 mg PO prn, max 150 mg/day.

PEDS – Esophagitis, GERD: 150 mg PO two times per day for age 12 yo or older.

UNAPPROVED ADULT – Has been used as adjunctive therapy with H1 antagonist for severe allergic reactions.

UNAPPROVED PEDS – 6 mo to 11 yo (limited data): 5 to 10 mg/kg/day PO in 2 divided doses.

FORMS – OTC Trade only (Axid AR): Tabs 75 mg. Rx Generic: Caps 150 mg. Oral soln 15 mg/mL (120, 480 mL). Generic: Caps 300 mg.

NOTES – May cause dizziness, headache, constipation, diarrhea. Decrease absorption of ketoconazole, itraconazole. Adjust dose if CrCl is less than 50 mL/min.

PEPCID COMPLETE **(famotidine + calcium carbonate + magnesium hydroxide)** ▶LK ♀B ▶? $
ADULT – Treatment of heartburn: 1 tab PO prn. Max 2 tabs/day.
PEDS – Not approved in children younger than 12 yo. In children 12 yo or older, use adult dosing for OTC product.
FORMS – OTC trade/generic: Chewable tab, famotidine 10 mg with calcium carbonate 800 mg and magnesium hydroxide 165 mg.

RANITIDINE (***Zantac, Zantac Efferdose, Zantac 75, Zantac 150, Peptic Relief***) ▶K ♀B ▶? $$$
ADULT – Treatment of duodenal ulcer: 150 mg PO two times per day or 300 mg at bedtime. Treatment of gastric ulcer or GERD: 150 mg PO two times per day. Maintenance of duodenal or gastric ulcer: 150 mg PO at bedtime. Treatment of erosive esophagitis: 150 mg PO four times per day. Maintenance of erosive esophagitis: 150 mg PO two times per day. Prevention/treatment of heartburn: (OTC product only approved for this indication) 75 to 150 mg PO prn, max 300 mg/day. Hypersecretory conditions: 150 mg PO two times per day. Patients unable to take oral meds: 50 mg IV/IM q 6 to 8 h or 6.25 mg/h continuous IV infusion.
PEDS – Treatment of duodenal or gastric ulcers: 2 to 4 mg/kg PO two times per day (max 300 mg) or 2 to 4 mg/kg/day IV q 6 to 8 h for ages 1 mo to 16 yo. GERD, erosive esophagitis: 2.5 to 5 mg/kg PO two times per day (max 200 mg/day) or 2 to 4 mg/kg/day IV divided q 6 to 8 h (max 200 mg/day). Maintenance of duodenal or gastric ulcers: 2 to 4 mg/kg/day PO daily (max 150 mg).
UNAPPROVED ADULT – Prevention of upper GI bleeding in critically ill patients: 6.25 mg/h continuous IV infusion (150 mg/day). Has been used as adjunctive therapy with H1 antagonist for severe allergic reactions.
UNAPPROVED PEDS – Treatment of duodenal or gastric ulcers, GERD, hypersecretory conditions: Premature and term infants younger than 2 weeks of age: 1 mg/kg/day PO two times per day or 1.5 mg/kg IV for one dose then 12 h later 0.75 to 1 mg/kg IV q 12 h. Continuous infusion 1.5 mg/kg for 1 dose then 0.04 to 0.08 mg/kg/h infusion. Neonates: 1 to 2 mg/kg PO two times per day or 2 mg/kg/24 h IV divided q 12 h. Infants and children: 2 to 4 mg/kg/24 h IV/IM divided q 6 to 12 h or 1 mg/kg IV loading dose followed by 0.08 to 0.17 mg/kg/h continuous IV infusion.
FORMS – Generic/Trade: Tabs 75 mg (OTC: Zantac 75), 150 mg (OTC and Rx: Zantac 150), 300 mg. Syrup 75 mg/5 mL. Rx Trade only: Effervescent tabs 25 mg. Rx Generic only: Caps 150, 300 mg.
NOTES – May cause dizziness, sedation, headache, drowsiness, rash, nausea, constipation, diarrhea. Elevations in SGPT have been observed when H2-antagonists have been administered IV in greater than recommended dosages for 5 days or longer. Bradycardia can occur if the IV form is injected too rapidly. Variable effects on warfarin, decreased absorption of ketoconazole, itraconazole. Dissolve effervescent tabs in water. Stagger doses of ranitidine and antacids. Adjust dose in patients with CrCl less than 50 mL/min.

GASTROENTEROLOGY: Antiulcer—*Helicobacter pylori* Treatment

HELIDAC **(bismuth subsalicylate + metronidazole + tetracycline)** ▶LK ♀D ▶– $$$$$
ADULT – Active duodenal ulcer associated with *H. pylori*: 1 dose (2 bismuth subsalicylate chewable tabs, 1 metronidazole tab, and 1 tetracycline cap) PO four times per day, at meals and at bedtime for 2 weeks with an H2 antagonist.
PEDS – Not approved in children.
UNAPPROVED ADULT – Active duodenal ulcer associated with *H. pylori*: Same dose as in "adult," but substitute proton pump inhibitor for H2 antagonist.
FORMS – Trade only: Each dose consists of bismuth subsalicylate 524 mg (2 × 262 mg) chewable tab + metronidazole 250 mg tab + tetracycline 500 mg cap.
NOTES – See components.

PREVPAC **(lansoprazole + amoxicillin + clarithromycin,** ✤ ***HP-Pac*****)** ▶LK ♀C ▶? $$$$$
ADULT – Active duodenal ulcer associated with *H. pylori*: 1 dose PO two times per day for 10 to 14 days.
PEDS – Not approved in children.
FORMS – Trade only: Each dose consists of lansoprazole 30 mg cap + amoxicillin 1 g (2 × 500 mg cap), + clarithromycin 500 mg tab.
NOTES – See components.

PYLERA **(bismuth subcitrate potassium + metronidazole + tetracycline)** ▶LK ♀D ▶– $$$$$
ADULT – Duodenal ulcer associated with *H. pylori*: 3 caps PO four times per day (after meals and at bedtime) for 10 days. To be given with omeprazole 20 mg PO two times per day.
PEDS – Not approved in children.

(cont.)

***HELICOBACTER PYLORI* THERAPY**

- Triple therapy PO for 10 to 14 days: clarithromycin 500 mg two times per day plus amoxicillin 1 g two times per day (or metronidazole 500 mg two times per day) plus PPI*
- Quadruple therapy PO for 14 days: bismuth subsalicylate 525 mg (or 30 mL) three to four times per day plus metronidazole 500 mg three to four times per day plus tetracycline 500 mg three to four times per day plus a PPI* or an H2 blocker†
- PPI or H2 blocker may need to be continued past 14 days to heal the ulcer.

*PPIs include esomeprazole 40 mg daily, lansoprazole 30 mg two times per day, omeprazole 20 mg two times per day, pantoprazole 40 mg two times per day, rabeprazole 20 mg two times per day.
†H2 blockers include cimetidine 400 mg two times per day, famotidine 20 mg two times per day, nizatidine 150 mg two times per day, ranitidine 150 mg two times per day. Adapted from *Medical Letter Treatment Guidelines* 2008:55.

***PYLERA** (cont.)*

FORMS – Trade only: Each cap contains bismuth subcitrate potassium 140 mg + metronidazole 125 mg + tetracycline 125 mg.

NOTES – See components.

GASTROENTEROLOGY: Antiulcer—Other

BELLERGAL-S **(phenobarbital + belladonna + ergotamine,** ✤ ***Bellergal Spacetabs*****)** ▶LK ♀X ▶– $

WARNING – Serious or life-threatening peripheral ischemia has been noted with ergotamine component when used with CYP3A4 inhibitors such as ritonavir, nelfinavir, indinavir, erythromycin, clarithromycin, ketoconazole, and itraconazole.

ADULT – Hypermotility/hypersecretion: 1 tab PO two times per day.

PEDS – Not approved in children.

FORMS – Generic: Tabs phenobarbital 40 mg, ergotamine 0.6 mg, belladonna 0.2 mg.

NOTES – May decrease INR in patients receiving warfarin. Variable effect on phenytoin levels. May cause sedation especially with alcohol, phenothiazines, opioids, or TCAs. Additive anticholinergic effects with TCAs.

DICYCLOMINE (***Bentyl,*** ✤ ***Bentylol***) ▶LK ♀B ▶– $

ADULT – Treatment of functional bowel/irritable bowel syndrome (irritable colon, spastic colon, mucous colon): Initiate with 20 mg PO four times per day and increase to 40 mg PO four times per day, if tolerated. Patients who are unable to take oral medications: 20 mg IM q 6 h.

PEDS – Not approved in children.

UNAPPROVED PEDS – Treatment of functional/irritable bowel syndrome: Infants 6 mo or older: 5 mg PO three to four times per day. Children: 10 mg PO three to four times per day.

FORMS – Generic/Trade: Tabs 20 mg. Caps 10 mg. Syrup 10 mg/5 mL.

NOTES – Although some use lower doses (ie, 10 to 20 mg PO four times per day), the only adult oral dose proven to be effective is 160 mg/day.

DONNATAL **(phenobarbital + hyoscyamine + atropine + scopolamine)** ▶LK ♀C ▶– $$$

ADULT – Adjunctive therapy of irritable bowel syndrome or adjunctive treatment of duodenal ulcers: 1 to 2 tabs/caps or 5 to 10 mL PO three to four times per day or 1 extended-release tab PO q 8 to 12 h.

PEDS – Adjunctive therapy of irritable bowel syndrome, adjunctive treatment of duodenal ulcers: 0.1 mL/kg/dose q 4 h, max 5 mL. Alternative dosing regimen: Give 0.5 mL PO q 4 h or 0.75 mL PO q 6 h for wt 4.5 kg, give 1 mL PO q 4 h or 1.5 mL PO q 6 h for wt 9.1 kg, give 1.5 mL PO q 4 h or 2 mL PO q 6 h for wt 13.6 kg, give 2.5 mL PO q 4 h or 3.75 mL PO q 6 h for wt 22.7 kg, give 3.75 mL PO q 4 h or 5 mL PO q 6 h for wt 34 kg, give 5 mL PO q 4 h or 7.5 mL PO q 6 h for wt 45 kg or greater.

FORMS – Generic/trade: Phenobarbital 16.2 mg + hyoscyamine 0.1 mg + atropine 0.02 mg + scopolamine 6.5 mcg in each tab or 5 mL. Trade only: Extended-release tab 48.6 + 0.3111 + 0.0582 + 0.0195 mg.

NOTES – The FDA has classified Donnatal as "possibly effective" for treatment of irritable bowel syndrome and duodenal ulcer. Heat stroke may occur in hot weather. Can cause anticholinergic side effects; use caution in narrow-angle glaucoma, BPH, etc.

GI COCKTAIL (**green goddess**) ▶LK ♀See individual ▶See individual $

UNAPPROVED ADULT – Acute GI upset: Mixture of Maalox/Mylanta 30 mL + viscous lidocaine (2%) 10 mL + Donnatal 10 mL administered PO in a single dose.

NOTES – Avoid repeat dosing due to risk of lidocaine toxicity.

✤**HYOSCINE** (***Buscopan***) ▶LK ♀C ▶? $$

ADULT – Canada: GI or bladder spasm: 10 to 20 mg PO/IV up to 60 mg daily (PO) or 100 mg daily (IV).

PEDS – Not approved in children.

FORMS – Canada Trade only: Tabs 10 mg.

NOTES – May cause dizziness, drowsiness, blurred vision, dry mouth, N/V, urinary retention. Contraindicated in glaucoma, obstructive conditions (eg, pyloric, duodenal, or other intestinal obstructive lesions, ileus, and obstructive uropathies), and myasthenia gravis.

HYOSCYAMINE (***Anaspaz, A-spaz, Cystospaz, ED Spaz, Hyosol, Hyospaz, Levbid, Levsin, Levsinex, Medispaz, NuLev, Spacol, Spasdel, Symax***) ▶LK ♀C ▶– $

ADULT – Bladder spasm, to control gastric secretion, GI hypermotility, irritable bowel syndrome: 0.125 to 0.25 mg PO/SL q 4 h or prn. Extended-release 0.375 to 0.75 mg PO q 12 h. Max 1.5 mg/day.

PEDS – Bladder spasm: Use adult dosing in age older than 12 yo. To control gastric secretion, GI hypermotility, irritable bowel syndrome, and others: Initial oral dose by wt for age younger than 2 yo: Give 12.5 mcg for 2.3 kg, give 16.7 mcg for 3.4 kg, give 20.8 mcg for 5 kg, give 25 mcg for 7 kg, give 31.3 to 33.3 mcg for 10 kg, give 45.8 mcg for 15 kg. Alternatively, if age younger than 2 yo: 3 gtts for wt 2.3 kg, give 4 gtts for 3.4 kg, give 5 gtts for 5 kg, give 6 gtts for 7 kg, give 8 gtts for 10 kg, give 11 gtts for 15 kg. Doses can be repeated q 4 h prn, but maximum daily dose is six times initial dose. Initial oral dose by wt for age 2 to 12 yo: Give 31.3 to 33.3 mcg for 10 kg, give 62.5 mcg for 20 kg, give 93.8 mcg for 40 kg, and give 125 mcg for 50 kg. Doses may be repeated q 4 h, but maximum daily dose should not exceed 750 mcg.

FORMS – Generic/Trade: Tabs 0.125. Sublingual tabs 0.125 mg. Chewable tabs 0.125 mg. Extended-release tabs 0.375 mg. Elixir 0.125 mg/5 mL. Gtts 0.125 mg/1 mL.

NOTES – May cause dizziness, drowsiness, blurred vision, dry mouth, N/V, urinary retention. Contraindicated in glaucoma, obstructive conditions (eg, pyloric, duodenal, or other intestinal obstructive lesions, ileus, achalasia, GI hemorrhage, and obstructive uropathies), unstable cardiovascular status, and myasthenia gravis.

MEPENZOLATE (***Cantil***) ▶K + gut ♀B ▶? $$$$$

ADULT – Adjunctive therapy in peptic ulcer disease: 25 to 50 mg PO four times per day, with meals and at bedtime.

PEDS – Not approved in children.

FORMS – Trade only: Tabs 25 mg.

NOTES – Contraindicated in glaucoma, obstructive uropathy, paralytic ileus, toxic megacolon, obstructive diseases of GI tract, intestinal atony in elderly/debilitated, myasthenia gravis, unstable CV status, acute GI bleed.

METHSCOPOLAMINE (***Pamine, Pamine Forte***) ▶LK ♀C ▶? $$$$

ADULT – Adjunctive therapy in peptic ulcer disease: 2.5 mg PO 30 min before meals and 2.5 to 5 mg PO at bedtime.

PEDS – Not approved in children.

FORMS – Generic/Trade: Tabs 2.5 mg (Pamine), 5 mg (Pamine Forte).

NOTES – Has not been shown to be effective in treating peptic ulcer disease.

MISOPROSTOL (***PGE1, Cytotec***) ▶LK ♀X ▶– $$$$

WARNING – Contraindicated in desired early or preterm pregnancy due to its abortifacient property. Pregnant women should avoid contact/exposure to the tabs. Uterine rupture reported with use for labor induction and medical abortion.

ADULT – Prevention of NSAID–induced gastric ulcers: 200 mcg PO four times per day. If not tolerated, use 100 mcg PO four times per day.

PEDS – Not approved in children.

UNAPPROVED ADULT – Cervical ripening and labor induction: 25 mcg intravaginally q 3 to 6 h (or 50 mcg q 6 h). First-trimester pregnancy failure: 800 mcg intravaginally, repeat on day 3 if expulsion incomplete. Medical abortion 63 days gestation or less: With mifepristone, see mifepristone; with methotrexate: 800 mcg intravaginally 5 to 7 days after 50 mg/m² IM methotrexate. Preop cervical ripening: 400 mcg intravaginally 3 to 4 h before mechanical cervical dilation. Postpartum hemorrhage: 400 mcg to 600 mcg PO or PR single dose. Treatment of duodenal ulcers: 100 mcg to 200 mcg PO four times per day. Alternatively, 400 mcg PO twice daily has been tried.

UNAPPROVED PEDS – Improvement in fat absorption in cystic fibrosis in children 8 to 16 yo: 100 mcg PO four times per day.

FORMS – Generic/Trade: Oral tabs 100, 200 mcg.

(cont.)

MISOPROSTOL (*cont.*)

NOTES – Contraindicated with prior C-section. Oral tabs can be inserted into the vagina for labor induction/cervical ripening. Monitor for uterine hyperstimulation and abnormal fetal heart rate. Risk factors for uterine rupture: Prior uterine surgery and 5 previous pregnancies or more.

PROPANTHELINE (***Pro-Banthine***) ▶LK ♀C ▶– $$$

ADULT – Adjunctive therapy in peptic ulcer disease: 7.5 to 15 mg PO 30 min before meals and 30 mg at bedtime.

PEDS – Not approved in children.

UNAPPROVED ADULT – Irritable bowel, pancreatitis, urinary bladder spasms: 7.5 to 15 mg PO three times per day and 30 mg at bedtime.

UNAPPROVED PEDS – Antisecretory effects: 1 to 2 mg/kg/day PO in 3 to 4 divided doses. Antispasmodic effects: 2 to 3 mg/kg/day PO divided q 4 to 6 h and at bedtime.

FORMS – Generic only: Tabs 15 mg.

NOTES – For elderly adults and those with small stature use 7.5 mg dose. May cause constipation, dry mucous membranes.

SIMETHICONE (***Mylicon, Gas-X, Phazyme,*** ♣ ***Ovol***) ▶Not absorbed ♀C but + ▶? $

ADULT – Excessive gas in GI tract: 40 to 360 mg PO after meals and at bedtime prn, max 500 mg/day.

PEDS – Excessive gas in GI tract: 20 mg PO four times per day prn, max 240 mg/day for age younger than 2 yo, 40 mg PO four times per day prn for age 2 to 12 yo (max 500 mg/day).

UNAPPROVED PEDS – Although used to treat infant colic (in approved dose for gas), several studies suggest no benefit.

FORMS – OTC Generic/Trade: Chewable tabs 80, 125 mg. Gtts 40 mg/0.6 mL. Trade only: Softgels 166 mg (Gas-X) 180 mg (Phazyme). Strips, oral (Gas-X) 62.5 mg (adults), 40 mg (children).

NOTES – For administration to infants, may mix dose in 30 mL of liquid. Chewable tabs should be chewed thoroughly.

SUCRALFATE (***Carafate,*** ♣ ***Sulcrate***) ▶Not absorbed ♀B ▶? $$

ADULT – Duodenal ulcer: 1 g PO four times per day, 1 h before meals and at bedtime. Maintenance therapy of duodenal ulcer: 1 g PO two times per day.

PEDS – Not approved in children.

UNAPPROVED ADULT – Gastric ulcer, reflux esophagitis, NSAID–induced GI symptoms, stress ulcer prophylaxis: 1 g PO four times per day 1 h before meals and at bedtime. Oral and esophageal ulcers due to radiation/chemo/sclerotherapy: (susp only) 5 to 10 mL swish and spit/swallow four times per day.

UNAPPROVED PEDS – Reflux esophagitis, gastric or duodenal ulcer, stress ulcer prophylaxis: 40 to 80 mg/kg/day PO divided q 6 h. Alternative dosing: 500 mg PO four times per day for age younger than 6 yo, give 1 g PO four times per day for age 6 yo or older.

FORMS – Generic/Trade: Tabs 1 g. Susp 1 g/10 mL.

NOTES – May cause constipation. May reduce the absorption of cimetidine, ciprofloxacin, digoxin, ketoconazole, levothyroxine, itraconazole, norfloxacin, phenytoin, ranitidine, tetracycline, theophylline, and warfarin; separate doses by at least 2 h. Antacids should be separated by at least 30 min. Hyperglycemia has been reported in patients with diabetes.

GASTROENTEROLOGY: Antiulcer—Proton Pump Inhibitors

NOTE: Long-term use may be associated with an increased risk of fractures, pneumonia, *C. difficile*–associated diarrhea and hypomagnesemia. Periodically reassess need and discontinue (taper dose to prevent rebound symptoms), if possible.

DEXLANSOPRAZOLE (***Dexilant***) ▶L ♀B ▶? $$$$

ADULT – Erosive esophagitis: 60 mg PO daily for up to 8 weeks. Maintenance therapy after healing of erosive esophagitis: 30 mg PO daily for up to 6 months. GERD: 30 mg PO daily for up to 4 weeks.

PEDS – Not approved in children.

FORMS – Trade only: Cap 30, 60 mg.

NOTES – May decrease absorption of atazanavir, ketoconazole, itraconazole, ampicillin, digoxin, and iron. Monitor INR in patients receiving warfarin. Swallow whole or mix with applesauce and take immediately.

ESOMEPRAZOLE (***Nexium***) ▶L ♀B ▶? $$$$

ADULT – Erosive esophagitis: 20 to 40 mg PO daily for 4 to 8 weeks. Maintenance of erosive esophagitis: 20 mg PO daily. Zollinger-Ellison: 40 mg PO two times per day. GERD: 20 mg PO daily for 4 weeks. GERD with esophagitis: 20 to 40 mg IV daily for 10 days until taking PO. Prevention of NSAID–associated gastric ulcer: 20 to 40 mg PO daily for up to 6 months. *H. pylori* eradication: 40 mg PO daily with amoxicillin 1000 mg PO two times per day and clarithromycin 500 mg PO two times per day for 10 days.

PEDS – GERD: wt less than 20 kg: 10 mg PO daily; wt 20 kg or more: 10 to 20 mg daily.

(cont.)

ESOMEPRAZOLE (*cont.*)

Alternatively, 10 to 20 mg PO daily for up to 8 weeks for age 1 to 11 yo, give 20 to 40 mg PO daily for up to 8 weeks for age 12 to 17 yo.

FORMS – Trade only: Caps delayed-release 20, 40 mg. Delayed-release granules for oral susp 10, 20, 40 mg per packet.

NOTES – Concomitant administration with voriconazole, an inhibitor of CYP2C19 and CYP3A4 may lead to a more than doubling of esomeprazole exposure. Esomeprazole may reduce the efficacy of clopidogrel. Use caution with high dose methotrexate.

LANSOPRAZOLE (***Prevacid***) ▶L ♀B ▶? $$$

ADULT – Heartburn: 15 mg PO daily. Erosive esophagitis: 30 mg PO daily or 30 mg IV daily for 7 days or until taking PO. Maintenance therapy following healing of erosive esophagitis: 15 mg PO daily. NSAID–induced gastric ulcer: 30 mg PO daily for 8 weeks (treatment), 15 mg PO daily for up to 12 weeks (prevention). GERD: 15 mg PO daily. Duodenal ulcer treatment and maintenance: 15 mg PO daily. Gastric ulcer: 30 mg PO daily. Part of a multidrug regimen for *H. pylori* eradication: 30 mg PO two times per day with amoxicillin 1000 mg PO two times per day and clarithromycin 500 mg PO two times per day for 10 to 14 days (see table) or 30 mg PO three times per day with amoxicillin 1000 mg PO three times per day for 14 days. Hypersecretory conditions: 60 mg PO daily.

PEDS – Not effective in patients with symptomatic GERD age 1 mo to younger than 1 yo. Esophagitis and GERD: 1 to 11 yo, less than 30 kg: 15 kg PO daily up to 12 weeks; 12 to 17 yo, 30 kg or greater: 30 mg PO daily up to 12 weeks.

FORMS – OTC Trade only: Caps 15 mg. Rx Generic/Trade: 15, 30 mg. Rx Trade only: Orally disintegrating tab 15, 30 mg. Prevacid NapraPac: 7 lansoprazole 15 mg caps packaged with 14 naproxen tabs 375 mg or 500 mg.

NOTES – Take before meals. Potential for PPIs to reduce the response to clopidogrel. Evaluate the need for a PPI in clopidogrel-treated patients and consider H2-blocker/antacid. Orally disintegrating tabs can be dissolved in water (15 mg tab in 4 mL, 30 mg tab in 10 mL) and administered via an oral syringe or nasogastric tube at least 8 French within 15 min. Delayed-release orally disintegrating tabs should not be broken or cut.

OMEPRAZOLE (***Prilosec***, ✤***Losec***) ▶L ♀C ▶? OTC $, Rx $$$$

ADULT – GERD, duodenal ulcer, erosive esophagitis: 20 mg PO daily. Heartburn (OTC): 20 mg PO daily for 14 days. Gastric ulcer: 40 mg PO daily. Hypersecretory conditions: 60 mg PO daily. Part of a multidrug regimen for *H. pylori* eradication: 20 mg PO two times per day with amoxicillin 1000 mg PO two times per day and clarithromycin 500 mg PO two times per day for 10 days, with additional 18 days of omeprazole 20 mg PO daily if ulcer present (see table); or 40 mg PO daily with clarithromycin 500 mg PO three times per day for 14 days, with additional 14 days of omeprazole 20 mg PO daily if ulcer present.

PEDS – GERD, acid-related disorders, maintenance of healing erosive esophagitis: 5 mg PO daily for wt 5 to 9 kg, 10 mg PO daily for wt 10 to 19 kg, give 20 mg PO daily for wt 20 kg or greater.

UNAPPROVED PEDS – Gastric or duodenal ulcers, hypersecretory states: 0.2 to 3.5 mg/kg/dose PO daily. GERD: 1 mg/kg/day PO one or two times per day.

FORMS – Rx Generic/Trade: Caps 10, 20, 40 mg. Trade only: Granules for oral susp 2.5 mg, 10 mg. OTC Trade only: Cap 20 mg.

NOTES – Take before meals. Caps contain enteric-coated granules; do not chew. Caps may be opened and administered in acidic liquid (eg, applejuice) or 1 tablespoon of applesauce. May increase levels of diazepam, warfarin, and phenytoin. May decrease absorption of ketoconazole, itraconazole, iron, ampicillin, and digoxin. Reduces plasma levels of atazanavir. Concomitant administration with voriconazole, an inhibitor of CYP2C19 and CYP3A4 may lead to a more than doubling of omeprazole exposure. Avoid administration with sucralfate. Use caution with high dose methotrexate. Omeprazole may reduce the efficacy of clopidogrel.

PANTOPRAZOLE (***Protonix***, ✤***Pantoloc***) ▶L ♀B ▶? $$$$

ADULT – GERD: 40 mg PO daily for 8 to 16 weeks. Maintenance therapy following healing of erosive esophagitis: 40 mg PO daily. Zollinger-Ellison syndrome: 80 mg IV q 8 to 12 h for 7 days until taking PO. GERD associated with a history of erosive esophagitis: 40 mg IV daily for 7 to 10 days until taking PO.

PEDS – Erosive esophagitis associated with GERD: 15 kg to less than 40 kg: 20 mg PO daily for up to 8 weeks. 40 kg or greater: 40 mg PO daily for up to 8 weeks.

UNAPPROVED ADULT – Has been studied as part of various multidrug regimens for *H. pylori* eradication. Decreases peptic ulcer rebleeding after hemostasis: 80 mg IV bolus,

(cont.)

PANTOPRAZOLE (*cont.*)

then 8 mg/h continuous IV infusion for 3 days, followed by oral therapy (or 40 mg IV q 12 h for 4 to 7 days if unable to tolerate PO).

UNAPPROVED PEDS – GERD associated with a history of erosive esophagitis: 0.5 to 1 mg/kg/day (max 40 mg/day).

FORMS – Generic/Trade: Tabs 20, 40 mg. Trade only: Granules for susp 40 mg/packet.

NOTES – Use caution with high dose methotrexate.

RABEPRAZOLE (***AcipHex***, ✤ ***Pariet***) ▶L ♀B ◗? $$$$

ADULT – GERD: 20 mg PO daily for 4 to 16 weeks. Duodenal ulcers: 20 mg PO daily for 4 weeks. Zollinger-Ellison syndrome: 60 mg PO daily, may increase up to 100 mg daily or 60 mg two times per day. Part of a multidrug regimen for *H. pylori* eradication: 20 mg PO two times per day, with amoxicillin 1000 mg PO two times per day and clarithromycin 500 mg PO two times per day for 7 days.

PEDS – 20 mg PO daily up to 8 weeks for age 12 yo or older.

FORMS – Trade: Tabs 20 mg.

ZEGERID **(omeprazole + bicarbonate)** ▶L ♀C ◗? $$$$$

ADULT – Duodenal ulcer, GERD, erosive esophagitis: 20 mg PO daily for 4 to 8 weeks. Gastric ulcer: 40 mg PO once daily for 4 to 8 weeks. Reduction of risk of upper GI bleed in critically ill (susp only): 40 mg PO, then 40 mg 6 to 8 h later, then 40 mg once daily thereafter for up to 14 days.

PEDS – Not approved in children.

FORMS – OTC Trade only: omeprazole/sodium bicarbonate caps 20 mg/1 g. Rx Trade only: 20 mg/1.1 g and 40 mg/1.68 g, powder packets for susp 20 mg/1.1 g and 40 mg/1.68 g.

NOTES – Omeprazole may reduce the efficiacy of clopidogrel.

GASTROENTEROLOGY: Laxatives—Bulk-Forming

METHYLCELLULOSE (***Citrucel***) ▶Not absorbed ♀+ ◗? $

ADULT – Laxative: 1 heaping tablespoon in 8 oz cold water PO daily (up to three times per day).

PEDS – Laxative: Age 6 to 12 yo: 1½ heaping teaspoons in 4 oz cold water daily (up to three times per day) PO prn.

FORMS – OTC Trade only: Regular and sugar-free packets and multiple-use canisters, Clear-mix soln, Caps 500 mg.

NOTES – Must be taken with water to avoid esophageal obstruction or choking.

POLYCARBOPHIL (***FiberCon, Konsyl Fiber, Equalactin***) ▶Not absorbed ♀+ ◗? $

ADULT – Laxative: 2 tabs (1250 mg) PO four times per day prn.

PEDS – Laxative: 6 to 12 yo: 625 mg PO up to four times per day prn; 12 yo or older: 2 tabs (1250 mg) PO four times per day prn.

UNAPPROVED ADULT – Diarrhea: 2 tabs (1250 mg) PO q 30 min prn. Max daily dose 6 g.

UNAPPROVED PEDS – Diarrhea: 500 mg PO q 30 min prn (up to 1 g polycarbophil/day for age 3 to 5 yo, and 2 g/day for age older than 6 yo).

FORMS – OTC Generic/Trade: Tabs/Caps 625 mg. OTC Trade only: Chewable tabs 625 mg (Equalactin).

NOTES – When used as a laxative, take dose with at least 8 oz of fluid. Do not administer concomitantly with tetracycline; separate by at least 2 h.

PSYLLIUM (***Metamucil, Fiberall, Konsyl, Hydrocil,*** ✤ ***Prodium Plain***) ▶Not absorbed ♀+ ◗? $

ADULT – Laxative: 1 rounded teaspoon in liquid, 1 packet in liquid or 1 wafer with liquid PO daily (up to three times per day).

PEDS – Laxative (children 6 to 11 yo): ½ to 1 rounded teaspoon in liquid, ½ to 1 packet in liquid or 1 wafer with liquid PO daily (up to three times per day).

UNAPPROVED ADULT – Reduction in cholesterol: 1 rounded teaspoon in liquid, 1 packet in liquid or 1 to 2 wafers with liquid PO three times per day. Prevention of GI side effects with orlistat: 6 g in liquid with each orlistat dose or 12 g in liquid at bedtime.

FORMS – OTC Generic/Trade: Regular and sugar-free powder, Granules, Caps, Wafers, including various flavors and various amounts of psyllium.

NOTES – Powders and granules must be mixed with 8 oz water/liquid prior to ingestion. Start with 1 dose/day and gradually increase to minimize gas and bloating. Can bind with warfarin, digoxin, potassium-sparing diuretics, salicylates, tetracycline, and nitrofurantoin; space at least 3 h apart.

GASTROENTEROLOGY: Laxatives—Osmotic

GLYCERIN (*Fleet*) ▶Not absorbed ♀C ▶? $

ADULT – Constipation: 1 adult suppository or 5 mL to 15 mL as an enema PR prn.

PEDS – Constipation: 0.5 mL/kg/dose as an enema PR prn in neonates, 1 infant suppository or 2 to 5 mL rectal soln as an enema PR prn for age younger than 6 yo, 1 adult suppository or 5 to 15 mL of rectal soln as enema PR prn for age 6 yo or older.

FORMS – OTC Generic/Trade: Supp infant and adult, Soln (Fleet Babylax) 4 mL/applicator.

LACTULOSE (*Enulose, Kristalose*) ▶Not absorbed ♀B ▶? $$

ADULT – Constipation: 15 to 30 mL (syrup) or 10 to 20 g (powder for oral soln) PO daily. Evacuation of barium following barium procedures: 15 to 30 mL (syrup) PO daily, may increase to 60 mL. Acute hepatic encephalopathy: 30 to 45 mL syrup/dose PO q 1 h until laxative effect observed or 300 mL in 700 mL water or saline PR as a retention enema q 4 to 6 h. Prevention of encephalopathy: 30 to 45 mL syrup PO three to four times per day.

PEDS – Prevention or treatment of encephalopathy: Infants: 2.5 to 10 mL/day (syrup) PO in 3 to 4 divided doses. Children/adolescents: 40 to 90 mL/day (syrup) PO in 3 to 4 divided doses.

UNAPPROVED ADULT – Restoration of bowel movements in hemorrhoidectomy patients: 15 mL syrup PO two times per day on days before surgery and for 5 days following surgery.

UNAPPROVED PEDS – Constipation: 7.5 mL syrup PO daily, after breakfast.

FORMS – Generic/Trade: Syrup 10 g/15 mL. Trade only (Kristalose): 10, 20 g packets for oral soln.

NOTES – May be mixed in water, juice, or milk to improve palatability. Packets for oral soln should be mixed in 4 oz of water or juice. Titrate dose to produce 2 to 3 soft stools/day.

MAGNESIUM CITRATE ▶K ♀B ▶? $

ADULT – Evacuate bowel prior to procedure: 150 to 300 mL PO once or in divided doses.

PEDS – Evacuate bowel prior to procedure: 2 to 4 mL/kg PO once or in divided doses for age younger than 6 yo. 100 to 150 mL PO once or in divided doses for age 6 to 12 yo.

FORMS – OTC Generic only: Soln 300 mL/bottle. Low-sodium and sugar-free available.

NOTES – Use caution with impaired renal function. May decrease absorption of phenytoin, ciprofloxacin, benzodiazepines, and glyburide. May cause additive CNS depression with CNS depressants. Chill to improve palatability.

MAGNESIUM HYDROXIDE (*Milk of Magnesia*) ▶K ♀+ ▶? $

ADULT – Laxative: 30 to 60 mL regular strength (400 mg per 5 mL), 15 to 30 mL (800 mg per 5 mL strength) or 10 to 20 mL (1200 mg per 5 mL) PO as a single dose or divided doses. Antacid: 5 to 15 mL/dose PO four times per day prn or 622 to 1244 mg PO four times per day prn.

PEDS – Laxative: 0.5 mL/kg regular strength (400 mg per 5 mL) PO as a single dose or in divided doses for age younger than 2 yo, 5 to 15 mL/day PO as a single dose or in divided doses for age 2 to 5 yo, 15 to 30 mL PO in a single dose or in divided doses for age 6 to 11 yo. Antacid: 5 to 15 mL/dose regular strength (400 mg per 5 mL) PO four times per day prn for age older than 12 yo.

FORMS – OTC Generic/Trade: Susp 400 mg/5 mL. Trade only: Chewable tabs 311, 400 mg. Generic only: Susp 800 mg/5 mL, (concentrated) 1200 mg/5 mL, sugar-free 400 mg/5 mL.

NOTES – Use caution with impaired renal function.

POLYETHYLENE GLYCOL (*MiraLax, GlycoLax*) ▶Not absorbed ♀C ▶? $

ADULT – Constipation: 17 g (1 heaping tablespoon) in 4 to 8 oz water, juice, soda, coffee, or tea PO daily.

PEDS – Not approved in children.

UNAPPROVED PEDS – Children older than 6 mo: 0.5 to 1.5 g/kg/day PO, maximum 17 g/day.

FORMS – OTC Trade only: Powder for oral soln 17 g/scoop. Rx Generic/Trade: Powder for oral soln 17 g/scoop.

NOTES – Takes 1 to 3 days to produce bowel movement. Indicated for up to 14 days.

POLYETHYLENE GLYCOL WITH ELECTROLYTES (*GoLYTELY, Colyte, TriLyte, NuLYTELY, Moviprep, HalfLytely, Bisacodyl Tablet Kit,* ♣ *Klean-Prep, Electropeg, Peg-Lyte*) ▶Not absorbed ♀C ▶? $

ADULT – Bowel cleansing prior to GI examination: 240 mL PO q 10 min or 20 to 30 mL/min NG until 4 L are consumed or rectal effluent is clear. Moviprep: 240 mL q 15 min for 4 doses (over 1 h) the night before plus 16 additional oz of clear liquid and 240 mL q 15 min for 4 doses (over 1 h) plus 16 additional oz of clear liquid on the morning of the colonoscopy. Alternatively, 240 mL q 15 min for 4 doses (over 1 h) at 6 pm on the evening

(cont.)

POLYETHYLENE GLYCOL WITH ELECTROLYTES (*cont.*)

before the colonoscopy and then 1.5 h later, 240 mL q 15 min for 4 doses (over 1 h) plus 32 additional oz of clear liquid on the evening before the colonoscopy (Moviprep only).

PEDS – Bowel prep (NuLYTELY, TriLyte): 25 mL/kg/h PO/NG, until rectal effluent is clear, maximum 4 L for age older than 6 mo.

UNAPPROVED ADULT – Chronic constipation: 125 to 500 mL/day PO daily (up to two times per day). Whole bowel irrigation in iron overdose: 1500 to 2000 mL/h.

UNAPPROVED PEDS – Bowel cleansing prior to GI examination: 25 to 40 mL/kg/h PO/NG for 4 to 10 h or until rectal effluent is clear or 20 to 30 mL/min NG until 4 L are consumed or rectal effluent is clear. Whole bowel irrigation in iron overdose: 9 mo to 6 yo: 500 mL/h; 6 yo to 12 yo 1000 mL/h; older than 12 yo, use adult dose.

FORMS – Generic/Trade: Powder for oral solution in disposable jug 4 L or 2 L (Moviprep). Also, as a kit of 2 L bottle of polyethylene glycol with electrolytes and 2 or 4 bisacodyl tabs 5 mg (HalfLytely and Bisacodyl Tablet Kit). Trade only (GoLYTELY): Packet for oral solution to make 3.785 L.

NOTES – Solid food should not be given within 2 h of soln. Effects should occur within 1 to 2 h. Chilling improves palatability.

SODIUM PHOSPHATE (***Fleet enema, Fleet Phospho-Soda, Fleet EZ-Prep, Accu-Prep, Osmoprep, Visicol, ♣ Enemol, Phoslax***) ▸Not absorbed ♀C ◗? $

WARNING – Phosphate-containing bowel cleansing regimens have been reported to cause acute phosphate nephropathy. Risk factors include advanced age, kidney disease or decreased intravascular volume, bowel obstruction or active colitis, and medications that affect renal perfusion or function such as diuretics, ACE inhibitors, ARBs, and maybe NSAIDs. Use extreme caution in bowel cleansing.

ADULT – 1 adult or pediatric enema PR or 20 to 30 mL of oral soln PO prn (max 45 mL/24 h). Visicol: Evening before colonoscopy: 3 tabs with 8 oz clear liquid q 15 min until 20 tabs are consumed. Day of colonoscopy: Starting 3 to 5 h before procedure, 3 tabs with 8 oz clear liquid q 15 min until 20 tabs are consumed.

PEDS – Laxative: 2 to 11 yo: one pediatric enema (67.5 mL) PR prn; 5 to 9 yo: 5 mL of oral soln PO prn; 10 to 12 yo: 10 mL of oral soln PO prn.

UNAPPROVED ADULT – Visicol: Evening before colonoscopy: 3 tabs with 8 oz clear liquid q 15 min until 20 tabs are consumed. Day of colonoscopy: Starting 3 to 5 h before procedure, 3 tabs with 8 oz clear liquid q 15 min until 8 to 12 tabs are consumed.

FORMS – OTC Generic/Trade: Adult enema, oral soln. OTC Trade only: Pediatric enema, bowel prep. Rx Trade only: Visicol, Osmoprep tab ($$$$) 1.5 g.

NOTES – Taking the last 2 doses of Visicol with ginger ale appears to minimize residue. Excessive doses (more than 45 mL/24 h) of oral products may lead to serious electrolyte disturbances. Use with caution in severe renal impairment.

SORBITOL ▸Not absorbed ♀C ◗? $

ADULT – Laxative: 30 to 150 mL (of 70% soln) PO or 120 mL (of 25 to 30% soln) PR. Cathartic: 4.3 mL/kg PO.

PEDS – Laxative: Children 2 to 11 yo: 2 mL/kg (of 70% soln) PO or 30 to 60 mL (of 25 to 30% soln) PR.

UNAPPROVED PEDS – Cathartic: 4.3 mL/kg of 35% soln (diluted from 70% soln) PO single dose.

FORMS – Generic only: Soln 70%.

NOTES – When used as a cathartic, can be given with activated charcoal to improve taste and decrease gastric transit time of charcoal. May precipitate electrolyte changes.

SUPREP **(sodium sulfate + potassium sulfate + magnesium sulfate)** ▸not absorbed ♀C ◗? $

ADULT – Evening before colonoscopy: Dilute 1 bottle to 16 oz with water and drink, then drink 32 oz water over next h. Next morning, repeat both steps. Complete 1 h before colonoscopy.

PEDS – Not approved in children.

FORMS – Trade: Two 6 oz bottles for dilution.

GASTROENTEROLOGY: Laxatives—Other or Combinations

LUBIPROSTONE (*Amitiza*) ▸Gut ♀C ◗? $$$$$

WARNING – Avoid if symptoms or history of mechanical GI obstruction.

ADULT – Chronic idiopathic constipation: 24 mcg PO two times per day with food and water. Irritable bowel syndrome with constipation in age 18 yo or older: 8 mcg PO two times per day.

PEDS – Not approved in children.

FORMS – Trade only: Cap 8, 24 mcg.

NOTES – Reduce dose with moderate to severe hepatic dysfunction.

MINERAL OIL (***Kondremul, Fleet Mineral Oil Enema, Liqui-Doss,*** ✤ ***Lansoyl***) ▶Not absorbed ♀C ▶? $
ADULT – Laxative: 15 to 45 mL PO in a single dose or in divided doses, 60 to 150 mL PR.
PEDS – Laxative: Children 6 to 11 yo: 5 to 15 mL PO in a single dose or in divided doses. Children 2 to 11 yo: 30 to 60 mL PR.
FORMS – OTC Generic/Trade: Oil (30, 480 mL), Enema (Fleet). OTC Trade only: Oral liquid (Liqui-Doss) 13.5 mg/15 mL. Oral microemulsion (Kondremul) 2.5 mg/5 mL.
NOTES – Use with caution in children younger than 4 yo and elderly or debilitated patients due to concerns for aspiration pneumonitis. Although usual directions for plain mineral oil are to administer at bedtime, this increases risk of lipid pneumonitis. Mineral oil emulsions may be administered with meals.

PERI-COLACE **(docusate + sennosides)** ▶L ♀C ▶? $
ADULT – Constipation: 2 to 4 tabs PO once daily or in divided doses prn.
PEDS – Constipation 6 to 12 yo: 1 to 2 tabs PO daily prn. 2 to 6 yo: Up to 1 tab PO daily prn.
FORMS – OTC Generic/Trade: Tabs 50 mg docusate + 8.6 mg sennosides.
NOTES – Chronic use of stimulant laxatives (casanthranol) may be habit forming.

SENOKOT-S **(senna + docusate)** ▶L ♀C ▶+ $
ADULT – 2 tabs PO daily, maximum 4 tabs two times per day.
PEDS – 6 to 12 yo: 1 tab PO daily, max 2 tabs two times per day. 2 to 6 yo: ½ tab PO daily, max 1 tab two times per day.
FORMS – OTC Generic/Trade: Tabs 8.6 mg senna concentrate + 50 mg docusate.
NOTES – Effects occur 6 to 12 h after oral administration. Use caution in renal dysfunction. Chronic use of stimulant laxatives may be habit forming.

GASTROENTEROLOGY: Laxatives—Stimulant

BISACODYL (***Correctol, Dulcolax, Feen-a-Mint, Fleet***) ▶L ♀C ▶? $
ADULT – Constipation/colonic evacuation prior to a procedure: 5 to 15 mg PO daily prn, 10 mg PR daily prn.
PEDS – Constipation/colonic evacuation prior to a procedure: 0.3 mg/kg/day PO daily prn. Children younger than 2 yo, 5 mg PR prn; 2 to 11 yo, 5 to 10 mg PO or PR prn; 12 yo or older: 10 mg PO or PR prn.
FORMS – OTC Generic/Trade: Tabs 5 mg, suppository 10 mg. OTC Trade only (Fleet): Enema, 10 mg/30 mL.
NOTES – Oral tab has onset of 6 to 10 h. Onset of action of suppository is approximately 15 to 60 min. Do not chew tabs, swallow whole. Do not give within 1 h of antacids or dairy products. Chronic use of stimulant laxatives may be habit forming.

CASCARA ▶L ♀C ▶+ $
ADULT – Constipation: 325 mg PO at bedtime prn or 5 mL/day of aromatic fluid extract PO at bedtime prn.
PEDS – Constipation: Infants: 1.25 mL/day of aromatic fluid extract PO daily prn. Children 2 to 11 yo: 2.5 mL/day of aromatic fluid extract PO daily prn.
FORMS – OTC Generic only: Tabs 325 mg, liquid aromatic fluid extract.
NOTES – Cascara sagrada fluid extract is 5 times more potent than cascara sagrada aromatic fluid extract. Chronic use of stimulant laxatives may be habit forming.

CASTOR OIL ▶Not absorbed ♀– ▶? $
ADULT – Constipation: 15 to 60 mL PO daily prn. Colonic evacuation prior to procedure: 15 to 60 mL of castor oil or 30 to 60 mL emulsified castor oil PO as a single dose 16 h prior to procedure.
PEDS – Colonic evacuation prior to procedure: 1 to 5 mL of castor oil or 2.5 to 7.5 mL emulsified castor oil PO as a single dose 16 h prior to procedure for age younger than 2 yo. 5 to 15 mL of castor oil or 7.5 to 30 mL of emulsified castor oil PO as a single dose 16 h prior to procedure for age 2 to 11 yo.
FORMS – OTC Generic only: Oil 60, 120, 180, 480 mL.
NOTES – Emulsions somewhat mask the bad taste. Onset of action approximately 2 to 6 h. Do not give at bedtime. Chill or administer with juice to improve taste.

SENNA (***Senokot, SenokotXTRA, Ex-Lax, Fletcher's Castoria,*** ✤ ***Glysennid***) ▶L ♀C ▶+ $
ADULT – Laxative or evacuation of the colon for bowel or rectal examinations: 1 teaspoon granules in water or 10 to 15 mL or 2 tabs PO at bedtime. Max daily dose 4 tsp of granules, 30 mL of syrup or 8 tabs.
PEDS – Laxative: 10 to 20 mg/kg/dose PO at bedtime. Alternative regimen: 1 mo to 2 yo: 1.25 to 2.5 mL syrup PO at bedtime, max 5 mL/day; 2 to 5 yo: 2.5 to 3.75 mL syrup PO at bedtime, max 7.5 mL/day; 6 to 12 yo: 5 to 7.5 mL syrup PO at bedtime, max 15 mL/day.

(cont.)

SENNA (*cont.*)

FORMS – OTC Generic/Trade (All dosing is based on sennosides content; 1 mg sennosides is equivalent to 21.7 mg standardized senna concentrate): Syrup 8.8 mg/5 mL, Liquid 33.3 mg senna concentrate/mL (Fletcher's Castoria), Tabs 8.6, 15, 17, 25 mg, Chewable tabs 10, 15 mg.

NOTES – Effects occur 6 to 24 h after oral administration. Use caution in renal dysfunction. Chronic use of stimulant laxatives may be habit forming.

GASTROENTEROLOGY: Laxatives—Stool Softener

DOCUSATE (***Colace, Surfak, Kaopectate Stool Softener, Enemeez***) ▸L ♀C ▸? $

ADULT – Constipation: Docusate calcium: 240 mg PO daily. Docusate sodium: 50 to 500 mg/day PO in 1 to 4 divided doses.

PEDS – Constipation: Docusate sodium: 10 to 40 mg/day for age younger than 3 yo, 20 to 60 mg/day for age 3 to 6 yo, 40 to 150 mg/day for age 6 to 12 yo. In all cases doses are divided up to four times per day.

UNAPPROVED ADULT – Docusate sodium, Constipation: Can be given as a retention enema: Mix 50 to 100 mg docusate liquid with saline or water retention enema for rectal use. Cerumen removal: Instill 1 mL liquid (not syrup) in affected ear; allow to remain for 10 to 15 min, then irrigate with 50 mL lukewarm NS if necessary.

UNAPPROVED PEDS – Docusate sodium: Cerumen removal: Instill 1 mL liquid (not syrup) in affected ear; allow to remain for 10 to 15 min, then irrigate with 50 mL lukewarm NS if necessary.

FORMS – Docusate calcium OTC Generic/Trade: Caps 240 mg. Docusate sodium OTC Generic/Trade: Caps 50, 100, 250 mg. Liquid 50 mg/5 mL. Syrup 20 mg/5 mL. Docusate sodium OTC Trade only (Enemeez): Enema, rectal 283 mg/5 mL.

NOTES – Takes 1 to 3 days to notably soften stools.

GASTROENTEROLOGY: Ulcerative Colitis

BALSALAZIDE (***Colazal, Giazo***) ▸Minimal absorption ♀B ▸? $$$$$

ADULT – Ulcerative colitis: 2.25 g PO three times per day (Colazal) for 8 to 12 weeks or 1.1 g PO twice per day (Giazo) for 8 weeks.

PEDS – 5 to 17 yo (Colazal): Mild to moderately active ulcerative colitis: 2.25 g PO three times per day for 8 weeks. Alternatively, 750 mg PO three times per day for 8 weeks.

FORMS – Generic/Trade (Colazal): Caps 750 mg. Trade (Giazo): Tabs 1.1 g.

NOTES – Contraindicated in salicylate allergy. Caution with renal insufficiency.

MESALAMINE (**5-aminosalicylic acid,** ***Apriso, 5-Aspirin, Asacol, Lialda, Pentasa, Canasa, Rowasa,*** ♣***Mesasal, Salofalk, Mezavant***) ▸Gut ♀C ▸? $$$$$

ADULT – Ulcerative colitis: Asacol: 800 to 1600 mg PO three times per day. Pentasa: 1 g PO four times per day. Lialda: 2.4 to 4.8 g PO daily with a meal for 8 weeks. Rectal susp: 4 g (60 mL) PR retained for 8 h at bedtime. Asacol: maintenance of remissiopn of ulcerative colitis: 1600 mg/day PO in divided doses. Apriso: 1.5 g (4 caps) PO q am. Lialda: 2.4 g PO daily. Ulcerative proctitis: Canasa suppository: 500 mg PR two to three times per day or 1000 mg PR at bedtime.

PEDS – Not approved in children.

UNAPPROVED ADULT – Active Crohn's: 0.4 to 4.8 g/day PO in divided doses. Maintenance of remission of Crohn's: 2.4 g/day in divided doses.

UNAPPROVED PEDS – Tabs: 50 mg/kg/day PO divided q 8 to 12 h. Caps: 50 mg/kg/day PO divided q 6 to 12 h.

FORMS – Trade only: Delayed-release tab 400 mg (Asacol), 800 mg (Asacol HD). Controlled-release cap 250, 500 mg (Pentasa). Delayed-release tab 1200 mg (Lialda). Rectal suppository 1000 mg (Canasa). Controlled-release cap 0.375 g (Apriso). Generic/Trade: Rectal susp 4 g/60 mL (Rowasa).

NOTES – Avoid in salicylate sensitivity or hepatic dysfunction. Reports of hepatic failure in patients with preexisting liver disease. May decrease digoxin levels. May discolor urine yellow-brown. Most common adverse effects include headache, abdominal pain, fever, rash. The coating of Asacol and Asacol HD contain the inactive chemical, dibutyl phthalate (DBP) In animal studies at doses more than 190 times the human dose, maternal DBP was associated with external and skeletal malformations and adverse effects on the male reproductive system.

OLSALAZINE (***Dipentum***) ▶L ♀C ▶– $$$$$

ADULT – Maintenance of remission of ulcerative colitis in patients intolerant to sulfasalazine: 500 mg PO two times per day with food.

PEDS – Not approved in children.

UNAPPROVED ADULT – Crohn's: 1.5 to 3 g/day PO in divided doses with food.

FORMS – Trade only: Caps 250 mg.

NOTES – Diarrhea in up to 17%. Avoid in salicylate sensitivity.

SULFASALAZINE (***Azulfidine, Azulfidine EN-tabs, ✤ Salazopyrin En-tabs***) ▶L ♀D ▶– $$

WARNING – Beware of hypersensitivity, marrow suppression, renal and liver damage, central nervous system effects, irreversible neuromuscular and CNS changes, fibrosing alveolitis.

ADULT – Ulcerative colitis: Initially 500 to 1000 mg PO four times per day. Maintenance: 500 mg PO four times per day. RA: 500 mg PO two times per day after meals to start. Increase to 1 g PO two times per day.

PEDS – JRA: initially 10 mg/kg/day and increase to 30 to 50 mg/kg/day (EN-tabs) PO divided two times per day to max of 2 g/day for age 6 yo or older. Ulcerative colitis: Initially 30 to 60 mg/kg/day PO divided into 3 to 6 doses for age older than 2 yo. Maximum 75 mg/kg/day. Maintenance: 30 to 50 mg/kg/day PO divided q 4 to 8 h, max 2 g/day.

UNAPPROVED ADULT – Ankylosing spondylitis: 1 to 1.5 g PO two times per day. Psoriasis: 1.5 to 2 g PO two times per day. Psoriatic arthritis: 1 g PO two times per day.

FORMS – Generic/Trade: Tabs 500 mg, scored. Enteric-coated, delayed-release (EN-tabs) 500 mg.

NOTES – Contraindicated in children younger than 2 yo. Avoid with hepatic or renal dysfunction, intestinal or urinary obstruction, porphyria, sulfonamide, or salicylate sensitivity. Monitor CBC q 2 to 4 weeks for 3 months then q 3 months. Monitor LFTs and renal function. Oligospermia and infertility, and photosensitivity may occur. May decrease folic acid, digoxin, cyclosporine, and iron levels. May turn body fluids, contact lenses, or skin orange-yellow. Enteric-coated (Azulfidine EN, Salazopyrin EN) tabs may cause fewer GI adverse effects. Pregnancy category B, except D at term.

GASTROENTEROLOGY: Other GI Agents

ALOSETRON (***Lotronex***) ▶L ♀B ▶? $$$$$

WARNING – Can cause severe constipation and ischemic colitis. Concomitant use with fluvoxamine, a potent CYP1A2 inhibitor, is contraindicated. Use caution with moderate CYP1A2 inhibitors such as quinolone antibiotics and cimetidine. Use caution with strong inhibitors of CYP3A4 such as ketoconazole, clarithromycin, protease inhibitors, voriconazole, and itraconazole. Can be prescribed only by drug company–authorized clinicians using special sticker and written informed consent.

ADULT – Diarrhea-predominant irritable bowel syndrome in women who have failed conventional therapy: 0.5 mg PO twice a day for 4 weeks; discontinue in patients who become constipated. If well tolerated and symptoms not controlled after 4 weeks, may increase to 1 mg PO two times per day. Discontinue if symptoms not controlled in 4 weeks on 1 mg PO two times per day.

PEDS – Not approved in children.

FORMS – Trade only: Tabs 0.5, 1 mg.

NOTES – Specific medication guide must be distributed with prescriptions.

ALPHA-GALACTOSIDASE (***Beano***) ▶Minimal absorption ♀? ▶? $

ADULT – 5 gtts or 1 tab per ½ cup gassy food, 2 to 3 tabs PO (chew, swallow, or crumble) or 1 melt-away tab or 10 to 15 gtts per typical meal.

PEDS – Not approved in age younger than 12 yo.

FORMS – OTC Trade only: Oral gtts, tabs, melt-away tabs.

NOTES – Beano produces 2 to 6 g of carbohydrates for every 100 g of food treated by Beano; may increase glucose levels.

ALVIMOPAN (***Entereg***) ▶Intestinal flora ♀B ▶? ?

ADULT – Short-term (up to 15 doses) in hospitalized patients undergoing partial large or small bowel resection surgery with primary anastomosis: 12 mg PO 30 min to 5 h prior to surgery, then 12 mg PO two times per day starting the day after surgery for up to 7 days.

PEDS – Not approved in children.

FORMS – Trade only: Caps 12 mg.

NOTES – Only available to hospitals who are authorized to use the medication (requires hospital DEA number to be dispensed). Contraindicated in patients who have taken therapeutic doses of opioids for more than 7 consecutive days. Serum concentrations in patients of Japanese descent may be up to 2-fold greater than Caucasian subjects with same dose. Monitor Japanese patients for adverse events.

BUDESONIDE (*Entocort EC*) ▸L ♀C ▸? $$$$$

ADULT – Mild to moderate Crohn's, induction of remission: 9 mg PO daily for up to 8 weeks. May repeat 8-week course for recurring episodes. Maintenance: 6 mg PO daily for 3 months.

PEDS – Not approved in children.

UNAPPROVED PEDS – Mild to moderate Crohn's: 0.45 mg/kg up to 9 mg PO daily for 8 to 12 weeks for age 9 yo or older.

FORMS – Trade only: Caps 3 mg.

NOTES – May taper dose to 6 mg for 2 weeks prior to discontinuation.

CERTOLIZUMAB (*Cimzia*) ▸Plasma, K ♀B ▸? $$$$$

WARNING – Increased risk of serious infections leading to hospitalization or death including tuberculosis (TB), bacterial sepsis, invasive fungal infections (such as histoplasmosis), and infections due to other opportunistic pathogens.

ADULT – Crohn's: 400 mg SC at 0, 2, and 4 weeks. If response occurs, then 400 mg SC q 4 weeks. Rheumatoid arthritis: 400 mg SC at 0, 2, and 4 weeks. Maintenance of RA: 200 mg SC every other week or 400 mg SC q 4 weeks.

PEDS – Not approved in children.

FORMS – Trade only: 400 mg kit.

NOTES – Monitor patients for signs and symptoms of TB and other infections.

CHLORDIAZEPOXIDE—CLIDINIUM ▸K ♀D ▸– $$$

ADULT – Irritable bowel syndrome: 1 cap PO three to four times per day.

PEDS – Not approved in children.

FORMS – Generic: Caps, chlordiazepoxide 5 mg + clidinium 2.5 mg.

NOTES – May cause drowsiness. After prolonged use, gradually taper to avoid withdrawal symptoms. Contains ingredients formerly contained in Librax.

CISAPRIDE (*Propulsid*) ▸LK ♀C ▸? From manufacturer only

WARNING – Available only through limited-access protocol through manufacturer. Can cause potentially fatal cardiac arrhythmias. Many drug and disease interactions.

ADULT – 10 mg PO four times per day, at least 15 min before meals and at bedtime. Some patients may require 20 mg PO four times per day. Max 80 mg/day.

PEDS – Not approved in children.

UNAPPROVED PEDS – GERD: 0.15 mg/kg/dose PO three to four times per day. Max 0.8 mg/kg/day for neonates, 10 mg/dose for infants and children.

FORMS – Trade only: Tabs 10, 20 mg, Susp 1 mg/1 mL.

GLYCOPYRROLATE (*Robinul, Robinul Forte, Cuvposa*) ▸K ♀B ▸? $$$$

ADULT – Peptic ulcer disease: 1 to 2 mg PO two to three times per day. Preop/intraoperative respiratory antisecretory: 0.1 mg IV/IM prn.

PEDS – Chronic drooling in children 3 to 16 yo (Cuvposa): 0.02 mg/kg three times per day, 1 h before or 2 h after meals. Increase by 0.02 mg/kg q 5 to 7 days.

UNAPPROVED ADULT – Drooling: 0.1 mg/kg PO two to three times per day, max 8 mg/day.

FORMS – Trade: Solution 1 mg/5 mL (480 mL, Cuvposa). Generic/Trade: Tabs 1, 2 mg.

NOTES – Contraindicated in glaucoma, obstructive uropathy, paralytic ileus or GI obstruction, myasthenia gravis, severe ulcerative colitis, toxic megacolon, and unstable cardiovascular status in acute hemorrhage.

LACTASE (*Lactaid*) ▸Not absorbed ♀+ ▸+ $

ADULT – Swallow or chew 3 tabs/caps (Original-strength), 2 tabs/caps (Extra-strength), 1 caplet (Ultra) with first bite of dairy foods. Adjust dose based on response.

PEDS – Titrate dose based on response.

FORMS – OTC Generic/Trade: Caplets, Chewable tabs.

METHYLNALTREXONE (*Relistor*) ▸unchanged ♀B ▸? $$$$$

ADULT – Opioid-induced constipation in patients with advanced illness who are receiving palliative care, when response to laxative therapy has not been sufficient: For wt less than 38 kg: 0.15 mg/kg SC every other day; wt 38 kg to 61 kg: 8 mg SC every other day; wt 62 kg to 114 kg: 12 mg SC every other day: wt 115 kg or greater: 0.15 mg/kg SC every other day.

PEDS – Not approved in children.

FORMS – Injectable soln 12 mg/0.6 mL.

NOTES – Do not use with GI obstruction or lesions of GI tract. Usual dose every other day, but no more frequently than once daily.

NEOMYCIN—ORAL (*Neo-Fradin*) ▸Minimally absorbed ♀D ▸? $$$

ADULT – Suppression of intestinal bacteria (given with erythromycin): 1 g PO at 19 h, 18 h, and 9 h prior to procedure (ie, 1 pm, 2 pm, 11 pm on prior day). Alternative regimen 1 g PO q 1 h for 4 doses then 1 g PO q 4 h for 5 doses. Hepatic encephalopathy: 4 to 12 g/day PO divided q 4 to 6 h for 5 to 6 days. Diarrhea caused by enteropathogenic *E. coli:* 3 g/day PO divided q 6 h.

PEDS – Suppression of intestinal bacteria (given with erythromycin): 25 mg/kg PO at 19 h, 18 h, and 9 h prior to procedure (ie, 1 pm, 2 pm, 11 pm on prior day). Alternative

(cont.)

NEOMYCIN—ORAL (*cont.*)

regimen: 90 mg/kg/day PO divided q 4 h for 2 days. Hepatic encephalopathy: 50 to 100 mg/kg/day PO divided q 6 to 8 h for 5 to 6 days. Diarrhea caused by enteropathogenic *E. coli:* 50 mg/kg/day PO divided q 6 h for 2 to 3 days.

FORMS – Generic only: Tabs 500 mg. Trade only: Soln 125 mg/5 mL.

NOTES – Increased INR with warfarin, decreased levels of digoxin, methotrexate.

OCTREOTIDE (***Sandostatin, Sandostatin LAR***) ▶LK ♀B ▶? $$$$$

ADULT – Diarrhea associated with carcinoid tumors: 100 to 600 mcg/day SC/IV in 2 to 4 divided doses for 2 weeks or 20 mg IM (Sandostatin LAR) q 4 weeks for 2 months. Adjust dose based on response. Diarrhea associated with vasoactive intestinal peptide-secreting tumors: 200 to 300 mcg/day SC/IV in 2 to 4 divided doses for 2 weeks or 20 mg IM (Sandostatin LAR) q 4 weeks for 2 months. Adjust dose based on response.

PEDS – Not approved in children.

UNAPPROVED ADULT – Variceal bleeding: Bolus 25 to 50 mcg IV followed by 25 to 50 mcg/h continuous IV infusion. AIDS diarrhea: 25 to 250 mcg SC three times per day, max 500 mcg SC q 8 h. Irritable bowel syndrome: 100 mcg as a single dose to 125 mcg SC two times per day. GI and pancreatic fistulas: 50 to 200 mcg SC/IV q 8 h.

UNAPPROVED PEDS – Diarrhea: Initially 1 to 10 mcg/kg SC/IV q 12 h. Congenital hyperinsulinism: 1 to 40 mcg/kg SC daily. Hypothalamic obesity in children 6 to 17 yo: 40 mg IM q 4 weeks (Sandostatin LAR) or 5 to 15 mcg/kg SC daily.

FORMS – Generic/Trade: Injection vials 0.05, 0.1, 0.2, 0.5, 1 mg. Trade only: Long-acting injectable susp (Sandostatin LAR) 10, 20, 30 mg.

NOTES – For the treatment of variceal bleeding, most studies treat for 3 to 5 days. Individualize dose based on response. Dosage reduction often necessary in elderly. May cause hypoglycemia, hyperglycemia; caution especially in diabetes. May cause hypothyroidism, cardiac arrhythmias. Increases bioavailability of bromocriptine. Sandostatin LAR only indicated for patients who are stabilized on Sandostatin.

ORLISTAT (***Alli, Xenical***) ▶Gut ♀X ▶? $$$

ADULT – Weight loss and wt management: 60 mg to 120 mg PO three times per day with meals or up to 1 h after meals.

PEDS – Children 12 to 16 yo: 60 mg to 120 mg PO three times per day with meals. Not approved in age younger than 12 yo.

FORMS – OTC Trade only (Alli): Caps 60 mg. Rx Trade only (Xenical): Caps 120 mg.

NOTES – May cause fatty stools, fecal urgency, flatus with discharge, and oily spotting in more than 20% of patients. GI adverse effects greater when taken with high-fat diet. Has been associated with liver damage and increased urinary oxylate levels. Can reduce the effect of levothyroxine or increase the effects of warfarin. Administer orlistat and levothyroxine at least 4 h apart. Administer cyclosporine 3 h after orlistat.

PANCREATIN (***Creon, Ku-Zyme, ✤Entozyme***) ▶Gut ♀C ▶? $$$

ADULT – Enzyme replacement (initial dose): 8000 to 24,000 units lipase (1 to 2 caps/tabs) PO with meals and snacks.

PEDS – Enzyme replacement (initial dose): 2000 units lipase PO with meals for age younger than 1 yo, 4000 to 8000 units lipase PO with meals or 4000 units lipase with snacks for age 1 to 6 yo, 4000 to 12,000 units lipase PO with meals and snacks for age 7 to 12 yo.

FORMS – Tabs, Caps with varying amounts of lipase, amylase, and protease.

NOTES – Titrate dose to stool fat content. Products are not interchangeable. Avoid concomitant calcium carbonate and magnesium hydroxide since these may affect the enteric coating. Do not crush/chew microspheres or tabs. Possible association of colonic strictures and high doses of lipase (greater than 16,000 units/kg/meal) in pediatric patients.

PANCRELIPASE (***Creon, Pancreaze, Viokase, Pancrease, Pancrecarb, Cotazym, Ku-Zyme HP, Ultressa, Viokace, Zenpep***) ▶Gut ♀C ▶? $$$

ADULT – Enzyme replacement (initial dose): 500 lipase units/kg per meal, max 2500 lipase units/kg per meal.

PEDS – Enzyme replacement (initial dose, varies by wt): Infants (up to 12 mo): 2000 to 4000 lipase units per 120 mL of formula or per breastfeeding. 12 mo or older to younger than 4 yo: 1000 lipase units/kg, max 2500 lipase units/kg per meal. 4 yo or older: 500 lipase units/kg per meal, max 2500 lipase units/kg per meal.

FORMS – Tabs, Caps, Powder with varying amounts of lipase, amylase, and protease.

NOTES – Titrate dose to stool fat content. Products are not interchangeable. Avoid concomitant calcium carbonate and magnesium hydroxide since these may affect the enteric coating. Do not crush/chew. Possible association of colonic strictures and high doses of lipase (greater than 16,000 units/kg/meal) in pediatric patients.

♣PINAVERIUM ▶? ♀C ▶– $$$
ADULT – Canada only. Irritable bowel syndrome: 50 mg PO three times per day, may increase to maximum of 100 mg three times per day.
PEDS – Not for children.
FORMS – Trade only: tabs 50, 100 mg.
NOTES – Take with a full glass of water during meal or snack.

RECTIV (*nitroglycerin*) ▶L – ♀C ▶? $$$$$
ADULT – Chronic anal fisures: Apply 1 inch intra-anally q 12 for up to 3 weeks.
PEDS – Not approved in children younger than 18 yo.
FORMS – Ointment 0.4% 30 g.
NOTES – Use within 8 weeks of opening. Do not use with PDE5 inhibitors.

SECRETIN (*SecreFlo, ChiRhoStim*) ▶Serum ♀C ▶? $$$$$
ADULT – Stimulation of pancreatic secretions, to aid in diagnosis of exocrine pancreas dysfunction: Test dose 0.2 mcg IV. If tolerated, 0.2 mcg/kg IV over 1 min. Stimulation of gastrin to aid in diagnosis of gastrinoma: Test dose 0.2 mcg IV. If tolerated, 0.4 mcg/kg IV over 1 min. Identification of ampulla of Vater and accessory papilla during ERCP: 0.2 mcg/kg IV over 1 min.
PEDS – Not approved in children.
UNAPPROVED PEDS – Has been used in autism.
NOTES – Previously known as SecreFlo. Contraindicated in acute pancreatitis.

TEGASEROD (*Zelnorm*) ▶stomach/L ♀B ▶? Free (investigational)
WARNING – Restricted (investigational) use; contact manufacturer to obtain. Severe diarrhea leading to hypovolemia, hypotension, and syncope has been reported, as has ischemic colitis and other forms of intestinal ischemia; discontinue immediately if symptoms occur.
ADULT – Constipation-predominant irritable bowel syndrome in women younger than the age of 55 yo: 6 mg PO two times per day before meals for 4 to 6 weeks. May repeat for an additional 4 to 6 weeks.
PEDS – Not approved in children.
FORMS – Restricted use only. Trade only: Tabs 2, 6 mg.

URSODIOL (*Actigall, URSO, URSO Forte*) ▶Bile ♀B ▶? $$$$
ADULT – Radiolucent gallstone dissolution (Actigall): 8 to 10 mg/kg/day PO divided in 2 to 3 doses. Prevention of gallstones associated with rapid wt loss (Actigall): 300 mg PO two times per day. Primary biliary cirrhosis (URSO): 13 to 15 mg/kg/day PO divided in 2 to 4 doses.
PEDS – Not approved in children.
UNAPPROVED ADULT – Cholestasis of pregnancy: 300 to 600 mg PO two times per day.
UNAPPROVED PEDS – Biliary atresia: 10 to 15 mg/kg/day PO once daily. Cystic fibrosis with liver disease: 15 to 30 mg/kg/day PO divided two times per day. TPN-induced cholestasis: 30 mg/kg/day PO divided three times per day.
FORMS – Generic/Trade: Caps 300 mg, Tabs 250, 500 mg.
NOTES – Gallstone dissolution requires months of therapy. Complete dissolution does not occur in all patients and 5-year recurrence up to 50%. Does not dissolve calcified cholesterol stones, radiopaque stones, or radiolucent bile pigment stones. Avoid concomitant antacids, cholestyramine, colestipol, estrogen, oral contraceptives.

HEMATOLOGY: Anticoagulants—Direct Thrombin Inhibitors

ARGATROBAN ▶L ♀B ▶– $$$$$
ADULT – Prevention/treatment of thrombosis in HIT: Start 2 mcg/kg/min IV infusion. Get PTT at baseline and 2 h after starting infusion. Adjust dose (up to 10 mcg/kg/min) until PTT is 1.5 to 3 times baseline (but not more than 100 sec). Percutaneous coronary intervention in those with or at risk for HIT: Bolus 350 mcg/kg IV over 3 to 5 min then 25 mcg/kg/min infusion. Target activated clotting time (ACT): 300 to 450 sec. If ACT is less than 300 sec, give 150 mcg/kg bolus and increase infusion rate to 30 mcg/kg/min. If ACT is more than 450 sec, reduce infusion rate to 15 mcg/kg/min. Maintain ACT 300 to 450 sec for the duration of the procedure.
PEDS – Not approved in children.
NOTES – ACCP recommends starting max of 2 mcg/kg/min with lower doses of 0.5 to 1.2 mcg/kg/min in patients with heart failure, multiorgan failure, anasarca, or postcardiac surgery. Argatroban prolongs INR with warfarin; discontinue when INR is greater than 4 on combined therapy, recheck INR in 4 to 6 h and restart argatroban if INR subtherapeutic. Dosage reduction recommended in liver dysfunction.

BIVALIRUDIN (*Angiomax*) ▶proteolysis/K ♀B ▶? $$$$$
ADULT – Anticoagulation in patients undergoing PCI (including patients with or at risk of HIT or HIT and thrombosis syndrome): 0.75 mg/kg IV bolus prior to intervention, then 1.75 mg/kg/h for duration of procedure (with provisional

(cont.)

BIVALIRUDIN (*cont.*)

Gp IIb/IIIa inhibition) and optionally up to 4 h postprocedure. For CrCl less than 30 mL/min, reduce infusion dose to 1 mg/kg/h after bolus. For patients on dialysis, reduce infusion dose to 0.25 mg/kg/h after bolus. Use with aspirin 300 to 325 mg PO daily. Additional bolus of 0.3 mg/kg if activated clotting time is less than 225 sec. Can additionally infuse 0.2 mg/kg/h for up to 20 h more.

PEDS – Not approved in children.

UNAPPROVED ADULT – Acute coronary syndrome (with or without Gp IIb/IIIa inhibition): 0.1 mg/kg bolus followed by 0.25 mg/kg/h. If PCI, then additional bolus 0.5 mg/kg then 1.75 mg/kg/h. Use with aspirin.

NOTES – Contraindicated in active major bleeding. Monitor activated clotting time. Former trade name Hirulog.

DABIGATRAN (***Pradaxa, ♣ Pradax***) ▶K ♀C ▶? $$$$$

ADULT – Stroke prevention in atrial fibrillation: CrCl greater than 30 mL/min with no interactive medications: 150 mg PO two times per day; CrCL between 30 and 50 mL/min with P-glycoprotein inhibitors (dronedarone and ketoconazole) or CrCL between 15 and 30 mL/min without interactive agents: 75 mg PO two times per day; CrCl less than 15 mL/min or CrCl between 15 and 30 mL/min with P-glycoprotein: contraindicated. Per ACCP CHEST guidelines, not recommended if CrCl is less than 30 mL/min.

PEDS – Not approved in children.

UNAPPROVED ADULT – VTE prevention in knee replacement: Start 110 mg for one dose given 1 to 4 h after surgery or start 220 mg once if started on postop day 1, then 220 mg daily for 10 days. VTE prevention in hip replacement: 110 mg for one dose given 1 to 4 h after surgery or start 220 mg once if started on postop day 1, then 220 mg daily for 28 to 35 days. Start only after hemostasis has been achieved. Note: 110 mg dose not available in United States.

FORMS – Trade only: caps 75, 150 mg.

NOTES – Do not break, open, or chew capsules. Must be stored in original container and used within 4 months or discarded; protect from moisture. Check renal function at baseline and periodically to dose adjust appropriately. May cause gastritis. Avoid interruptions in therapy as this may increase risk of stroke. Avoid use with rifampin. Discontinue 1 to 2 days (if CrCl is 50 mL/min or greater) or 3 to 5 days (if CrCl is less than 50 mL/min) before invasive procedures. When transitioning from warfarin, stop warfarin and start dabigatran when INR is less than 2. When transitioning from heparin/LMWH, timing of initiation depends on renal function, see prescribing information. Serious, sometimes fatal, bleeding has been reported.

DESIRUDIN (***Iprivask***) ▶K ♀C ▶? $$$$$

WARNING – Contraindicated in active major bleeding. High risk of spinal/epidural hematoma if spinal puncture or neuraxial anesthesia before/during treatment. Risk increased by drugs that affect hemostasis including NSAIDs, antiplatelets, and other anticoagulants. Risk also increased by use of indwelling catheters, history of trauma or repeated epidural punctures, spinal deformity, or spinal surgery.

ADULT – DVT prophylaxis (hip replacement surgery): 15 mg SC q 12 h. If CrCl is 31 to 60 mL/min give 5 mg SC q 12 h; if CrCl is less than 31 mL/min give 1.7 mg SC q 12 h.

PEDS – Not approved in children.

NOTES – ACCP guidelines recommend against use if CrCl is less than 30 mL/min and against repeated use due to risk of anaphylaxis. Severe anaphylactic reactions resulting in death have been reported upon initial or reexposure.

LEPIRUDIN (***Refludan***) ▶K ♀B ▶? $$$$$

ADULT – Anticoagulation in HIT and associated thromboembolic disease: Bolus 0.4 mg/kg up to 44 mg IV over 15 to 20 sec, then infuse 0.15 mg/kg/h up to 16.5 mg/h for 2 to 10 days. Adjust dose to maintain PTT ratio of 1.5 to 2 times baseline. Adjunct to thrombolytic therapy: Bolus 0.2 mg/kg IV over 15 to 20 sec, then infuse 0.1 mg/kg/h.

PEDS – Not approved in children.

UNAPPROVED ADULT – Anticoagulation in HIT, dosing recommended by ACCP: Bolus 0.2 mg/kg IV then infuse 0.1 mg/kg/h or less. Adjust dose to maintain PTT ratio of 1.5 to 2 times baseline. Dose reduction for renal insufficiency.

NOTES – Dosing for HIT recommended by ACCP guidelines is lower than FDA-approved dosing due to higher rates of bleeding with FDA-approved dosing. Dosage adjustment for renal impairment per ACCP guidelines: Bolus 0.2 mg/kg IV (bolus only if life- or limb-threatening thrombosis) followed by 0.05 mg/kg/h for Cr 1.0 to 1.6 mg/dL, 0.01 mg/kg/h for Cr 1.7 to 4.5 mg/dL, 0.005 mg/kg/h for Cr greater than 4.5 mg/dL. Not recommended in dialysis. May increase INR. Severe anaphylactic reactions resulting in death have been reported upon initial or reexposure. Product has been discontinued by the manufacturer. Expected stock depletion in mid-2013.

HEMATOLOGY: Anticoagulants—Low Molecular Weight Heparins (LWMH)

NOTE: Contraindicated in active major bleeding. High risk of spinal/epidural hematoma if spinal puncture or neuraxial anesthesia before/during treatment [see *Reg Anesth Pain Med.* 2010;35(1):64-101]. Risk of bleeding increased by oral anticoagulants, aspirin, dipyridamole, dextran, glycoprotein IIb/IIIA inhibitors, NSAIDs (including ketorolac), ticlopidine, clopidogrel, and thrombolytics. Monitor platelets, Hb, stool for occult blood. Use caution and consider monitoring anti-Xa levels if CrCl is less than 30 mL/min, pregnancy, morbidly obese, underweight, or abnormal coagulation/bleeding. Contraindicated in patients with heparin or pork allergy, history of heparin-induced thrombocytopenia. Drug effect can be partially reversed with protamine.

DALTEPARIN (*Fragmin*) ▶KL ♀B ▶+ $$$$$

ADULT – DVT prophylaxis, acute medical illness with restricted mobility: 5000 units SC daily for 12 to 14 days. DVT prophylaxis, abdominal surgery: 2500 units SC 1 to 2 h preop and daily postop for 5 to 10 days. DVT prophylaxis, abdominal surgery in patients with malignancy: 5000 units SC evening before surgery and daily postop for 5 to 10 days. Alternatively, 2500 units SC 1 to 2 h preop and 12 h later, then 5000 units SC daily for 5 to 10 days. DVT prophylaxis, hip replacement: Give SC for up to 14 days. Preop start (day of surgery): 2500 units 2 h preop and 4 to 8 h postop, then 5000 units daily starting at least 6 h after second dose. Preop start (evening before surgery): 5000 units SC given evening before surgery then 5000 units daily starting at least 4 to 8 h postop (approximately 24 h between doses). Postop start regimen: 2500 units 4 to 8 h postop, then 5000 units daily starting at least 6 h after first dose. Treatment of DVT/PE in cancer: 200 units/kg SC daily for 1 month, then 150 units/kg SC daily for 5 months. Max 18,000 units/day, round to nearest commercially available syringe dose (if CrCl is less than 30 mL/min, target therapeutic anti-Xa level of 0.5 to 1.5

(cont.)

Enoxaparin Adult Dosing

Indication	Dose	Dosing in Renal Impairment (CrCl less than 30 mL/min)*
DVT prophylaxis		
Abdominal surgery	40 mg SC once daily	30 mg SC once daily
Knee replacement	30 mg SC q 12 h	30 mg SC once daily
Hip replacement	30 mg SC q12 h or 40 mg SC once daily	30 mg SC once daily
Medical patients	40 mg SC once daily	30 mg SC once daily
Acute DVT		
Inpatient treatment with or without PE	1 mg/kg SC q 12 h or 1.5 mg/kg SC once daily	1 mg/kg SC once daily
Outpatient treatment without PE	1 mg/kg SC q 12 h	1 mg/kg SC once daily
Acute coronary syndrome		
Unstable angina and non-Q-wave MI with aspirin	1 mg/kg SC q 12 h with aspirin	1 mg/kg SC once daily
Acute STEMI in patients age less than 75 yo with aspirin†	30 mg IV bolus with 1 mg/kg SC dose, then 1 mg/kg SC q 12 h (max 100 mg/dose for the first two doses)	30 mg IV bolus with 1 mg/kg SC dose, then 1 mg/kg SC once daily
Acute STEMI in patients age 75 yo or older with aspirin†	No IV bolus, 0.75 mg/kg SC q 12 h (max 75 mg/dose for the first two doses)	No IV bolus, 1 mg/kg SC once daily

DVT=Deep vein thrombosis, PE=pulmonary embolism.

*Not FDA-approved in dialysis.

†If used with thrombolytics, SC dose should be started between 15 min before and 30 min after thrombolytic dose.

DALTEPARIN (*cont.*)

units/mL; recheck 4 to 6 h after dose following at least 3 to 4 doses). Unstable angina or non-Q-wave MI: 120 units/kg up to 10,000 units SC q 12 h with aspirin (75 to 165 mg/day PO) until clinically stable.

PEDS – Not approved in children.

UNAPPROVED ADULT – Therapeutic anticoagulation: 200 units/kg SC daily or 100 to 120 units/kg SC two times per day. Venous thromboembolism in pregnancy. Prevention: 5000 units SC daily. Treatment: 100 units/kg SC q 12 h or 200 units/kg SC daily. To avoid unwanted anticoagulation during delivery, stop LMWH 24 h before elective induction of labor.

FORMS – Trade only: Single-dose syringes 2500, 5000 units/0.2 mL, 7500 units/0.3 mL, 10,000 units/1 mL, 12,500 units/0.5 mL, 15,000 units/0.6 mL, 18,000 units/0.72 mL; multidose vial 10,000 units/mL, 9.5 mL and 25,000 units/mL, 3.8 mL.

NOTES – Longer prophylaxis may be warranted based on individual thromboembolic risk. ACCP recommendations suggest that patients with total hip or knee replacement or hip fracture surgery receive prophylaxis for at least 10 days; consider extended prophylaxis (28 to 35 days) in hip replacement or hip fracture surgery.

ENOXAPARIN (***Lovenox***) ▶KL ♀B ▶+ $$$$$

ADULT – See table.

PEDS – Not approved in children.

UNAPPROVED ADULT – DVT prophylaxis after major trauma: 30 mg SC q 12 h starting 12 to 36 h postinjury if hemostasis achieved. DVT prophylaxis in acute spinal cord injury: 30 mg SC q 12 h. Venous thromboembolism in pregnancy: Prevention: 40 mg SC daily. Treatment: 1 mg/kg SC q 12 h. To avoid unwanted anticoagulation during delivery, stop LMWH 24 h before elective induction of labor.

UNAPPROVED PEDS – Therapeutic anticoagulation: Age younger than 2 mo: 1.5 mg/kg/dose SC q 12 h titrated to anti-Xa level of 0.5 to 1 units/mL. Age 2 mo or older: 1 mg/kg/dose SC q 12 h titrated to anti-Xa level of 0.5 to 1 units/mL. DVT prophylaxis: Age younger than 2 mo: 0.75 mg/kg/dose q 12 h. Age 2 mo or older: 0.5 mg/kg/dose q 12 h.

FORMS – Generic/Trade: Syringes 30, 40 mg; graduated syringes 60, 80, 100, 120, 150 mg. Concentration is 100 mg/mL except for 120, 150 mg, which are 150 mg/mL, All strengths also available preservative free. Trade only: Multidose vial 300 mg.

NOTES – Longer prophylaxis may be warranted based on individual thromboembolic risk. ACCP recommendations suggest that patients with total hip or knee replacement or hip fracture surgery receive prophylaxis for at least 10 days; consider extended prophylaxis (28 to 35 days) in hip replacement or hip fracture surgery. In PCI, if last enoxaparin administration was more than 8 h before balloon inflation, give 0.3 mg/kg IV bolus. Use caution in mechanical heart valves, especially in pregnancy; reports of valve thrombosis (maternal and fetal deaths reported). Congenital anomalies linked to enoxaparin use during pregnancy; causality unclear. Multidose formulation contains benzyl alcohol, which can cause hypersensitivity and cross placenta in pregnancy.

HEMATOLOGY: Anticoagulants—Other

HEPARIN ▶Reticuloendothelial system ♀C but + ▶+ $$

ADULT – Venous thrombosis/pulmonary embolus treatment: Load 80 units/kg IV, then initiate infusion at 18 units/kg/h. Adjust based on coagulation testing (PTT)—see Table. DVT prophylaxis: 5000 units SC q 8 to 12 h. Prevention of thromboembolism in pregnancy: 5000 to 10,000 units SC q 12 h. Treatment of thromboembolism in pregnancy: 80 units/kg IV load, then infuse 18 units/kg/h with dose titrated to achieve full anticoagulation for at least 5 days. Then continue via SC route with at least 10,000 units SC q 8 to 12 h adjusted to achieve PTT of 1.5 to 2.5× control. To avoid unwanted anticoagulation during delivery, stop SC heparin 24 h before elective induction of labor.

PEDS – Venous thrombosis/pulmonary embolus treatment: Load 50 units/kg IV, then 25 units/kg/h infusion.

UNAPPROVED ADULT – Venous thrombosis/pulmonary embolus treatment (unmonitored): Load 333 units/kg SC, then 250 units/kg SC q 12 h based on max 100 kg wt. Venous thrombosis/pulmonary embolus treatment (monitored): initial dose 17,500 units or 250 units/kg SC twice daily with dose adjustment to achieve and maintain an APTT prolongation that corresponds to plasma heparin levels of 0.3 to 0.7 units/mL anti-Xa activity when measured 6 h after injection. Acute coronary syndromes with or without PCI: 60 units/kg IV, then 12 units/kg/h infusion, adjust according to aPTT or antiXa. See Table.

(cont.)

HEPARIN DOSING FOR ACUTE CORONARY SYNDROME (ACS)

ST elevation myocardial infarction (STEMI)	Adjunct to thrombolytics: For use with alteplase, reteplase, or tenecteplase: Bolus 60 units/kg IV load (max 4000 units), then initial infusion 12 units/kg/h (max 1000 units/h) adjusted to achieve goal PTT 1.5 to 2 × control.
Unstable angina/Non-ST elevation myocardial infarction (UA/NSTEMI)	Initial treatment: Bolus 60 units/kg IV load (max 4000 units), then initiate infusion at 12 to 15 units/kg/h (max 1000 units) and adjust to achieve goal PTT 1.5 to 2.5 × control.
Percutaneous coronary intervention (PCI)	With prior anticoagulant therapy but *without* concurrent GPIIb/IIIa inhibitor planned: additional heparin as needed (2000 to 5000 units) to achieve target ACT 250–300 seconds for HemoTec or 300–350 seconds for Hemochron.
	With prior anticoagulant therapy and *with* planned concurrent GPIIb/IIIa inhibitor: additional heparin as needed (2000 to 5000 units) to achieve target 200–250 seconds.
	Without prior anticoagulant therapy and *without* concurrent GPIIb/IIIa inhibitor planned: Bolus 70–100 units/kg with target ACT 250–300 seconds for HemoTec or 300–350 seconds for Hemochron.
	Without prior anticoagulant therapy and *with* planned concurrent GPIIb/IIIa inhibitor: Bolus 50–70 units/kg with target ACT 200–250 seconds

References: *J Am Coll Cardiol* 2011;57:1946. *Circulation* 2011;124:e608. *Circulation* 2004;110;e82-292. *J Am Coll Cardiol* 2009;54:2235.

HEPARIN (*cont.*)

UNAPPROVED PEDS – Venous thrombosis/pulmonary embolus treatment: Load 75 units/kg IV over 10 min, then 28 units/kg/h if age younger than 1 yo, 20 units/kg/h if age 1 yo or older.

FORMS – Generic only: 1000, 5000, 10,000, 20,000 units/mL in various vial and syringe sizes.

NOTES – Beware of HIT, which may present as a serious thrombotic event. When HIT suspected/diagnosed, discontinue all heparin sources and use alternative anticoagulant. HIT can occur up to several weeks after heparin discontinued. Monitor for elevated LFTs, hyperkalemia/hypoaldosteronism. Osteoporosis with long-term use. Bleeding risk increased by high dose; concomitant thrombolytic or platelet GPIIb/IIIa receptor inhibitor; recent surgery, trauma, or invasive procedure; concomitant hemostatic defect. Monitor platelets, Hb, stool for occult blood. Anti-Xa is an alternative to PTT for monitoring. Drug effect can be reversed with protamine. Do not administer heparin preserved with benzyl alcohol to neonates, infants, or pregnant or lactating women. Do not use Heparin Sodium Injection product as a "catheter lock flush"; fatal medication errors have occurred.

WARFARIN (***Coumadin, Jantoven***) ▶L ♀X, (D for mechanical heart valve replacement) ▶+ $

WARNING – Major or fatal bleeding possible. Higher risk during initiation and when INR elevated. Additional risk factors include: High intensity of anticoagulation (INR greater than 4.0), age 65 yo or older, highly variable INRs, history of GI bleed, hypertension, cerebrovascular disease, heart disease, anemia, malignancy, trauma, renal insufficiency, and long duration of therapy. Regular monitoring of INR needed; monitor those at higher risk more frequently. Educate patients about signs and symptoms of bleeding, measures to reduce risk, and how to manage/seek treatment if bleeding occurs. Many important drug interactions that increase/decrease INR, see table.

ADULT – Oral anticoagulation for prophylaxis/treatment of DVT/PE, thromboembolic complications associated with A-fib, mechanical and bioprosthetic heart valves: Individualize dosing. Start 2 to 5 mg PO daily for 1 to 2 days, then adjust dose to maintain therapeutic PT/INR. Consider using an initial dose of less than 5 mg/day if elderly, malnourished, liver disease, or high bleeding risk. For healthy outpatients, 2012 ACCP CHEST guidelines recommend starting at 10 mg PO daily for 2 days, then adjust dose to maintain therapeutic INR. See product information if CYP2C9 or VKORIC genotypes are known. Target INR of 2 to 3 for most indications, 2.5 to 3.5 for mechanical mitral heart valve. See table for specific target INR.

(cont.)

WARFARIN *(cont.)*

PEDS – Not approved in children.

FORMS – Generic/Trade: Tabs 1, 2, 2.5, 3, 4, 5, 6, 7.5, 10 mg.

NOTES – Clinical factors that may affect maintenance dose needed to achieve target PT/INR include age, race, wt, sex, medications, and comorbidities. Many important drug interactions that increase/decrease INR, see table for significant drug interactions. Warfarin onset of action is within 24 h, peak effect delayed by 3 to 4 days. Most patients can begin warfarin at the same time as injectable (heparin/LMWH/fondaparinux) therapy. Continue injectable therapy until the INR has been in the therapeutic range for 24 h. Tissue necrosis in protein C or S deficiency. See phytonadione (vitamin K) entry for management of abnormally high INR.

HEMATOLOGY: Anticoagulants—Factor Xa Inhibitors

NOTE: See Cardiovascular section for antiplatelet drugs and thrombolytics. Contraindicated in active major bleeding. High risk of spinal/epidural hematoma if spinal puncture or neuraxial anesthesia before/during treatment (see *Reg Anesth Pain Med* 2010;35:64-101). Risk of bleeding increased by oral anticoagulants, aspirin, dipyridamole, dextran, glycoprotein IIb/IIIA inhibitors, NSAIDs (including ketorolac), ticlopidine, clopidogrel, and thrombolytics. Monitor platelets, Hb, stool for occult blood.

FONDAPARINUX (*Arixtra*) ▶K ♀B ▶? $$$$$

ADULT – DVT prophylaxis, hip/knee replacement or hip fracture surgery, abdominal surgery: 2.5 mg SC daily starting 6 to 8 h postop (giving earlier increases risk of bleeding). Usual duration is 5 to 9 days; extend prophylaxis up to 24 additional days (max 32 days) in hip fracture surgery. DVT/PE treatment based on wt: wt less than 50 kg: 5 mg SC daily; wt between 50 and 100 kg: 7.5 mg SC daily; wt greater than 100 kg: 10 mg SC daily for at least 5 days and therapeutic oral anticoagulation.

(cont.)

WEIGHT-BASED HEPARIN DOSING FOR DVT/PE*

Initial dose	80 units/kg IV bolus, then 18 units/kg/h. Check PTT in 6 h
PTT less than 35 sec (less than 1.2 × control)	80 units/kg IV bolus, then increase infusion rate by 4 units/kg/h
PTT 35–45 sec (1.2–1.5 × control)	40 units/kg IV bolus, then increase infusion by 2 units/kg/h
PTT 46–70 sec (1.5–2.3 × control)	No change
PTT 71–90 sec (2.3–3 × control)	Decrease infusion rate by 2 units/kg/h
PTT greater than 90 sec (greater than 3 × control)	Hold infusion for 1 h, then decrease infusion rate by 3 units/kg/h

*PTT = Activated partial thromboplastin time. Reagent-specific target PTT may differ; use institutional nomogram when available. Consider establishing a max bolus dose/max initial infusion rate or use an adjusted body wt in obesity. Monitor PTT 6 h after heparin initiation and 6 h after each dosage adjustment. When PTT is stable within therapeutic range, monitor every morning. Therapeutic PTT range corresponds to anti-factor Xa activity of 0.3–0.7 units/mL. Check platelets between days 3 and 5. Can begin warfarin on first day of heparin; continue heparin for at least 4 to 5 days of combined therapy. Adapted from *Ann Intern Med* 1993;119:874. *Chest* 2012:141:e28S, e154S. *Circulation* 2001;103:2994.

THERAPEUTIC GOALS FOR ANTICOAGULATION

INR Range*	Indication
2.0–3.0	Atrial fibrillation, deep venous thrombosis, pulmonary embolism, bioprosthetic heart valve (mitral position), mechanical prosthetic heart valve (aortic position)
2.5–3.5	Mechanical prosthetic heart valve (mitral position)

*Aim for an INR in the middle of the INR range (eg, 2.5 for range of 2 to 3 and 3.0 for range of 2.5 to 3.5). Adapted from: *Chest* 2012; 141:e422S, e425S, e533S, e578S; see these guidelines for additional information and other indications.

FONDAPARINUX (*cont.*)

PEDS – Not approved in children. Since risk for bleeding is increased if wt less than 50 kg, bleeding may be a particular concern in pediatrics.

UNAPPROVED ADULT – Unstable angina or non-ST-elevation MI: 2.5 mg SC daily until hospital discharge or for up to 8 days. ST-elevation MI and creatinine less than 3 mg/dL: 2.5 mg IV loading dose, then 2.5 mg SC daily until hospital discharge or for up to 8 days. Heparin-induced thrombocytopenia with thrombosis: 5 mg SC daily if less than 50 kg; 7.5 mg SC daily if 50 to 100 kg; 10 mg SC daily if more than 100 kg.

FORMS – Generic/Trade: Prefilled syringes 2.5 mg/0.5 mL, 5 mg/0.4 mL, 7.5 mg/0.6 mL, 10 mg/0.8 mL.

NOTES – May cause thrombocytopenia; however, lacks in vitro cross-reactivity with heparin-induced thrombocytopenia antibodies. Risk of major bleeding increased in elderly. Contraindicated if CrCl is less than 30 mL/min due to increased bleeding risk. Caution advised if CrCl is 30 to 50 mL/min. Monitor renal function in all patients; discontinue if severely impaired or labile. In DVT prophylaxis, contraindicated if body wt less than 50 kg. Protamine ineffective for reversing anticoagulant effect. Factor VIIa partially reverses anticoagulant effect in small studies. Risk of catheter thrombosis in PCI; use in conjunction with anticoagulant with anti-IIa activity. Store at room temperature.

RIVAROXABAN (*Xarelto*) ▶K – ♀C ▶? $$$$$

WARNING – Discontinuation in atrial fibrillation increases risk of thrombotic events. Unless pathological bleeding, consider administering another anticoagulant during periods of interruption. Spinal or epidural hematomas reported; consider risk/benefit if neuraxial intervention required.

ADULT – DVT prophylaxis in knee or hip replacement: 10 mg PO daily, if CrCl is less than 30 mL/min avoid use. Start at least 6 to 10 h post-surgery after hemostasis. Continue for 35 days in hip replacement and 12 days in knee replacement. Nonvalvular atrial fibrillation: 20 mg PO daily if CrCl is greater than 50 mL/min; reduce dose to 15 mg PO daily if CrCl is 15 to 50 mL/min, avoid use if CrCl is less than 15 mL/min.

UNAPPROVED ADULT – DVT treatment: 15 mg PO twice daily for 3 weeks, then 20 mg PO daily. If CrCl is 30 to 49 mL/min: 15 mg PO twice daily for 3 weeks, then 15 mg PO daily

FORMS – Trade only: Tabs 10, 15, 20 mg.

NOTES – Concomitant use with anticoagulants, clopidogrel NSAIDs, and other drugs impacting hemostasis may increase risk of bleeding. For DVT prophylaxis, avoid if CrCl is less than 30 mL/min; caution if CrCl is 30 to 50 mL/min due to increased rivaroxaban exposure. For atrial fibrillation, when transitioning from warfarin, start rivaroxaban when INR is below 3.0. Rivaroxaban affects INR; initial measurements of INR during transition may be unreliable. When transitioning from LMWH or other oral anticoagulant, start rivaroxaban 0 to 2 h before next scheduled evening administration of the anticoagulant. When transitioning from heparin, start rivaroxaban when heparin drip infusion is discontinued.

HEMATOLOGY: Antihemophilic Agents

ANTI-INHIBITOR COAGULANT COMPLEX (*Feiba VH, Feiba NF,* ♣ *Feiba VH Immuno*) ▶L ♀C ▶? $$$$$

ADULT – Hemophilia A or B with factor VIII inhibitors, XI and XII (if surgery or active bleeding): 50 to 100 units/kg IV; specific dose and frequency based on site of bleeding, max 200 units/kg/day.

PEDS – Not approved in children.

FORMS – Trade only: Single-dose vials 500, 1000, 2500 units/vial.

NOTES – Contraindicated if normal coagulation. Human plasma product, thus risk of infectious agent transmission. Avoid in active or impending disseminated intravascular coagulation (DIC).

FACTOR VIIA (*NovoSeven, NovoSeven RT,* ♣ *Niastase*) ▶L ♀C ▶? $$$$$

WARNING – Serious thrombotic events reported when used outside of labeled indications, including fatal arterial and venous events. Thrombotic events also reported when used for labeled uses. Monitor all patients for thrombosis. Patients with DIC, advanced atherosclerotic disease, crush injury, or septicemia may be at increased thrombotic risk. Use with caution in those with thromboembolic risk factors. If DIC or thrombosis confirmed, reduce dose or stop treatment depending on symptoms.

ADULT – Hemophilia A or B: Individualize factor VIIa dose.

(cont.)

WARFARIN—SELECTED DRUG INTERACTIONS
Assume possible interactions with any new medication. When starting/stopping a medication, the INR should be checked at least weekly for at least 2 to 3 weeks and dose adjusted accordingly. For further information regarding mechanism or management, refer to the *Tarascon Pocket Pharmacopoeia* drug interactions database (mobile or web edition). Similarly monitor if significant change in diet (including supplements) or illness resulting in decreased oral intake.
Increased Anticoagulant Effect of warfarin / Increased Risk of Bleeding
Monitor INR when agents below started, stopped, or dosage changed. Consider alternative agent. acetaminophen 2 g/day or more for 3 to 4 days or longer, allopurinol, amiodarone*, amprenavir, **anabolic steroids**, ASA¶, cefixime, cefoperazone, cefotetan, celecoxib, chloramphenicol, cimetidine†, **corticosteroids**, danazol, danshen, disulfiram, dong quai, erlotinib, etravirine, **fibrates,** fish oil, fluconazole,**fluoroquinolones**, fluorouracil, fluvoxamine, fosphenytoin (acute), garlic supplements, gemcitabine, gemfibrozil, glucosamine-chondroitin, ginkgo, ifosfamide, imatinib, isoniazid, itraconazole, ketoconazole, leflunomide, lepirudin, levothyroxine#, **macrolides**‡, metronidazole, miconazole (intravaginal), neomycin (PO for 1 to 2 daysor longer), **NSAIDs**¶, (acute), olsalazine, omeprazole, paroxetine, penicillin (high-dose IV), pentoxifylline, phenytoin propafenone,propoxyphene, quinidine, quinine, **statins**§, sulfinpyrazone (with later inhibition), **sulfonamides**, tamoxifen, **testosterones tetracyclines**, tramadol, tigecycline, tipranavir, **TCAs,** valproate, voriconazole, vorinostat, vitamin A (high-dose), vitamin E, zafirlukast, zileuton
Decreased Anticoagulant Effect of Warfarin/Increased Risk of Thrombosis
Monitor INR when agents below started, stopped, or dosage changed. Consider alternative agent. Aprepitant, cefotetan, azathioprine, barbiturates, bosentan, carbamazepine, coenzyme Q-10, dicloxacillin, fosphenytoin (chronic), ginseng (American), griseofulvin, mercaptopurine, mesalamine, methimazole#, mitotane, nafcillin, oral contraceptives**, phenytoin (chronic), primidone, propylthiouracil#, raloxifene, ribavirin, rifabutin, rifampin, rifapentine, ritonavir, St. John's wort, vitamin C (high-dose). *Use alternative to agents below, or give at different times of day and monitor INR when agent started, stopped, or dose/dosing schedule changed.* cholestyramine, colestipol††, sucralfate

*Interaction may be delayed; monitor INR for several weeks after starting and several months after stopping amiodarone. May need to decrease warfarin dose by 33% to 50%.

† Famotidine, nizatidine, and ranitidine are alternatives.

‡ Azithromycin appears to have lower risk of interaction than clarithromycin or erythromycin.

§ Pravastatin appears to have lower risk of interaction.

Hyperthyroidism/thyroid replacement increases metabolism of clotting factors, increasing response to warfarin therapy and increased bleed risk (typically requires lowering warfarin dose). Reversal of hyperthyroidism (as with methimazole, propylthiouracil) will decrease metabolism of clotting factors and decrease response to warfarin (typically requires increasing warfarin dose).

¶ Does not necessarily increase INR, but increases bleeding risk. Check INR frequently and monitor for GI bleeding.

**Does not necessarily decrease INR, but may induce hypercoagulability.

†† Likely lower risk than cholestyramine

Table Adapted from: Coumadin product information; Am Fam Phys 1999;59:635; Chest 2004;126:204S; Hansten and Horn's Drug Interactions Analysis and Management; *Ann Intern Med* 2004;141:23; *Arch Intern Med* 2005;165:1095. *Tarascon Pocket Pharmacopoeia* drug interactions database (mobile or web edition).

FACTOR VIIA (*cont.*)

PEDS – Hemophilia A or B: Individualize factor VIIa dose.

UNAPPROVED ADULT – Serious bleeding with INR elevation or life-threatening bleeding (ACCP guidelines): Varying doses have been shown effective (10 mcg/kg to max cumulative dose 400 mcg/kg). Factor VIIa has a short half-life; monitor for desired effect. Intracerebral hemorrhage (within 4 h of symptom onset): 40 to 160 mcg/kg IV over 1 to 2 min. Perioperative blood loss in retropubic prostatectomy: 20 or 40 mcg/kg IV bolus.

FORMS – Trade only: NovoSeven: 1200, 2400, 4800 mcg/vial. NovoSeven RT: 1, 2, 5, 8 mg/vial.

NOTES – Caution if hypersensitivity to mouse, hamster, or bovine proteins.

FACTOR VIII (***Advate, Alphanate, Helixate, Hemofil M, Humate P, Koate, Kogenate, Monoclate P, Monarc-M, Recombinate, ReFacto, Xyntha***) ▶L ♀C ▶? $$$$$

ADULT – Hemophilia A: Individualize factor VIII dose. Surgical procedures in patients with von Willebrand disease (Alphanate, Humate P): Individualized dosing. Bleeding in patients with von Willebrand disease (Humate P): Individualized dosing.

PEDS – Hemophilia A: Individualize factor VIII dose.

FORMS – Specific formulation usually chosen by specialist in Hemophilia Treatment Center. Recombinant formulations: Advate, Helixate, Kogenate, Recombinate, ReFacto, Xyntha. Human plasma-derived formulations: Alphanate, Hemofil M, Humate P, Koate, Monoclate P, Monarc-M.

NOTES – Risk of HIV/hepatitis transmission varies by product; no such risk with recombinant product. Reduced response with development of factor VIII inhibitors. Hemolysis with large/repeated doses in patients with A, B, AB blood type.

FACTOR IX (***AlphaNine SD, Benefix, Mononine, ♣ Immunine VH***) ▶L ♀C ▶? $$$$$

ADULT – Hemophilia B: Individualize factor IX dose.

PEDS – Hemophilia B: Individualize factor IX dose.

FORMS – Specific formulation usually chosen by specialist in Hemophilia Treatment Center.

NOTES – Risk of HIV/hepatitis transmission varies by product. Products that contain factors II, VII, and X may cause thrombosis in at-risk patients. Stop infusion if signs of DIC.

HEMATOLOGY: Colony–Stimulating Factors

DARBEPOETIN (***Aranesp, NESP***) ▶cellular sialidases, L ♀C ▶? $$$$$

WARNING – Increased risk of death and serious cardiovascular events, including arterial and venous thrombotic events; may shorten time to tumor progression in cancer patients. To minimize risks in cancer patients, use lowest effective dose to avoid blood transfusion. To minimize risks in chronic renal failure, individualize dosing to maintain Hb 10 to 12 g/dL; risks have not been excluded with targeted Hb less than 12 g/dL. Consider antithrombotic DVT prophylaxis, especially in perioperative period. Not approved for use in cancer patients unless anemia is caused by concurrent myelosuppressive chemotherapy; discontinue when chemotherapy completed. Not for patients receiving myelosuppressive chemotherapy in whom anticipated outcome is cure.

ADULT – Anemia of chronic renal failure: 0.45 mcg/kg IV/SC q week, or 0.75 mcg/kg SC q 2 weeks for some nondialysis patients. Maintenance dose may be lower in predialysis patients than dialysis patients. Initiate when Hb is less than 10 g/dL, decrease dose or discontinue when Hb approaches or exceeds 11 g/dL if on dialysis or 10 g/dL if not on dialysis. Anemia in cancer chemo patients: Initially 2.25 mcg/kg SC q week, or 500 mcg SC q 3 weeks. For weekly administration, max 4.5 mcg/kg/dose. Adjust dose based on Hb to maintain lowest level to avoid transfusion. Weekly dose conversion to darbepoetin (D) from erythropoietin (E): 6.25 mcg D for less than 2500 units E; 12.5 mcg D for 2500 to 4999 units E; 25 mcg D for 5000 to 10,999 units E; 40 mcg D for 11,000 to 17,999 units E; 60 mcg D for 18,000 to 33,999 units E; 100 mcg D for 34,000 to 89,999 units E; 200 mcg D for 90,000 units E or greater. Give D once a week for patients taking E 2 to 3 times per week; give D once q 2 weeks for patients taking E once a week. Monitor Hb weekly until stable, then at least monthly.

PEDS – Not approved in children.

UNAPPROVED ADULT – Chemotherapy-induced anemia: 3 mcg/kg or 200 mcg SC q 2 weeks.

FORMS – Trade only: All forms are available with or without albumin. Single-dose vials: 25, 40, 60, 100, 200, 300, 500 mcg/1 mL, and 150 mcg/0.75 mL. Single-dose prefilled

(cont.)

DARBEPOETIN (*cont.*)

syringes or autoinjectors: 25 mcg/0.42 mL, 40 mcg/0.4 mL, 60 mcg/0.3 mL, 100 mcg/0.5 mL, 150 mcg/0.3 mL, 200 mcg/0.4 mL, 300 mcg/0.6 mL, 500 mcg/1 mL.

NOTES – May exacerbate HTN; contraindicated if uncontrolled HTN. Not for immediate correction of anemia. Evaluate iron stores before and during treatment; most patients eventually require iron supplements. Consider other causes of anemia if no response. Use only 1 dose per vial/syringe; discard any unused portion. Do not shake. Protect from light.

EPOETIN ALFA (***Epogen, Procrit,*** **erythropoietin alpha,** ***Eprex***) ▶L ♀C ▶? $$$$$

WARNING – Increased risk of death and serious cardiovascular events, including myocardial infarction, stroke, venous thromboembolism, and vascular access thrombosis; in controlled trials, these events were demonstrated when Hb of greater than 11 g/dL was targeted. May shorten time to tumor progression in cancer patients. To minimize risks, use lowest dose to minimum level to avoid blood transfusion. Consider antithrombotic DVT prophylaxis, especially in the perioperative period. Not approved for use in cancer patients unless anemia is caused by concurrent myelosuppressive chemotherapy; discontinue when chemotherapy completed. Not for patients receiving myelosuppressive chemotherapy in whom anticipated outcome is cure.

ADULT – Anemia of chronic renal failure: Initial dose 50 to 100 units/kg IV/SC 3 times per week. Initiate when Hb is less than 10 g/dL, decrease dose or discontinue when Hb approaches or exceeds 11 g/dL if on dialysis or 10 g/dL if not on dialysis. Maintain lowest level to avoid transfusion. Zidovudine-induced anemia in HIV-infected patients: 100 to 300 units/kg IV/SC 3 times per week. Anemia in cancer chemo patients: 150 to 300 units/kg SC 3 times per week or 40,000 units SC once a week. Start only if Hb is less than 10 g/dL and two additional months of mylosuppression therapy planned. Adjust dose based on Hb to maintain lowest level to avoid transfusion. Reduction of allogeneic blood transfusion in surgical patients: 300 units/kg/day SC for 10 days preop, on the day of surgery, and 4 days postop. Or 600 units/kg SC once a week starting 21 days preop and ending on day of surgery (4 doses).

PEDS – Anemia in cancer chemo: 600 Units/kg IV q week until completion of chemo.

UNAPPROVED PEDS – Anemia of chronic renal failure: Initial dose 50 to 100 units/kg IV/SC 3 times per week. Zidovudine-induced anemia in HIV-infected patients: 100 units/kg SC 3 times per week; max of 300 units/kg/dose.

FORMS – Trade only: Single-dose 1-mL vials 2000, 3000, 4000, 10,000, 40,000 units/mL. Multidose vials 10,000 units/mL 2 mL, 20,000 units/mL 1 mL.

NOTES – May exacerbate HTN; contraindicated if uncontrolled HTN. Not for immediate correction of anemia. Evaluate iron stores before and during treatment; most patients eventually require iron supplements. Consider other causes of anemia if no response. Single-dose vials contain no preservatives. Use 1 dose per vial; do not re-enter vial. Discard unused portion.

FILGRASTIM (***G-CSF, Neupogen***) ▶L ♀C ▶? $$$$$

ADULT – Neutropenia from myelosuppressive chemotherapy: 5 mcg/kg/day SC/IV until postnadir ANC is at least 10,000/mm^3 for no more than 2 weeks. Can increase by 5 mcg/kg/day with each cycle prn. Bone Marrow Transplant: 10 mcg/kg/day IV infusion over 4 to 24 h or 24-h SC infusion. Administer 1st dose at least 24 h after cytotoxic chemotherapy and at least 24 h after bone marrow. Adjust to neutrophil response (see prescribing information). Peripheral blood progenitor cell collection: 10 mcg/kg/day in donors for at least 4 days (usually 6 to 7 days) before the 1st leukapheresis and continued until the final leukapheresis. Consider decreased dose if WBC is greater than 100,000/mm^3. Severe chronic neutropenia (congenital): Start 6 mcg/kg SC two times per day. Severe chronic neutropenia (idiopathic or cyclic): Start 5 mcg/kg SC daily.

PEDS – Neutropenia from myelosuppressive chemotherapy: 5 mcg/kg/day SC/IV for no more than 2 weeks until postnadir ANC is at least 10,000/mm^3. 10,000/mm^3 for no more than 2 weeks. Can increase by 5 mcg/kg/day with each cycle prn. Bone marrow transplant: 10 mcg/kg/day IV infusion over 4 to 24 h or 24-h SC infusion. Administer 1st dose at least 24 h after cytotoxic chemotherapy and at least 24 h after bone marrow. Adjust to neutrophil response (see product information). Peripheral blood progenitor cell collection: 10 mcg/kg/day in donors for at least 4 days (usually 6 to 7 days) before the first leukapheresis and continued until the final leukapheresis. Consider decreased dose if WBC is greater than 100,000/mm^3. Severe chronic neutropenia (congenital): Start 6 mcg/kg SC two times per day. Severe chronic neutropenia (idiopathic or cyclic): Start 5 mcg/kg SC daily.

(cont.)

FILGRASTIM (*cont.*)

UNAPPROVED ADULT – AIDS: 0.3 to 3.6 mcg/kg/day.

FORMS – Trade only: Single-dose vials: 300 mcg/1 mL, 480 mcg/1.6 mL. Single-dose syringes: 300 mcg/0.5 mL, 480 mcg/0.8 mL.

NOTES – Allergic-type reactions, bone pain, cutaneous vasculitis. Do not give within 24 h before/after cytotoxic chemotherapy. Store in refrigerator; use within 24 h when kept at room temperature.

OPRELVEKIN (***Neumega***) ▸K ♀C ▸? $$$$$

WARNING – Risk of allergic reactions and anaphylaxis.

ADULT – Prevention of severe thrombocytopenia after chemo for nonmyeloid malignancies: 50 mcg/kg SC daily starting 6 to 24 h after chemo and continuing until postnadir platelet count is at least 50,000 cells/mcL (usual duration 10 to 21 days).

PEDS – Not approved in children. Safe and effective dose not established. Papilledema with 100 mcg/kg; 50 mcg/kg ineffective.

FORMS – Trade only: 5 mg single-dose vials with diluent.

NOTES – Fluid retention: Monitor fluid and electrolyte balance. Transient atrial arrhythmias, visual blurring, papilledema.

PEGFILGRASTIM (***Neulasta***) ▸Plasma ♀C ▸? $$$$$

ADULT – To reduce febrile neutropenia after chemo for nonmyeloid malignancies: 6 mg SC once each chemo cycle.

PEDS – Not approved in children.

FORMS – Trade only: Single-dose syringes 6 mg/0.6 mL.

NOTES – Do not use if wt less than 45 kg. Bone pain common. Do not give in the time period between 14 days prior to and 24 h after cytotoxic chemo. Store in refrigerator. Stable at room temperature for no more than 48 h. Protect from light.

PEGINESATIDE (***Omontys***) ▸K – ♀C ▸? $$$$$

WARNING – Increased risk of death and serious cardiovascular events, including myocardial infarction, stroke, venous thromboembolism, and vascular access thrombosis; in controlled trials, these events were demonstrated when Hb of greater than 11 g/dL was targeted. To minimize risks, use lowest dose to minimum level to avoid blood transfusion.

ADULT – Anemia of chronic kidney disease on dialysis: 0.04 mg/kg SC once monthly. Initiate when Hb is less than 10 g/dL, decrease dose or discontinue when Hb approaches or exceeds 11 g/dL. Dose adjust based on response.

PEDS – Not approved in children.

FORMS – Trade only: 2, 3, 4, 5, 6 mg/0.5 mL single-use vials; 1, 2, 3, 4, 5, 6 mg/0.5 mL single-use prefilled syringes; 10 mg/mL, 20 mg/2 mL multiple-use vials.

NOTES – Monitor Hb q 2 weeks until stable, then monthly. Not indicated if not on dialysis or in cancer-related anemia. May exacerbate HTN; contraindicated if uncontrolled HTN. Not for immediate correction of anemia. Evaluate iron stores before and during treatment; most patients eventually require iron supplements. Consider other causes of anemia if no response. Single-dose vials contain no preservatives. Use 1 dose per vial; do not re-enter vial. Discard unused portion.

SARGRAMOSTIM (***GM-CSF, Leukine***) ▸L ♀C ▸? $$$$$

ADULT – Specialized dosing for leukemia, bone marrow transplantation.

PEDS – Not approved in children.

HEMATOLOGY: Other Hematological Agents

AMINOCAPROIC ACID (***Amicar***) ▸K ♀D ▸? $ IV $$$$$ Oral

ADULT – To improve hemostasis when fibrinolysis contributes to bleeding: 4 to 5 g IV/PO over 1 h, then 1 g/h for 8 h or until bleeding controlled.

PEDS – Not approved in children.

UNAPPROVED ADULT – Prevention of recurrent subarachnoid hemorrhage: 6 g IV/PO q 4 h (6 doses/day). Reduction of postop bleeding after cardiopulmonary bypass: 5 g IV, then 1 g/h for 6 to 8 h.

UNAPPROVED PEDS – To improve hemostasis when fibrinolysis contributes to bleeding: 100 mg/kg or 3 g/m^2 IV infusion during 1st h, then continuous infusion of 33.3 mg/kg/h or 1 g/m^2/h. Max dose of 18 g/m^2/day. IV prep contains benzyl alcohol; do not use in newborns.

FORMS – Generic/Trade: Syrup 250 mg/mL, Tabs 500 mg. Trade only: Tabs 1000 mg.

NOTES – Contraindicated in active intravascular clotting. Do not use in DIC without heparin. Can cause intrarenal thrombosis, hyperkalemia. Skeletal muscle weakness, necrosis with prolonged use; monitor CPK. Use with estrogen/oral contraceptives can cause hypercoagulability. Rapid IV administration can cause hypotension, bradycardia, arrhythmia.

ANAGRELIDE (*Agrylin*) ▶LK ♀C ▶? $$$$$

ADULT – Thrombocythemia due to myeloproliferative disorders (including essential thrombocythemia): Start 0.5 mg PO four times per day or 1 mg PO two times per day, then after 1 week adjust to lowest effective dose that maintains platelet count less than 600,000/mcL. Max 10 mg/day or 2.5 mg as a single dose. Usual dose 1.5 to 3 mg/day.

PEDS – Limited data. Thrombocythemia due to myeloproliferative disorders (including essential thrombocythemia): Start 0.5 mg PO daily, then after 1 week adjust to lowest effective dose that maintains platelet count less than 600,000/mcL. Max 10 mg/day or 2.5 mg as a single dose. Usual dose 1.5 to 3 mg/day.

FORMS – Generic/Trade: Caps 0.5 mg. Generic only: Caps 1 mg.

NOTES – Caution with heart disease, may cause vasodilation, tachycardia, palpitations, heart failure. Contraindicated in severe hepatic impairment, use with caution in mild to moderate hepatic impairment. Monitor LFTs baseline and during therapy. Caution in lung disease and renal insufficiency. Dosage should be increased by not more than 0.5 mg/day in any 1 week.

DEFERASIROX (*Exjade*) ▶L ♀B ▶? $$$$$

WARNING – Monitor renal and hepatic function closesly. Renal impairment, including failure, has been reported; assess serum creatinine and creatinine clearance before therapy and monthly thereafter. Fatal hepatic failure has been reported; monitor LFTs and bilirubin baseline, q 2 weeks for 1 month, then monthly. Gastrointestinal bleeding reported.

ADULT – Chronic iron overload: 20 mg/kg PO daily; adjust dose q 3 to 6 months based on ferritin trends. Max 40 mg/kg/day.

PEDS – Chronic iron overload, age 2 yo or older: 20 mg/kg PO daily; adjust dose q 3 to 6 months based on ferritin trends. Max 40 mg/kg/day.

FORMS – Trade only: Tabs for dissolving into oral susp 125, 250, 500 mg.

NOTES – Do not use if CrCl is less than 40 mL/min, serum creatinine greater than twice upper limit of normal. Do not use if severe (Child-Pugh C) hepatic impairment. Reduce starting dose by 50% in moderate (Child-Pugh B) hepatic impairment. Closely monitor patients with mild hepatic impairment. Contraindicated if high risk for myelodysplastic syndrome, advanced malignancy, or poor performance status. Give on an empty stomach, 30 min or more before eating. Reports of fatal cytopenias, monitor CBC regularly. Perform auditory and ophthalmic testing before initiation of therapy and yearly thereafter. Do not take with aluminum-containing antacids. May decrease serum ferritin and liver iron concentrations.

ECULIZUMAB (*Soliris*) ▶Serum ♀C ▶? $$$$$

WARNING – Increased risk of meningococcal infections. Administer meningococcal vaccine at least 2 weeks prior to therapy and revaccinate according to current guidelines. Monitor patients for early signs of meningococcal infections, evaluate, and treat with antibiotics as necessary.

ADULT – Reduction of hemolysis in paroxysmal nocturnal hemoglobinuria: 600 mg IV infusion q 7 days for 4 weeks, then 900 mg for fifth dose 7 days later, then 900 mg q 14 days. Atypical hemolytic uremic syndrome: 900 mg IV infusion weekly for 4 weeks, then 1200 mg for fifth dose 1 week later, then 1200 mg q 14 days. Administer infusion over 35 minutes.

PEDS – Not approved in children.

NOTES – Contraindicated if active meningococcal infection or without current meningococcal vaccination. Increases risk of infection with encapsulated bacteria, including *Streptococcus pneumoniae* and *Haemophilus influenzae* type b (Hib). Consider appropriate immunization. Caution if systemic infection. Dose may be given within 2 days of scheduled dosing date. Give supplemental dose after plasmapheresis, plasma exchange, or fresh frozen plasma infusion; see product information for dosing. Monitor LDH (if used for paroxysmal nocturnal hemoglobinuria) or LDH, platelets, and serum creatnine (if used for atypical hemolytic uremic syndrome) during therapy. Monitor following discontinuation for hemolysis for 8 weeks (if used for paroxysmal nocturnal hemoglobinuria) or thrombotic microangiopathy for 12 weeks (if used for atypical hemolytic uremic syndrome).

ELTROMBOPAG (*Promacta*) ▶LK ♀C ▶? $$$$$

WARNING – Hepatotoxicity. Obtain serum transaminases and bilirubin at baseline and q 2 weeks during dose adjustment, then monthly. If abnormal, repeat LFTs within 3 to 5 days. If LFTs remain abnormal, monitor weekly until LFTs return to baseline, stabilize, or resolve. Discontinue if ALT is 3 or more times upper limit of normal and increasing, persistent for at least 4 weeks, hepatotoxicity symptoms or with increased direct bilirubin. Available only through restricted access program.

(cont.)

ELTROMBOPAG (*cont.*)

ADULT – Thrombocytopenia in ITP (unresponsive to steroids, immunoglobulins, or splenectomy): Start 50 mg daily. In hepatic insufficiency or East Asian ancestry, start 25 mg daily. Adjust to achieve platelet count of 50,000; max 75 mg daily. Discontinuation may worsen thrombocytopenia, monitor CBC weekly for 4 weeks after discontinuation.

PEDS – Not approved in children.

FORMS – Trade only: Tabs, 25, 50, 75 mg.

NOTES – Available through restricted distribution program. Give on empty stomach (1 h before or 2 h after meal); separate from medications and food containing iron, Ca, Mg, selenium, and zinc. Monitor CBC weekly until platelet counts stabilize, then monthly. Discontinue if no response after 4 weeks on 75 mg daily. Not for use to normalize platelet count; goal is increase platelet count to a level that reduces bleeding. Monitor peripheral blood for signs of marrow fibrosis. Do not use for thrombocytopenia in chronic liver disease, possible risk of portal vein thrombosis.

HYDROXYUREA (***Hydrea, Droxia***) ▶LK ♀D ▶– $ varies by therapy

WARNING – Mutagenic and clastogenic; may cause secondary leukemia. Instruct patients to report promptly fever, sore throat, signs of local infection, bleeding from any site, or symptoms suggestive of anemia. Cutaneous vasculitic toxicities, including vasculitic ulcerations and gangrene, have been reported most often in patients on interferon therapy.

ADULT – Sickle cell anemia (Droxia): Start 15 mg/kg PO daily while monitoring CBC q 2 weeks. If WBC is $2500/mm^3$ or greater, platelet count is $95{,}000/mm^3$ or greater, and Hb is above 5.3 g/dL, then increase dose q 12 weeks by 5 mg/kg/day (max 35 mg/kg/day). Solid tumors (Hydrea): Intermittent therapy: 80 mg/kg PO for a single dose q 3 days. Continuous therapy: 20 to 30 mg/kg PO daily. Head and neck cancer with radiation (Hydrea): 80 mg/kg PO for a single dose q 3 days. Resistant chronic myelocytic leukemia: 20 to 30 mg/kg PO daily. Give concomitant folic acid.

PEDS – Not approved in children.

UNAPPROVED ADULT – Essential thrombocythemia at high risk for thrombosis: 0.5 to 1 g PO daily adjusted to keep platelets under $400/mm^3$. Also has been used for HIV, psoriasis, polycythemia vera.

UNAPPROVED PEDS – Sickle cell anemia.

FORMS – Generic/Trade: Caps 500 mg. Trade only: (Droxia) Caps 200, 300, 400 mg.

NOTES – Reliable contraception is recommended. Monitor CBC and renal function. Elderly may need lower doses. Minimize exposure to the drug by wearing gloves during handling.

PLERIXAFOR (***Mozobil***) ▶K ♀D ▶? $$$$$

ADULT – Hematopoietic stem cell mobilization with G-CSF for autologous transplantation in non-Hodgkin's lymphoma and multiple myeloma: 0.24 mg/kg (actual body wt) SC once daily for up to 4 days, max 40 mg/day.

PEDS – Not approved in children.

FORMS – Trade only: Single-dose vials 20 mg/mL, 1.2 mL vial.

NOTES – Use with G-CSF; initiate after patient has received G-CSF daily for 4 days. Administer 11 h prior to apheresis. If CrCl is less than 50 mL/min, decrease dose to 0.16 mg/kg. Do not use in leukemia. Monitor CBC, may increase WBC and decrease platelets. May mobilize tumor cells from marrow. Evaluate for splenic rupture if left upper abdominal, scapular, or shoulder pain.

PROTAMINE ▶Plasma ♀C ▶? $

WARNING – Hypotension, cardiovascular collapse, pulmonary edema/vasoconstriction/hypertension may occur. May be more common with higher doses, overdose, or repeated doses, including previous exposure to protamine or protamine-containing drugs (including insulin). Other risk factors include fish allergy, vasectomy, LV dysfunction, and pulmonary hemodynamic instability.

ADULT – Heparin overdose: Within 30 minutes of IV heparin: 1 mg antagonizes about 100 units heparin. If greater than 30 minutes since heparin: 0.5 mg antagonizes about 100 units heparin. Due to short half-life of heparin (60 to 90 min), use IV heparin doses only from last several hours to calculate dose of protamine. SC heparin may require prolonged administration of protamine. Give IV over 10 min in doses of no greater than 50 mg.

PEDS – Not approved in children.

UNAPPROVED ADULT – Reversal of low-molecular-weight heparin: If within 8 h of LMWH dose: Give 1 mg protamine per 100 anti-Xa units of dalteparin or 1 mg protamine per 1 mg enoxaparin. Smaller doses advised if greater than 8 h since LMWH administration. Give additional 0.5 mg protamine per 100 anti-Xa units dalteparin or 0.5 mg protamine per 1 mg enoxaparin if PTT remains prolonged 2 to 4 h after first infusion of protamine.

UNAPPROVED PEDS – Heparin overdose: Within 30 min of last heparin dose, give 1 mg protamine per 100 units of heparin received;

(cont.)

PROTAMINE (*cont.*)

between 30 to 60 min since last heparin dose, give 0.5 to 0.75 mg protamine per 100 units of heparin received; between 60 to 120 min since last heparin dose, give 0.375 to 0.5 mg protamine per 100 units of heparin; more than 120 min since last heparin dose, give 0.25 to 0.375 mg protamine per 100 units of heparin.

NOTES – Severe hypotension/anaphylactoid reaction possible with too rapid administration. Additional doses of protamine may be required in some situations (neutralization of SC heparin, heparin rebound after cardiac surgery). Monitor APTT to confirm. Incomplete neutralization of LMWHs.

PROTEIN C CONCENTRATE (*Ceprotin*) ▶Serum ♀C ▶? $$$$$

ADULT – Severe congenital protein C deficiency (prevention and treatment of venous thrombosis and purpura fulminans): Individualized dosing.

PEDS – Severe congenital protein C deficiency (prevention and treatment of venous thrombosis and purpura fulminans): Individualized dosing.

NOTES – Product contains heparin; do not use if history of heparin induced thrombocytopenia. Check platelets and discontinue if heparin induced thrombocytopenia suspected. Product contains sodium. Made from pooled human plasma, may transmit infectious agents.

ROMIPLOSTIN (*Nplate*) ▶L ♀C ▶? $$$$$

ADULT – Chronic immune idiopathic thrombocytopenic purpura: 1 mcg/kg SC weekly. Adjust by 1 mcg/kg weekly to achieve and maintain platelet count at least 50,000 cells/mcL; max 10 mcg/kg weekly. Hold dose if platelet count is 400,000 cells/mcL or greater.

PEDS – Not approved in children.

NOTES – Use only for chronic ITP; do not use if low platelets from other causes. Use only if increased risk of bleeding and insufficient response to corticosteroids, immunoglobulins, or splenectomy. Do not use to normalize platelet counts; excessive therapy may increase risk of thrombosis. May increase risk for fibrous deposits in bone marrow. Monitor CBC (platelets and peripheral blood smears) weekly until stable dose; then monthly. Platelet counts may drop below baseline following discontinuation; monitor CBC for 2 weeks following cessation of therapy. May increase risk of hematologic malignancies, especially if myelodysplastic syndrome. Available only through restricted distribution program.

THROMBIN—TOPICAL (*Evithrom, Recothrom, Thrombin-JMI*) ▶? ♀C ▶? $$$

WARNING – The bovine form (Thrombin-JMI) has been associated with rare but potentially fatal abnormalities in hemostasis ranging from asymptomatic alterations in PT and/or aPTT to severe bleeding or thrombosis. Hemostatic abnormalities are likely due to antibody formation, may cause factor V deficiency, and are more likely with repeated applications. Consult hematologist if abnormal coagulation, bleeding, or thrombosis after topical thrombin use.

ADULT – Hemostatic aid for minor bleeding: Apply topically to site of bleeding; dose depends on area to be treated.

PEDS – Hemostatic aid for minor bleeding (Evithrom): Apply topically to site of bleeding; dose depends on area to be treated. Recothrom/Thrombin-JMI not approved in children.

NOTES – Do not inject; for topical use only. Do not use for severe or brisk arterial bleeding. Thaw Evithrom prior to use. Reconstitute Recothrom and Thrombin-JMI prior to use. Evithrom is human-derived and carries risk of viral transmission. Recothrom is a recombinant product; risk of allergic reaction in known hypersensitivity to snake proteins; contraindicated in hypersensitivity to hamster proteins. Thrombin-JMI is a bovine origin product; contraindicated in hypersensitivity to products of bovine origin.

TRANEXAMIC ACID (*Cyklokapron, Lysteda*) ▶K ♀B ▶– $$$

ADULT – Prophylaxis/reduction of bleeding during tooth extraction in hemophilia patients: 10 mg/kg IV immediately before surgery, then 25 mg/kg PO 3 to 4 times per day for 2 to 8 days following surgery. Additional regimens include: 10 mg/kg IV 3 to 4 times per day if intolerant of oral therapies or 25 mg/kg PO 3 to 4 times per day beginning 1 day before surgery. Heavy menstrual bleeding (Lysteda): 1300 mg PO three times per day for up to 5 days during menstruation.

PEDS – Not approved in children.

FORMS – Oral: Trade only, tab: 650 mg.

NOTES – Dose adjust in renal impairment. Thromboembolic risk greater in women on oral contraceptives, especially if over 35 years of age, obese, and/or smoker.

HERBAL AND ALTERNATIVE THERAPIES

NOTE: In the United States, herbal and alternative therapy products are regulated as dietary supplements, not drugs. Premarketing evaluation and FDA approval are not required unless specific therapeutic claims are made. Because these products are not required to demonstrate efficacy, it is unclear whether many of them have health benefits. In addition, there may be considerable variability in content from lot to lot or between products.

ALOE VERA (**acemannan, burn plant**) ▶LK ♀oral– topical+? ◗oral– topical+? $

UNAPPROVED ADULT – Topical: Efficacy unclear for seborrheic dermatitis, psoriasis, genital herpes, partial-thickness skin burns. Does not prevent radiation-induced skin injury. Do not apply to surgical incisions; impaired healing reported. Oral: Efficacy unclear for active ulcerative colitis or type 2 diabetes.

UNAPPROVED PEDS – Not for use in children.

FORMS – Not by prescription.

NOTES – OTC laxatives containing aloe latex were removed from the US market due to concerns about increased risk of colon cancer. Cases of Henoch-Schonlein purpura and hepatotoxicity reported with oral administration.

ANDROSTENEDIONE (***andro***) ▶L, peripheral conversion to estrogens and androgens ♀– ◗– $

UNAPPROVED ADULT – Was marketed as anabolic steroid to enhance athletic performance. Advise patients against use because of potential for androgenic (primarily in women) and estrogenic (primarily in men) side effects.

UNAPPROVED PEDS – Not for use in children.

FORMS – Not by prescription.

NOTES – Banned as dietary supplement by FDA. Also banned by many athletic organizations. In theory, chronic use may increase risk of hormone-related cancers (prostate, breast, endometrial, ovarian). Increase in androgen levels could exacerbate hyperlipidemia.

ARISTOLOCHIC ACID (***Aristolochia, Asarum, Bragantia, Mu Tong, Fangchi***) ▶? ♀– ◗– $

UNAPPROVED ADULT – Do not use due to well documented risk of nephrotoxicity. Was promoted for wt loss.

UNAPPROVED PEDS – Do not use.

FORMS – Not by prescription.

NOTES – Banned by FDA due to risk of nephrotoxicity and cancer. Possible adulterant in other Chinese herbal products like Akebia, Clematis, Stephania, and others. Rule out aristolochic acid nephrotoxicity in cases of unexplained renal failure.

ARNICA (***Arnica montana,*** **leopard's bane, wolf's bane**) ▶? ♀– ◗– $

UNAPPROVED ADULT – Toxic if taken by mouth. Topical preparations promoted for treatment of bruises, aches, and sprains; but insufficient data to assess efficacy. Do not use on open wounds.

UNAPPROVED PEDS – Not for use in children.

FORMS – Not by prescription.

NOTES – Repeated topical application can cause skin reactions.

ARTICHOKE LEAF EXTRACT (***Cynara scolymus***) ▶? ♀? ◗? $

UNAPPROVED ADULT – May reduce total cholesterol, but clinical significance is unclear. Possibly effective for functional dyspepsia. Does not appear to prevent alcohol-induced hangover.

UNAPPROVED PEDS – Not for use in children.

FORMS – Not by prescription.

NOTES – Advise against use by patients with bile duct obstruction or gallstones.

ASTRAGALUS (***Astragalus membranaceus,*** **huang qi, Jin Fu Kang, vetch**) ▶? ♀? ◗? $

UNAPPROVED ADULT – Used in combination with other herbs in traditional Chinese medicine for CHD, CHF, chronic kidney disease, viral infections, upper respiratory tract infections. Early studies suggested that astragalus might improve efficacy of platinum-based chemotherapy for non-small cell lung cancer. However, an astragalus-based herbal formula (Jin Fu Kang) did not affect survival in phase II study of non-small cell lung cancer.

UNAPPROVED PEDS – Not for use in children.

FORMS – Not by prescription.

NOTES – Not used for more than 3 weeks without close follow-up in traditional Chinese medicine. In theory, may enhance activity of drugs for diabetes, HTN, and anticoagulation.

BILBERRY (***Vaccinium myrtillus,*** **huckleberry,** ***Tegens, VMA extract***) ▶Bile, K ♀– ◗– $

UNAPPROVED ADULT – Insufficient data to evaluate efficacy for macular degeneration or cataracts. Does not appear to improve night vision.

UNAPPROVED PEDS – Supplements not for use in children.

FORMS – Not by prescription.

NOTES – High doses may impair platelet aggregation, affect clotting time, and cause GI distress.

BITTER MELON (***Momordica charantia,*** **ampalaya, karela**) ▶? ♀– ▶– $$
UNAPPROVED ADULT – Efficacy unclear for type 2 diabetes.
UNAPPROVED PEDS – Not for use in children. Two cases of hypoglycemic coma in children ingesting bitter melon tea.
FORMS – Not by prescription.

BITTER ORANGE (***Citrus aurantium,*** **Seville orange**) ▶K ♀– ▶– $
UNAPPROVED ADULT – Marketed as substitute for ephedra in weight-loss dietary supplements; safety and efficacy not established.
UNAPPROVED PEDS – Not for use in children.
FORMS – Not by prescription.
NOTES – Contains sympathomimetics including synephrine and octopamine. Synephrine banned by some sports organizations. Do not use within 14 days of an MAOI. Juice may inhibit intestinal CYP3A4.

BLACK COHOSH (***Cimicifuga racemosa, Remifemin, Menofem***) ▶Bile + Feces ♀– ▶– $
UNAPPROVED ADULT – Ineffective for relief of menopausal symptoms.
UNAPPROVED PEDS – Not for use in children.
FORMS – Not by prescription.
NOTES – *US Pharmacopeia* concluded black cohosh is possible cause of hepatotoxicity in 30 case reports. Does not alter vaginal epithelium, endometrium, or estradiol levels in postmenopausal women.

BUTTERBUR (***Petasites hybridus, Petadolex***) ▶? ♀– ▶– $$
UNAPPROVED ADULT – Migraine prophylaxis (effective): Petadolex 50 to 75 mg PO two times per day. Am Acad Neurology and Am Headache Society recommend for migraine prophylaxis. Allergic rhinitis prophylaxis (possibly effective): Petadolex 50 mg PO two times per day. Efficacy unclear for asthma.
UNAPPROVED PEDS – Not for children.
FORMS – Not by prescription. Standardized pyrrolizidine-free extracts: Petadolex tabs 50, 75 mg.
NOTES – Do not use raw butterbur; it may contain hepatotoxic pyrrolizidine alkaloids which are removed by processing. Butterbur is related to Asteraceae and Compositae; consider the potential for cross-allergenicity between plants in these families.

CESIUM CHLORIDE ▶K ♀– ▶– $$$
UNAPPROVED ADULT – Health Canada and the FDA are taking action against Internet sellers promoting cesium chloride as alternative treatment of late-stage cancer. Evidence for benefit as cancer treatment is lacking.
FORMS – Not by prescription.
NOTES – Can prolong QT interval and cause torsades de pointes. Toxicity can be prolonged due to extremely long half-life (approximately 200 days to reach steady-state). Prussian blue has been used to speed cesium chloride elimination.

CHAMOMILE (***Matricaria recutita*****—German chamomile,** ***Anthemis nobilis*****—Roman chamomile**) ▶? ♀– ▶? $
UNAPPROVED ADULT – Oral extract: Modest benefit in study for generalized anxiety disorder, but little to no benefit in study for primary chronic insomnia. Topical: Efficacy unclear for skin infections or inflammation. Does not appear to reduce mucositis caused by 5-fluorouracil or radiation.
UNAPPROVED PEDS – Supplements not for use in children. Efficacy and safety unclear for treatment of infant colic with multi-ingredient teas/extracts of chamomile, fennel, and lemon balm.
FORMS – Not by prescription.
NOTES – Theoretical concern (no clinical evidence) for interactions due to increased sedation, increased risk of bleeding (contains coumarin derivatives), delayed GI absorption of other drugs (due to antispasmodic effect). Increased INR with warfarin attributed to chamomile in single case report.

CHASTEBERRY (***Vitex agnus castus fruit extract, Femaprin***) ▶? ♀– ▶– $
UNAPPROVED ADULT – Premenstrual syndrome (possibly effective): 20 mg PO daily of extract ZE 440 (ratio 6–12:1; standardized for casticin).
UNAPPROVED PEDS – Not for use in children.
FORMS – Not by prescription.
NOTES – Liquid formulations may contain alcohol. Avoid concomitant dopamine antagonists such as haloperidol or metoclopramide.

CHONDROITIN ▶K ♀? ▶? $
UNAPPROVED ADULT – Appears ineffective overall for OA pain, but glucosamine 500 mg plus chondroitin 400 mg both PO three times per day may improve pain in moderate to severe knee OA.
UNAPPROVED PEDS – Not for use in children.
FORMS – Not by prescription.
NOTES – Chondroitin content not standardized and known to vary. Cosamin DS contains 3 mg manganese/cap; tolerable upper limit of manganese is 11 mg/day. Some products made from bovine cartilage. Case reports of increased INR/bleeding with warfarin in patient taking chondroitin with glucosamine.

CINNAMON (***Cinnamomum Cassia, Aromaticum***) ▶? ♀+ in food, – in supplements ◗+ in food, – in supplements $

UNAPPROVED ADULT – Doses of 1 to 6 g/day do not appear to substantially reduce HgA1c, fasting glucose, or lipids in type 2 diabetes.

UNAPPROVED PEDS – Does not appear to improve glycemic control in adolescents with type 1 diabetes.

FORMS – Not by prescription.

NOTES – A ½ teaspoon of powdered cinnamon from grocery store is approximately 1 g.

COENZYME Q10 (***CoQ-10,* ubiquinone**) ▶Bile ♀– ◗– $

UNAPPROVED ADULT – Heart failure: 100 mg/day PO divided two to three times per day (conflicting clinical trials; may reduce hospitalization, dyspnea, edema, but AHA does not recommend). Statin-induced myalgia: 100 to 200 mg PO daily (efficacy unclear; conflicting clinical trials). Parkinson's disease: 1200 mg/day PO divided four times per day at meals and at bedtime ($$$$; efficacy unclear; might slow progression slightly, but Am Academy of Neurology does not recommend). Study for progression of Huntington's disease was inconclusive. Prevention of migraine (possibly effective): 100 mg PO three times per day. May be considered for migraine prevention per Am Academy Neurology and Am Headache Society. Efficacy unclear for hypertension and improving athletic performance. Appears ineffective for diabetes, amyotrophic lateral sclerosis.

UNAPPROVED PEDS – Not for use in children.

FORMS – Not by prescription.

NOTES – Case reports of increased INR with warfarin; but a crossover study did not find an interaction.

CRANBERRY (***Cranactin, Vaccinium macrocarpon***) ▶? ♀+ in food, – in supplements ◗+ in food, – in supplements $

UNAPPROVED ADULT – Prevention of UTI (possibly effective): 300 mL/day PO cranberry juice cocktail. Usual dose of cranberry juice extract caps/tabs is 300 to 400 mg PO two times per day. Insufficient data to assess efficacy for treatment of UTI. Does not appear to prevent UTI in spinal cord injury; IDSA advises against routine use to reduce bacteriuria/UTI in neurogenic bladder managed with intermittent/indwelling catheter.

UNAPPROVED PEDS – Insufficient data to assess efficacy for prevention/treatment of UTI in children. Does not appear to prevent UTI in spinal cord injury; IDSA advises against routine use to reduce bacteriuria/UTI in neurogenic bladder managed with intermittent/indwelling catheter.

FORMS – Not by prescription.

NOTES – Numerous case reports of increased INRs and bleeding with warfarin. However, most clinical trials did not find an increase in the INR with cranberry. Approximately 100 calories/6 oz of cranberry juice cocktail. Advise diabetics that some products have high sugar content. Increases urinary oxalate excretion; may increase risk of oxalate kidney stones.

CREATINE ▶LK ♀– ◗– $

UNAPPROVED ADULT – Promoted to enhance athletic performance. No benefit for endurance exercise, but modest benefit for intense anaerobic tasks lasting less than 30 sec. Usually taken as loading dose of 20 g/day PO for 5 days, then 2 to 5 g/day. Possibly effective for increasing muscle strength in Duchenne muscular dystrophy, polymyositis/dermatomyositis. Does not appear effective for myotonic dystrophy Type 1, amyotrophic lateral sclerosis. Research ongoing in Huntington's disease and Parkinson's disease.

UNAPPROVED PEDS – Not usually for use in children. The AAP strongly discourages performance-enhancing substances by athletes. Possibly effective for increasing muscle strength in Duchenne muscular dystrophy.

FORMS – Not by prescription.

NOTES – Caffeine may antagonize the ergogenic effects of creatine. Creatine is metabolized to creatinine. In young healthy adults, large doses can increase serum creatinine slightly without affecting CrCl. The effect in elderly is unknown.

DANSHEN (***Salvia miltiorrhiza***) ▶? ♀? ◗? $

UNAPPROVED ADULT – Used for treatment of cardiovascular diseases in traditional Chinese medicine.

UNAPPROVED PEDS – Not for use in children.

FORMS – Not by prescription.

NOTES – Case reports of increased INR with warfarin.

DEHYDROEPIANDROSTERONE (***DHEA, Aslera, Fidelin, Prasterone***) ▶Peripheral conversion to estrogens and androgens ♀– ◗– $

UNAPPROVED ADULT – Does not improve cognition, quality of life, or sexual function in elderly. Not recommended as androgen replacement in late-onset male hypogonadism. To improve well being in women with adrenal insufficiency: 50 mg PO daily (possibly effective; conflicting clinical trials). Used by athletes as a substitute for anabolic steroids, but no convincing evidence of enhanced athletic performance or increased muscle mass. Banned by many sports organizations.

(cont.)

DEHYDROEPIANDROSTERONE (*cont.*)

UNAPPROVED PEDS – Not for use in children.
FORMS – Not by prescription.
NOTES – In theory, chronic use may increase risk of hormone-related cancers (prostate, breast, ovarian). But epidemiologic studies found no link between sex hormone serum levels and prostate cancer.

DEVIL'S CLAW (***Harpagophytum procumbens, Doloteffin, Harpadol***) ▶? ♀– ▶– $
UNAPPROVED ADULT – OA, acute exacerbation of chronic low-back pain (possibly effective): 2400 mg extract/day (50 to 100 mg harpagoside/day) PO divided two to three times per day.
UNAPPROVED PEDS – Not for children.
FORMS – Not by prescription. Extracts standardized to harpagoside (iridoid glycoside) content.

DONG QUAI (***Angelica sinensis***) ▶? ♀– ▶– $
UNAPPROVED ADULT – Appears ineffective for postmenopausal symptoms; North American Menopause Society recommends against use. Used with other herbs for treatment and prevention of dysmenorrhea, TIA, CVA, PAD, and cardiovascular conditions in traditional Chinese medicine.
UNAPPROVED PEDS – Not for use in children.
FORMS – Not by prescription.
NOTES – Increased risk of bleeding with warfarin with/without increase in INR; avoid concurrent use.

ECHINACEA (***E. purpurea, E. angustifolia, E. pallida,* cone flower, *EchinaGuard, Echinacin Madaus***) ▶L ♀– ▶– $
UNAPPROVED ADULT – Promoted as immune stimulant. Conflicting clinical trials for prevention or treatment of upper respiratory infections. Does not appear effective for treatment of common cold.
UNAPPROVED PEDS – Not for use in children. Appears ineffective for treatment of upper respiratory tract infections in children.
FORMS – Not by prescription.
NOTES – Single case reports of eosinophilia, precipitation of thrombotic thrombocytopenic purpura, and exacerbation of pemphigus vulgaris; causality unclear. Rare allergic reactions including anaphylaxis. Cross-hypersensitivity possible with other plants in Compositae family. Photosensitivity possible. Could interact with immunosuppressants due to immunomodulating effects. Some experts limit use to no more than 8 weeks and recommend against use in patients with autoimmune disorders.

ELDERBERRY (***Sambucus nigra, Rubini, Sambucol, Sinupret***) ▶? ♀– ▶– $
UNAPPROVED ADULT – Efficacy unclear for influenza, sinusitis, and bronchitis.
UNAPPROVED PEDS – Not for use in children.
FORMS – Not by prescription.
NOTES – Sinupret and Sambucol also contain other ingredients. Eating uncooked elderberries may cause nausea or cyanide toxicity.

EPHEDRA (***Ephedra sinica,* ma huang**) ▶K ♀– ▶– $
UNAPPROVED ADULT – Little evidence of efficacy for obesity, other than modest short-term wt loss. Traditional use as a bronchodilator.
UNAPPROVED PEDS – Not for use in children.
FORMS – Not by prescription.
NOTES – FDA banned ephedra supplements in 2004 because of link to CVA, MI, sudden death, HTN, palpitations, tachycardia, seizures. Risk of serious reactions may increase with dose, strenuous exercise, or concomitant use of other stimulants like caffeine. Country mallow (*Sida cordifolia*) contains ephedrine.

EVENING PRIMROSE OIL (***Oenothera biennis***) ▶? ♀? ▶? $
UNAPPROVED ADULT – Appears ineffective for premenstrual syndrome, postmenopausal symptoms, atopic dermatitis. Inadequate data to evaluate efficacy for cervical ripening.
UNAPPROVED PEDS – Not for use in children.
FORMS – Not by prescription.

FENUGREEK (***Trigonelle foenum-graecum***) ▶? ♀– ▶? $$
UNAPPROVED ADULT – Efficacy unclear for diabetes or hyperlipidemia. Insufficient data to evaluate efficacy as galactagogue.
UNAPPROVED PEDS – Not for use in children.
FORMS – Not by prescription.
NOTES – Case report of increased INR with warfarin possibly related to fenugreek. Can cause maple syrup–like body odor. Fiber content could decrease GI absorption of some drugs.

FEVERFEW (***Chrysanthemum parthenium, MIG-99, MigraLief, Tanacetum parthenium L.***) ▶? ♀– ▶– $
UNAPPROVED ADULT – Prevention of migraine (probably effective): 50 to 100 mg extract PO daily. May take 1 to 2 months to be effective. Inadequate data to evaluate efficacy for acute migraine. Should be considered for migraine prevention per Am Academy Neurology and Am Headache Society.
UNAPPROVED PEDS – Not for use in children.
FORMS – Not by prescription.
NOTES – May cause uterine contractions; avoid in pregnancy. MigraLief contains feverfew,

(cont.)

FEVERFEW (*cont.*)

riboflavin, and magnesium. MigraSpray and Gelstat are homeopathic products that are unlikely to be beneficial.

FLAVOCOXID (***Limbrel, UP446***) ▶L ♀– ▶– $$$

UNAPPROVED ADULT – OA (efficacy unclear): 250 to 500 mg PO two times per day. Max 2000 mg/day short-term. Taking 1 h before or after meals may increase absorption.

UNAPPROVED PEDS – Not for use in children.

FORMS – Caps 250, 500 mg. Marketed as medical food by prescription only (not all medical foods require a prescription).

NOTES – Hepatotoxicity reported. Be alert for confusion between the brand names, Limbrel and Enbrel, as well as misidentification of flavocoxid as a COX-2 inhibitor. Baicalin, a component of Limbrel, may reduce exposure to rosuvastatin in some patients. Each cap contains 10 mg elemental zinc.

GARCINIA (***Garcinia cambogia, Citri Lean***) ▶? ♀– ▶– $

UNAPPROVED ADULT – Appears ineffective for wt loss.

UNAPPROVED PEDS – Not for use in children.

FORMS – Not by prescription.

GARLIC SUPPLEMENTS (***Allium sativum, Kwai, Kyolic***) ▶LK ♀– ▶– $

UNAPPROVED ADULT – Ineffective for hyperlipidemia; American College of Cardiology does not recommend for this indication. Small reduction in BP, but efficacy in HTN unclear. Does not appear effective for diabetes.

UNAPPROVED PEDS – Not for use in children.

FORMS – Not by prescription.

NOTES – Topical application of garlic can cause burn/rash. Significantly decreases saquinavir levels; may also interact with other protease inhibitors. May increase bleeding risk with warfarin with/without increase in INR. However, Kyolic (aged garlic extract) and enteric-coated garlic did not affect the INR in clinical studies.

GINGER (***Zingiber officinale***) ▶bile ♀? ▶? $

UNAPPROVED ADULT – American College of Obstetrics and Gynecology considers ginger 250 mg PO four times per day a nonpharmacologic option for N/V in pregnancy. Some experts advise pregnant women to limit dose to usual dietary amount (no more than 1 g/day). Acute chemotherapy-induced nausea (possibly effective adjunct to standard antiemetics): 250 to 500 mg PO two times per day for 6 days, starting 3 days before chemo. No benefit for chemo-induced acute vomiting, or delayed N/V. Possibly ineffective for prevention of motion sickness. Does not appear effective for postoperative N/V. Efficacy unclear for relief of OA pain.

UNAPPROVED PEDS – Not for use in children.

FORMS – Not by prescription.

NOTES – Increased INR attributed to ginger in a phenprocoumon-treated patient, but study in healthy volunteers found no effect of ginger on INR or pharmacokinetics of warfarin. Some European countries advise pregnant women to avoid ginger in supplements because it is cytotoxic in vitro. A ½ teaspoon of ground ginger is about 1 g of ginger.

GINKGO BILOBA (***EGb 761, Ginkgold, Ginkoba***) ▶K ♀– ▶– $

UNAPPROVED ADULT – Dementia (efficacy unclear): 40 mg PO three times per day of standardized extract containing 24% ginkgo flavone glycosides and 6% terpene lactones. American Psychiatric Association and others find evidence too weak to recommend for Alzheimer's or other dementias. Does not prevent dementia in elderly with normal or mildly impaired cognitive function. Does not improve cognition in healthy younger people. Does not appear effective for intermittent claudication or prevention of acute altitude sickness.

UNAPPROVED PEDS – Not for use in children.

FORMS – Not by prescription.

NOTES – Possible increased risk of stroke. Case reports of intracerebral, subdural, and ocular bleeding; but no increase in major bleeding in large clinical trial. Does not appear to increase INR with warfarin, but monitoring for bleeding is advised. May reduce efficacy of efavirenz. Ginkgo seeds contain a neurotoxin. A few reports attributing exacerbation or precipitation of seizures to ginkgo supplements have raised concern about possible contamination with the neurotoxin. Some experts advise caution or avoidance of ginkgo by those with seizures or taking drugs that lower the seizure threshold.

GINSENG—AMERICAN (***Panax quinquefolius L., Cold-fX***) ▶K ♀– ▶– $

UNAPPROVED ADULT – Reduction of postprandial glucose in type 2 diabetes (possibly effective): 3 g PO taken with or up to 2 h before meal. Cold-fX (1 cap PO two times per day) may modestly reduce the frequency of colds/flu; approved in Canada to strengthen immune system. Cancer-related fatigue (possibly effective): 500 to 1000 mg PO two times per day in am and midafternoon with food.

UNAPPROVED PEDS – Usually not for use in children. Cold-fX (1 cap PO two times per day) may modestly reduce the frequency of colds/

(cont.)

GINSENG—AMERICAN (*cont.*)

flu; approved in Canada for children 12 yo and older to strengthen immune system.

FORMS – Not by prescription.

NOTES – Ginseng content varies widely and some products are mislabeled or adulterated with caffeine. American, Asian, and Siberian ginseng are often misidentified. Decreased INR with warfarin.

GINSENG—ASIAN (***Panax ginseng, Ginsana, G115,* Korean red ginseng**) ▶? ♀– ▶– $

UNAPPROVED ADULT – Promoted to improve vitality and wellbeing: 200 mg PO daily. Ginsana: 2 caps PO daily or 1 cap PO two times per day. Preliminary evidence of efficacy for erectile dysfunction. Efficacy unclear for improving physical or psychomotor performance, diabetes, herpes simplex infections, cognitive or immune function. American College of Obstetrics and Gynecologists and North American Menopause Society recommend against use for postmenopausal hot flashes.

UNAPPROVED PEDS – Not for use in children.

FORMS – Not by prescription.

NOTES – Some formulations may contain up to 34% alcohol. Reports of an interaction with the MAOI, phenelzine. May decrease INR with warfarin. Ginseng content varies widely and some products are mislabeled or adulterated with caffeine. American, Asian, and Siberian ginseng are often misidentified. May interfere with some digoxin assays.

GINSENG—SIBERIAN (***Eleutherococcus senticosus, Ci-wu-jia***) ▶? ♀– ▶– $

UNAPPROVED ADULT – Does not appear to improve athletic endurance. Did not appear effective in single clinical trial for chronic fatigue syndrome.

UNAPPROVED PEDS – Not for use in children.

FORMS – Not by prescription.

NOTES – May interfere with some digoxin assays. A case report of thalamic CVA attributed to Siberian ginseng plus caffeine.

GLUCOSAMINE (***Cosamin DS, Dona***) ▶L ♀– ▶– $

UNAPPROVED ADULT – OA: Glucosamine HCl 500 mg PO three times per day or glucosamine sulfate (Dona $$) 1500 mg PO once daily. Appears ineffective overall for OA pain, but glucosamine 500 mg plus chondroitin 400 mg both PO three times per day may improve pain in moderate to severe knee OA.

UNAPPROVED PEDS – Not for use in children.

FORMS – Not by prescription.

NOTES – Use cautiously or avoid in patients with shellfish allergy. Case reports of increased INR/bleeding with warfarin in patient taking chondroitin plus glucosamine.

GOLDENSEAL (***Hydrastis canadensis***) ▶? ♀– ▶– $

UNAPPROVED ADULT – Often used in attempts to achieve false-negative urine test for illicit drug use (efficacy unclear). Often combined with echinacea in cold remedies; but insufficient data to assess efficacy of goldenseal for the common cold or URIs.

UNAPPROVED PEDS – Not for use in children.

FORMS – Not by prescription.

NOTES – Alkaloids in goldenseal with antibacterial activity not well absorbed orally. Oral use contraindicated in pregnancy (may cause uterine contractions), newborns (may cause kernicterus), and HTN (high doses may cause peripheral vasoconstriction). Adding goldenseal directly to urine turns it brown. May inhibit CYP2D6 and 3A4. Berberine, a component of goldenseal, may increase cyclosporine levels.

GRAPE SEED EXTRACT (***Vitis vinifera L.,* procyanidolic oligomers, *PCO***) ▶? ♀? ▶? $

UNAPPROVED ADULT – Small clinical trials suggest benefit in chronic venous insufficiency. No benefit in single study of seasonal allergic rhinitis. Insufficient evidence to evaluate for treatment of hypertension.

UNAPPROVED PEDS – Not for use in children.

FORMS – Not by prescription.

NOTES – Pine bark (pycnogenol) and grape seed extract are often confused; they both contain oligomeric proanthocyanidins.

GREEN TEA (***Camellia sinensis, Polyphenon E***) ▶LK ♀+ in moderate amount in food, – in supplements ▶+ in moderate amount in food, – in supplements $

UNAPPROVED ADULT – Some population studies suggest a reduction in adenomatous polyps and chronic atrophic gastritis in green tea drinkers. Efficacy unclear for cancer prevention, wt loss, hypercholesterolemia. Green tea catechins (Polyphenon E) under evaluation for chronic lymphocytic leukemia and prevention of prostate cancer in men with high-grade prostate intraepithelial neoplasia.

UNAPPROVED PEDS – Not for children.

FORMS – Not by prescription. Green tea extract available in caps standardized to polyphenol content.

NOTES – Case report of decreased INR with warfarin attributed to drinking large amounts of green tea (due to vitamin K content). The vitamin K content of green tea is low with usual consumption. Case reports of hepatotoxicity with supplements (not tea).

GUARANA (***Paullinia cupana***) ▶? ♀+ in food, – in supplements ▶+ in food, – in supplements $

UNAPPROVED ADULT – Marketed as a source of caffeine in weight-loss dietary supplements. Guarana in weight-loss dietary supplements may provide high doses of caffeine.

UNAPPROVED PEDS – Not for children.

FORMS – Not by prescription.

GUGGULIPID (***Commiphora mukul extract,*** **guggul**) ▶? ♀– ▶– $$

UNAPPROVED ADULT – Does not appear effective for hyperlipidemia with doses up to 2000 mg PO three times per day.

UNAPPROVED PEDS – Not for use in children.

FORMS – Not by prescription.

NOTES – May decrease levels of propranolol and diltiazem. A randomized controlled trial conducted in the United States with 1000 mg or 2000 mg PO three times per day reported no change in total cholesterol, triglycerides, or HDL, and a small increase in LDL. Earlier studies of weaker design reported reductions in total cholesterol of up to 27%.

HAWTHORN (***Crataegus laevigata,*** **monogyna, oxyacantha, standardized extract WS 1442—*Crataegutt novo, HeartCare***) ▶? ♀– ▶– $

UNAPPROVED ADULT – Symptomatic improvement of mild CHF (NYHA I–II; possibly effective): 80 mg PO two times per day to 160 mg PO three times per day of standardized extract (19% oligomeric procyanidins; WS 1442; HeartCare 80 mg tabs); doses as high as 900 to 1800 mg/day have been studied. Initial presentation of SPICE study found no benefit for primary outcome (composite of cardiac death/hospitalization) but possible reduction of sudden cardiac death for LVEF 25 to 35%. American College of Cardiology found evidence insufficient to recommend for mild heart failure. Does not appear effective for HTN.

UNAPPROVED PEDS – Not for use in children.

FORMS – Not by prescription.

NOTES – Unclear whether hawthorn and digoxin should be used together; mechanisms of action may be similar.

HONEY (***Medihoney***) ▶? ♀+ ▶+ $ for oral $$$ for Medihoney

UNAPPROVED ADULT – Topical for burn/wound care (including pressure ulcers, 1st- and 2nd-degree partial thickness burns, donor sites, surgical/traumatic wounds): Apply Medihoney to wound for 12 to 24 h/day. Efficacy of topical honey unclear for prevention of dialysis catheter infections. Oral. Constipation (efficacy unclear): 1 to 2 tbsp (30 to 60 g) in glass of water.

UNAPPROVED PEDS – Topical for burn/wound care (including pressure ulcers, 1st- and 2nd-degree partial thickness burns, donor sites, surgical/traumatic wounds): Apply Medihoney to wound for 12 to 24 h/day. Do not feed honey to children younger than 1 yo due to risk of infant botulism. Nocturnal cough due to upper RTI in children (possibly effective): Give PO within 30 min before sleep. Give ½ tsp for 2 to 5 yo, 1 tsp for 6 to 11 yo, 2 tsp for 12 to 18 yo. WHO considers honey a cheap, popular, and safe demulcent for children.

FORMS – Mostly not by prescription. Medihoney is FDA approved.

NOTES – Honey may contain trace amounts of antimicrobials used to treat infection in honeybee hives. Medihoney sterile dressings contain Leptospermum (Manuka) honey that is irradiated to inactivate C botulinum spores.

HORSE CHESTNUT SEED EXTRACT (***Aesculus hippocastanum,*** **buckeye,** ***HCE50, Venastat***) ▶? ♀– ▶– $

UNAPPROVED ADULT – Chronic venous insufficiency (effective): 1 cap Venastat PO two times per day with water before meals. Response within 1 month. Venastat is 16% escin in standardized extract. American College of Cardiology found evidence insufficient to recommend for peripheral arterial disease.

UNAPPROVED PEDS – Not for use in children.

FORMS – Not by prescription.

NOTES – Venastat does not contain aesculin, a toxin in horse chestnuts.

KAVA (***Piper methysticum***) ▶K ♀– ▶– $

UNAPPROVED ADULT – Promoted as anxiolytic (possibly effective) or sedative; recommend against use due to hepatotoxicity.

UNAPPROVED PEDS – Not for use in children.

FORMS – Not by prescription.

NOTES – Reports of severe hepatotoxicity leading to liver transplantation. May potentiate CNS effects of benzodiazepines and other sedatives, including alcohol. Reversible yellow skin discoloration with long-term use.

KOMBUCHA TEA (**Manchurian or Kargasok tea**) ▶? ♀– ▶– $

UNAPPROVED ADULT – Promoted for many indications, but no scientific evidence to support benefit for any condition. FDA advises caution due to a case of fatal acidosis.

UNAPPROVED PEDS – Not for use in children.

FORMS – Not by prescription.

NOTES – Acidic fermented drink made from addition of bacterial and yeast culture to sweetened black or green tea. It may contain alcohol, ethyl acetate, acetic acid, and lactate.

LICORICE (*Cankermelt, Glycyrrhiza glabra, Glycyrrhiza uralensis*) ▶Bile ♀– ◗– $

UNAPPROVED ADULT – Insufficient data to assess efficacy for postmenopausal vasomotor symptoms. Cankermelt dissolving oral patch for pain relief and healing of aphthous stomatitis (efficacy unclear). Apply patch to ulcer for 16 h/day until ulcer is healed.

UNAPPROVED PEDS – Not for use in children.

FORMS – Not by prescription.

NOTES – Chronic high doses can cause pseudoprimary aldosteronism (with hypertension, edema, hypokalemia). Case reports of myopathy. Diuretics or stimulant laxatives could potentiate licorice-induced hypokalemia. In the United States, "licorice" candy usually does not contain licorice. Deglycyrrhizinated licorice does not have mineralocorticoid effects.

MELATONIN (**N-acetyl-5-methoxytryptamine**) ▶L ♀– ◗– $

UNAPPROVED ADULT – To reduce jet lag after flights across more than 5 time zones (effective; especially traveling East; may also help for 2 to 4 time zones): 0.5 to 5 mg PO at bedtime (10 pm to midnight) for 3 to 6 nights starting on day of arrival. Faster onset and better sleep quality with 5 mg. No benefit with use before departure or slow-release formulations. Do not take earlier in day (may cause drowsiness and delay adaptation to local time). To promote daytime sleep in night shift workers: 1.8 to 3 mg PO prior to daytime sleep. Delayed sleep phase disorder: 0.3 to 5 mg PO 1.5 to 6 h before habitual bedtime. Orphan drug for treatment of circadian rhythm-related sleep disorders in blind patients with no light perception. Possibly effective for difficulty falling asleep but not for staying asleep. American Academy of Sleep Medicine does not recommend for chronic insomnia but does recommend for jet lag.

UNAPPROVED PEDS – Not usually used in children. Sleep-onset insomnia in ADHD, age 6 yo or older (possibly effective): 3 to 6 mg PO at bedtime. Orphan drug treatment of circadian rhythm-related sleep disorders in blind patients with no light perception.

FORMS – Not by prescription.

NOTES – High melatonin levels linked to nocturnal asthma; some experts advise patients with nocturnal asthma to avoid melatonin supplements until more data available.

METHYLSULFONYLMETHANE (*MSM*, **dimethyl sulfone, crystalline DMSO2**) ▶? ♀– ◗– $

UNAPPROVED ADULT – Insufficient data to assess efficacy of oral and topical MSM for arthritis pain.

UNAPPROVED PEDS – Not for use in children.

FORMS – Not by prescription.

NOTES – Can cause nausea, diarrhea, headache. DMSO metabolite promoted as a source of sulfur without odor.

MILK THISTLE (*Silybum marianum, Legalon, silymarin, Thisylin*) ▶LK ♀– ◗– $

UNAPPROVED ADULT – Hepatic cirrhosis (efficacy unclear): 100 to 200 mg PO three times per day of standardized extract with 70 to 80% silymarin. Guidelines for management of alcoholic liver disease recommend against use. Hepatitis C: Does not appear to improve viral load, serum transaminases, or liver histology; the American Gastroenterological Association recommends against use. Used in Europe to treat Amanita mushroom poisoning.

UNAPPROVED PEDS – Not for use in children.

FORMS – Not by prescription.

NOTES – May inhibit CYP2C9. May decrease blood glucose in patients with cirrhosis and diabetes.

NETTLE ROOT (**stinging nettle,** *Urtica dioica radix*) ▶? ♀– ◗– $

UNAPPROVED ADULT – Efficacy unclear for treatment of BPH or osteoarthritis.

UNAPPROVED PEDS – Not for use in children.

FORMS – Not by prescription.

NOTES – Can cause allergic skin reactions, mild GI upset, sweating. Case reports of gynecomastia in a man and galactorrtea in a woman.

NONI (*Morinda citrifolia*) ▶? ♀– ◗– $$$

UNAPPROVED ADULT – Promoted for many medical disorders; but insufficient data to assess efficacy.

UNAPPROVED PEDS – Supplements not for use in children.

FORMS – Not by prescription.

NOTES – Potassium content comparable to orange juice. Hyperkalemia reported in a patient with chronic renal failure. Case reports of hepatotoxicity.

PEPPERMINT OIL (*Mentha x piperita oil*) ▶LK ♀+ in food, ? in supplements ◗+ in food, ? in supplements $

UNAPPROVED ADULT – Irritable bowel syndrome (possibly effective): 0.2 to 0.4 mL enteric-coated caps PO three times per day before meals. Efficacy of peppermint oil plus caraway seed is unclear for dyspepsia.

UNAPPROVED PEDS – Irritable bowel syndrome, age 8 yo or older (possibly effective): 0.1 to 0.2 mL enteric-coated capsules PO three times per day before meals.

FORMS – Not by prescription.

NOTES – Generally regarded as safe as food by FDA. May exacerbate GERD. For irritable

(cont.)

PEPPERMINT OIL (*cont.*)

bowel syndrome, use enteric-coated caps that deliver peppermint oil to lower GI tract. Drugs that increase gastric pH (antacids, H2 blockers, proton pump inhibitors) may dissolve enteric-coated capsules too soon, causing heart burn and reducing benefit. Separate peppermint oil and antacid doses by at least 2 h.

POLICOSANOL (***CholeRx, Cholestin***) ▸? ♀– ◗– $

UNAPPROVED ADULT – Ineffective for hyperlipidemia. A Cuban formulation (unavailable in the United States) 5 mg two times per day reduced LDL cholesterol in studies by a single group of researchers, but studies by other groups found no benefit. Clinical study of a US formulation also found no benefit.

UNAPPROVED PEDS – Not for use in children.

FORMS – Not by prescription.

NOTES – An old formulation of Cholestin contained red yeast rice; the current formulation contains policosanol.

PROBIOTICS (***Acidophilus, Align, Bifantis, Bifidobacteria, Lactobacillus, Bacid, Culturelle, Florastor, IntestiFlora, LiveBac, Power-Dophilus, Primadophilus, Saccharomyces boulardii, VSL#3***) ▸? ♀+ ◗+ $

ADULT – VSL#3 approved as medical food. Ulcerative colitis (possibly effective); 1 to 2 packets or 4 to 8 caps/day. Active ulcerative colitis: 4 to 8 packets or 16 to 32 caps/day. Pouchitis (effective): 2 to 4 packets or 6 to 18 caps/day. Irritable bowel syndrome (may relieve gas and bloating): ½ to 1 packet PO daily or 2 to 4 caps daily. Mix powder from packets with at least 4 oz of cold water before taking.

PEDS – VSL#3 approved as medical food for ulcerative colitis (possibly effective) or pouchitis (effective), for age 3 mo or older: Dose based on wt and number of bowel movements/day. See www.vsl3.com. Use adult dose for age 15 yo or older. Mix powder with at least 4 oz of cold water before taking.

UNAPPROVED ADULT – Antibiotic-associated diarrhea (effective): *Saccharomyces boulardii* 500 mg PO two times per day (Florastor 2 caps PO two times per day). IDSA recommends against probiotics to prevent *C. difficile*–associated diarrhea; safety and efficacy are unclear. Probiotics may reduce GI side effects of *H. pylori* eradication regimens. Bifido bacterium and some combo products improve abdominal pain and bloating in irritable bowel syndrome (eg, Align 1 cap PO once daily), but *Lactobacillus* alone did not improve symptoms. Efficacy of probiotics unclear for traveler's diarrhea (conflicting evidence), Crohn's disease, *H. pylori*, radiation enteritis. *Lactobacillus* GG appears ineffective for prevention of postantibiotic vulvovaginitis.

UNAPPROVED PEDS – Prevention of antibiotic-associated diarrhea (effective): *Lactobacillus* GG 10 to 20 billion cells/day PO (Culturelle 1 cap PO once daily or two times per day) or *S. boulardii* 250 mg PO two times per day (Floraster 1 cap PO two times per day). IDSA recommends against probiotics to prevent *C. difficile*–associated diarrhea; safety and efficacy are unclear. Rotavirus gastroenteritis: *Lactobacillus* GG at least 10 billion cells/day PO started early in illness. Efficacy of probiotics unclear for travelers' diarrhea (conflicting evidence), radiation enteritis. *Lactobacillus* GG does not appear effective for Crohn's disease in children. Research ongoing for prevention and treatment of atopic dermatitis.

FORMS – Not by prescription. Culturelle contains *Lactobacillus* GG 10 billion cells/cap. Florastor contains *Saccharomyces boulardii* 5 billion cells/250 mg cap. VSL#3 (nonprescription medical food) contains 450 billion cells/packet, 225 billion cells/2 caps (*Bifidobacterium breve, longum, infantis; Lactobacillus acidophilus, plantarum, casei, bulgaricus; Streptococcus thermophilus*). Align contains *Bifidobacterium infantis* 35624, 1 billion cells/cap.

NOTES – Do not use probiotics in patients with acute pancreatitis; increased mortality and bowel ischemia reported in clinical trial. Acquired infection possible, especially in immunocompromised or critically ill patients; bacteremia, endocarditis, abscess reported, with possible contamination of central venous access port in some cases. Microbial type and content varies by product. Pick yogurt products labeled "Live and active cultures." Refrigerate packets of VSL#3; can store at room temp for 1 week.

PYCNOGENOL (**French maritime pine tree bark**) ▸L ♀? ◗? $

UNAPPROVED ADULT – Promoted for many medical disorders, but efficacy unclear for chronic venous insufficiency, sperm dysfunction, melasma, OA, HTN, type 2 diabetes, diabetic retinopathy, and ADHD.

UNAPPROVED PEDS – Not for use in children.

FORMS – Not by prescription.

NOTES – Pine bark (pycnogenol) and grape seed extract are often confused; they both contain oligomeric proanthocyanidins.

PYGEUM AFRICANUM (**African plum tree**) ▶? ♀– ◗– $

UNAPPROVED ADULT – Benign prostatic hypertrophy (may have modest efficacy): 50 to 100 mg PO two times per day or 100 mg PO daily of standardized extract containing 14% triterpenes.

UNAPPROVED PEDS – Not for use in children.

FORMS – Not by prescription.

NOTES – Appears well tolerated. Self-treatment could delay diagnosis of prostate cancer.

RED CLOVER (**red clover isoflavone extract, *Trifolium pratense*, trefoil, *Promensil, Trinovin***) ▶Gut, L, K ♀– ◗– $$

UNAPPROVED ADULT – Promensil (1 tab PO one to two times per day with meals) marketed for menopausal symptoms; Trinovin (1 tab PO daily) for maintaining prostate health and urinary function in men. Conflicting evidence of efficacy for postmenopausal vasomotor symptoms. Does not appear effective overall, but may have modest benefit for severe symptoms. Efficacy unclear for prevention of osteoporosis and treatment of hyperlipidemia in postmenopausal women, and for BPH symptoms in men.

UNAPPROVED PEDS – Not for use in children.

FORMS – Not by prescription. Isoflavone content (genistein, daidzein, biochanin, formononetin) is 40 mg/tab in Promensil and Trinovin.

NOTES – Does not appear to stimulate endometrium. Effect on breast cancer risk is unclear; some experts recommend against use of isoflavone supplements by women with breast cancer. No effect on breast density in women with Wolfe P2 or DY mammographic breast density patterns. H2 blockers, proton pump inhibitors, and antibiotics may decrease metabolic activation of isoflavones in GI tract. Ingesting large amounts of red clover can cause bleeding in cattle; bleeding risk of supplements in humans is theoretical.

RED YEAST RICE (***Monascus purpureus, Xuezhikang, Zhibituo, Hypocol***) ▶L ♀– ◗– $$

UNAPPROVED ADULT – Hyperlipidemia: Usual dose is 1200 mg PO two times per day. Efficacy for hyperlipidemia depends on whether formulation contains lovastatin or other statins. In the United States, red yeast rice should not contain more than trace amounts of statins, but some products contain up to 10 mg lovastatin per cap. Some clinicians consider red yeast rice an alternative for patients who develop myalgia with prescription statins. In China, red yeast rice was effective for secondary prevention of CAD events.

UNAPPROVED PEDS – Not for use in children.

FORMS – Not by prescription. Xuezhikang marketed in Asia, Norway (HypoCol).

NOTES – In 1997, a red yeast rice product called Cholestin was marketed in the United States as a cholesterol-lowering supplement. It was removed from the market in 2001 after a judge ruled it an unapproved drug because it contained lovastatin. Cholestin later returned to the market; it now contains policosanol (ineffective for hyperlipidemia). Current red yeast rice products should not contain more than trace amounts of statins, but tests show they may contain up to 10 mg lovastatin per capsule. Can cause myopathy. Case reports of hepatotoxicity. Consider the potential for lovastatin drug interactions.

S-ADENOSYLMETHIONINE (***SAM-e***) ▶L ♀? ◗? $$$

UNAPPROVED ADULT – Mild to moderate depression (effective): 800 to 1600 mg/day PO in divided doses with meals. Efficacy unclear for OA and alcoholic liver disease.

UNAPPROVED PEDS – Not for use in children.

FORMS – Not by prescription.

NOTES – Serotonin syndrome possible when coadministered with SSRIs. Do not use within 2 weeks of an MAOI or in bipolar disorder.

SAINT JOHN'S WORT (***Hypericum perforatum, Kira, LI-160***) ▶L ♀– ◗– $

UNAPPROVED ADULT – Mild to moderate depression (effective): 300 mg PO three times per day of standardized extract (0.3% hypericin).

UNAPPROVED PEDS – Not for use in children. Does not appear effective for ADHD.

FORMS – Not by prescription.

NOTES – Photosensitivity possible with more than 1800 mg/day. Inducer of hepatic CYP3A4, CYP2C9, CYP2C19, and P-glycoprotein. May decrease efficacy of drugs with hepatic metabolism including alprazolam, cyclosporine, methadone, nonnucleoside reverse transcriptase inhibitors, omeprazole, oral contraceptives, oxycodone, protease inhibitors, statins, tacrolimus, voriconazole, zolpidem. May need increased dose of digoxin, theophylline, TCAs. Decreased INR with warfarin. Administration with SSRIs, SNRIs, triptans may cause serotonin syndrome. Do not use within 14 days of an MAOI.

SAW PALMETTO (***Serenoa repens***) ▶? ♀– ◗– $

UNAPPROVED ADULT – Ineffective for BPH symptoms.

UNAPPROVED PEDS – Not for use in children.

FORMS – Not by prescription.

(cont.)

SAW PALMETTO (*cont.*)

NOTES – Not for use by women of childbearing potential. Does not interfere with PSA test. Self-treatment could delay diagnosis of prostate cancer.

SHARK CARTILAGE (*Cartilade*) ▶? ♀– ▶– $$$$$

UNAPPROVED ADULT – Appears ineffective for palliative care of advanced cancer. A derivative of shark cartilage was ineffective in a phase III clinical trial for non-small cell lung cancer.

UNAPPROVED PEDS – Not for use in children.

FORMS – Not by prescription.

NOTES – Case reports of hypercalcemia linked to high calcium content up to 600 to 780 mg/day elemental calcium in Cartilade. Contamination with *Salmonella* was reported in some shark cartilage caps.

SILVER—COLLOIDAL (mild and strong silver protein, silver ion) ▶tissues ♀– ▶– $

UNAPPROVED ADULT – The FDA does not recognize OTC colloidal silver products as safe or effective for any use.

UNAPPROVED PEDS – Not for use in children.

FORMS – Not by prescription. May come as silver chloride, cyanide, iodide, oxide, or phosphate.

NOTES – Silver accumulates in skin (leads to permanent grey tint), conjunctiva, and internal organs with chronic use.

SOY (***Genisoy, Healthy Woman, Novasoy, Phytosoya, Supro***) ▶Gut, L, K ♀+ for food, ? for supplements ▶+ for food, ? for supplements $

UNAPPROVED ADULT – Soy protein or isoflavone supplements do not substantially reduce hyperlipidemia or HTN. Postmenopausal vasomotor symptoms (modest benefit): Per North Am Menopause Society, consider 50 mg/day or more of soy isoflavones for at least 12 weeks. There is not enough data to make recommendations about soy or isoflavone consumption by breast cancer survivors. Conflicting clinical trials for reducing postmenopausal bone loss. AHA recommends against isoflavone supplements for treatment or prevention of hyperlipidemia, or breast, endometrial, or prostate cancer.

UNAPPROVED PEDS – Soy foods are regarded as safe for children.

FORMS – Not by prescription.

NOTES – Effect of soy supplements on breast cancer risk is unclear. Per North Am Menopause Society, there is not enough data to make recommendations about soy or isoflavone consumption by breast cancer survivors. Some experts recommend against use of isoflavone or phytoestrogen supplements by women with endometrial or breast cancer (especially estrogen receptor–positive tumor or receiving tamoxifen). Case report of decreased INR with ingestion of soy milk by patient taking warfarin. Report of decreased levothyroxine absorption with soy protein.

STEVIA (***Stevia rebaudiana***) ▶L ♀– ▶? $

ADULT – Rebaudioside A (a component of stevia) is FDA approved as a general purpose sweetener.

PEDS – Rebaudioside A (a component of stevia) is FDA approved as a general purpose sweetener.

UNAPPROVED ADULT – Leaves traditionally used as a sweetener but not enough safety data for FDA approval as such. WHO acceptable daily intake of up to 4 mg/kg/day of steviol glycosides. Health Canada advises a max of 280 mg/day of stevia leaf powder in adults.

UNAPPROVED PEDS – Stevia leaves not for use in children.

FORMS – Not by prescription. Rebaudioside A available as Rebiana, Truvia, PureVia.

NOTES – Unrefined stevia is available as a dietary supplement in the United States, but is not FDA approved as a food sweetener. In 2008, FDA approved rebaudioside A (a component of stevia) as a general purpose sweetener. Rebaudioside A lacks bitter aftertaste of unrefined stevia. Canadian labeling advises against use by pregnant women, children, or those with low BP.

TEA TREE OIL (melaleuca oil, *Melaleuca alternifolia*) ▶? ♀– ▶– $

UNAPPROVED ADULT – Not for oral use; CNS toxicity reported. Efficacy unclear for topical treatment of onychomycosis, tinea pedis, acne vulgaris, dandruff, pediculosis.

UNAPPROVED PEDS – Not for use in children.

FORMS – Not by prescription.

NOTES – Can cause allergic contact dermatitis, especially with concentration of 2% or greater.

VALERIAN (***Valeriana officinalis, Alluna***) ▶? ♀– ▶– $

UNAPPROVED ADULT – Insomnia (possibly modestly effective; conflicting clinical trials): 400 to 900 mg of standardized extract PO 30 min before bedtime. Response reported in 2 to 4 weeks. Alluna (valerian plus hops): 2 tabs PO 1 h before bedtime. American Academy of Sleep Medicine does not recommend for chronic insomnia due to inadequate safety and efficacy data.

UNAPPROVED PEDS – Not for use in children.

FORMS – Not by prescription.

(cont.)

VALERIAN (*cont.*)

NOTES – Do not combine with CNS depressants. Withdrawal symptoms reported after long-term use. Some products have unpleasant smell.

WILD YAM (*Dioscorea villosa*) ▶L ♀? ▶? $

UNAPPROVED ADULT – Ineffective as topical "natural progestin."

UNAPPROVED PEDS – Not for use in children.

FORMS – Not by prescription.

WILLOW BARK EXTRACT (*Salix alba, Salicis cortex,* **salicin**) ▶K ♀– ▶– $

UNAPPROVED ADULT – OA, low-back pain (possibly effective): 60 to 240 mg/day salicin PO divided two to three times per day. Onset of pain relief is approximately 2 h. Often included in multi-ingredient wt-loss supplements based on preliminary research suggesting that aspirin increases thermogenesis.

UNAPPROVED PEDS – Not for use in children.

FORMS – Not by prescription. Some products standardized to 15% salicin content.

NOTES – Contraindicated in 3rd trimester of pregnancy and in patients with intolerance or allergy to aspirin or other NSAIDs. Consider contraindications and precautions that apply to other salicylates. Avoid concomitant use of NSAIDs.

YOHIMBE (*Corynanthe yohimbe, Pausinystalia yohimbe*) ▶L ♀– ▶– $

UNAPPROVED ADULT – Promoted for impotence and as aphrodisiac, but some products contain little yohimbine (active constituent). FDA considers yohimbe bark in herbal remedies an unsafe herb.

UNAPPROVED PEDS – Not for use in children.

FORMS – Not by prescription.

NOTES – Can cause CNS stimulation. High doses of yohimbine have MAOI activity and can increase BP. Avoid in patients with hypotension, diabetes, heart, liver, or kidney disease. Reports of renal failure, seizures, death in patients taking products containing yohimbe.

IMMUNOLOGY: Immunizations

NOTE: For vaccine info see CDC website (www.cdc.gov).

AVIAN INFLUENZA VACCINE H5N1—INACTIVATED INJECTION ▶Immune system ♀C ▶? ?

ADULT – 18 to 64 yo: 1 mL IM for 2 doses, separated by 21 to 35 days.

PEDS – Not approved for use in children.

NOTES – Caution if hypersensitivity to chicken or egg proteins. The immunocompromised may have a blunted immune response.

BCG VACCINE (✤ *Oncotice, Immucyst*) ▶Immune system ♀C ▶? $$$$

WARNING – BCG infections reported in healthcare workers following exposure from accidental needle sticks or skin lacerations. Nosocomial infections reported in patients receiving parenteral drugs that were prepared in areas in which BCG was reconstituted. Serious infections, including fatal infections, have been reported in patients receiving intravesical BCG.

ADULT – 0.2 to 0.3 mL percutaneously (using 1 mL sterile water for reconstitution).

PEDS – Decrease concentration by 50% using 2 mL sterile water for reconstitution, then 0.2 to 0.3 mL percutaneously for age younger than 1 mo. May revaccinate with full dose (adult dose) after 1 yo if necessary. Use adult dose for age older than 1 mo.

COMVAX **(haemophilus B vaccine + hepatitis B vaccine)** ▶Immune system ♀C ▶? $$$

ADULT – Do not use in adults.

PEDS – Infants born of HBsAg-negative mothers: 0.5 mL IM for 3 doses at 2, 4, and 12 to 15 mo.

NOTES – Combination is made of PedvaxHIB (haemophilus b vaccine) plus Recombivax HB (hepatitis B vaccine). For infants 8 weeks of age or older.

DIPHTHERIA, TETANUS, AND ACELLULAR PERTUSSIS VACCINE (*DTaP, Tdap, Tripedia, Infanrix, Daptacel, Boostrix, Adacel,* ✤ *Tripacel*) ▶Immune system ♀C ▶– $$

ADULT – 0.5 mL IM in deltoid as a single dose, 2 to 5 years since last tetanus dose one time only.

PEDS – Check immunization history: DTaP is preferred for all DTP doses. Give 1st dose of 0.5 mL IM at approximately 2 mo, 2nd dose at 4 mo, 3rd dose at 6 mo, 4th dose at 15 to 18 mo, and 5th dose (booster) at 4 to 6 yo. Use Boostrix only if 10 yo or older, and at least 2 to 5 years after the last childhood dose of DTaP. Use Adacel only in 11 to 64 yo and at least 2 to 5 years after last childhood dose of DTaP or Td.

NOTES – When feasible, use same brand for first 3 doses. Do not give if prior DTaP vaccination caused anaphylaxis or encephalopathy within 7 days. Avoid Tripedia in thimerosal-allergic patients. Do not use Boostrix or Adacel for primary childhood vaccination series, if prior DTaP vaccination caused anaphylaxis

(cont.)

DIPHTHERIA, TETANUS, AND ACELLULAR PERTUSSIS VACCINE (*cont.*)

or encephalopathy, or if progressive neurologic disorders (eg, encephalopathy) or uncontrolled epilepsy. For adolescents and adults, only 1 dose should be given, at least 2 to 5 years after last tetanus dose. Specify Adacel/Boostrix vaccine for adolescent and adult booster as pediatric formulations have increased pertussis concentrations and may increase local reaction. No information available on repeat doses in adolescents or adults.

DIPHTHERIA-TETANUS TOXOID (***Td, DT, ♣ D2T5***) ▶Immune system ♀C ▶? $

ADULT – 0.5 mL IM, 2nd dose 4 to 8 weeks later, and 3rd dose 6 to 12 months later. Give 0.5 mL booster dose at 10-year intervals. Use adult formulation (Td) for adults and children at least 7 yo.

PEDS – 0.5 mL IM for age 6 weeks to 6 yo, 2nd dose 4 to 8 weeks later, and 3rd dose 6 to 12 months later using DT for pediatric use. If immunization of infants begins in the first year of life using DT rather than DTP (ie, pertussis is contraindicated), give three 0.5 mL doses 4 to 8 weeks apart, followed by a fourth dose 6 to 12 months later.

FORMS – Injection DT (pediatric: 6 weeks to 6 yo). Td (adult and children at least 7 yo).

NOTES – DTaP is preferred for most children age younger than 7 yo. Td is preferred for adults and children at least 7 yo. Avoid in thimerosal allergy.

HAEMOPHILUS B VACCINE (***ActHIB, Hiberix, PedvaxHIB***) ▶Immune system ♀C ▶? $$

PEDS – Doses vary depending on formulation used and age at first dose. ActHIB/OmniHIB/Hiberix: Give 0.5 mL IM for 3 doses at 2-month intervals for age 2 to 6 mo, give 0.5 mL IM for 2 doses at 2-month intervals for age 7 to 11 mo, give 0.5 mL IM for 1 dose for age 12 to 14 mo. A single 0.5 mL IM booster dose is given to previously immunized children at least 15 mo, and at least 2 months after the previous injection. For children age 15 mo to 5 yo at age of 1st dose, give 0.5 mL IM for 1 dose (no booster). PedvaxHIB: 0.5 mL IM for 2 doses at 2-month intervals for age 2 to 14 mo. If the 2 doses are given before age 12 mo, a 3rd 0.5 mL IM (booster) dose is given at least 2 months after the 2nd dose. 0.5 mL IM for 1 dose (no booster) for age 15 mo to 5 yo.

UNAPPROVED ADULT – Asplenia, at least 14 days prior to elective splenectomy, or immunodeficiency: 0.5 mL IM for 1 dose of any Hib conjugate vaccine.

UNAPPROVED PEDS – Asplenia, at least 14 days prior to elective splenectomy, or immunodeficiency age 5 yo or older: 0.5 mL IM for 1 dose of any Hib vaccine.

NOTES – Not for IV use. No data on interchangeability between brands; AAP and ACIP recommend use of any product in children age 12 to 15 mo.

HEPATITIS A VACCINE (***Havrix, Vaqta, ♣ Avaxim, Epaxal***) ♀C ▶+ $$$

ADULT – Havrix: 1 mL (1440 ELU) IM, then 1 mL (1440 ELU) IM booster dose 6 to 12 months later. Vaqta: 1 mL (50 units) IM, then 1 mL (50 units) IM booster 6 months later for age 18 yo or older.

PEDS – Havrix: 0.5 mL (720 ELU) IM for 1 dose, then 0.5 mL (720 ELU) IM booster 6 to 12 months after 1st dose for age 1 to 18 yo. Vaqta: 0.5 mL (25 units) IM for 1 dose, then 0.5 mL (25 units) IM booster 6 to 18 months later for age 1 to 18 yo.

FORMS – Single-dose vial (specify pediatric or adult).

NOTES – Do not inject IV, SC, or ID. Brands may be used interchangeably. Need for boosters is unclear. Postexposure prophylaxis with hepatitis A vaccine alone is not recommended. Should be given 4 weeks prior to travel to endemic area. May be given at the same time as immune globulin, but preferably at different site.

TETANUS WOUND CARE (www.cdc.gov)

	Unknown or less than 3 prior tetanus immunizations	*3 or more prior tetanus immunizations*
Non-tetanus-prone wound (eg, clean and minor)	Td (DT age younger than 7 yo)	Td if more than 10 years since last dose
Tetanus-prone wound (eg, dirt, contamination, punctures, crush components)	Td (DT age younger than 7 yo), tetanus immune globulin 250 units IM at site other than Td	Td if more than 5 years since last dose

If patient age 10 yo or older has never received a pertussis booster consider DTaP (Boostrix if 10 yo or older, Adacel if 11–64 yo).

CHILDHOOD IMMUNIZATION SCHEDULE*

	Months								Years		
Age	*Birth*	*1*	*2*	*4*	*6*	*12*	*15*	*18*	*2*	*4–6*	*11–12*
Hepatitis B	HB	HB		HB							
Rotavirus			Rota	Rota	Rota®						
DTP			DTaP	DTaP	DTaP		DTaP		DTaP	DTaP***	
H influenza b			Hib	Hib	Hib	Hib					
Pneumococci**			PCV	PCV	PCV	PCV					
Polio			IPV	IPV	IPV		IPV#				
Influenza†					Influ-enza (yearly)†						
MMR						MMR			MMR		
Varicella						Vari-cella	Vari				
Hepatitis A¶						Hep A × 2¶					
Papillomavirus§										Hep A × 3¶	
Meningococcal^										MCV^	MCV^

*2011 schedule from the CDC, ACIP, AAP, & AAFP, see CDC website
**Administer 1 dose Prevnar 13 to all healthy children 24 to 59 mo having an incomplete schedule.
***When immunizing adolescents 10 yo or older, consider DTaP if patient has never received a pertussis booster (Boostrix if 10 yo or older, Adacel if 11 to 64 yo).
®If using Rotarix at 2 and 4 months, dose at 6 months is not indicated. Max age for final dose is 8 mo.
#Last IPV on or after 4th birthday, and at least 6 months since last dose. If 4 doses given before 4th birthday, give 5th dose at ages 4 to 6 yo.
†For healthy patients age 2 yo or older can use intranasal form. If age younger than 9 yo and receiving for first time, administer 2 doses 4 or more weeks apart for injected form and 6 or more weeks apart for intranasal form. FluLaval not indicated for younger than 18 yo. Use Afluria only if 9 yo or older due to risk of febrile reaction
¶Two doses at least 6 months apart.
§Second and third doses 2 and 6 months after first dose. Also approved (Gardasil) for males 9 to 18 yo to reduce risk of genital warts.
^Vaccinate all children at 11 to 12 yo, booster at 16 yo. Give one dose between 13 yo and 18 yo, if previously unvaccinated. For children 2–10 yo at high risk for meningococcal disease, vaccinate with meningococcal polysaccharide vaccine (*Menactra*). Revaccinate after 3 years (if first dose was at 2 to 6 yo) for children who remain at high risk or after 5 years (if first dose was a 7 yo or older).

HEPATITIS B VACCINE (***Engerix-B, Recombivax HB***) ♀C ▶+ $$$

ADULT – Engerix-B: 1 mL (20 mcg) IM, repeat in 1 and 6 months for age 20 yo or older. Hemodialysis: Give 2 mL (40 mcg) IM, repeat in 1, 2, and 6 months. Give 2 mL (40 mcg) IM booster when antibody levels decline to less than 10 mIU/mL. Recombivax HB: 1 mL (10 mcg) IM, repeat in 1 and 6 months. Hemodialysis: 1 mL (40 mcg) IM, repeat in 1 and 6 months. Give 1 mL (40 mcg) IM booster when antibody levels decline to less than 10 mIU/mL.

PEDS – Specialized dosing based on age and maternal HBsAg status. Engerix-B 10 mcg (0.5 mL) IM 0, 1, 6 months for infants of hepatitis B–negative and –positive mothers and children age 15 to 20 yo. Recombivax 5 mcg (0.5 mL) IM 0, 1, 6 months for infants of hepatitis B–negative and –positive mothers and children age 15 to 20 yo. A 2-dose schedule can be used (Recombivax HB) 10 mcg (1 mL) IM at 0 and 4 to 6 months for age 11 to 15 yo.

NOTES – Infants born to hepatitis B–positive mothers should also receive hepatitis B immune globulin and hepatitis B vaccine within 12 h of birth. Not for IV or ID use. May interchange products. Recombivax HB Dialysis Formulation is intended for adults only. Avoid if yeast allergy.

HUMAN PAPILLOMAVIRUS RECOMBINANT VACCINE (***Gardasil, Cervarix***) ♀B ▶? $$$$$

ADULT – Prevention of cervical cancer, vulvar and vaginal cancer in females 9 to 26 yo: 0.5 mL IM at time 0, 2, and 6 months. Prevention of anal cancer, genital warts, anal intraepithelial neoplasia in males 9 to 26 yo: 0.5 mL IM at time 0, 2, and 6 months.

(cont.)

HUMAN PAPILLOMAVIRUS RECOMBINANT VACCINE (*cont.*)

PEDS – Prevention of cervical cancer, vulvar and vaginal cancer in females 9 to 26 yo: 0.5 mL IM at time 0, 2, and 6 months. Prevention of anal cancer, genital warts, anal intraepithelial neoplasia in males 9 to 26 yo: 0.5 mL IM at time 0, 2, and 6 months.

NOTES – Patients must be counseled to continue to use condoms. Immunosuppression may reduce response. Fainting and falling may occur after vaccination; observe patient for 15 min after vaccination.

INFLUENZA VACCINE—INACTIVATED INJECTION (***Afluria, Agriflu Fluarix, FluLaval, Fluzone, Fluzone HD, Fluvirin, ♣ Fluviral, Vaxigrip***) ▶Immune system ♀C ▶+ $

ADULT – 0.5 mL IM single dose once a year.

PEDS – FluLaval is not indicated for age younger than 18 yo, Fluvirin not indicated for age younger than 4 yo. Fluarix not indicated for age younger than 3 yo. Alfuria should only be used for 9 yo or older due to febrile reactions. Give 0.25 mL IM for age 6 to 35 mo, repeat dose after 4 weeks if previously unvaccinated. Give 0.5 mL IM for age 3 to 8 yo, repeat dose after 4 weeks if previously unvaccinated. Give 0.5 mL IM once a year for age 9 to 12 yo. Fluzone intradermal 0.1 mL IM for ages 18 to 64 yo only. Fluzone HD for 65 yo or older only.

NOTES – Avoid in Guillain-Barré syndrome, chicken egg allergy, aspirin therapy in children (Reye's risk), thimerosal allergy (Fluzone is thimerosal-free). Optimal administration October to November.

INFLUENZA VACCINE—LIVE INTRANASAL (***FluMist***) ▶Immune system ♀C ▶+ $

ADULT – 1 dose (0.2 mL) intranasally once a year for healthy adults age 18 to 49 yo.

PEDS – 1 dose (0.2 mL) intranasally for healthy children age 2 to 17 yo, repeat dose after 4 weeks if previously unvaccinated and age 2 to 8 yo.

NOTES – Avoid in Guillain-Barré syndrome, chicken egg allergy, aspirin therapy in children (Reye's risk), pregnancy, chronic illness that could increase vulnerability to influenza complications (CHF, asthma, diabetes, renal failure), recurrent wheezing and in children younger than 2 yo. Optimal administration October to November. Since FluMist is a live vaccine, do not use with immune deficiencies (eg, HIV, malignancy) or altered immune status (eg, taking systemic corticosteroids, chemotherapy, radiation).

JAPANESE ENCEPHALITIS VACCINE (***JE-Vax***) ♀C ▶? $$$$

ADULT – 1 mL SC for 3 doses on days 0, 7, and 30.

PEDS – 0.5 mL SC for 3 doses on days 0, 7, and 30 for age 1 to 3 yo. Give 1 mL SC for 3 doses on days 0, 7, and 30 for age 3 yo or older.

NOTES – Give at least 10 days before travel to endemic areas. An abbreviated schedule on days 0, 7, and 14 can be given if time limits. A booster dose may be given after 2 years. Avoid in thimerosal allergy.

MEASLES VACCINE (***Attenuvax***) ▶Immune system ♀C ▶+ $

ADULT – 0.5 mL (1 vial) SC.

PEDS – Age 12 to 15 mo: 0.5 mL (1 vial) SC. Revaccinate prior to elementary school. If measles outbreak, may immunize infants age 6 to 12 mo with 0.5 mL SC; then start 2-dose regimen (usually with MMR) between age 12 to 15 mo.

NOTES – Do not inject IV. Contraindicated in pregnancy. Advise women to avoid pregnancy for 4 weeks following vaccination. Live virus contraindicated in immunocompromised patients. Avoid if allergic to neomycin or gelatin; caution in patients with egg allergies.

MEASLES, MUMPS, & RUBELLA VACCINE (***M-M-R II, ♣ Priorix***) ▶Immune system ♀C ▶+ $$$

ADULT – 0.5 mL (1 vial) SC.

PEDS – 0.5 mL (1 vial) SC for age 12 to 15 mo. Revaccinate prior to elementary and/or middle school according to local health guidelines. If measles outbreak, may immunize infants 6 to 12 mo with 0.5 mL SC; then start 2-dose regimen between 12 to 15 mo.

NOTES – Do not inject IV. Contraindicated in pregnancy. Advise women to avoid pregnancy for 4 weeks following vaccination. Live virus, contraindicated in immunocompromised patients. Avoid if allergic to neomycin or gelatin; caution in egg allergy.

MENINGOCOCCAL VACCINE (***Menomune-A/C/Y/W-135, Menveo Menactra, ♣ Menjugate***) ♀C ▶? $$$$

WARNING – Reports of associated Guillain-Barré syndrome; avoid if prior history of this condition.

ADULT – 0.5 mL SC (Menomune) or IM (Menactra, Menveo).

PEDS – 0.5 mL SC for age 2 yo or older. Vaccinate all children 11 to 12 yo and give booster at 16 yo.

UNAPPROVED PEDS – 0.5 mL SC for 2 doses separated by 3 months for age 3 to 18 mo.

(cont.)

MENINGOCOCCAL VACCINE (*cont.*)

NOTES – Give 2 weeks before elective splenectomy or travel to endemic areas. May consider revaccination q 3 to 5 years in high-risk patients. Do not inject IV. Contraindicated in pregnancy. Vaccinate all 1st-year college students living in dormitories who are unvaccinated. Avoid in thimerosal allergy (except Menactra which is thimerosal-free).

MUMPS VACCINE (***Mumpsvax***) ▶Immune system ♀C ◗+ $$

ADULT – 0.5 mL (1 vial) SC.

PEDS – Age 12 to 15 mo: 0.5 mL (1 vial) SC. Revaccinate prior to elementary school.

NOTES – Do not inject IV. Contraindicated in pregnancy. Advise women to avoid pregnancy for 4 weeks following vaccination. Live virus, contraindicated in immunocompromised patients. Avoid if allergic to neomycin or gelatin; caution in patients with egg allergies.

PEDIARIX **(diphtheria tetanus and acellular pertussis vaccine + hepatitis B vaccine + polio vaccine)** ▶Immune system ♀C ◗? $$$

PEDS – 0.5 mL at 2, 4, 6 mo IM.

NOTES – Do not administer before 6 weeks of age.

PLAGUE VACCINE ▶Immune system ♀C ◗+ $

ADULT – 1 mL IM for 1 dose, then 0.2 mL IM 1 to 3 months after the 1st injection, then 0.2 mL IM 5 to 6 months after the 2nd injection for age 18 to 61 yo.

PEDS – Not approved in children.

NOTES – Up to 3 booster doses (0.2 mL) may be administered at 6-month intervals in high-risk patients. Jet injector gun may be used for IM administration.

PNEUMOCOCCAL 13-VALENT CONJUGATE VACCINE (***Prevnar 13***) ♀C ◗? $$$

ADULT – Not approved in adults.

PEDS – 0.5 mL IM for 3 doses at 2 mo, 4 mo and 6 mo followed by a fourth dose of 0.5 mL IM at 12 to 15 mo. For previously unvaccinated older infants and children age 7 to 11 mo: 0.5 mL for 2 doses 4 weeks apart, followed by a third dose of 0.5 mL at 12 to 15 mo. For previously unvaccinated older infants and children age 12 to 23 mo: Give 0.5 mL for 2 doses 8 weeks apart. For previously unvaccinated children 24 mo to 5 yo, give a single 0.5 mL dose IM before the 6th birthday.

NOTES – For IM use only; do not inject IV. Shake susp vigorously prior to administration.

PNEUMOCOCCAL 23-VALENT VACCINE (***Pneumovax, ✤Pneumo 23***) ▶Immune system ♀C ◗+ $$

ADULT – All adults 65 yo or older: 0.5 mL IM/SC for 1 dose. Vaccination also recommended for high-risk individuals younger than age 65 yo. Routine revaccination in immunocompetent patients is not recommended. Consider revaccination once in patients age 65 yo or older who were vaccinated before the age of 65 or patients at high risk of developing serious pneumococcal infection if more than 5 years from initial vaccine.

PEDS – 0.5 mL IM/SC for age 2 yo or older. Consider revaccination once in patients at high risk of developing serious pneumococcal infection after 3 to 5 years from initial vaccine in patients who would be 10 yo or younger at time of revaccination.

NOTES – Do not give IV or ID. May be given in conjunction with influenza virus vaccine at different site. OK for high-risk children at least 2 yo who received Prevnar series already to provide additional serotype coverage.

POLIO VACCINE (***IPOL***) ♀C ◗? $$

ADULT – Previously unvaccinated adults at increased risk of exposure should receive a complete primary immunization series of 3 doses (2 doses at intervals of 4 to 8 weeks; a third dose at 6 to 12 months after the second dose). Accelerated schedules are available. Travelers to endemic areas who have received primary immunization should receive a single booster in adulthood.

PEDS – 0.5 mL IM or SC at age 2 mo, with second dose at 4 mo, third dose at 6 to 18 mo, and fourth dose at 4 to 6 yo.

NOTES – Oral polio vaccine no longer available.

PROQUAD **(measles mumps & rubella vaccine + varicella vaccine, MMRV)** ▶Immune system ♀C ◗? $$$$

ADULT – Not indicated in adults.

PEDS – 0.5 mL (1 vial) SC for age 12 mo to 12 yo.

NOTES – Give at least 1 month after a MMR-containing vaccine and at least 3 months after a varicella-containing vaccine. Do not inject IV. Contraindicated in pregnancy. Following vaccination avoid pregnancy for 3 months and aspirin/salicylates for 6 weeks. Live virus, contraindicated in immunocompromise or untreated TB. Avoid if allergic to neomycin; caution with egg allergies.

RABIES VACCINE (***RabAvert, Imovax Rabies, BioRab, Rabies Vaccine Adsorbed***) ♀C ◗? $$$$$

ADULT – Postexposure prophylaxis: Give rabies immune globulin (20 international units/kg) immediately after exposure, then give rabies vaccine 1 mL IM in deltoid region on days 0, 3, 7, 14, and 28. If patients have received

(cont.)

RABIES VACCINE (*cont.*)

pre-exposure immunization, give 1 mL IM rabies vaccine on days 0 and 3 only, without rabies immune globulin. Pre-exposure immunization: 1 mL IM rabies vaccine on days 0, 7, and between days 21 and 28. Or 0.1 mL intradermally on days 0, 7, and between days 21 and 28. (Imovax Rabies ID vaccine formula only). Repeat q 2 to 5 years based on antibody titer.

PEDS – Same as adults.

NOTES – Do not use ID preparation for postexposure prophylaxis.

ROTAVIRUS VACCINE (***RotaTeq, Rotarix***) ▶? $$$$$

ADULT – Not recommended.

PEDS – RotaTeq: Give the first dose (2 mL PO) between 6 to 12 weeks of age, and then the second and third doses at 4- to 10-week intervals thereafter (last dose no later than 32 weeks). Rotarix: Give first dose (1 mL) at 6 weeks of age, and second dose (1 mL) at least 4 weeks later, and prior to 24 weeks of age.

FORMS – Trade only: Oral susp 2 mL (RotaTeq), 1 mL (Rotarix).

NOTES – Live vaccine so potential for transmission, especially to immunodeficient close contacts. Safety unclear in immunocompromised infants.

RUBELLA VACCINE (***Meruvax II***) ▶Immune system ♀C ▶+ $

ADULT – 0.5 mL (1 vial) SC.

PEDS – Age 12 to 15 mo: 0.5 mL (1 vial) SC. Revaccinate prior to elementary school according to local health guidelines.

NOTES – Do not inject IV. Contraindicated in pregnancy. Advise women to avoid pregnancy for 4 weeks following vaccination. Live virus, contraindicated in immunocompromised patients. Avoid if allergic to neomycin or gelatin.

SMALLPOX VACCINE (***ACAM 2000*, vaccinia vaccine**) ▶Immune system ♀C ▶– Not available to civilians.

ADULT – Prevention of smallpox or monkeypox: Specialized administration using bifurcated needle SC for 1 dose.

PEDS – Specialized administration using bifurcated needle SC for 1 dose for children older than 1 yo.

NOTES – Caution in polymyxin, neomycin, tetracycline, or streptomycin allergy. Avoid in those (or household contacts of those) with eczema or a history of eczema, those with a rash due to other causes (eg, burns, zoster, impetigo, psoriasis), immunocompromised, or pregnancy. Persons with known cardiac disease or at least 3 risk factors for cardiac disease should not be vaccinated.

TETANUS TOXOID ▶Immune system ♀C ▶+ $$

WARNING – Td is preferred in adults and children age 7 yo or older. DTaP is preferred in children younger than 7 yo. Use fluid tetanus toxoid in assessing cell-mediated immunity only.

ADULT – 0.5 mL IM (adsorbed) for 2 doses 4 to 8 weeks apart. Give third dose 6 to 12 months after second injection. Give booster q 10 years. Assess cell-mediated immunity: 0.1 mL of 1:100 diluted skin-test reagent or 0.02 mL of 1:10 diluted skin-test reagent injected intradermally.

PEDS – 0.5 mL IM (adsorbed) for 2 doses 4 to 8 weeks apart. Give third dose 6 to 12 months after second injection. Give booster q 10 years.

NOTES – May use tetanus toxoid fluid for active immunization in patients hypersensitive to the aluminum adjuvant of the adsorbed formulation: 0.5 mL IM or SC for 3 doses at 4- to 8-week intervals. Give fourth dose 6 to 12 months after third injection. Give booster dose q 10 years. Avoid in thimerosal allergy.

TRIHIBIT **(haemophilus B vaccine + diphtheria tetanus and acellular pertussis vaccine)** ▶Immune system ♀C ▶– $$$

PEDS – For fourth dose only, 15 to 18 mo: 0.5 mL IM.

NOTES – Tripedia (DTaP) is used to reconstitute ActHIB (Haemophilus b) to make TriHIBit and will appear whitish in color. Use within 30 min. Avoid in thimerosal allergy.

TWINRIX **(hepatitis A vaccine + hepatitis B vaccine)** ▶Immune system ♀C ▶? $$$$

ADULT – 1 mL IM in deltoid only for age 18 yo or older, repeat at 1 and 6 months. Accelerated dosing schedule: 0, 7, 21, and 30 days and booster dose at 12 months.

PEDS – Not approved in children.

NOTES – Not for IV or intradermal use. 1 mL is equivalent to 720 ELU inactivated hepatitis A + 20 mcg hepatitis B surface antigen.

TYPHOID VACCINE—INACTIVATED INJECTION (***Typhim Vi***, ✤ ***Typherix***) ▶Immune system ♀C ▶? $$

ADULT – 0.5 mL IM for 1 dose given at least 2 weeks prior to potential exposure. May consider revaccination q 2 years in high-risk patients.

PEDS – Same as adult dose for age 2 yo or older.

NOTES – Recommended for travel to endemic areas.

TYPHOID VACCINE—LIVE ORAL (***Vivotif Berna***) ▶Immune system ♀C ▶? $$

ADULT – 1 cap 1 h before a meal with cold or lukewarm drink every other day for 4 doses to be completed at least 1 week prior to potential

(cont.)

TYPHOID VACCINE—LIVE ORAL *(cont.)*

exposure. May consider revaccination q 5 years in high-risk patients.

PEDS – Give adult dose for age 6 yo or older.

FORMS – Trade only: Caps.

NOTES – Recommended for travel to endemic areas. Oral vaccine may be inactivated by antibiotics, including antimalarials.

VARICELLA VACCINE (*Varivax*, ♣ *Varilrix*) ♀C ◗+ $$$$

ADULT – 0.5 mL SC. Repeat 4 to 8 weeks later.

PEDS – 0.5 mL SC for 1 dose for age 1 to 12 yo. Repeat at ages 4 yo, 6 yo. Use adult dose for age 13 yo or older. Not recommended for infants younger than 1 yo.

UNAPPROVED PEDS – Postexposure prophylaxis: 0.5 mL SC within 3 to 5 days of exposure.

NOTES – Do not inject IV. Following vaccination avoid pregnancy for 3 months and aspirin/salicylates for 6 weeks. This live vaccine is contraindicated in immunocompromised. Vaccine is stored in freezer; thawed vaccine must be used within 30 min.

YELLOW FEVER VACCINE (*YF-Vax*) ♀C ◗+ $$$

ADULT – 0.5 mL SC.

PEDS – 0.5 mL SC into thigh (6 mo to 3 yo) or deltoid region for age 3 yo or older.

NOTES – Must be accredited site to administer vaccination. International Certificate of Vaccination obligatory for some travel destinations. Consult CDC traveler's health website for accredited sites or to apply for accreditation. A booster dose (0.5 mL) may be administered q 10 years.

ZOSTER VACCINE—LIVE (*Zostavax*) ▶Immune system ♀C ◗? $$$$

ADULT – 0.65 mL SC for 1 dose for age 50 yo or older. However, ACIP recommends immunizing those 60 yo and older.

PEDS – Not approved in children.

NOTES – Avoid if history of anaphylactic/anaphylactoid reaction to gelatin or neomycin, if primary or acquired immunodeficiency states, or if taking immunosuppressives. Do not administer if active untreated TB or in possible pregnancy. Theoretically possible to transmit to pregnant household contact who has not had varicella infection or immunocompromised contact. Do not substitute for Varivax in children.

IMMUNOLOGY: Immunoglobulins

NOTE: Adult IM injections should be given in the deltoid region; injection in the gluteal region may result in suboptimal response.

ANTIVENIN—CROTALIDAE IMMUNE FAB OVINE POLYVALENT (*CroFab*) ▶? ♀C ◗? $$$$$

ADULT – Rattlesnake envenomation: Give 4 to 6 vials IV infusion over 60 min, within 6 h of bite if possible. Administer 4 to 6 additional vials if no initial control of envenomation syndrome, then 2 vials q 6 h for up to 18 h (3 doses) after initial control has been established.

PEDS – Same as adults, although specific studies in children have not been conducted.

NOTES – Contraindicated in allergy to papaya or papain. Start IV infusion slowly over the first 10 min at 25 to 50 mL/h and observe for allergic reaction, then increase to full rate of 250 mL/h.

ANTIVENIN—CROTALIDAE POLYVALENT ▶L ♀C ◗? $$$$$

ADULT – Pit viper envenomation: 20 to 40 mL (2 to 4 vials) IV infusion for minimal envenomation, 50 to 90 mL (5 to 9 vials) IV infusion for moderate envenomation; give at least 100 to 150 mL (10 to 15 vials) IV infusion for severe envenomation. Administer within 4 h of bite, less effective after 8 h, and of questionable value after 12 h. May give additional 10 to 50 mL (1 to 5 vials) IV infusion based on clinical assessment and response to initial dose.

PEDS – Larger relative doses of antivenin are needed in children and small adults because of small volume of body fluid to dilute the venom. The dose is not based on wt.

NOTES – Test first for sensitivity to horse serum. Serum sickness may occur 5 to 24 days after dose. IV route is preferred. May give IM.

ANTIVENIN—LATRODECTUS MACTANS ▶L ♀C ◗? $$

ADULT – Specialized dosing for black widow spider toxicity; consult poison center.

PEDS – Specialized dosing for black widow spider toxicity; consult poison center.

NOTES – Test first for horse serum sensitivity. Serum sickness may occur 5 to 24 days after dose.

BOTULISM IMMUNE GLOBULIN (*BabyBIG*) ▶L ♀? ◗? $$$$$

ADULT – Not approved in age 1 yo or older.

PEDS – Infant botulism: 1 mL (50 mg)/kg IV for age younger than 1 yo.

ADULT IMMUNIZATION SCHEDULE*
Tetanus, diphtheria (Td): For all ages, 1 dose booster q 10 years.
Pertussis: Consider single dose of pertussis in adults younger than 65 yo (as part of Tdap), at least 10 years since last tetanus dose. If patient has never received a pertussis booster use Boostrix if 10 to 18 yo, Adacel if 11 to 64 yo.
Influenza: 1 yearly dose if age 50 yo or older. If younger than 50 yo, then 1 yearly dose if healthcare worker, pregnant, chronic underlying illness, household contact of person with chronic underlying illness or household contact with children younger than 5 yo, or those who request vaccination. Intranasal vaccine indicated for healthy adults younger than 50 yo.
Pneumococcal (polysaccharide): 1 dose if age 65 yo or older. If younger than 65 yo, consider immunizing if chronic underlying illness, nursing home resident. Consider revaccination 5 years later if high risk or if age 65 yo or older and received primary dose before age 65 yo.
Hepatitis A: For all ages with clotting factor disorders, chronic liver disease, or exposure risk (travel to endemic areas, illegal drug use, men having sex with men), 2 doses (0, 6 to 12 months).
Hepatitis B: For all ages with medical (hemodialysis, clotting factor recipients, chronic liver disease), occupational (healthcare or public safety workers with blood exposure), behavioral (illegal drug use, multiple sex partners, those seeking evaluation or treatment of sexually transmitted disease, men having sex with men), or other (household/sex contacts of those with chronic HBV or HIV infections, clients/staff of developmentally disabled, more than 6 months of travel to high-risk areas, inmates of correctional facilities) indications, 3 doses (0, 1–2, 4–6 months). Hemodialysis patients require 4 doses and higher dose (40 mcg).
Measles, mumps, rubella (MMR): If born during or after 1957 and immunity in doubt, see www.cdc.gov.
Varicella: For all ages if immunity in doubt, age 13 yo or older, 2 doses separated by 4 to 8 weeks.
Meningococcal (conjugate vaccine is preferred for age 55 or younger): For all ages with medical indications (complement deficiency, anatomic or functional asplenia) or other indications (travel to endemic regions, college dormitory residents, military recruits), administer 1 dose. Consider revaccination in 3 to 5 years if high risk.
Human papillomavirus: Consider HPV vaccine in women 9 to 26 yo at 0, 2, and 6 months. Can be used in males 9 to 26 yo to decrease risk of genital warts.
Herpes zoster: Consider single dose of HZ vaccine in individuals for 60 or older.
Haemophilus influezae type b (Hib): 1 dose in high-risk adults (sickle cell, leukemia, HIV, splenectomy), if not previously immunized.

*2010 schedule from the CDC, ACIP, & AAFP, see: www.cdc.gov/vaccines/schedules

CYTOMEGALOVIRUS IMMUNE GLOBULIN HUMAN (***Cytogam***) ▶L ♀C ▶? $$$$$

ADULT – Specialized dosing based on indication and time since transplant.

PEDS – Specialized dosing based on indication and time since transplant.

HEPATITIS B IMMUNE GLOBULIN (***H-BIG, HyperHep B, HepaGam B, NABI-HB***) ▶L ♀C ▶? $$$

ADULT – Postexposure prophylaxis for needlestick, ocular, mucosal exposure: 0.06 mL/kg IM (usual dose 3 to 5 mL) within 24 h of exposure. Initiate hepatitis B vaccine series within 7 days. Consider a second dose of hepatitis B immune globulin (HBIG) 1 month later if patient refuses hepatitis B vaccine series. Postexposure prophylaxis for sexual exposure: 0.06 mL/kg IM within 14 days of sexual contact. Initiate hepatitis B vaccine series. Prevention of hepatitis B recurrence following liver transplantation in HBsAg-positive (HepaGam B): first dose given during transplantation surgery. Subsequent doses daily for 7 days, then biweekly up to 3 months and monthly thereafter. Doses adjusted based on regular monitoring of HBsAg, HBV-DNA, HBeAg, and anti-HBs antibody levels.

PEDS – Prophylaxis of infants born to HBsAg-positive mothers: 0.5 mL IM within 12 h of birth. Initiate hepatitis B vaccine series within 7 days. If hepatitis B vaccine series is refused, repeat HBIG dose at 3 and 6 mo. Household

(cont.)

HEPATITIS B IMMUNE GLOBULIN (*cont.*)

exposure age younger than 12 mo: Give 0.5 mL IM within 14 days of exposure. Initiate hepatitis B vaccine series.

NOTES – HBIG may be administered at the same time or up to 1 month prior to hepatitis B vaccine without impairing the active immune response from hepatitis B vaccine.

IMMUNE GLOBULIN—INTRAMUSCULAR (***Baygam, ✤ Gamastan***) ▶L ♀C ▶? $$$$

ADULT – Hepatitis A postexposure prophylaxis for household or institutional contacts: 0.02 mL/kg IM within 2 weeks of exposure. Hepatitis A pre-exposure prophylaxis (ie, travel to endemic area): Give 0.02 mL/kg IM for length of stay less than 3 months, give 0.06 mL/kg IM and repeat q 4 to 6 months for length of stay longer than 3 months. Measles: 0.2 to 0.25 mL/kg IM within 6 days of exposure, max 15 mL. Varicella zoster (if VariZIG unavailable): 0.6 to 1.2 mL/kg IM. Rubella exposure in pregnant, susceptible women: 0.55 mL/kg IM. Immunoglobulin deficiency: 0.66 mL/kg IM q 3 to 4 weeks.

PEDS – Not approved in children.

UNAPPROVED PEDS – Measles: 0.2 to 0.25 mL/kg IM within 6 days of exposure. In susceptible immunocompromised children use 0.5 mL/kg IM (max 15 mL) immediately after exposure. Varicella zoster (if VariZIG unavailable): 0.6 to 1.2 mL/kg IM.

NOTES – Human-derived product, increased infection risk. Hepatitis A vaccine preferred over immune globulin for age 2 yo or older who plan to travel to high-risk areas repeatedly or for long periods of time.

IMMUNE GLOBULIN—INTRAVENOUS (***Carimune, Flebogamma, Gammagard, Gammaplex, Gamunex, Octagam, Privigen***) ▶L ♀C ▶? $$$$$

WARNING – Renal dysfunction, acute renal failure, osmotic nephrosis, and death may be associated with IV immune globulins, especially those containing sucrose. Administer at the minimum concentration available and the minimum practical infusion rate.

ADULT – Idiopathic thrombocytopenic purpura (induction): 400 mg/kg IV daily for 5 days (or 1 g/kg IV daily for 1 to 2 days). Bone marrow transplant: 500 mg/kg IV daily, given 7 and 2 days before transplant, and then weekly until 90 days post transplant for age older than 20 yo. Primary humoral immunodeficiency: 200 to 300 mg/kg IV each month; increase prn to max 400 to 800 mg/kg/month. B-cell chronic lymphocytic leukemia: Specialized dosing. Chronic inflammatory demyelinating polyneuropathy (CIDP): (Gamunex) 2 g/kg IV loading dose followed by 1 g/kg IV q 3 weeks.

PEDS – Pediatric HIV: 400 mg/kg IV q 28 days. Idiopathic thrombocytopenic purpura (induction): 400 mg/kg IV daily for 5 days (or 1 g/kg IV daily for 1 to 2 days). Kawasaki syndrome (acute): 400 mg/kg IV daily for 4 days (or 2 g/kg IV for 1 dose over 10 h). Primary humoral immunodeficiency: 200 to 300 mg/kg IV each month; increase prn to max 400 to 800 mg/kg/month.

UNAPPROVED ADULT – First-line therapy in severe Guillain-Barré syndrome, chronic inflammatory demyelinating polyneuropathy, multifocal motor neuropathy, severe post-transfusion purpura, inclusion body myositis, fetomaternal alloimmune thrombocytopenia; 2nd-line therapy in stiff-person syndrome, dermatomyositis, myasthenia gravis, and Lambert-Eaton myasthenic syndrome. Various dosing regimens have been used; a common one is myasthenia gravis (induction): 400 mg/kg IV daily for 5 days (total 2 g/kg). Has been used in multiple sclerosis and inflammatory myositis (polymyositis and dermatomyositis), renal transplant rejection, systemic lupus erythematosus, toxic epidermal necrolysis and Stevens-Johnson syndrome, *Clostridium difficile* colitis, Graves' ophthalmopathy, pemphigus, Wegener's granulomatosis, Churg-Strauss syndrome, and Duchenne muscular dystrophy.

UNAPPROVED PEDS – Myasthenia gravis (induction): 400 mg/kg IV daily for 5 days. Other dosing regimens have been used.

NOTES – Indications and doses vary by product. Follow LFTs, renal function, vital signs, and urine output closely. Contraindicated in IgA deficiency. Use caution (and lower infusion rates) if risk factors for thrombosis, heart failure, or renal insufficiency. Use slower infusion rates for initial doses. Consider pretreatment with acetaminophen and/or diphenhydramine to minimize some infusion-related adverse effects. Human-derived product; although donors are carefully screened there is risk of transmission of infectious agents.

IMMUNE GLOBULIN—SUBCUTANEOUS (***Vivaglobulin, Hizentra***) ▶L ♀C ▶? $$$$$

ADULT – Primary immune deficiency: 100 to 200 mg/kg SC weekly. In patients already receiving IV immune globulin: SC dose is equivalent to previous IV dose multiplied by 1.37 then divided by frequency of IV regimen in weeks.

PEDS – Limited information. Dosing appears to be same as in adults.

(cont.)

IMMUNE GLOBULIN—SUBCUTANEOUS (*cont.*)

NOTES – Do not administer IV. Contraindicated in IgA deficiency. Human-derived product, increased infection risk.

LYMPHOCYTE IMMUNE GLOBULIN (*Atgam*) ▶L ♀C ▶? $$$$$

ADULT – Renal allograft recipients: 10 to 30 mg/kg IV daily. Delaying onset of allograft rejection: 15 mg/kg IV daily for 14 days, then every other day for 14 days. Treatment of renal transplant rejection: 10 to 15 mg/kg IV for 14 days. Aplastic anemia: 10 to 20 mg/kg IV daily for 8 to 14 days, then every other day prn, max 21 total doses.

PEDS – Limited experience. Has been safely administered to a limited number of children with renal transplant and aplastic anemia at doses comparable to adults.

NOTES – Equine product. Doses should be administered over at least 4 h.

RABIES IMMUNE GLOBULIN HUMAN (*Imogam Rabies-HT, HyperRAB S/D*) ▶L ♀C ▶? $$$$$

ADULT – Postexposure prophylaxis: 20 units/kg (0.133 mL/kg), with as much as possible infiltrated around the bite and the rest given IM. Give as soon as possible after exposure. Administer with the first dose of vaccine, but in a different extremity.

PEDS – Not approved in children.

UNAPPROVED PEDS – Use adult dosing.

NOTES – Do not repeat dose once rabies vaccine series begins. Do not give to patients who have been completely immunized with rabies vaccine. Do not administer IV.

RSV IMMUNE GLOBULIN (*RespiGam*) ▶Plasma ♀C ▶? $$$$$

PEDS – RSV prophylaxis: 1.5 mL/kg/h for 15 min for age younger than 24 mo. Increase rate as clinical condition permits to 3 mL/kg/h for 15 min, then to a maximum rate of 6 mL/kg/h. Max total dose/month is 750 mg/kg.

NOTES – May cause fluid overload; monitor vital signs frequently during IV infusion. RSV season is typically November through April.

TETANUS IMMUNE GLOBULIN (*BayTet*) ▶L ♀C ▶? $$$$

ADULT – See tetanus wound management table. Postexposure prophylaxis in tetanus-prone wounds for age 7 yo or older: If less than 3 doses of tetanus vaccine have been administered or if history is uncertain, give 250 units IM for 1 dose along with dT. If at least 3 doses of tetanus vaccine have been administered in the past, do not give tetanus immune globulin. Tetanus treatment: 3000 to 6000 units IM in combination with other therapies.

PEDS – 4 units/kg IM or 250 units IM for age younger than 7 yo. Initiate tetanus toxoid vaccine (DTP or DT).

NOTES – Do not give tetanus immune globulin for clean, minor wounds. May be given at the same time as tetanus toxoid active immunization. Do not inject IV.

VARICELLA-ZOSTER IMMUNE GLOBULIN (*VariZIG, VZIG*) ▶L ♀C ▶? $$$$$

ADULT – Specialized dosing for postexposure prophylaxis.

PEDS – Specialized dosing for postexposure prophylaxis.

IMMUNOLOGY: Immunosuppression

BASILIXIMAB (*Simulect*) ▶Plasma ♀B ▶? $$$$$

WARNING – To be used only by trained physicians. To be given only in facility with adequate laboratory and supportive medical resources.

ADULT – Specialized dosing for organ transplantation.

PEDS – Specialized dosing for organ transplantation.

BELATACEPT (*Nulojix*) ▶serum – ♀C ▶– $$$$$

WARNING – Should only be prescribed by physicians who are knowledgeable about the drug. Serious adverse effects have been reported.

ADULT – Specialized dosing for organ transplantation.

PEDS – Not approved in children.

FORMS – Injection.

CYCLOSPORINE (*Sandimmune, Neoral, Gengraf*) ▶L ♀C ▶– $$$$$

WARNING – Should only be prescribed by physicians who are knowledgeable about the drug. Serious adverse effects can occur.

ADULT – Specialized dosing for organ transplantation, RA, and psoriasis.

PEDS – Not approved in children.

UNAPPROVED ADULT – Specialized dosing for autoimmune eye disorders, vasculitis, inflammatory myopathies, Behcet's disease, psoriatic arthritis, chronic refractory idiopathic thrombocytopenia.

UNAPPROVED PEDS – Specialized dosing for organ transplantation, chronic refractory idiopathic thrombocytopenia.

FORMS – Generic/Trade: Microemulsion Caps 25, 100 mg. Generic/Trade: Caps (Sandimmune)

(cont.)

CYCLOSPORINE (*cont.*)

25, 100 mg. Soln (Sandimmune) 100 mg/mL. Microemulsion soln (Neoral, Gengraf) 100 mg/mL.

NOTES – Monitor cyclosporine blood concentrations closely. Many drug interactions including atorvastatin, azithromycin, lovastatin, oral contraceptives, rosuvastatin, simvastatin, sirolimus, terbinafine, voriconazole. Use caution when combining with methotrexate or potassium sparing drugs such as ACE inhibitors. Reduce dose in renal dysfunction. Monitor BP and renal function closely. Avoid excess UV light exposure. Monitor patients closely when switching from Sandimmune to microemulsion formulations.

DACLIZUMAB (*Zenapax*) ▸L ♀C ▸? $$$$$

WARNING – Should only be prescribed by physicians who are knowledgeable about the drug. Serious adverse effects have been reported.

ADULT – Specialized dosing for organ transplantation.

PEDS – Not approved in children.

UNAPPROVED PEDS – Specialized dosing for organ transplantation.

MYCOPHENOLATE MOFETIL (*Cellcept, Myfortic*) ▸? ♀D ▸? $$$$$

WARNING – Has been associated with lymphoma, malignancy, increased risk of infection, and progressive multifocal leukoencephalopathy (PML).

ADULT – Specialized dosing for organ transplantation.

PEDS – Not approved in children.

UNAPPROVED ADULT – Lupus nephritis: 1000 mg PO two times per day. Has been used in pemphigus, bullous pemphigoid, and refractory uveitis.

UNAPPROVED PEDS – Specialized dosing for organ transplantation.

FORMS – Generic/Trade: Caps 250 mg. Tabs 500 mg. Trade only (CellCept): Susp 200 mg/mL (175 mL). Trade only (Myfortic): Tabs extended-release: 180, 360 mg.

NOTES – Increased risk of 1st trimester pregnancy loss and increased risk of congenital malformations, especially external ear and facial abnormalities.

SIROLIMUS (*Rapamune*) ▸L ♀C ▸– $$$$$

WARNING – Increased risk of infection and lymphoma. Combination of sirolimus plus cyclosporine or tacrolimus is associated with hepatic artery thrombosis in liver transplant patients. Combination with tacrolimus and corticosteroids in lung transplant patients may cause bronchial anastomotic dehiscence. Possible increased mortality in stable liver transplant patients after conversion from a calcineurin inhibitor (CNI)–based immunosuppressive regimen to sirolimus. Can cause hypersensitivity reactions including anaphylactic and/or anaphylactoid reactions, angioedema, vasculitis. Avoid with strong inhibitors of CYP3A4 and/or P-glycoprotein (ketoconazole, voriconazole, itraconazole, erythromycin, clarithromycin) or strong inducers of CYP3A4 and/or P-glycoprotein (rifampin, rifabutin). Monitor level if cyclosporine is discontinued or dose has markedly changed.

ADULT – Specialized dosing for organ transplantation.

PEDS – Not approved in children.

UNAPPROVED PEDS – Specialized dosing for organ transplantation.

FORMS – Trade only: Soln 1 mg/mL (60 mL). Tabs 1, 2 mg.

NOTES – Wear protective clothing and sunscreen when exposed to sunlight to reduce the risk of skin cancer. Be aware of site-specific assay method, as this may affect reported serum concentrations. Adjust dose by ⅓ to ½ in liver dysfunction. Monitor trough levels, particularly in patients likely to have altered drug metabolism, age 13 yo or older with wt less than 40 kg, hepatic impairment, when changing doses, or with interacting medications. Do not adjust dose more frequently than q 1 to 2 weeks. Oral soln and tabs are clinically equivalent from a dosing standpoint at the 2 mg level; however, this is unknown at higher doses.

TACROLIMUS (*Prograf, FK 506*) ▸L ♀C ▸– $$$$$

WARNING – Has been associated with lymphoma, malignancy, increased risk of infection, Should only be prescribed by physicians who are knowledgeable about the drug. To be given only in facility with adequate laboratory and supportive medical resources.

ADULT – Specialized dosing for organ transplantation.

PEDS – Specialized dosing for organ transplantation.

UNAPPROVED ADULT – RA (approved in Canada), active vasculitis, systemic lupus erythematosus nephritis, and vasculitis.

FORMS – Generic/Trade: Caps 0.5, 1, 5 mg.

NOTES – Reduce dose in renal dysfunction. Monitor BP and renal function closely. Neurotoxic, especially in high doses. Many drug interactions. Increased risk of infections.

IMMUNOLOGY: Other

HYMENOPTERA VENOM ▶Serum ♀C ▶? $$$$

ADULT – Specialized desensitization dosing protocol.

PEDS – Specialized desensitization dosing protocol.

NOTES – Venom products available: Honey bee (*Apis mellifera*) and yellow jacket (*Vespula* sp.), yellow hornet (*Dolichovespula arenaria*), white-faced hornet (*D. maculata*) and wasp (*Polistes* sp.). Mixed vespid venom protein (yellow jacket, yellow hornet, and white-faced hornet) is also available.

RILONACEPT (***Arcalyst***) ▶? ♀? ▶? $$$$$

ADULT – Familial cold auto-inflammatory syndrome (FCAS) and Muckle-Wells syndrome (MWS): Begin therapy with a loading dose of 320 mg (160 mg SC on the same day at two different sites), then 160 mg SC once weekly.

PEDS – Familial cold auto-inflammatory syndrome (FCAS) and Muckle-Wells syndrome (MWS): Begin therapy with a loading dose of 4.4 mg/kg (to a maximum of 320 mg) SC in one or two doses, then 2.2 mg/kg (to a max of 160 mg) SC once weekly.

NOTES – Increased risk of infections.

TUBERCULIN PPD (***Aplisol, Tubersol, Mantoux, PPD***) ▶L ♀C ▶+ $

ADULT – 5 tuberculin unites (0.1 mL) intradermally.

PEDS – Same as adult dose. AAP recommends screening at 12 mo, 4 to 6 yo, and 14 to 16 yo.

NOTES – Avoid SC injection. Read 48 to 72 h after intradermal injection. Repeat testing in patients with known prior positive PPD; may cause scarring at injection site.

NEUROLOGY: Alzheimer's Disease—Cholinesterase Inhibitors

NOTE: Avoid concurrent use of anticholinergic agents. Use caution in asthma/COPD. May be co-administered with memantine.

DONEPEZIL (***Aricept***) ▶LK ♀C ▶? $$$$

ADULT – Alzheimer's disease: Start 5 mg PO at bedtime. May increase to 10 mg PO at bedtime in 4 to 6 weeks. Max 10 mg/day for mild to moderate disease. For moderate to severe disease (MMSE 10 or less), may increase after 3 months to 23 mg/day.

PEDS – Not approved in children.

UNAPPROVED ADULT – Dementia in Parkinson's disease: 5 to 10 mg/day.

FORMS – Generic/Trade: Tabs 5, 10 mg, Orally disintegrating tabs 5, 10 mg. Trade only: Tab 23 mg.

NOTES – Some clinicians start with 5 mg PO every other day to minimize GI side effects.

GALANTAMINE (***Razadyne, Razadyne ER,*** ✤ ***Reminyl***) ▶LK ♀B ▶? $$$$

ADULT – Alzheimer's disease: Extended-release: Start 8 mg PO q am with food; increase to 16 mg q am after 4 weeks. May increase to 24 mg q am after another 4 weeks. Immediate-release: Start 4 mg PO two times per day with food; increase to 8 mg two times per day after 4 weeks. May increase to 12 mg PO two times per day after another 4 weeks.

PEDS – Not approved in children.

UNAPPROVED ADULT – Dementia in Parkinson's disease: 4 to 8 mg PO two times per day (immediate-release).

FORMS – Generic/Trade: Tabs 4, 8, 12 mg. Extended-release caps 8, 16, 24 mg. Oral soln 4 mg/mL. Prior to April 2005 was called Reminyl in the United States.

NOTES – Do not exceed 16 mg/day in renal or hepatic impairment. Use caution with CYP3A4 and CYP2D6 inhibitors. Avoid abrupt discontinuation. If therapy has been interrupted for several days or more, then restart at the lowest dose.

RIVASTIGMINE (***Exelon, Exelon Patch***) ▶K ♀B ▶? $$$$$

ADULT – Alzheimer's disease: Start 1.5 mg PO two times per day with food. Increase to 3 mg two times per day after 2 weeks. Usual effective dose is 6 to 12 mg/day. Max 12 mg/day. Patch: Start 4.6 mg/24 h once daily; may increase after 1 month or more to max 9.5 mg/24 h. Rotate sites. Dementia in Parkinson's disease: Start 1.5 mg PO two times per day with food. Increase by 3 mg/day at intervals more than 4 weeks to max 12 mg/day. Patch: Use dosing for Alzheimer's disease.

PEDS – Not approved in children.

FORMS – Trade only: Caps 1.5, 3, 4.5, 6 mg. Oral soln 2 mg/mL (120 mL). Transdermal patch: 4.6 mg/24 h (9 mg/patch), 9.5 mg/24 h (18 mg/patch).

NOTES – Restart treatment with the lowest daily dose (ie, 1.5 mg PO two times per day) if discontinued for several days to reduce the risk of severe vomiting. When changing from PO to patch, patients taking less than 6 mg/day can be placed on 4.6 mg/24 h patch. For

(cont.)

RIVASTIGMINE (*cont.*)

those taking 6 to 12 mg/day, may start with 9.5 mg/24 h patch. Have patient start the day after stopping oral dosing. Rotate application sites and do not apply to same spot for 14 days.

TACRINE (***Cognex***) ▶L ♀C ▶? $$$$$

ADULT – Alzheimer's disease (not first line): Start 10 mg PO four times per day for 4 weeks, then increase to 20 mg four times per day. Titrate to higher doses q 4 weeks as tolerated. Max 160 mg/day.

PEDS – Not approved in children.

FORMS – Trade only: Caps 10, 20, 30, 40 mg.

NOTES – Hepatotoxicity may occur. Monitor LFTs q 2 weeks for 16 weeks, then q 3 months.

NEUROLOGY: Alzheimer's Disease—NMDA Receptor Antagonists

MEMANTINE (***Namenda, Namenda XR,*** ✣ ***Ebixa***) ▶KL ♀B ▶? $$$$$

ADULT – Alzheimer's disease (moderate to severe): Start 5 mg PO daily. Increase by 5 mg/day at weekly intervals to max 20 mg/day. Doses greater than 5 mg/day should be divided two times per day. Extended-release: Start 7 mg once daily. Increase at weekly intervals to target dose of 28 mg/day. Reduce to 14 mg/day in renal impairment.

PEDS – Not approved in children.

FORMS – Generic/Trade: Tabs 5, 10 mg. Trade only: Oral soln 2 mg/mL. Extended-release caps 7, 14, 21, 28 mg.

NOTES – May be used in combination with acetylcholinesterase inhibitors. Reduce target dose to 5 mg PO two times per day in severe renal impairment (CrCl 5 to 29 mL/min). No dosage adjustment needed for mild to moderate renal impairment. When switching to extended-release caps patients taking 10 mg two times per day can be changed to 28 mg/day of ER after last regular dose. Patients switched from 5 mg two times per day can be changed to 14 mg/day of ER.

NEUROLOGY: Anticonvulsants

NOTE: Avoid rapid discontinuation of anticonvulsants, since this can precipitate seizures or other withdrawal symptoms. Recent data suggest an increased risk of suicidal ideation or behaviors with antiepileptic drugs. Monitor closely for signs of depression, anxiety, hostility, hypomania/mania, or suicidality. Symptoms may develop within 1 week of initiation, and risk continues for at least 24 weeks.

CARBAMAZEPINE (***Tegretol, Tegretol XR, Carbatrol, Epitol, Equetro***) ▶LK ♀D ▶+ $$

WARNING – Risk of aplastic anemia, agranulocytosis, and hyponatremia; contraindicated if prior bone marrow depression. Monitor CBC and serum sodium at baseline and periodically.

ADULT – Epilepsy: Start 200 mg PO twice per day. Increase by 200 mg/day at weekly intervals, divided into two to four doses per day (immediate-release), or two times per day (extended-release), or four times per day (susp) to max 1600 mg/day. Trigeminal neuralgia: Start 100 mg PO twice per day or 50 mg PO four times per day (susp); increase by 200 mg/day until pain relief. Max 1200 mg/day. Bipolar disorder, acute manic/mixed episodes (Equetro): Start 200 mg PO two times per day; increase by 200 mg/day to max 1600 mg/day. See UNAPPROVED ADULT for alternative bipolar dosing.

PEDS – Epilepsy, age younger than 6 yo: Start 10 to 20 mg/kg/day PO divided two to three doses per day or four times per day (susp). Increase weekly prn. Max 35 mg/kg/day. Epilepsy, age 6 to 12 yo: Start 100 mg PO twice per day or 50 mg PO four times per day (susp); increase by 100 mg/day at weekly intervals divided into three or four doses per day (immediate-release), two times per day (extended-release), or four times per day (susp) to max 1000 mg/day. Epilepsy, age 13 yo or older: Start 200 mg PO twice per day or 100 mg PO four times per day (susp); increase by 200 mg/day at weekly intervals, divided into three or four doses per day (immediate release), two times per day (extended-release), or four times per day (susp) to max 1000 mg/day (age 13 to 15 yo) or 1200 mg/day (age older than 15 yo).

UNAPPROVED ADULT – Neuropathic pain: Start 100 mg PO two times per day; usual effective dose is 200 mg PO two to four times per day. Max 1200 mg/day.

UNAPPROVED PEDS – Bipolar disorder (manic or mixed phase): Start 100 to 200 mg PO daily

(cont.)

CARBAMAZEPINE (*cont.*)

or two times per day; titrate to usual effective dose of 200 to 600 mg/day for children and up to 1200 mg/day for adolescents.

FORMS – Generic/Trade: Tabs 200 mg, Chewable tabs 100 mg, Susp 100 mg/5 mL. Extended-release tabs (Tegretol XR) 100, 200, 400 mg. Generic only: Tabs 100, 300, 400 mg, Chewable tabs 200 mg. Trade only: Extended-release caps (Carbatrol and Equetro): 100, 200, 300 mg.

NOTES – Usual therapeutic level is 4 to 12 mcg/mL. Stevens-Johnson syndrome, hepatitis, aplastic anemia, and hyponatremia may occur. Monitor CBC and LFTs. Many drug interactions. Should not be used for absence or atypical absence seizures. Dangerous and possibly fatal skin reactions are more common with the HLA-B*1502 allele (most common in people of Asian and Indian ancestry); screen new patients for this allele prior to starting therapy.

CLOBAZAM (*ONFI*, ✤*Frisium*) ▶L ♀X (first trimester) D (second/third trimesters) ▶–©IV $

WARNING – Use caution in the elderly; may accumulate and cause side effects such as psychomotor impairment.

ADULT – Canada only. Epilepsy, adjunctive: Start 5 to 15 mg PO daily. Gradually increase prn to max 80 mg/day.

PEDS – United States, epilepsy, adjunctive. Adults and children 2 yo and older, weight greater than 30 kg: Start 5 mg PO twice per day. Increase to 10 mg PO twice daily after 1 week then to 20 mg PO twice daily after 2 weeks. Weight 30 kg or less: Start 5 mg PO daily. Increase to 5 mg PO twice per day after 1 week, then 10 mg PO twice per day after 2 weeks. Canada, epilepsy, adjunctive: Start 0.5 to 1 mg/kg PO daily for age younger than 2 yo or 5 mg daily for age 2 to 16 yo: Then may increase prn to max 40 mg/day.

FORMS – Generic/Trade: Tabs 10 mg.

NOTES – Reduce dose in hepatic or renal dysfunction. Drug interactions with enzyme-inducing anticonvulsants such as carbamazepine and phenytoin; may need to adjust dose.

ETHOSUXIMIDE (*Zarontin*) ▶LK ♀C ▶+ $$$$

ADULT – Absence seizures: Start 500 mg PO given once daily or divided twice per day. Increase by 250 mg/day q 4 to 7 days prn. Max 1.5 g/day.

PEDS – Absence seizures: Start 250 mg PO daily or divided two times per day(up to 500 mg/day) for age 3 to 6 yo. Use adult dosing for age older than 6 yo.

UNAPPROVED PEDS – Absence seizures, age younger than 3 yo: Start 15 mg/kg/day PO divided two times per day. Increase q 4 to 7 days prn. Usual effective dose is 15 to 40 mg/kg/day divided two times per day. Max 500 mg/day.

FORMS – Generic/Trade: Caps 250 mg. Syrup 250 mg/5 mL.

NOTES – Usual therapeutic level is 40 to 100 mcg/mL. Monitor CBC for blood dyscrasias. Use caution in hepatic and renal impairment. May increase the risk of grand mal seizures in some patients.

ETHOTOIN (*Peganone*) ▶L ♀C ▶+ $$$$

ADULT – Generalized tonic-clonic or complex partial seizures: Start 1 g or less per day given in 4 to 6 divided doses. Usual effective dose is 2 to 3 g/day.

PEDS – Generalized tonic-clonic or complex partial seizures: Star 750 mg/day or less in 4 to 6 divided doses. Usual effective dose is 0.5 to 1 g/day. Max 2 to 3 g/day.

FORMS – Trade only: Tabs 250 mg.

NOTES – Usual therapeutic level is 15 to 50 mcg/mL. Doses less than 2 g/day are usually ineffective in adults. Give after food to reduce GI side effects.

EZOGABINE (*POTIGA*) ▶KL – ♀C ▶?

ADULT – Partial-onset seizures, adjunctive: Start 100 mg PO three times per day. Increase weekly by no more than 50 mg three times daily to usual maintenance dose of 200 to 400 mg PO three times daily or max of 250 mg three times daily if older than 65 yo.

PEDS – Not approved for use in children or adolescents.

FORMS – Trade: Tabs 50, 200, 300, 400 mg.

NOTES – Taper dose over at least 3 weeks when discontinuing. Reduce dose to max of 200 mg three times daily for CrCl less than 50 mL/min or severe hepatic impairment, or 250 mg three times daily for moderate hepatic impairment.

FELBAMATE (*Felbatol*) ▶KL ♀C ▶– $$$$$

WARNING – Aplastic anemia and fatal hepatic failure have occurred.

ADULT – Severe, refractory epilepsy: Start 400 mg PO three times per day. Increase by 600 mg/day q 2 weeks to max 3600 mg/day.

PEDS – Lennox-Gastaut syndrome, adjunctive therapy, age 2 to 14 yo: Start 15 mg/kg/day PO in 3 to 4 divided doses. Increase by 15 mg/kg/day at weekly intervals to max 45 mg/kg/day.

FORMS – Generic/Trade: Tabs 400, 600 mg, Oral susp 600 mg/5 mL.

NOTES – Not a first-line agent. Use only after discussing the risks and obtaining written informed consent. Many drug interactions.

Dermatomes

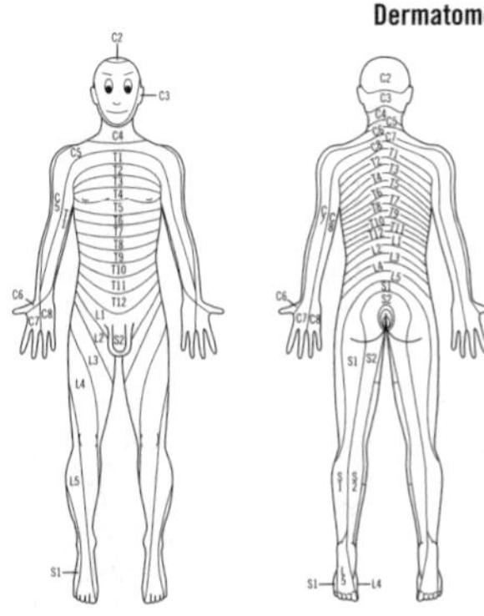

MOTOR FUNCTION BY NERVE ROOTS

Level	*Motor Function*
C3/C4/C5	Diaphragm
C5/C6	Deltoid/biceps
C7/C8	Triceps
C8/T1	Finger flexion/ intrinsics
T1–T12	Intercostal/ abd muscles
L2/L3	Hip flexion
L2/L3/L4	Hip adductor/quads
L4/L5	Ankle dorsiflexion
S1/S2	Ankle plantarflexion
S2/S3/S4	Rectal tone

LUMBOSACRAL NERVE ROOT COMPRESSIONS	*Root*	*Motor*	*Sensory*	*Reflex*
	L4	quadriceps	medial foot	knee-jerk
	L5	dorsiflexors	dorsum of foot	medial hamstring
	S1	plantarflexors	lateral foot	ankle-jerk

GLASGOW COMA SCALE

Eye Opening	*Verbal Activity*	*Motor Activity*
		6. Obeys commands
	5. Oriented	5. Localizes pain
4. Spontaneous	4. Confused	4. Withdraws to pain
3. To command	3. Inappropriate	3. Flexion to pain
2. To pain	2. Incomprehensible	2. Extension to pain
1. None	1. None	1. None

FOSPHENYTOIN (***Cerebyx***) ▶L ♀D ▶+ $$$$$

ADULT – Status epilepticus: Load 15 to 20 mg "phenytoin equivalents" (PE) per kg IV no faster than 100 to 150 mg PE/min. Nonemergent loading dose: 10 to 20 mg PE/kg IM/IV at rate no greater than 150 mg/min. Maintenance: 4 to 6 mg PE/kg/day.

PEDS – Not approved in children.

UNAPPROVED PEDS – Status epilepticus: 15 to 20 mg PE/kg IV at a rate less than 2 mg PE/kg/min. Nonemergent use age older than 7 yo: 4 to 6 mg PE/kg/24 h IV/IM no faster than 100 to 150 mg PE/min.

NOTES – Fosphenytoin is dosed in phenytoin equivalents (PE). Use beyond 5 days has not been systematically studied. Monitor ECG and vital signs continuously during and after infusion. Contraindicated in cardiac conduction block. Many drug interactions. Usual therapeutic level is 10 to 20 mcg/mL in normal hepatorenal function. Renal/hepatic disease may change protein binding and levels. Low albumin levels may increase free fraction.

GABAPENTIN (***Neurontin, Horizant, Gralise***) ▶K ♀C ▶? $$$$

ADULT – Partial seizures, adjunctive therapy: Start 300 mg PO at bedtime. Increase gradually to usual effective dose of 300 to 600 mg PO three times per day. Max 3600 mg/day divided three times per day. Partial seizures, initial monotherapy: Titrate as above. Usual effective dose is 900 to 1800 mg/day. Postherpetic neuralgia, immediate-release tabs: Start 300 mg PO on day 1. Increase to 300 mg twice per day on day 2, and to 300 mg three times per day on day 3. Max 1800 mg/day divided three times per day. Postherpetic neuralgia (Gralise): Start 300 mg PO once daily with evening meal. Increase to 600 mg on day 2, 900 mg on days 3 to 6, 1200 mg on days 7 to 10, 1500 mg on days 11 to 14, and 1800 mg on day 15. Max 1800 mg/day.

(cont.)

GABAPENTIN (*cont.*)

Restless legs syndrome (Horizant): 600 mg PO once daily around 5 pm taken with food.

PEDS – Partial seizures, adjunctive therapy: Start 10 to 15 mg/kg/day PO divided three times per day for age 3 to 12 yo. Titrate over 3 days to usual effective dose of 25 to 40 mg/kg/day divided three times per day. Max 50 mg/kg/day. Use adult dosing for age older than 12 yo.

UNAPPROVED ADULT – Partial seizures, initial monotherapy: Titrate as indicated in ADULTS. Usual effective dose is 900 to 1800 mg/day. Neuropathic pain: 300 mg PO three times per day, max 3600 mg/day in 3 to 4 divided doses. Migraine prophylaxis: Start 300 mg PO daily, then gradually increase to 1200 to 2400 mg/day in 3 to 4 divided doses. Restless legs syndrome: Start 300 mg PO at bedtime. Max 3600 mg/day divided three times per day. Hot flashes: 300 mg PO three times per day.

UNAPPROVED PEDS – Neuropathic pain: Start 5 mg/kg PO at bedtime. Increase to 5 mg/kg twice per day on day 2, and 5 mg/kg three times per day on day 3. Titrate to usual effective level of 8 to 35 mg/kg/24 h.

FORMS – Generic only: Tabs 100, 300, 400 mg. Generic/Trade: Caps 100, 300, 400 mg. Tabs scored 600, 800 mg. Soln 50 mg/mL. Trade only: Tabs, extended release 600 mg (gabapentin enacarbil, Horizant). Trade only (Gralise): Tabs 300, 600 mg.

NOTES – Reduce dose in renal impairment (CrCl less than 60 mL/min); table in prescribing information. Discontinue gradually over 1 week or longer. Do not substitute other brands for Gralise because of bioavailability differences.

LACOSAMIDE (*Vimpat*) ▶KL ♀C ▶? $$$$$

ADULT – Partial onset seizures, adjunctive (17 yo and older): Start 50 mg PO/IV two times per day. Increase by 50 mg two times per day to recommended dose of 100 to 200 mg two times per day. Max 600 mg/day or 300 mg/day in mild to moderate hepatic failure or severe renal impairment (CrCl less than 30 mL/min).

PEDS – Not approved in children.

FORMS – Trade only: Tabs 50, 100, 150, 200 mg.

NOTES – Use caution in patients with cardiac conduction problems or on drugs that increase the PR interval.

LAMOTRIGINE (*Lamictal, Lamictal CD, Lamictal ODT*) ▶LK ♀C (see notes) ▶– $$$$

WARNING – Potentially life-threatening rashes (eg, Stevens-Johnson syndrome) have been reported in 0.3% of adults and 0.8% of children, usually within 2 to 8 weeks of initiation; discontinue at first sign of rash. Drug interaction with valproate; see adjusted dosing guidelines.

ADULT – Partial seizures, Lennox-Gastaut syndrome, or generalized tonic-clonic seizures, adjunctive therapy with an enzyme-inducing anticonvulsant (age older than 12 yo): Start 50 mg PO daily for 2 weeks, then 50 mg PO twice per day for 2 weeks. Increase by 100 mg/day q 1 to 2 weeks to usual maintenance dose of 150 to 250 mg PO twice per day. Partial seizures, conversion to monotherapy from adjunctive therapy with a single enzyme-inducing anticonvulsant (age 16 yo and older): Use above guidelines to gradually increase the dose to 250 mg PO twice per day; then taper the enzyme-inducing anticonvulsant by 20% per week over 4 weeks. Partial seizures, Lennox-Gastaut syndrome, or generalized tonic-clonic seizures, adjunctive therapy with valproate (age older than 12 yo): Start 25 mg PO every other day for 2 weeks, then 25 mg PO daily for 2 weeks. Increase by 25 to 50 mg/day q 1 to 2 weeks to usual maintenance dose of 100 to 400 mg/day (when used with valproate and other anticonvulsants) or 100 to 200 mg/day (when used with valproate alone) given once daily or divided twice per day. Partial seizures, conversion to monotherapy from adjunctive therapy with valproate (age 16 yo and older): Use above guidelines to gradually increase the dose to 200 mg/day PO given daily or divided twice per day; then decrease valproate weekly in increments less than or equal to 500 mg/day to an initial goal of 500 mg/day. After 1 week at these doses, increase lamotrigine to 300 mg/day and decrease valproate to 250 mg/day divided twice per day. A week later, discontinue valproate; then increase lamotrigine weekly by 100 mg/day to usual maintenance dose of 500 mg/day. Partial seizures, Lennox-Gastaut syndrome, or generalized tonic-clonic seizures, adjunctive therapy with other anticonvulsants (not valproate or enzyme inducers; age older than 12 yo): Start 25 mg PO daily for 2 weeks, then 50 mg PO daily for 2 weeks. Increase by 50 mg/day q 1 to 2 weeks to usual maintenance dose of 225 to 375 mg/day divided twice per day. See psychiatry section for bipolar disorder dosing.

PEDS – Partial seizures, Lennox-Gastaut syndrome or generalized tonic-clonic seizures, adjunctive therapy with an enzyme-inducing anticonvulsant, age 2 to 12 yo: Start 0.6 mg/kg/day PO divided twice per day for 2 weeks,

(cont.)

LAMOTRIGINE (*cont.*)

then 1.2 mg/kg/day PO divided twice per day for 2 weeks. Increase q 1 to 2 weeks by 1.2 mg/kg/day (rounded down to the nearest whole tab) to usual maintenance dose of 5 to 15 mg/kg/day. Max 400 mg/day. Partial seizures, Lennox-Gastaut syndrome, or generalized tonic-clonic seizures, adjunctive therapy with valproate, age 2 to 12 yo: Start 0.15 mg/kg/day PO (given daily or divided twice per day) for 2 weeks, then 0.3 mg/kg/day PO (given daily or divided twice per day) for 2 weeks. Increase every 1 to 2 weeks by 0.3 mg/kg/day (rounded down to nearest whole tab) to usual maintenance dose of 1 to 5 mg/kg/day (lamotrigine + valproate and other anticonvulsants) or 1 to 3 mg/kg/day if used with valproate alone. Max 200 mg/day. Partial seizures, Lennox-Gastaut syndrome, or generalized tonic-clonic seizures, adjunctive therapy with other anticonvulsants (not valproate or enzyme inducers), age 2 to 12 yo: Start 0.3 mg/kg/day (given daily or divided twice per day) for 2 weeks, then 0.6 mg/kg/day for 2 weeks. Increase every 1 to 2 weeks by 0.6 mg/kg/day (rounded down to nearest whole tab) to usual maintenance dose of 4.5 to 7.5 mg/kg/day. Max 300 mg/day. Age older than 12 yo: Use adult dosing for all of the above indications.

UNAPPROVED ADULT – Initial monotherapy for partial seizures: Start 25 mg PO daily. Usual maintenance dose is 100 to 300 mg/day divided twice per day. Max 500 mg/day.

UNAPPROVED PEDS – Initial monotherapy for partial seizures: Start 0.5 mg/kg/day given daily or divided twice per day. Max 10 mg/kg/day. Newly diagnosed absence seizures: Titrate as indicated in PEDS section. Usual effective dose is 2 to 15 mg/kg/day.

FORMS – Generic/Trade: Tabs, 25, 100, 150, 200 mg. Trade only: Chewable dispersible tabs (Lamictal CD) 2, 5, 25 mg. Trade only: Orally disintegrating tabs (Lamictal ODT) 25, 50, 100, 200 mg. Chewable dispersible tabs (Lamictal CD) 2 mg may not be available in all pharmacies; obtain through manufacturer representative, or by calling 888-825-5249.

NOTES – Drug interactions with valproate and enzyme-inducing antiepileptic drugs (ie, carbamazepine, phenobarbital, phenytoin, primidone); may need to adjust dose. May increase carbamazepine toxicity. Women taking estrogen-containing oral contraceptives without an enzyme-inducing anticonvulsant will generally require an increase of the lamotrigine maintenance dose by up to 2-fold. Consider increasing the lamotrigine dose when the contraceptive is started. Taper lamotrigine by 25% or less of daily dose q week over a 2-week period if the contraceptive is stopped. Preliminary evidence suggests that exposure during the first trimester of pregnancy is associated with a risk of cleft palate and/or cleft lip.

LEVETIRACETAM (*Keppra, Keppra XR*) ▶K ♀C ▶? $$$$$

ADULT – Partial seizures, juvenile myoclonic epilepsy (JME), or primary generalized tonic-clonic seizures (GTC), adjunctive therapy: Start 500 mg PO/IV twice per day (Keppra, IV route not approved for GTC) or 1000 mg PO daily (Keppra XR, partial seizures only); increase by 1000 mg/day q 2 weeks prn to max 3000 mg/day (partial seizures) or to target dose of 3000 mg/day (JME or GTC).

PEDS – Partial seizures, adjunctive therapy for age older than 4 yo: Start 20 mg/kg/day PO (or IV if 16 yo or older) divided twice per day. Increase q 2 weeks as tolerated to target dose of 60 mg/kg/day. Juvenile myoclonic epilepsy, adjunctive therapy, age 12 yo or older: See adult dosing (IV approved for 16 yo or older only). Primary generalized tonic-clonic seizures (GTC), adjunctive therapy, age 6 to 15 yo: Start 20 mg/kg/day PO (or IV if 16 yo or older) divided twice per day. Increase by 20 mg/kg/day q 2 weeks to target dose of 60 mg/kg/day.

UNAPPROVED ADULT – Myoclonus: Start 500 to 1000 mg/day in divided doses. May increase to max 1500 to 3000 mg/day or 50 mg/kg/day.

FORMS – Generic/Trade: Tabs 250, 500, 750, 1000 mg, Oral soln 100 mg/mL, Tabs extended-release 500, 750 mg.

NOTES – Drug interactions unlikely. Decrease dose in renal dysfunction (CrCl less than 80 mL/min). Emotional lability, hostility, and depression may occur. Use same dose when switching between IV and PO forms.

METHSUXIMIDE (*Celontin*) ▶L ♀C ▶? $$$

ADULT – Refractory absence seizures: Start 300 mg PO daily; increase weekly by 300 mg/day. Max 1200 mg/day.

PEDS – Refractory absence seizures: Start 10 to 15 mg/kg/day PO in 3 to 4 divided doses; increase weekly prn. Max 30 mg/kg/day.

FORMS – Trade only: Caps 150, 300 mg.

NOTES – Monitor CBC, UA, and LFTs.

OXCARBAZEPINE (*Trileptal*) ▶LK ♀C ▶– $$$$$

WARNING – Serious multiorgan hypersensitivity reactions and life-threatening rashes (eg, Stevens-Johnson syndrome, toxic epidermal necrolysis) have occurred, with some

(cont.)

OXCARBAZEPINE (*cont.*)

fatalities. Consider discontinuation if skin reactions occur.

ADULT – Partial seizures, monotherapy: Start 300 mg PO two times per day. Increase by 300 mg/day q 3 days to usual effective dose of 1200 mg/day. Max 2400 mg/day. Partial seizures, adjunctive: Start 300 mg PO two times per day. Increase by no more than 600 mg/day at weekly intervals to usual effective dose of 1200 mg/day. Max 2400 mg/day.

PEDS – Partial seizures, adjunctive, age 2 to 16 yo: Start 8 to 10 mg/kg/day PO divided two times per day (max starting dose 600 mg/day). Titrate to max 60 mg/kg/day for age 2 to younger than 4 yo, titrate to max 900 mg/day for wt 20 to 29 kg, titrate to max 1200 mg/day for wt 29.1 to 39 kg, titrate to max 1800 mg/day for wt greater than 39 kg. Consider using a starting dose of 16 to 20 mg/kg for children age 2 to younger than 4 yo who weigh less than 20 kg to account for more rapid clearance. Partial seizures, initial monotherapy, age 4 to 16 yo: Start 8 to 10 mg/kg/day divided two times per day. Increase by 5 mg/kg/day q 3 days to recommended dose (in mg/day based on wt rounded to nearest 5 kg) as follows: 600 to 900 for wt 20 kg, 900 to 1200 for wt 25 and 30 kg, 900 to 1500 for wt 35 and 40 kg, 1200 to 1500 for wt 45 kg, 1200 to 1800 for wt 50 and 55 kg, 1200 to 2100 for wt 60 and 65 kg, 1500 to 2100 for wt 70 kg. Partial seizures, conversion to monotherapy, age 4 to 16 yo: Start 8 to 10 mg/kg/day divided two times per day. Increase at weekly intervals by no more than 10 mg/kg/day to target dose listed for initial monotherapy.

FORMS – Generic/Trade: Tabs (scored) 150, 300, 600 mg. Trade only: Oral susp 300 mg/5 mL.

NOTES – Monitor serum sodium. Decrease initial dose by ½ in renal dysfunction (CrCl less than 30 mL/min). Inhibits CYP2C19 and induces CYP3A4/5. Interactions with other antiepileptic drugs, oral contraceptives, and dihydropyridine calcium channel blockers.

PHENOBARBITAL (***Luminal***) ▶L ♀D ▶– ©IV $

ADULT – Epilepsy: 100 to 300 mg/day PO divided one to two times per day. Status epilepticus: 20 mg/kg IV at rate no faster than 60 mg/min.

PEDS – Epilepsy: 3 to 5 mg/kg/day PO divided two to three times per day. Status epilepticus: 20 mg/kg IV at rate no faster than 60 mg/min.

UNAPPROVED ADULT – Status epilepticus: May give up to a total dose of 30 mg/kg IV.

UNAPPROVED PEDS – Status epilepticus: 15 to 20 mg/kg IV load; may give additional 5 mg/kg doses q 15 to 30 mins to max total dose of 30 mg/kg. Epilepsy: Give 3 to 5 mg/kg/day given once daily or divided two times per day for neonates, give 5 to 6 mg/kg/day once daily or divided two times per day for infants, give 6 to 8 mg/kg/day given once daily or divided two times per day for age 1 to 5 yo, give 4 to 6 mg/kg/day once daily or divided two times per day for age 6 to 12 yo, give 1 to 3 mg/kg/day once daily or divided two times per day for age older than 12 yo.

FORMS – Generic only: Tabs 15, 16.2, 30, 32.4, 60, 100 mg. Elixir 20 mg/5 mL.

NOTES – Usual therapeutic level is 15 to 40 mcg/mL. Monitor cardiopulmonary function closely when administering IV. Decrease dose in renal or hepatic dysfunction. Many drug interactions.

PHENYTOIN (***Dilantin, Phenytek***) ▶L ♀D ▶+ $$

ADULT – Status epilepticus: 15 to 20 mg/kg IV at rate no faster than 50 mg/min, then 100 mg IV/PO q 6 to 8 h. Epilepsy, oral loading dose: 400 mg PO initially, then 300 mg in 2 h and 4 h. Epilepsy, maintenance dose: 300 mg/day PO given once daily (extended release) or divided three times per day (susp and chew tabs) and titrated to a therapeutic level.

PEDS – Epilepsy, age older than 6 yo: 5 mg/kg/day PO divided two to three times per day, to max 300 mg/day. Status epilepticus: 15 to 20 mg/kg IV at a rate no faster than 1 mg/kg/min.

FORMS – Generic/Trade: Extended-release caps 30, 100 mg (Dilantin). Susp 125 mg/5 mL. Trade only: Extended-release caps 200, 300 mg (Phenytek). Chewable tabs 50 mg (Dilantin Infatabs). Generic only: Extended-release caps 200, 300 mg.

NOTES – Usual therapeutic level is 10 to 20 mcg/mL. Limit dose increases to 10% or less due to saturable metabolism. Monitor ECG and vital signs when administering IV. Many drug interactions. Monitor serum levels closely when switching between forms (free acid vs sodium salt). The free fraction may be increased in patients with low albumin levels. IV loading doses of 15 to 20 mg/kg have also been recommended. May need to reduce loading dose if patient is already on phenytoin. Avoid in patients known to be positive for HLA-B*1502 due to possible increased risk of Stevens-Johnson syndrome.

PREGABALIN (*Lyrica*) ▶K ♀C ▶?©V $$$$$

ADULT – Painful diabetic peripheral neuropathy: Start 50 mg PO three times per day; may increase within 1 week to max 100 mg PO three times per day. Postherpetic neuralgia: Start 150 mg/day PO divided two to three times per day; may increase within 1 week to 300 mg/day divided two to three times per day; max 600 mg/day. Partial seizures (adjunctive): Start 150 mg/day PO divided two to three times per day; may increase prn to max 600 mg/day divided two to three times per day. Fibromyalgia: Start 75 mg PO two times per day; may increase to 150 mg two times per day within 1 week; max 225 mg two times per day. Neuropathic pain associated with spinal cord injury: Start 75 mg PO two times per day; may increase to 150 mg two times per day within 1 week and then to 300 mg two times per day after 2 to 3 weeks if tolerated.

PEDS – Not approved in children.

FORMS – Trade only: Caps 25, 50, 75, 100, 150, 200, 225, 300 mg. Oral solution 20 mg/mL (480 mL).

NOTES – Adjust dose if CrCl is less than 60 mL/min; refer to prescribing information. Warn patients to report changes in visual acuity and muscle pain. May increase creatine kinase. Must taper if discontinuing to avoid withdrawal symptoms. Increased risk of peripheral edema when used in conjunction with thiazolidinedione antidiabetic agents.

PRIMIDONE (*Mysoline*) ▶LK ♀D ▶– $$$$

ADULT – Epilepsy: Start 100 to 125 mg PO at bedtime. Increase over 10 days to usual maintenance dose of 250 mg PO three to four time per day. Max 2 g/day.

PEDS – Epilepsy, age younger than 8 yo: Start 50 mg PO at bedtime. Increase over 10 days to usual maintenance dose of 125 to 250 mg PO three times per day or 10 to 25 mg/kg/day.

UNAPPROVED ADULT – Essential tremor: Start 12.5 to 25 mg PO at bedtime. May increase weekly prn by 50 mg/day to 250 mg/day given once daily or in divided doses. Max 750 mg/day.

FORMS – Generic/Trade: Tabs 50, 250 mg.

NOTES – Usual therapeutic level is 5 to 12 mcg/mL. Metabolized to phenobarbital.

RUFINAMIDE (*Banzel*) ▶K ♀C ▶? $$$$$

ADULT – Epilepsy, Lennox-Gastaut syndrome (adjunctive): Start 400 to 800 mg/day PO divided two times per day. Increase by 400 to 800 mg/day q 2 days to max 3200 mg/day divided two times per day.

PEDS – Epilepsy, Lennox-Gastaut syndrome (adjunctive) age 4 yo or older: Start 10 mg/kg/day PO given two times per day. Increase by 10 mg/kg every other day to target of 45 mg/kg/day or 3200 mg/day divided two times per day.

FORMS – Trade only: Tabs 200, 400 mg.

NOTES – Give with food. Use caution for patients with mild to moderate hepatic impairment and avoid in severe hepatic impairment and short QT syndrome.

TIAGABINE (*Gabitril*) ▶L ♀C ▶? $$$$$

WARNING – New onset seizures and status epilepticus may occur when used in patients without epilepsy, particularly when combined with other medications that lower the seizure threshold. Avoid off-label use.

ADULT – Partial seizures, adjunctive therapy with an enzyme-inducing anticonvulsant: Start 4 mg PO daily. Increase by 4 to 8 mg/day prn at weekly intervals to max 56 mg/day divided two to four times per day.

PEDS – Partial seizures, adjunctive therapy with an enzyme-inducing anticonvulsant (age 12 to 18 yo): Start 4 mg PO daily. Increase by 4 mg/day prn q 1 to 2 weeks to max 32 mg/day divided two to four times per day.

FORMS – Trade only: Tabs 2, 4, 12, 16 mg.

NOTES – Take with food. Dosing is for patients on enzyme-inducing anticonvulsants such as carbamazepine, phenobarbital, phenytoin, or primidone. Reduce dosage in patients who are not taking enzyme-inducing medications, and in those with liver dysfunction.

TOPIRAMATE (*Topamax*) ▶K ♀D ▶? $$$$$

ADULT – Partial seizures or primary generalized tonic-clonic seizures, monotherapy: Start 25 mg PO two times per day (week 1), 50 mg two times per day (week 2), 75 mg two times per day (week 3), 100 mg two times per day (week 4), 150 mg two times per day (week 5), then 200 mg two times per day as tolerated. Partial seizures, primary generalized tonic-clonic seizures, or Lennox-Gastaut syndrome, adjunctive therapy: Start 25 to 50 mg PO at bedtime. Increase weekly by 25 to 50 mg each day to usual effective dose of 100 to 200 mg PO two times per day (partial seizures and LGS) or 200 mg PO two times per day (generalized tonic-clonic seizures). Doses greater than 400 mg per day not shown to be more effective. Migraine prophylaxis: Start 25 mg PO at bedtime (week 1), then 25 mg two times per day (week 2), then 25 mg q am and 50 mg q pm (week 3), then 50 mg two times per day (week 4 and thereafter).

(cont.)

TOPIRAMATE (*cont.*)

PEDS – Partial seizures or primary generalized tonic-clonic seizures, monotherapy age older than 10 yo: Use adult dosing. Ages 2 to less than 10 yo: Start 25 mg PO nightly (week 1), 25 mg two times daily (week 2), then increase by 25 to 50 mg/day weekly as tolerated to maintenance range of 75 to 125 mg twice daily based on wt (up to 11 kg), 100 to 150 mg twice daily (for wt 12 to 22 kg), 100 to 175 mg twice daily (for wt 23 to 31 kg), 125 to 175 mg twice daily (for wt 32 to 38 kg), or 125 to 200 mg twice daily (for wt greater than 38 kg). Partial seizures, primary generalized tonic-clonic seizures, or Lennox-Gastaut syndrome, adjunctive therapy, age 2 to 16 yo: Start 1 to 3 mg/kg (max 25 mg) PO at bedtime. Increase by 1 to 3 mg/kg/day q 1 to 2 weeks to usual effective dose of 5 to 9 mg/kg/day divided twice a day.

UNAPPROVED ADULT – Essential tremor: Start 25 mg PO daily. Increase by 25 mg/day at weekly intervals to 100 mg/day; max 400 mg/day. Bipolar disorder: Start 25 to 50 mg PO daily. Titrate prn to max 400 mg/day. Alcohol dependence: Start 25 mg PO q day; increase by 25 mg/day at weekly intervals as tolerated to 300 mg/day for up to 14 weeks total.

FORMS – Trade: Tabs 25, 50, 100, 200 mg. Sprinkle Caps 15, 25 mg.

NOTES – Give ½ usual adult dose in renal impairment (CrCl less than 70 mL/min). Confusion, nephrolithiasis, glaucoma, and wt loss may occur. Risk of oligohidrosis and hyperthermia, particularly in children; use caution in warm ambient temperatures and/or with vigorous physical activity. Hyperchloremic, nonanion gap metabolic acidosis may occur; monitor serum bicarbonate and either reduce dose or taper off entirely if this occurs. Max dose tested was 1600 mg/day. Use during pregnancy associated with cleft palate/lip. Report fetal exposure to North American Antiepileptic Drug Pregnancy Registry (888-233-2334).

VALPROIC ACID—NEURO (***Depakene, Depakote, Depakote ER, Depacon, Stavzor, divalproex,*** **sodium valproate,** ✤ ***Epival, Deproic***) ▶L ♀D ▶+ $$$$

WARNING – Fatal hepatic failure has occurred; monitor LFTs during first 6 months of treatment. Should not be used in children under 2 yo. Life-threatening pancreatitis has been reported after initial or prolonged use. Evaluate for abdominal pain, N/V, and/or anorexia. Discontinue if pancreatitis occurs. May be more teratogenic than other anticonvulsants (eg, carbamazepine, lamotrigine, and phenytoin). Hepatic failure and clotting disorders have occurred when used during pregnancy.

ADULT – Epilepsy: 10 to 15 mg/kg/day (for absence seizures start 15 mg/kg/day) PO or IV infusion over 60 min (rate no faster than 20 mg/min) divided two to four times per day (standard-release, delayed-release, or IV) or given once daily (Depakote ER). Increase dose by 5 to 10 mg/kg/day at weekly intervals to max 60 mg/kg/day. Migraine prophylaxis: Start 250 mg PO two times per day (Depakote or Stavzor) or 500 mg PO daily (Depakote ER) for 1 week, then increase to max 1000 mg/day PO divided two times per day (Depakote or Stavzor) or given once daily (Depakote ER).

PEDS – Seizures, age older than 2 yo: 10 to 15 mg/kg/day PO or IV infusion over 60 min (rate no faster than 20 mg/min). Increase dose by 5 to 10 mg/kg/day at weekly intervals to max 60 mg/kg/day. Divide doses greater than 250 mg/day into two to four times per day; may give once daily (Depakote ER) if age older than 10 yo. For complex partial seizures: Stavzor used for age 10 yo older.

UNAPPROVED ADULT – Status epilepticus (not first line): Load 20 to 40 mg/kg IV (rate no faster than 6 mg/kg/min), then continue 4 to 8 mg/kg IV three times per day to achieve therapeutic level. May use lower loading dose if already on valproate.

UNAPPROVED PEDS – Status epilepticus, age older than 2 yo (not first line): Load 20 to 40 mg/kg IV over 1 to 5 min, then 5 mg/kg/h adjusted to achieve therapeutic level. May use lower loading dose if already on valproate.

FORMS – Generic/Trade: Immediate-release caps 250 mg (Depakene), syrup (Depakene, valproic acid) 250 mg/5 mL. Delayed-release tabs (Depakote) 125, 250, 500 mg, Extended-release tabs (Depakote ER) 250, 500 mg, Delayed-release sprinkle caps (Depakote) 125 mg. Trade only (Stavzor): Delayed-release caps 125, 250, 500 mg.

NOTES – Contraindicated in urea cycle disorders or hepatic dysfunction. Usual therapeutic trough level is 50 to 100 mcg/mL. Depakote and Depakote ER are not interchangeable. Depakote ER is approximately 10% less bioavailable than Depakote. Depakote-releases divalproex sodium over 8 to 12 h (daily to four times per day dosing); Depakote ER-releases divalproex sodium over 18 to 24 h (daily dosing). Many drug interactions. Patients receiving other anticonvulsants may require higher doses of valproic acid. Reduce dose in the

(cont.)

VALPROIC ACID—NEURO *(cont.)*

elderly. Hyperammonemia, GI irritation, or thrombocytopenia may occur.

VIGABATRIN ▸K ♀C ▸– $$$$

WARNING – Ophthalmologic abnormalities have been reported. Visual field testing should be performed prior to treatment and q 3 months thereafter. Given the limitations of visual field testing in children younger than 9 yo, vigabatrin should be used in this age group only if clearly indicated. Do not use with other retinotoxic drugs.

ADULT – Canada only. Epilepsy, adjunctive treatment: Start: 1 g/day in divided doses. Maintenance: 2 to 3 g/day in divided doses.

PEDS – Canada only. Epilepsy, adjunctive treatment, or infantile spasms, monotherapy: Start: 40 mg/kg/day, maintenance: 50 to 100 mg/kg/day in divided doses.

FORMS – Trade only: Tabs 500 mg. Oral powder 500 mg/sachet.

ZONISAMIDE (*Zonegran*) ▸LK ♀C ▸? $$$$

ADULT – Partial seizures, adjunctive: Start 100 mg PO daily for 2 weeks, then increase to 200 mg PO daily. May increase prn q 2 weeks to 300 to 400 mg/day, given once daily or divided two times per day. Max 600 mg/day.

PEDS – Not approved in children.

FORMS – Generic/Trade: Caps 25, 50, 100 mg.

NOTES – This is a sulfonamide; contraindicated in sulfa allergy. Fatalities and severe reactions including Stevens-Johnson syndrome, toxic epidermal necrolysis, fulminant hepatic necrosis, and blood dyscrasias have occurred with sulfonamides. Clearance is affected by CYP3A4 inhibitors or inducers such as phenytoin, carbamazepine, phenobarbital, and valproic acid. Nephrolithiasis may occur. Oligohidrosis and hyperthermia may occur, and are more common in children. Patients with renal disease may require slower titration.

NEUROLOGY: Migraine Therapy—Triptans (5-HT1 Receptor Agonists)

NOTE: May cause vasospasm. Avoid in ischemic or vasospastic heart disease, cerebrovascular syndromes, peripheral arterial disease, uncontrolled HTN, and hemiplegic or basilar migraine. Do not use within 24 h of ergots or other triptans. Risk of serotonin syndrome if used with SSRIs or MAOIs. Contraindicated with MAOIs.

ALMOTRIPTAN (*Axert*) ▸LK ♀C ▸? $$

ADULT – Migraine treatment: 6.25 to 12.5 mg PO. May repeat in 2 h prn. Max 25 mg/day.

PEDS – Migraine treatment for age 12 to 17 yo: 6.25 to 12.5 mg PO. May repeat in 2 h prn. Max 25 mg/day.

FORMS – Trade only: Tabs 6.25, 12.5 mg.

NOTES – MAOIs inhibit almotriptan metabolism; use together only with extreme caution. Use lower doses (6.25 mg) in renal and/or hepatic dysfunction. Use with caution in patients with known hypersensitivity to sulfonamides.

ELETRIPTAN (*Relpax*) ▸LK ♀C ▸? $$$

ADULT – Migraine treatment: 20 to 40 mg PO at onset. May repeat after 2 h prn. Max 40 mg/dose or 80 mg/day.

PEDS – Not approved in children.

FORMS – Trade only: Tabs 20, 40 mg.

NOTES – Do not use within 72 h of potent CYP3A4 inhibitors such as ketoconazole, itraconazole, nefazodone, troleandomycin, clarithromycin, ritonavir, or nelfinavir.

FROVATRIPTAN (*Frova*) ▸LK ♀C ▸? $

ADULT – Migraine treatment: 2.5 mg PO. May repeat in 2 h prn. Max 7.5 mg/24 h.

PEDS – Not approved in children.

FORMS – Trade only: Tabs 2.5 mg.

NARATRIPTAN (*Amerge*) ▸KL ♀C ▸? $$$

ADULT – Migraine treatment: 1 to 2.5 mg PO. May repeat in 4 h prn. Max 5 mg/24 h.

PEDS – Not approved in children.

FORMS – Generic/Trade: Tabs 1, 2.5 mg.

NOTES – Contraindicated in severe renal or hepatic impairment.

RIZATRIPTAN (*Maxalt, Maxalt MLT*) ▸LK ♀C ▸? $$

ADULT – Migraine treatment: 5 to 10 mg PO; May repeat in 2 h prn. Max 30 mg/24 h.

PEDS – Migraine treatment: Children 6 to 17 yo, 5 mg PO if wt less than 40 kg and 10 mg PO for wt 40 kg and above. Do not give more than one dose in 24 h.

FORMS – Trade only: Tabs 5, 10 mg. Orally disintegrating tabs (MLT) 5, 10 mg.

NOTES – MLT form dissolves on tongue without liquids. Adult patients receiving propranolol should only receive 5 mg dose and not more than 3 doses per 24 h. For pediatric patients taking propranolol and weighing more than 40 kg, only a 5 mg dose one time in 24 h should be used. Do not give to children weighing less than 40 kg and taking propranolol.

SUMATRIPTAN (*Imitrex, Alsuma*) ▶LK ♀C ▶+ $

ADULT – Migraine treatment: 4 to 6 mg SC. May repeat in 1 h prn. Max 12 mg/24 h. Tabs: 25 to 100 mg PO (50 mg most common). May repeat q 2 h prn with 25 to 100 mg doses. Max 200 mg/24 h. Intranasal spray: 5 to 20 mg. May repeat q 2 h prn. Max 40 mg/24 h. Cluster headache treatment: 6 mg SC. May repeat after 1 h or longer prn. Max 12 mg/24 h. Initial oral dose of 50 mg appears to be more effective than 25 mg. If HA returns after initial SC injection, then tabs may be used q 2 h prn, max 100 mg/24 h.

PEDS – Not approved in children.

UNAPPROVED PEDS – Acute migraine, intranasal spray, for age 8 to 17 yo: Give 20 mg for wt 40 kg or greater or 10 mg for wt 20 to 39 kg intranasally at headache onset. May repeat after 2 h prn.

FORMS – Generic/Trade: Tabs 25, 50, 100 mg. Nasal Spray 5 mg and 20 mg (box of #6). Injection (STATdose System) 4, 6 mg prefilled cartridges. Trade only (Alsuma): Injection 6 mg prefilled cartridge.

NOTES – Avoid IM/IV route.

TREXIMET **(sumatriptan + naproxen)** ▶LK ♀C ▶– $$

WARNING – Risk of GI bleeding and perforation. Do not use ergots within 24 h of Treximet.

ADULT – Migraine treatment: 1 tab PO at onset. Efficacy of more than one tablet not established. Max 2 tabs/24 h separated by at least 2 h.

PEDS – Not approved in children.

FORMS – Trade only: Tabs 85 mg sumatriptan + 500 mg naproxen sodium.

NOTES – Avoid if CrCl is less than 30 mL/min, hepatic impairment; cerebrovascular, cardiovascular, or peripheral vascular disease; uncontrolled HTN. Contraindicated with MAOIs.

ZOLMITRIPTAN (*Zomig, Zomig ZMT*) ▶L ♀C ▶? $$

ADULT – Migraine treatment: Tabs: 1.25 to 2.5 mg PO q 2 h. Max 10 mg/24 h. Orally disintegrating tabs (ZMT): 2.5 mg PO. May repeat in 2 h prn. Max 10 mg/24 h. Nasal spray: 5 mg (1 spray) in 1 nostril. May repeat in 2 h prn. Max 10 mg/24 h.

PEDS – Not approved in children.

FORMS – Trade only: Tabs 2.5, 5 mg. Orally disintegrating tabs (ZMT) 2.5, 5 mg. Nasal spray 5 mg/spray.

NOTES – Use lower doses (less than 2.5 mg) in hepatic dysfunction. May break 2.5 mg tabs in half.

NEUROLOGY: Migraine Therapy—Other

CAFERGOT (ergotamine + caffeine) ▶L ♀X ▶– $

WARNING – Contraindicated with concomitant use of potent CYP3A4 inhibitors (eg, macrolides, protease inhibitors) due to risk of serious/life-threatening peripheral ischemia. Ergots have been associated with potentially life-threatening fibrotic complications.

ADULT – Migraine and cluster headache treatment: 2 tabs PO at onset, then 1 tab q 30 min prn to max 6 tabs/attack or 10 tabs/week.

PEDS – Not approved in children.

UNAPPROVED PEDS – Migraine treatment: 1 tab PO at onset, then 1 tab q 30 min prn to max 3 tabs/attack.

FORMS – Trade only: Tabs 1/100 mg ergotamine/caffeine.

NOTES – Contraindicated in sepsis, CAD, peripheral arterial disease, HTN, impaired hepatic or renal function, malnutrition, or severe pruritus.

DIHYDROERGOTAMINE (*D.H.E. 45, Migranal*) ▶L ♀X ▶– $$

WARNING – Contraindicated with concomitant use of potent CYP3A4 inhibitors (eg, macrolides, protease inhibitors) due to risk of serious/life-threatening peripheral ischemia. Ergots have been associated with potentially life-threatening fibrotic complications.

ADULT – Migraine treatment: Soln (DHE 45): 1 mg IV/IM/SC; may repeat q 1 h prn to max 2 mg (IV) or 3 mg (IM/SC) per 24 h. Nasal spray (Migranal): 1 spray (0.5 mg) in each nostril; may repeat in 15 min prn to max 6 sprays (3 mg)/24 h or 8 sprays (4 mg)/week.

PEDS – Not approved in children.

FORMS – Trade only: Nasal spray 0.5 mg/spray (Migranal). Self-injecting soln (D.H.E 45): 1 mg/mL.

NOTES – Contraindicated in basilar or hemiplegic migraine, sepsis, ischemic or vasospastic cardiac disease, peripheral vascular

(cont.)

DIHYDROERGOTAMINE (*cont.*)

disease, vascular surgery, impaired hepatic or renal function, or uncontrolled HTN. Avoid concurrent ergotamine, methysergide, or triptan use.

ERGOTAMINE (***Ergomar***) ▶L ♀X ▶– $$

ADULT – Vascular headache: Start 2 mg SL; may repeat q 30 min to max 6 mg/24 h. Drug interactions. Fibrotic complications.

PEDS – Not approved in children.

FORMS – Trade only: Sublingual tabs (ergotamine tartrate) 2 mg.

NOTES – Avoid use with potent CYP3A4 inhibitors (eg, ritonavir, nelfinavir, indinavir, erythromycin, clarithromycin, troleandomycin); severe peripheral vasoconstriction may result.

♣ **FLUNARIZINE** ▶L ♀C ▶– $$

ADULT – Canada only. Migraine prophylaxis: 10 mg PO at bedtime; if side effects occur, then reduce dose to 5 mg at bedtime. Safety of long-term use (more than 4 months) has not been established.

PEDS – Not approved in children.

FORMS – Generic/Trade: Caps 5 mg.

NOTES – Gradual onset of benefit, over 6 to 8 weeks. Not for acute therapy. Contraindicated if history of depression or extrapyramidal disorders.

NEUROLOGY: Multiple Sclerosis

DALFAMPRIDINE (***Ampyra***) ▶K – ♀C ▶?

WARNING – Risk of drug-induced seizures.

ADULT – Multiple sclerosis: 10 mg PO two times per day.

PEDS – Not approved for use in children or adolescents.

FORMS – Trade: Extended-release tabs 10 mg.

NOTES – Contraindicated with moderate to severe renal impairment and history of seizures. Obtained from a specialty pharmacy (Ampyra Patient Support Service 888-883-3053). Do not exceed recommended dose. Do not combine with other forms of 4-aminopyridine.

FINGOLIMOD (***Gilenya***) ▶L - ♀C ▶?

ADULT – Relapsing remitting multiple sclerosis: 0.5 mg PO once daily.

PEDS – Not approve for use in children or adolescents.

FORMS – Trade only: Caps 0.5 mg.

NOTES – Do not use within 6 months of MI, stroke/TIA, unstable angina, AV block, decompensated or Class III or IV heart failure. Observe all patients for bradycardia for 6 h after the first dose. Obtain baseline ECG for patients on drugs such as beta-blockers and antiarrhythmics that can cause bradycardia. Obtain CBC prior to initiation. Monitor for infection and consider stopping if a serious infection occurs. Obtain baseline ophthalmic exam and after 3 to 4 months of therapy to monitor for macular edema. Obtain baseline LFTs. Use effective contraception during and for 2 months following therapy. Avoid live attenuated vaccines during and for 2 months following therapy. Avoid use with ketoconazole.

GLATIRAMER (***Copaxone***) ▶Serum ♀B ▶? $$$$$

ADULT – Multiple sclerosis (relapsing-remitting): 20 mg SC daily.

PEDS – Not approved in children.

FORMS – Trade only: Injection 20 mg single-dose vial.

NOTES – Do not inject IV.

INTERFERON BETA-1A (***Avonex, Rebif***) ▶L ♀C ▶? $$$$$

WARNING – Risk of severe hepatic injury and failure, possibly greater when used with other hepatotoxic drugs. Monitor LFTs. Suicidality risk; use caution in depression.

ADULT – Relapsing-remitting multiple sclerosis forms: Avonex 30 mcg (6 million units) IM q week. Rebif start 8.8 mcg SC 3 times weekly; titrate over 4 weeks to maintenance dose of 44 mcg 3 times weekly.

PEDS – Not approved in children.

FORMS – Trade only (Avonex): Injection 30 mcg single-dose vial with or without albumin. Prefilled syringe 30 mcg. Trade only (Rebif): Starter kit 20 mcg prefilled syringe. Prefilled syringe 22, 44 mcg.

NOTES – Use caution in patients with depression, seizure disorders, or cardiac disease. Follow LFTs and CBC. Avonex: Indicated for the first attack of MS. Rebif: Give same dose 3 days each week, with at least 48 h between doses.

INTERFERON BETA-1B (*Betaseron*) ▶L ♀C ▶? $$$$$

ADULT – Multiple sclerosis (relapsing-remitting): Start 0.0625 mg SC every other day; titrate over 6 weeks to 0.25 mg (8 million units) SC every other day.

PEDS – Not approved in children.

FORMS – Trade only: Injection 0.3 mg (9.6 million units) single-dose vial.

NOTES – Suicidality risk; use caution in depression. Check LFTs after 1, 3, and 6 months and then periodically. Product can be stored at room temp until reconstituted; then refrigerate and use within 3 h.

NATALIZUMAB (*Tysabri*) ▶Serum ♀C ▶? $$$$$

WARNING – May cause progressive multifocal leukoencephalopathy; avoid concomitant use of other immunomodulators. Risk of severe hepatotoxicity; discontinue if jaundice or evidence of liver injury. Risk of anaphylaxis or other hypersensitivity reactions; permanently discontinue if they occur.

ADULT – Refractory, relapsing multiple sclerosis (monotherapy) and Crohn's disease: 300 mg IV infusion over 1 h q 4 weeks.

PEDS – Not approved in children.

NOTES – Not first line; recommended only when there has been an inadequate response or failure to tolerate other therapies. Available only through the MS-TOUCH or CD-TOUCH prescribing programs at 800-456-2255. Observe closely for infusion reactions. Avoid other immunosuppressants when using for Crohn's disease; discontinue if no response by 12 weeks. For patients on steroids, taper them as soon as a benefit is noted and discontinue natalizumab if steroids cannot be tapered off within 6 months. Consider stopping natalizumab in patients who require steroids more than 3 months/year.

NEUROLOGY: Myasthenia Gravis

AMBENONIUM (*Mytelase*) ▶L ♀C ▶? $$$$$

ADULT – Myasthenia gravis: Start 5 mg PO three to four times per day. Adjust q 1 to 2 days to usual effective dose of 5 to 25 mg three to four times per day. Usual max 200 mg/day. Narrow therapeutic window. Doses greater than 200 mg/day require close supervision.

PEDS – Not approved in children.

FORMS – Trade only: Tabs 10 mg

NOTES – Avoid concomitant use of atropine, ganglionic blocking agents, or other cholinergic drugs. Narrow therapeutic window and variable individual dose requirements, so titrate slowly. Extended or high-dose (more than 200 mg/day) therapy requires close supervision. Cholinergic crisis may be treated by discontinuing the drug and giving atropine 0.5 to 1.0 mg IV plus supportive care.

EDROPHONIUM (*Tensilon, Enlon*) ▶Plasma ♀C ▶? $

ADULT – Evaluation for myasthenia gravis (diagnostic purposes only): 2 mg IV over 15 to 30 sec (test dose) while on cardiac monitor, then 8 mg IV after 45 sec. Reversal of neuromuscular blockade: 10 mg IV over 30 to 45 sec; repeat prn to max 40 mg.

PEDS – Evaluation for myasthenia gravis (diagnostic purposes only): Give 1 mg IV (test dose), then 1 mg IV q 30 to 45 sec to max 5 mg for wt 34 kg or less, give 2 mg IV (test dose), then 2 mg IV q 30 to 45 sec to max 10 mg for wt greater than 34 kg.

UNAPPROVED ADULT – Reversal of nondepolarizing neuromuscular blocking agents: 0.5 to 1 mg/kg IV together with atropine 0.007 to 0.014 mg/kg.

FORMS – 10 mg/mL MDV vial.

NOTES – Not for maintenance therapy of myasthenia gravis because of short duration of action (5 to 10 min). May give IM. Monitor cardiac function. Atropine should be readily available in case of cholinergic reaction. Contraindicated in mechanical urinary or intestinal obstruction.

NEOSTIGMINE (*Prostigmin*) ▶L ♀C ▶? $$$$

ADULT – Myasthenia gravis: 15 to 375 mg/day PO in divided doses, or 0.5 mg IM/SC when oral therapy is not possible. Reversal of nondepolarizing neuromuscular blocking agents: 0.5 to 2 mg slow IV (preceded by atropine 0.6 to 1.2 mg or glycopyrrolate 0.2 to 0.6 mg); repeat prn to max 5 mg.

PEDS – Not approved in children.

UNAPPROVED PEDS – Myasthenia gravis: 7.5 to 15 mg PO three to four times per day; or 0.03 mg/kg IM q 2 to 4 h. Reversal of nondepolarizing neuromuscular blocking agents: 0.025 to 0.08 mg/kg/dose slow IV, preceded by either atropine (0.4 mg for each mg of neostigmine) or glycopyrrolate (0.2 mg for each mg of neostigmine).

FORMS – Trade only: Tabs 15 mg.

NOTES – Oral route preferred when possible.

PYRIDOSTIGMINE (*Mestinon, Mestinon Timespan, Regonol*) ▶Plasma, K ♀C ▶+ $$

ADULT – Myasthenia gravis, standard-release tabs: Start 60 mg PO three times per day; gradually increase to usual therapeutic dose of 200 mg PO three times per day. Extended-release tabs: Start 180 mg PO daily or divided two times per day. Max 1500 mg/day. May give 2 mg IM or slow IV injection q 2 to 3 h.

PEDS – Not approved in children.

UNAPPROVED PEDS – Myasthenia gravis, neonates: 5 mg PO q 4 to 6 h or 0.05 to 0.15 mg/kg IM/IV q 4 to 6 h. Myasthenia gravis, children: 7 mg/kg/day PO in 5 to 6 divided doses, or 0.05 to 0.15 mg/kg/dose IM/IV q 4 to 6 h. Max 10 mg IM/IV single dose.

FORMS – Generic/Trade: Tabs 60 mg. Trade only: Extended-release tabs 180 mg. Syrup 60 mg/ 5 mL.

NOTES – Give injection at 1/30 oral dose when oral therapy is not possible.

NEUROLOGY: Parkinsonian Agents—Anticholinergics

NOTE: Anticholinergic medications may cause memory loss, delirium, or psychosis, particularly in elderly patients or those with baseline cognitive impairment. Contraindicated in narrow-angle glaucoma, bowel obstruction, and megacolon.

BENZTROPINE MESYLATE (*Cogentin*) ▶LK ♀C ▶? $

ADULT – Parkinsonism: Start 0.5 to 2 mg/day PO/IM/IV. Increase in 0.5-mg increments at weekly intervals to max 6 mg/day. May divide doses one to four times per day. Drug-induced extrapyramidal disorders: 1 to 4 mg PO/IM/IV given once daily or divided two times per day.

PEDS – Not approved in children.

UNAPPROVED PEDS – Parkinsonism in age older than 3 yo: 0.02 to 0.05 mg/kg/dose given once daily or divided two times per day. Use caution; potential for undesired anticholinergic effects.

FORMS – Generic only: Tabs 0.5, 1, 2 mg.

NOTES – Contraindicated in narrow-angle glaucoma. Avoid concomitant use of donepezil, rivastigmine, galantamine, or tacrine.

BIPERIDEN (*Akineton*) ▶LK ♀C ▶? $$$

ADULT – Parkinsonism: 2 mg PO three to four times per day. Titrate to max 16 mg/day. Drug-induced extrapyramidal disorders: 2 mg PO daily to three times per day to max 8 mg/24 h.

PEDS – Not approved in children.

FORMS – Trade only: Tabs 2 mg.

NOTES – Contraindicated in narrow-angle glaucoma, bowel obstruction, and megacolon.

TRIHEXYPHENIDYL (*Artane*) ▶LK ♀C ▶? $

ADULT – Parkinsonism: 1 mg PO daily. Increase by 2 mg/day at 3- to 5-day intervals to usual therapeutic dose of 6 to 10 mg/day divided three times per day with meals. Max 15 mg/day.

PEDS – Not approved in children.

FORMS – Generic only: Tabs 2, 5 mg. Elixir 2 mg/5 mL.

NEUROLOGY: Parkinsonian Agents—COMT Inhibitors

ENTACAPONE (*Comtan*) ▶L ♀C ▶? $$$$$

ADULT – Parkinson's disease, adjunctive: Start 200 mg PO with each dose of carbidopa-levodopa. Max 8 tabs (1600 mg)/day.

PEDS – Not approved in children.

FORMS – Trade only: Tabs 200 mg.

NOTES – Adjunct to carbidopa-levodopa in patients who have end-of-dose "wearing off." Has no antiparkinsonian effect on its own. Avoid concomitant use of nonselective MAOIs. Use caution in hepatobiliary dysfunction. Avoid rapid withdrawal, which may precipitate neuroleptic malignant syndrome.

TOLCAPONE (*Tasmar*) ▶LK ♀C ▶? $$$$$

WARNING – Fatal hepatic failure has occurred. Use only in patients on carbidopa-levodopa who fail alternative therapies and provide written informed consent. Monitor LFTs at baseline, q 2 to 4 weeks for 6 months, and then periodically. Discontinue if LFT elevation is more than 2 times upper limit of normal or if there is no clinical benefit after 3 weeks of therapy.

ADULT – Parkinson's disease, adjunctive (not first line): Start 100 mg PO three times per day. Increase to 200 mg PO three times per day only if expected benefit justifies the risk. Max 600 mg/day. Only effective when used in combination with carbidopa-levodopa.

PEDS – Not approved in children.

FORMS – Trade only: Tabs 100, 200 mg.

NOTES – Adjunct to carbidopa-levodopa in patients who have refractory end-of-dose "wearing off." Has no antiparkinsonian effect

(cont.)

TOLCAPONE (*cont.*)

on its own. Contraindicated in hepatic dysfunction. Monitor LFTs. Avoid concomitant use of nonselective MAOIs. Avoid rapid withdrawal, which may precipitate neuroleptic malignant syndrome. Informed consent forms are available from the manufacturer (www.tasmar.com).

NEUROLOGY: Parkinsonian Agents—Dopaminergic Agents and Combinations

NOTE: Dopaminergic medications may cause hallucinations, particularly when used in combination. They have also been associated with sudden-onset episodes of sleep without warning ("sleep attacks"), and with the development of impulse control disorders such as compulsive gambling, eating, or shopping, and hypersexuality. This is more common with dopamine agonists than L-dopa. Avoid rapid discontinuation of dopamine agonists, which may precipitate a syndrome similar to neuroleptic malignant syndrome.

APOMORPHINE (***Apokyn***) ▸L ♀C ▸? $$$$$

WARNING – Never administer IV due to risk of severe adverse effects including pulmonary embolism.

ADULT – Acute, intermittent treatment of hypomobility ("off episodes") in Parkinson's disease: Start 0.2 mL SC test dose in the presence of medical personnel. May increase dose by 0.1 mL every few days as tolerated. Max 0.6 mL/dose or 2 mL/day. Monitor for orthostatic hypotension after initial dose and with dose escalation. Potent emetic; pretreat with trimethobenzamide 300 mg PO three times per day (or domperidone 20 mg PO three times per day) starting 3 days prior to use, and continue for at least 6 weeks before weaning.

PEDS – Not approved in children.

FORMS – Trade only: Cartridges (for injector pen, 10 mg/mL) 3 mL. Ampules (10 mg/mL) 2 mL.

NOTES – Write doses exclusively in mL rather than mg to avoid errors. Most effective when administered at (or just prior to) the onset of an "off" episode. Avoid concomitant use of 5HT3 antagonists (eg, ondansetron, granisetron, dolasetron, palonosetron, alosetron), which can precipitate severe hypotension and loss of consciousness. Inform patients that the dosing pen is labeled in mL (not mg), and that it is possible to dial in a dose of medication even if the cartridge does not contain sufficient drug. Rotate injection sites. Restart at 0.2 mL/day if treatment is interrupted for 1 week or more. Use cautiously with hepatic impairment. Reduce starting dose to 0.1 mL in patients with mild or moderate renal failure. Contains sulfites.

CARBIDOPA (***Lodosyn***) ▸LK ♀C ▸? $$$

ADULT – Parkinson's disease, adjunct to carbidopa-levodopa: Start 25 mg PO daily with 1st daily dose of carbidopa-levodopa. May give an additional 12.5 to 25 mg with each dose of carbidopa-levodopa prn. Max 200 mg/day.

PEDS – Not approved in children.

FORMS – Trade only: Tabs 25 mg.

NOTES – Adjunct to carbidopa-levodopa to reduce peripheral side-effects such as nausea. Also increases the CNS availability of levodopa. Monitor for CNS side effects such as dyskinesias and hallucinations when initiating therapy, and reduce the dose of levodopa as necessary.

CARBIDOPA-LEVODOPA (***Sinemet, Sinemet CR, Parcopa***) ▸L ♀C ▸– $$$$

ADULT – Parkinsonism: Standard-release and orally disintegrating tab: Start 1 tab (25/100 mg) PO three times per day. Increase by 1 tab/day q 1 to 2 days prn. Use 1 tab (25/250 mg) PO three to four times per day when higher levodopa doses are needed. Sustained-release: Start 1 tab (50/200 mg) PO twice per day; separate doses by at least 4 h. Increase prn at intervals of 3 days or more. Typical max dose is 1600 to 2000 mg/day of levodopa, but higher doses have been used.

PEDS – Not approved in children.

UNAPPROVED ADULT – Restless legs syndrome: Start ½ tab (25/100 mg) PO at bedtime; increase q 3 to 4 days to max 50/200 mg (two 25/100 tabs) at bedtime. If symptoms recur during the night, then a combination of standard-release (25/100 mg, 1 to 2 tabs at bedtime) and sustained-release (25/100 or 50/200 mg at bedtime) tabs may be used. Dopa-responsive dystonia: Start 1 tab (25/100) PO daily and titrate to max 1000 mg of levodopa daily.

FORMS – Generic/Trade: Tabs (carbidopa-levodopa) 10/100, 25/100, 25/250 mg. Tabs, sustained-release (Sinemet CR, carbidopa-levodopa ER) 25/100, 50/200 mg. Trade only: Orally disintegrating tab (Parcopa) 10/100, 25/100, 25/250 mg.

NOTES – Motor fluctuations and dyskinesias may occur. The 25/100 mg tabs are preferred

(cont.)

CARBIDOPA-LEVODOPA (*cont.*)

as initial therapy, since most patients require at least 70 to 100 mg/day of carbidopa to reduce the risk of N/V. The 10/100 mg tabs have limited clinical utility. Extended-release formulations have a lower bioavailability than conventional preparations. Do not use within 2 weeks of a nonselective MAOI. When used for restless legs syndrome, may precipitate rebound (recurrence of symptoms during the night) or augmentation (earlier daily onset of symptoms). Orally disintegrating tab is placed on top of the tongue and does not require water or swallowing, but is absorbed through the GI tract (not sublingually). Use caution in patients with undiagnosed skin lesions or a history of melanoma. Intense urges (gambling and sexual for example) have been reported. Consider discontinuing the medication or reducing the dose if these occur.

PRAMIPEXOLE (***Mirapex, Mirapex ER***) ▶K ♀C ▶? $$$$$

ADULT – Parkinson's disease: Start 0.125 mg PO three times per day for 1 week, then 0.25 mg for 1 week; after that, increase by 0.75 mg/week divided three times per day. Usual effective dose is 0.5 to 1.5 mg PO three times per day. Extended release: Start 0.375 mg daily. May increase after 5 to 7 days to 0.75 mg/day then by 0.75 mg/day increments q 5 to 7 days to max 4.5 mg/day. Restless legs syndrome: Start 0.125 mg PO 2 to 3 h prior to bedtime. May increase q 4 to 7 days to 0.25 mg then 0.5 mg if needed.

PEDS – Not approved in children.

FORMS – Generic/Trade: Tabs 0.125, 0.25, 0.5, 0.75, 1, 1.5 mg. Trade only: Tabs extended release 0.375, 0.75, 1.5, 3, 4.5 mg.

NOTES – Decrease dose in renal impairment. Titrate slowly. May change to extended-release tabs at same daily dose as regular tabs overnight.

ROPINIROLE (***Requip, Requip XL***) ▶L ♀C ▶? $$$$$

ADULT – Parkinson's disease: Start 0.25 mg PO three times per day. Increase by 0.25 mg/dose (0.75 mg/day) at weekly intervals to 1 mg PO three times daily. If needed after week 4 may increase dose by 1.5 mg/day weekly up to 9 mg/day and then 3 mg/day weekly to max 24 mg/day. Extended-release: Start 2 mg PO daily, then increase by 2 mg daily at weekly or longer intervals. Max 24 mg/day. Restless legs syndrome: Start 0.25 mg PO 1 to 3 h before bedtime for 2 days, then increase to 0.5 mg/day on days 3 to 7. Increase by 0.5 mg/day at weekly intervals prn to max 4 mg/day given 1 to 3 h before bedtime.

PEDS – Not approved in children.

FORMS – Generic/Trade: Tabs, immediate-release 0.25, 0.5, 1, 2, 3, 4, 5 mg. Trade only: Tabs, extended-release (Requip XL) 2, 3, 4, 6, 8, 12 mg.

NOTES – Retitrate if significant interruption of therapy occurs.

ROTIGOTINE (***Neupro***) ▶L – ♀C ▶?

ADULT – Early stage Parkinson's disease: Start 2 mg/24 h patch daily; may increase by 2 mg/24 h at weekly intervals to max 6 mg/24 h. Advanced-stage Parkinson's disease: Start 4 mg/24 h patch daily; may increase by 2 mg/24 h at weekly intervals to max 8 mg/24 h. Restless legs syndrome: Start 1 mg/24 h patch daily; may be increased by 1 mg/24 h at weekly intervals to max 3 mg/24 h.

PEDS – Not approved for use in children.

FORMS – Trade: Transdermal patch 1, 2, 3, 4, 6, 8 mg/24 h.

NOTES – Contains sulfites. Remove prior to MRI or cardioversion to avoid burns. Apply to clean, dry intact skin of the abdomen, thigh, flank, shoulder, or upper arm and hold in place for 20 to 30 seconds. Rotate application sites daily, and wash skin after removal. Taper by 2 mg/24 h every other day when discontinuing.

STALEVO **(carbidopa + levodopa + entacapone)** ▶L ♀C ▶– $$$$$

ADULT – Parkinson's disease (conversion from carbidopa-levodopa with or without entacapone): Start Stalevo tab that contains the same amount of carbidopa-levodopa as the patient was previously taking, and titrate to desired response. May need to lower the dose of levodopa in patients not already taking entacapone. Max 1600 mg/day of entacapone or 1600 to 2000 mg/day of levodopa.

PEDS – Not approved in children.

FORMS – Trade only: Tabs (carbidopa-levodopa-entacapone): Stalevo 50 (12.5/50/200 mg), Stalevo 75 (18.75/75/200 mg), Stalevo 100 (25/100/200 mg), Stalevo 125 (31.25/125/200 mg), Stalevo 150 (37.5/150/200 mg), Stalevo 200 (50/200/200 mg).

NOTES – Patients who are not currently taking entacapone may benefit from titration of the individual components of this medication before conversion to this fixed-dose preparation. Avoid concomitant use of nonselective MAOIs. Use caution in hepatobiliary dysfunction. Motor fluctuations and dyskinesias may occur.

NEUROLOGY: Parkinsonian Agents—Monoamine Oxidase Inhibitors (MAOIs)

RASAGILINE (*Azilect*) ▶L ♀C ▶? $$$$$

ADULT – Parkinson's disease, monotherapy: 1 mg PO q am. Parkinson's disease, adjunctive: 0.5 mg PO q am. Max 1 mg/day.

PEDS – Not approved in children.

FORMS – Trade only: Tabs 0.5, 1 mg.

NOTES – Requires an MAOI diet. Contraindicated (risk of hypertensive crisis) with meperidine, methadone, tramadol, propoxyphene, dextromethorphan, sympathomimetic amines (eg, pseudoephedrine, phenylephrine, ephedrine), antidepressants, other MAOIs, cyclobenzaprine, and general anesthesia. Discontinue at least 14 days before liberalizing diet, starting one of these medications, or proceeding with elective surgery that requires general anesthesia. May need to reduce levodopa dose when used in combination. Reduce dose to 0.5 mg when used with CYP1A2 inhibitors (eg, ciprofloxacin) and in mild hepatic impairment. Do not use in moderate or severe liver disease. Parkinson's disease and drugs used to treat it have been associated with an increased risk of melanoma. Consider periodic skin exams for melanoma.

SELEGILINE (*Eldepryl, Zelapar*) ▶LK ♀C ▶? $$$$

ADULT – Parkinsonism (adjunct to levodopa): 5 mg PO q am and q noon; max 10 mg/day. Zelapar ODT: Start 1.25 mg sublingual q am for at least 6 weeks, then increase prn to max 2.5 mg q am.

PEDS – Not approved in children.

UNAPPROVED ADULT – Parkinsonism (monotherapy): 5 mg PO q am and q noon; max 10 mg/day.

FORMS – Generic/Trade: Caps 5 mg. Tabs 5 mg. Trade only: Oral disintegrating tabs (Zelapar ODT) 1.25 mg.

NOTES – Should not be combined with meperidine or other opioids. Do not exceed max recommended dose; risk of nonselective MAO inhibition. Zelapar should be taken in the morning before food and without water. Intense urges (eg, gambling and sexual) have been reported. Consider discontinuing the medication or reducing the dose if these occur. Parkinson's disease and drugs used to treat it have been associated with an increased risk of melanoma.

NEUROLOGY: Other Agents

ABOBOTULINUMTOXIN A (*DYSPORT*) ♀C ▶?

WARNING – Symptoms of systemic botulism have been reported, particularly in children treated for spasticity due to cerebral palsy.

ADULT – Cervical dystonia: 500 units IM total dose divided among affected muscles. May repeat q 12 weeks or longer. Max dose 1000 units per treatment. Glabellar line (age younger than 65 yo): 50 units IM total dose divided into 10 unit injections at 5 sites (see prescribing information). May repeat q 12 weeks or longer.

PEDS – Not approved for use in children.

FORMS – Trade: vials 300, 500 units for reconstitution.

NOTES – Refer to prescribing information for injection sites and technique. Use caution in peripheral motor neuropathic diseases, amyotrophic lateral sclerosis, or neuromuscular junction disorders (eg, myasthenia gravis or Lambert-Eaton syndrome) and monitor closely when given botulinum toxin due to increased risk of severe dysphagia or respiratory compromise. Contains trace amounts of cow's milk protein: Do not use in patients allergic to milk. Use cautiously with neuromuscular blocking drugs (eg, aminoglycosides and curare-like drugs).

♣BETAHISTINE ▶LK ♀? ▶? $

ADULT – Canada only. Vertigo of Meniere's disease: 8 to 16 mg PO three times per day.

PEDS – Not approved in children.

FORMS – Trade only: Tabs 8, 16 mg.

NOTES – Contraindicated in peptic ulcer disease and pheochromocytoma; use caution in asthmatics.

BOTULINUM TOXIN TYPE B (*Myobloc*) ▶Not significantly absorbed ♀+ ▶? $$$$$

WARNING – Symptoms of systemic botulism have been reported, particularly in children treated for spasticity due to cerebral palsy.

ADULT – Cervical dystonia: Start 2500 to 5000 units IM in affected muscles. Use lower initial dose if no prior history of botulinum toxin therapy. Benefits usually last for 12 to 16 weeks when a total dose of 5000 to 10,000 units has been administered. Titrate to effective dose. Give treatments at least 3 months apart to decrease the risk of producing neutralizing antibodies.

PEDS – Not approved in children.

NOTES – Low systemic concentrations are expected with IM injection; monitor closely for dysphagia. Contraindicated in peripheral motor neuropathic disease (eg, ALS, motor neuropathy), neuromuscular junction disease

(cont.)

BOTULINUM TOXIN TYPE B (*cont.*)

(eg, myasthenia gravis, Lambert-Eaton syndrome due to an increased risk of systemic effects) and with other drugs that block neuromuscular function (eg, aminoglycosides, curare-like compounds).

DEXTROMETHORPHAN/QUINIDINE (***Nuedexta***) ▶LK - ♀C ▶?

ADULT – Pseudobulbar affect: Start 1 cap PO daily. Increase after 7 days to maintenance dose of 1 cap two times per day.

PEDS – Not approved for use in children.

FORMS – Trade only: cap 10 mg dextromethorphan plus 20 mg quinidine.

NOTES – Contraindicated with prolonged QT interval, a history of torsades de pointes, with drugs that prolong the QT interval and metabolized by CYP2D6, or with MAOIs. Contraindicated with complete AV block. Obtain EKG at baseline and at 4 h post-dose to evaluate effect on QT in the presence of CYP3A4 inhibitors, or patients with left ventricular hypertrophy or left ventricular dysfunction. May cause serotonin syndrome if used with serotonergic drugs. Clinical trials were only conducted in patients with PBA secondary to Alzheimer's disease. Response in other subgroups has not been assessed.

INCOBOTULINUMTOXIN A (***Xeomin***) ▶not absorbed – ♀C ▶?

WARNING – Symptoms of systemic botulism have been reported.

ADULT – Cervical dystonia: Total of 120 units IM divided among the sternocleidomastoid, levator scapulae, splenis capitis, scalenus, and trapezius muscles as indicated. Repeat at intervals of at least 12 weeks with dose individualized according to response. Blepharospasm in patients previously treated with Botox: Start with same dose as Botox used before. If prior Botox dose unknown, start with 1.25 to 2.5 units per injection site. Usual number of injections is 6 per eye. Average dose 33 units/eye. Do not exceed initial dose of 35 units/eye. May repeat at intervals of at least 12 weeks.

PEDS – Not approved for use in children or adolescents.

FORMS – Trade only: 50 and 100 unit single-use vials.

NOTES – Cannot convert units of Xeomin to other botulinum toxins. The max dose in trials for blepharospasm was 50 units/eye. Toxin effects may become systemic and produce asthenia, muscle weakness, diplopia, ptosis, dysphagia, dysphonia, urinary incontinence, and breathing difficulties.

MANNITOL (***Osmitrol, Resectisol***) ▶K ♀C ▶? $$

ADULT – Intracranial HTN: 0.25 to 2 g/kg IV over 30 to 60 min as a 15, 20, or 25% soln.

PEDS – Not approved in children.

UNAPPROVED ADULT – Increased ICP or head trauma: 0.25 to 1 g/kg IV push over 20 min. Repeat q 4 to 6 h prn.

UNAPPROVED PEDS – Increased ICP, cerebral edema: 0.25 to 1 g/kg/dose IV push over 20 to 30 min, then 0.25 to 0.5 g/kg/dose IV q 4 to 6 h prn.

NOTES – Monitor fluid and electrolyte balance and cardiac function. Filter IV solns with concentrations at least 20%; crystals may be present.

MILNACIPRAN (***Savella***) ▶KL ♀C ▶? $$$$

ADULT – Fibromyalgia: Start day 1: 12.5 mg PO once, then days 2 to 3: 12.5 mg two times per day, days 4 to 7: 25 mg two times per day, then 50 mg two times per day. Max 200 mg/day.

PEDS – Not approved for use in children.

FORMS – Trade only: Tabs 12.5, 25, 50, 100 mg.

NOTES – Reduce dose by 50% for severe renal impairment with CrCl less than 30 mL/min. Taper if discontinued.

NIMODIPINE (***Nimotop***) ▶L ♀C ▶– $$$$$

ADULT – Subarachnoid hemorrhage: 60 mg PO q 4 h for 21 days.

PEDS – Not approved in children.

FORMS – Generic only: Caps 30 mg.

NOTES – Begin therapy within 96 h. Give 1 h before or 2 h after meals. May give cap contents SL or via NG tube. Reduce dose in hepatic dysfunction.

ONABOTULINUM TOXIN TYPE A (***Botox, Botox Cosmetic***) ▶Not absorbed ♀C ▶? $$$$$

WARNING – Symptoms of systemic botulism have been reported, particularly in children treated for spasticity due to cerebral palsy.

ADULT – Moderate to severe glabellar lines in patients no older than age 65 yo: Inject 0.1 mL into each of 5 sites. Blepharospasm: 1.25 to 5 units IM into each of several sites in the orbicularis oculi of upper and lower lids q 3 months; use lower doses at initial visit. Strabismus: 1.25 to 5 units depending on diagnosis, injected into extraocular muscles. Cervical dystonia: 15 to 100 units IM (with or without EMG guidance) into affected muscles q 3 months (eg, splenius capitis/cervicis, sternocleidomastoid, levator scapulae, trapezius, semispinalis, scalene, longissimus); usual total dose is 200 to 300 units/treatment. Primary axillary hyperhidrosis: 50 units/axilla intradermally, divided over 10 to 15 sites. Upper limb spasticity: Biceps brachii, 100 to 200 units IM divided into 4 sites (with or without EMG guidance) q 3 months; flexor carpi

(cont.)

ONABOTULINUM TOXIN TYPE A (*cont.*)

radialis, 12.5 to 50 units IM in 1 site; flexor carpi ulnaris, 12.5 to 50 units IM in 1 site; flexor digitorum profundus, 30 to 50 units IM in 1 site; flexor digitorum sublimis, 30 to 50 units IM in 1 site. Chronic migraine headache: Dilute to 5 units/0.1 mL then inject 155 units total as a series of 0.1 mL (5 units) IM injections at 7 specific head/neck sites. Refer to prescribing information for locations of injections and amount per site. Repeat q 12 weeks. Botulinum toxin products are not interchangeable.

PEDS – Not approved in children younger than 12 yo for blepharospasm and strabismus, younger than 16 yo for cervical dystonia, or younger than 18 yo for hyperhidrosis, spasticity, or chronic migraine headahce.

UNAPPROVED ADULT – Hemifacial spasm: 1.25 to 2.5 units IM into affected muscles q 3 to 4 months (eg, corrugator, orbicularis oculi, zygomaticus major, buccinator, depressor anguli oris, platysma); usual total dose is 10 to 34 units/treatment.

FORMS – Trade only: 100 unit single-use vials.

NOTES – Clinical benefit occurs within 2 weeks (2 to 3 days for facial injections), peaks at 1 to 6 weeks, and wears off in approximately 3 months. Contraindicated in peripheral motor neuropathic disease (eg, ALS, motor neuropathy) or neuromuscular junction disease (eg, myasthenia gravis, Lambert-Eaton syndrome). The use of lower doses and longer dosing intervals may decrease the risk of producing neutralizing antibodies. Increased risk of dysphagia when more than 100 units are injected into the sternocleidomastoid or with bilateral sternocleidomastoid injections. Potency units of Botox cannot be interchanged with other products. For chronic migraine headache the amount injected varies by muscle site. Refer to prescribing information for specific amounts to inject at each stie.

OXYBATE (***XYREM GHB,*** **gamma hydroxybutyrate**) ▶L ♀B ▶?©III $$$$$

WARNING – CNS depressant with abuse potential; avoid concurrent alcohol or sedative use.

ADULT – Cataplexy or excessive daytime sleepiness in narcolepsy: 2.25 g PO at bedtime. Repeat in 2.5 to 4 h. May increase by 1.5 g/day at 2-week intervals to max 9 g/day. Dilute each dose in 60 mL water.

PEDS – Not approved in children.

FORMS – Trade only: Soln 180 mL (500 mg/mL) supplied with measuring device and child-proof dosing cups.

NOTES – Available only through the XYREM Success Program centralized pharmacy (866-997-3688). Adjust dose in hepatic dysfunction. Prepare doses just prior to bedtime, and use within 24 h. May need an alarm to signal 2nd dose.

RILUZOLE (***Rilutek***) ▶LK ♀C ▶– $$$$$

ADULT – Amyotrophic lateral sclerosis: 50 mg PO q 12 h.

PEDS – Not approved in children.

FORMS – Trade only: Tabs 50 mg.

NOTES – Take 1 h before or 2 h after meals. Monitor LFTs.

TETRABENAZINE (***Xenazine,*** ✱***Nitoman***) ▶L ♀C ▶? ? $$$$$

WARNING – Contraindicated with untreated or inadequately responding depression or suicidality; monitor closely and discontinue at the first signs thereof.

ADULT – Chorea associated with Huntington's disease: Start 12.5 mg PO q am. Increase after 1 week to 12.5 mg PO two times per day. May increase by 12.5 mg/day weekly. For doses greater than 37.5 to 50 mg/day divide doses three times per day. For doses greater than 50 mg/day genotype the patient for CYP2D6 activity, titrate by 12.5 mg/day weekly and divide doses three times per day to max 37.5 mg/dose and 100 mg/day (extensive/intermediate metabolizers) or 25 mg/dose and 50 mg/day (poor metabolizers).

PEDS – Not approved in children.

UNAPPROVED ADULT – Hyperkinetic movement disorders such as tic disorders (including Tourette's syndrome), tardive syndromes, hemiballismus, dystonia, and other choreas (approved dosing in Canada): Start 12.5 mg PO two to three times per day. May increase by 12.5 mg/day q 3 to 5 days to usual dose of 25 mg PO three times per day. Max 200 mg/day, but most patients do not tolerate more than 75 mg/day. Discontinue if there is no benefit after 7 days of treatment at max tolerated dose.

UNAPPROVED PEDS – Limited data suggest that ½ of the adult dose may be used and titrated as tolerated.

FORMS – Trade only: Tabs 12.5, 25 mg.

NOTES – Contraindicated in hepatic impairment, suicidality, untreated/inadequately responding depression, and with MAOIs. Reduce dose by 50% if used with potent CYP2D6 inhibitors. Monitor patient for depression, akathisia, sedation/somnolence, and parkinsonism, which may respond to dose reduction. Retitrate dose if interrupted longer than 5 days. Use caution when combined with antipsychotics and other dopamine receptor–blocking agents. May attenuate the effects of levodopa and antidepressants. Increases QTc by approximately 8 msec.

OB/GYN: Contraceptives—Oral Monophasic

NOTE: Not recommended in women older than 35 yo who smoke or have complex migraine headaches. Increased risk of thromboembolism, CVA, MI, hepatic neoplasia, and gallbladder disease. Nausea, breast tenderness, and breakthrough bleeding are common transient side effects. Nighttime dosing may minimize nausea. Effectiveness is reduced by hepatic enzyme-inducing drugs such as certain anticonvulsants and barbiturates, rifampin, rifabutin, griseofulvin, and protease inhibitors. Additionally, products that contain St. John's wort may decrease efficacy. Vomiting or diarrhea may also increase the risk of contraceptive failure. An additional form of birth control may be advisable. Advise patients to take at the same time every day. See prescribing information for instructions on missing doses. Most available in 21- and 28-day packs. Although not approved by the FDA, combined OCPs are used for dysfunctional uterine bleeding, emergency contraception, dysmenorrhea, pelvic pain, and hirsutism (with spironolactone): 1 tab PO daily. Wait 6 weeks postpartum to initiate combination OCPs to decrease the risk of thromboembolism and to support lactation.

AMETHYST **(ethinyl estradiol + levonorgestrel)** ▶L – ♀X ▶–
ADULT – Contraception: 1 tab PO daily.
PEDS – Not approved in children.
FORMS – Trade only: Tabs 20 mcg ethinyl estradiol/90 mcg levonorgestrel
NOTES – Approved for continuous use without a "pill-free" period. May cause breakthrough bleeding. Same as Lybrel.

APRI **(ethinyl estradiol + desogestrel, *♣Marvelon*)** ▶L ♀X ▶– $$
ADULT – Contraception: 1 tab PO daily.
PEDS – Not approved in children.
FORMS – Trade only: Tabs 30 mcg ethinyl estradiol/0.15 mg desogestrel.
NOTES – Same as Desogen, Ortho-Cept, and Reclipsen.

AVIANE **(ethinyl estradiol + levonorgestrel)** ▶L ♀X ▶– $$
ADULT – Contraception: 1 tab PO daily.
PEDS – Not approved in children.
UNAPPROVED ADULT – Emergency contraception: See table.
FORMS – Trade only: Tabs 20 mcg ethinyl estradiol/0.1 mg levonorgestrel.
NOTES – May cause less nausea and breast tenderness and may increase breakthrough bleeding due to lower estrogen content. Same as Lessina, Lutera, and Sronyx.

BALZIVA **(ethinyl estradiol + norethindrone)** ▶L ♀X ▶– $$
ADULT – Contraception: 1 tab PO daily.
PEDS – Not approved in children.
FORMS – Trade only: Tabs 35 mcg ethinyl estradiol/0.4 mg norethindrone.
NOTES – Same as Ovcon-35.

BEYAZ **(ethinyl estradiol + drospirenone + levomefolate calcium)** ▶L – ♀X ▶– $$$
ADULT – Contraception, premenstrual dysphoric disorder, acne, folate supplementation. 1 tab PO daily.
PEDS – Not approved in children.
FORMS – Trade only. Tabs 0.02 mg ethinyl estradiol, 2 mg drospirenone, 0.451 mg levomefolate calcium. 24 active pills followed by 4 inert pills.
NOTES – May cause hyperkalemia due to antimineralcorticoid activity of drospirenone (equal to 25 mg spironolactone). Monitor potassium in patients on ACE inhibitors, ARBs. potassium-sparing diuretics, heparin, aldosterone antagonists, and NSAIDs.

BREVICON **(ethinyl estradiol + norethindrone)** ▶L ♀X ▶– $$$
ADULT – Contraception: 1 tab PO daily.
PEDS – Not approved in children.
FORMS – Trade only: Tabs 35 mcg ethinyl estradiol/0.5 mg norethindrone.
NOTES – Same as Modicon, Necon 0.5/35, Nortrel 0.5/35.

CRYSELLE **(ethinyl estradiol + norgestrel)** ▶L ♀X ▶– $$
ADULT – Contraception: 1 tab PO daily.
PEDS – Not approved in children.
UNAPPROVED ADULT – Emergency contraception: See table.
FORMS – Trade only: Tabs: 30 mcg ethinyl estradiol/0.3 mg norgestrel.
NOTES – Same as Lo/Ovral and Low-Ogestrel.

DEMULEN **(ethinyl estradiol + ethynodiol)** ▶L ♀X ▶– $$
WARNING – Multiple strengths; see FORMS and write specific product on Rx.
ADULT – Contraception: 1 tab PO daily.
PEDS – Not approved in children.
FORMS – Trade only: Tabs 35 mcg ethinyl estradiol/1 mg ethynodiol (Demulen 1/35); 50 mcg ethinyl estradiol/1 mg ethynodiol (Demulen 1/50).
NOTES – 50 mcg estrogen component rarely necessary.

DESOGEN **(ethinyl estradiol + desogestrel, *♣Marvelon*)** ▶L ♀X ▶– $$
ADULT – Contraception: 1 tab PO daily.

(cont.)

DESOGEN *(cont.)*

PEDS – Not approved in children.

FORMS – Trade only: Tabs 30 mcg ethinyl estradiol/0.15 mg desogestrel.

NOTES – Same as Apri, Ortho-Cept, and Reclipsen.

FEMCON FE **(ethinyl estradiol + norethindrone, *Zeosa*)** ▶L ♀X ▶– $$$

ADULT – Contraception: 1 tab PO daily.

PEDS – Not approved in children.

FORMS – Trade only: Chewable tabs 35 mcg ethinyl estradiol/0.4 mg norethindrone. Placebo tabs are ferrous fumarate 75 mg.

NOTES – Chewable formulation may be swallowed whole or chewed. If chewed, follow with 8 oz liquid. Same as Zeosa.

GENERESS FE **(ethinyl estradiol + norethindrone + ferrous fumarate)** ▶L – ♀X ▶–

ADULT – Contraception: 1 tab PO daily.

PEDS – Not approved in children.

FORMS – Trade only: Tabs 0.8 mgnorethindrone and 25 mcg ethinyl estradiol with 4 days 75 mg ferrous fumarate.

JUNEL **(ethinyl estradiol + norethindrone)** ▶L ♀X ▶– $$

WARNING – Multiple strengths; see FORMS and write specific product on Rx.

ADULT – Contraception: 1 tab PO daily.

PEDS – Not approved in children.

FORMS – Trade only: Tabs 1 mg norethindrone/20 mcg ethinyl estradiol (Junel 1/20). 1.5 mg norethindrone/30 mcg ethinyl estradiol (Junel 1.5/30).

NOTES – Junel 1/20 may cause less nausea and breast tenderness and may increase breakthrough bleeding due to lower estrogen content. Same as Loestrin.

JUNEL FE **(ethinyl estradiol + norethindrone + ferrous fumarate)** ▶L ♀X ▶– $$

WARNING – Multiple strengths; see FORMS and write specific product on Rx.

ADULT – Contraception: 1 tab PO daily.

PEDS – Not approved in children.

FORMS – Trade only: Tabs 1 mg norethindrone/20 mcg ethinyl estradiol with 7 days 75 mg ferrous fumarate (Junel Fe 1/20). 1.5 mg norethindrone/30 mcg ethinyl estradiol with 7 days 75 mg ferrous fumarate (1.5/30).

NOTES – Junel Fe 1/20 may cause less nausea and breast tenderness and may increase breakthrough bleeding due to lower estrogen content. Same as Loestrin Fe.

KARIVA **(ethinyl estradiol + desogestrel)** ▶L ♀X ▶– $$$

ADULT – Contraception: 1 tab PO daily.

PEDS – Not approved in children.

FORMS – Trade only: Tabs 20 mcg ethinyl estradiol/0.15 mg desogestrel (21 tabs), 10 mcg ethinyl estradiol (5 tabs).

NOTES – May have less breakthrough bleeding. All 28 tabs must be taken. Same as Mircette.

KELNOR **(ethinyl estradiol + ethynodiol)** ▶L ♀X ▶– $$

ADULT – Contraception: 1 tab PO daily.

PEDS – Not approved in children.

FORMS – Generic/Trade: Tabs 35 mcg ethinyl estradiol/1 mg ethynodiol.

NOTES – Same as Demulen 1/35.

LESSINA **(ethinyl estradiol + levonorgestrel)** ▶L ♀X ▶– $$

ADULT – Contraception: 1 tab PO daily.

PEDS – Not approved in children.

UNAPPROVED ADULT – Emergency contraception: See table.

FORMS – Generic/Trade: Tabs 20 mcg ethinyl estradiol/0.1 mg levonorgestrel.

NOTES – May cause less nausea and breast tenderness and may increase breakthrough bleeding due to lower estrogen content. Same as Aviane, Lutera, and Sronyx.

LEVORA **(ethinyl estradiol + levonorgestrel, ✤*Min-Ovral*)** ▶L ♀X ▶– $$

ADULT – Contraception: 1 tab PO daily.

PEDS – Not approved in children.

UNAPPROVED ADULT – Emergency contraception: See table.

FORMS – Trade only: Tabs 30 mcg ethinyl estradiol/0.15 mg levonorgestrel.

NOTES – Same as Nordette, Portia, and Solia.

LO/OVRAL **(ethinyl estradiol + norgestrel)** ▶L ♀X ▶– $$

ADULT – Contraception: 1 tab PO daily.

PEDS – Not approved in children.

UNAPPROVED ADULT – Emergency contraception: See table.

FORMS – Trade only: Tabs: 30 mcg ethinyl estradiol/0.3 mg norgestrel.

NOTES – Same as Cryselle and Low-Ogestrel.

LOESTRIN **(ethinyl estradiol + norethindrone, ✤*Minestrin 1/20*)** ▶L ♀X ▶– $$$

WARNING – Multiple strengths; see FORMS and write specific product on Rx.

ADULT – Contraception: 1 tab PO daily.

PEDS – Not approved in children.

FORMS – Trade only: Tabs 1 mg norethindrone/20 mcg ethinyl estradiol (Loestrin 1/20). 1.5 mg norethindrone/30 mcg ethinyl estradiol (Loestrin 1.5/30).

NOTES – Loestrin 1/20 may cause less nausea and breast tenderness and may increase breakthrough bleeding due to lower estrogen content. Same as Junel.

LOESTRIN 24 FE **(ethinyl estradiol + norethindrone + ferrous fumarate)** ▶L ♀X ▶– $$$
ADULT – Contraception: 1 tab PO daily.
PEDS – Not approved in children.
FORMS – Trade only: Tabs 1 mg norethindrone/20 mcg ethinyl estradiol (24 days) with 4 days 75 mg ferrous fumarate.
NOTES – Loestrin 24 Fe 1/20 may cause less nausea and breast tenderness and may increase breakthrough bleeding due to lower estrogen content.

LOESTRIN FE **(ethinyl estradiol + norethindrone + ferrous fumarate)** ▶L ♀X ▶– $$$
WARNING – Multiple strengths; see FORMS and write specific product on Rx.
ADULT – Contraception: 1 tab PO daily.
PEDS – Not approved in children.
FORMS – Trade only: Tabs 1 mg norethindrone/20 mcg ethinyl estradiol with 7 days 75 mg ferrous fumarate (Loestrin Fe 1/20); 1.5 mg norethindrone/30 mcg ethinyl estradiol with 7 days 75 mg ferrous fumarate (1.5/30).
NOTES – Loestrin Fe 1/20 may cause less nausea and breast tenderness and may increase breakthrough bleeding due to lower estrogen content. All 28 tabs must be taken. Same as Junel Fe.

LOSEASONIQUE **(ethinyl estradiol + levonorgestrel)** ▶L ♀X ▶– $$$
ADULT – Contraception: 1 tab PO daily.
PEDS – Not approved in children.
FORMS – Trade only: Tabs 20 mcg ethinyl estradiol/0.1 mg levonorgestrel. 84 orange active pills followed by 7 yellow pills with 10 mcg ethinyl estradiol.
NOTES – Decreases menstrual periods from q month to q 3 months; however, intermenstrual bleeding and spotting is more frequent than with 28-day regimens. All 91 tabs must be taken.

LOW-OGESTREL **(ethinyl estradiol + norgestrel)** ▶L ♀X ▶– $$
ADULT – Contraception: 1 tab PO daily.
PEDS – Not approved in children.
UNAPPROVED ADULT – Emergency contraception: See table.
FORMS – Trade only: Tabs: 30 mcg ethinyl estradiol/0.3 mg norgestrel.
NOTES – Same as Cryselle and Lo/Ovral.

LUTERA **(ethinyl estradiol + levonorgestrel)** ▶L ♀X ▶– $$
ADULT – Contraception: 1 tab PO daily.
PEDS – Not approved in children.
UNAPPROVED ADULT – Emergency contraception: See table.
FORMS – Trade only: Tabs 20 mcg ethinyl estradiol/0.1 mg levonorgestrel.
NOTES – May cause less nausea and breast tenderness and may increase breakthrough bleeding due to lower estrogen content. Same as Aviane, Lessina, and Sronyx.

LYBREL **(ethinyl estradiol + levonorgestrel)** ▶L ♀X ▶– $$$
ADULT – Contraception: 1 tab PO daily.
PEDS – Not approved in children.
FORMS – Trade only: Tabs 20 mcg ethinyl estradiol/90 mcg levonorgestrel.
NOTES – Approved for continuous use without a "pill-free" period. May cause breakthrough bleeding. Same as Amethyst.

MICROGESTIN FE **(ethinyl estradiol + norethindrone + ferrous fumarate)** ▶L ♀X ▶– $$
WARNING – Multiple strengths; see FORMS and write specific product on Rx.
ADULT – Contraception: 1 tab PO daily.
PEDS – Not approved in children.
FORMS – Trade only: Tabs 1 mg norethindrone/20 mcg ethinyl estradiol with 7 days 75 mg ferrous fumarate (Microgestin Fe 1/20). 1.5 mg norethindrone/30 mcg ethinyl estradiol with 7 days 75 mg ferrous fumarate (1.5/30).
NOTES – Microgestin Fe 1/20 may cause less nausea and breast tenderness and may increase breakthrough bleeding due to lower estrogen content. All 28 tabs must be taken. Same as Loestrin Fe.

MIRCETTE **(ethinyl estradiol + desogestrel, Azurette)** ▶L ♀X ▶– $$$
ADULT – Contraception: 1 tab PO daily.
PEDS – Not approved in children.
FORMS – Tabs 20 mcg ethinyl estradiol/0.15 mg desogestrel (21 tabs), 10 mcg ethinyl estradiol (5 tabs).
NOTES – May have less breakthrough bleeding. All 28 tabs must be taken. Same as Kariva.

MODICON **(ethinyl estradiol + norethindrone)** ▶L ♀X ▶– $$$
ADULT – Contraception: 1 tab PO daily.
PEDS – Not approved in children.
FORMS – Trade only: Tabs 35 mcg ethinyl estradiol/0.5 mg norethindrone.
NOTES – Same as Brevicon.

MONONESSA **(ethinyl estradiol + norgestimate)** ▶L ♀X ▶– $$
ADULT – Contraception: 1 tab PO daily.
PEDS – Not approved in children.
FORMS – Trade only: Tabs: 35 mcg ethinyl estradiol/0.25 mg norgestimate.
NOTES – Same as Ortho-Cyclen.

NECON **(ethinyl estradiol + norethindrone, ♣ *Select 1/35, Brevicon 1/35*)** ▶L ♀X ▶– $$
WARNING – Multiple strengths; see FORMS and write specific product on Rx.
ADULT – Contraception: 1 tab PO daily.

(cont.)

NECON *(cont.)*

PEDS – Not approved in children.
FORMS – Trade only: Tabs 0.5 mg norethindrone/35 mcg ethinyl estradiol (Necon 0.5/35). 1 mg norethindrone/35 mcg ethinyl estradiol (Necon 1/35).
NOTES – Same as Brevicon (0.5/35), Ortho-Novum 1/35 (1/35).

NECON 1/50 **(mestranol + norethindrone)** ▶L ♀X ▶– $$
ADULT – Contraception: 1 tab PO daily.
PEDS – Not approved in children.
FORMS – Trade only: Tabs: 1 mg norethindrone/50 mcg mestranol.
NOTES – 50 mcg estrogen component rarely necessary. Same as Norinyl 1+50.

NORDETTE **(ethinyl estradiol + levonorgestrel,** ✤ ***Min-Ovral*****)** ▶L ♀X ▶– $$$
ADULT – Contraception: 1 tab PO daily.
PEDS – Not approved in children.
UNAPPROVED ADULT – Emergency contraception: See table.
FORMS – Trade only: Tabs 30 mcg ethinyl estradiol/0.15 mg levonorgestrel.
NOTES – Same as Levlen.

NORINYL 1+35 **(ethinyl estradiol + norethindrone,** ✤ ***Select 1/35, Brevicon 1/35*****)** ▶L ♀X ▶– $$
ADULT – Contraception: 1 tab PO daily.
PEDS – Not approved in children.
FORMS – Trade only: Tabs 1 mg norethindrone/35 mcg ethinyl estradiol.
NOTES – Same as Ortho-Novum 1/35.

NORINYL 1+50 **(mestranol + norethindrone)** ▶L ♀X ▶– $$
ADULT – Contraception: 1 tab PO daily.
PEDS – Not approved in children.
FORMS – Trade only: Tabs: 1 mg norethindrone/50 mcg mestranol.
NOTES – 50 mcg estrogen component rarely necessary. Same as Necon 1/50.

NORTREL **(ethinyl estradiol + norethindrone)** ▶L ♀X ▶– $$
WARNING – Multiple strengths; see FORMS and write specific product on Rx.
ADULT – Contraception: 1 tab PO daily.
PEDS – Not approved in children.
FORMS – Trade only: Tabs 35 mcg ethinyl estradiol/1 mg norethindrone (Nortrel 1/35). 35 mcg ethinyl estradiol/0.5 mg norethindrone (Nortrel 0.5/35).
NOTES – Same as Brevicon (0.5/35), Ortho-Novum 1/35 (1/35).

OGESTREL **(ethinyl estradiol + norgestrel)** ▶L ♀X ▶– $$
ADULT – Contraception: 1 tab PO daily.
PEDS – Not approved in children.
UNAPPROVED ADULT – Emergency contraception: See table.
FORMS – Trade only: Tabs: 50 mcg ethinyl estradiol/0.5 mg norgestrel.
NOTES – 50 mcg estrogen component rarely necessary. Same as Ovral.

ORTHO-CEPT **(ethinyl estradiol + desogestrel,** ✤ ***Marvelon*****)** ▶L ♀X ▶– $$$
ADULT – Contraception: 1 tab PO daily.
PEDS – Not approved in children.
FORMS – Trade only: Tabs 30 mcg ethinyl estradiol/0.15 mg desogestrel.
NOTES – Same as Desogen.

ORTHO-CYCLEN **(ethinyl estradiol + norgestimate,** ✤ ***Cyclen*****)** ▶L ♀X ▶– $$
ADULT – Contraception: 1 tab PO daily.
PEDS – Not approved in children.
FORMS – Generic/Trade: Tabs: 35 mcg ethinyl estradiol/0.25 mg norgestimate.

ORTHO-NOVUM 1/35 **(ethinyl estradiol + norethindrone)** ▶L ♀X ▶– $$$
ADULT – Contraception: 1 tab PO daily.
PEDS – Not approved in children.
FORMS – Trade only: Tabs 1 mg norethindrone/35 mcg ethinyl estradiol.

OVCON-35 **(ethinyl estradiol + norethindrone)** ▶L ♀X ▶– $$$
ADULT – Contraception: 1 tab PO daily.
PEDS – Not approved in children.
FORMS – Trade only: Tabs 35 mcg ethinyl estradiol/0.4 mg norethindrone.
NOTES – Same as Balziva and Zenchent

OVCON-50 **(ethinyl estradiol + norethindrone)** ▶L ♀X ▶– $$$
ADULT – Contraception: 1 tab PO daily.
PEDS – Not approved in children.
FORMS – Trade only: Tabs 50 mcg ethinyl estradiol/0.4 mg norethindrone.
NOTES – 50 mcg estrogen component rarely necessary.

PORTIA **(ethinyl estradiol + levonorgestrel)** ▶L ♀X ▶– $$
ADULT – Contraception: 1 tab PO daily.
PEDS – Not approved in children.
UNAPPROVED ADULT – Emergency contraception: See table.
FORMS – Trade only: Tabs 30 mcg ethinyl estradiol/0.15 mg levonorgestrel.
NOTES – Same as Levora, Nordette, and Solia.

PREVIFEM **(ethinyl estradiol + norgestimate)** ▶L ♀X ▶– $$
ADULT – Contraception: 1 tab PO daily.
PEDS – Not approved in children.
FORMS – Trade only: Tabs: 35 mcg ethinyl estradiol/0.25 mg norgestimate.

QUASENSE **(ethinyl estradiol + levonorgestrel)** ▶L ♀X ▶– $$$

ADULT – Contraception: 1 tab PO daily.

PEDS – Not approved in children.

UNAPPROVED ADULT – Emergency contraception: See table.

FORMS – Generic/Trade: Tabs 30 mcg ethinyl estradiol/0.15 mg levonorgestrel. 84 white active pills followed by 7 peach placebo pills.

NOTES – Decreases menstrual periods from q month to q 3 months; however, intermenstrual bleeding and spotting is more frequent than with 28-day regimens. Same as Jolessa and Seasonale.

RECLIPSEN **(ethinyl estradiol + desogestrel)** ▶L ♀X ▶– $$

ADULT – Contraception: 1 tab PO daily.

PEDS – Not approved in children.

FORMS – Trade only: Tabs 30 mcg ethinyl estradiol/0.15 mg desogestrel.

NOTES – Same as Apri, Desogen, and Ortho-Cept.

SAFYRAL **(ethinyl estradiol + drospirenone + levomefolate calcium)** ▶L – ♀C ▶–©V

ADULT – Contraception and folate supplementation: 1 tab PO daily.

PEDS – Not approved in children

FORMS – Trade only. 0.03 mg ethinyl estradiol, 3 mg drospirenone, 0.451 mg levomefolate calcium. 24 active pills are followed by 4 inert pills.

NOTES – May cause hyperkalemia due to antimineralcorticoid activity of drospirenone (equal to 25mg spironolactone). Monitor potassium in patients on ACE inhibitors, ARBs, potassium-sparing diuretics, heparin, aldosterone antagonists, and NSAIDs.

SEASONALE **(ethinyl estradiol + levonorgestrel)** ▶L ♀X ▶– $$$

ADULT – Contraception: 1 tab PO daily.

PEDS – Not approved in children.

UNAPPROVED ADULT – Emergency contraception: See table.

FORMS – Generic/Trade: Tabs 30 mcg ethinyl estradiol/0.15 mg levonorgestrel. 84 pink active pills followed by 7 white placebo pills.

NOTES – Decreases menstrual periods from q month to q 3 months; however, intermenstrual bleeding and spotting is more frequent than with 28-day regimens. Same as Jolessa and Quasense.

SEASONIQUE **(ethinyl estradiol + levonorgestrel, *Amethia*)** ▶L ♀X ▶– $$$

ADULT – Contraception: 1 tab PO daily.

PEDS – Not approved in children.

UNAPPROVED ADULT – Emergency contraception: See table.

FORMS – Trade only: Tabs 30 mcg ethinyl estradiol/0.15 mg levonorgestrel. 84 active pills followed by 7 pills with 10 mcg ethinyl estradiol.

NOTES – Decreases menstrual periods from q month to q 3 months; however, intermenstrual bleeding and spotting is more frequent than with 28-day regimens. All 91 tabs must be taken.

SPRINTEC **(ethinyl estradiol + norgestimate)** ▶L ♀X ▶– $$

ADULT – Contraception: 1 tab PO daily.

PEDS – Not approved in children.

FORMS – Trade only: Tabs: 35 mcg ethinyl estradiol/0.25 mg norgestimate.

NOTES – Same as Ortho-Cyclen.

YASMIN **(ethinyl estradiol + drospirenone)** ▶L ♀X ▶– $$$

ADULT – Contraception: 1 tab PO daily.

PEDS – Not approved in children.

FORMS – Trade only: Tabs: 30 mcg ethinyl estradiol/3 mg drospirenone.

NOTES – May cause hyperkalemia due to antimineralocorticoid activity of drospirenone (equal to 25 mg spironolactone). Monitor potassium in patients on ACE inhibitors, ARBs, potassium-sparing diuretics, heparin, aldosterone antagonists, and NSAIDs. Same as Ocella, Safyral, and Zarah.

YAZ **(ethinyl estradiol + drospirenone)** ▶L ♀X ▶– $$$

ADULT – Contraception, premenstrual dysphoric disorder, acne: 1 tab PO daily.

PEDS – Not approved in children.

FORMS – Generic/Trade: Tabs 20 mcg ethinyl estradiol/3 mg drospirenone. 24 active pills are followed by 4 inert pills.

NOTES – May cause hyperkalemia due to antimineralocorticoid activity of drospirenone (equal to 25 mg spironolactone). Monitor potassium in patients on ACE inhibitors, ARBs, potassium-sparing diuretics, heparin, aldosterone antagonists, and NSAIDs. Same as Gianvi, Loryna, Vestura.

ZARAH **(ethinyl estradiol + drospirenone)** ▶L – ♀X ▶–

ADULT – Contraception: 1 tab PO daily.

PEDS – Not approved in children.

FORMS – Trade only: Tabs: 30 mcg ethinyl estradiol/3 mg drospirenone.

NOTES – May cause hyperkalemia due to antimineralcorticoid activity of drospirenone (equal to 25 mg of spironolactone). Monitor potassium in patients on ACE inhibitors, ARBs, potassium-sparing diuretics, heparin, aldosterone antagonists, and NSAIDs. Same as Ocella, Safyral, and Yasmin.

ZOVIA **(ethinyl estradiol + ethynodiol)** ▶L ♀X ▶– $$

WARNING – Multiple strengths; see FORMS and write specific product on Rx.

ADULT – Contraception: 1 tab PO daily.

PEDS – Not approved in children.

FORMS – Trade only: Tabs 1 mg ethynodiol/35 mcg ethinyl estradiol (Zovia 1/35E). 1 mg ethynodiol/50 mcg ethinyl estradiol (Zovia 1/50E).

NOTES – 50 mcg estrogen component rarely necessary. Same as Demulen.

OB/GYN: Contraceptives—Oral Biphasic

NOTE: Not recommended in women older than 35 yo who smoke or have complex migraine headaches. Increased risk of thromboembolism, CVA, MI, hepatic neoplasia, and gallbladder disease. Nausea, breast tenderness, and breakthrough bleeding are common transient side effects. Nighttime dosing may minimize nausea. Effectiveness is reduced by hepatic enzyme-inducing drugs such as certain anticonvulsants and barbiturates, rifampin, rifabutin, griseofulvin, and protease inhibitors. Additionally, products that contain St. John's wort may decrease efficacy. Vomiting or diarrhea may also increase the risk of contraceptive failure. An additional form of birth control may be advisable. Advise patients to take at the same time every day. See prescribing information for instructions on missing doses. Most available in 21- and 28-day packs. Although not approved by the FDA, combined OCPs are used for dysfunctional uterine bleeding, dysmenorrhea, pelvic pain, and hirsutism (with spironolactone): 1 tab PO daily. Wait 6 weeks postpartum to initiate combination OCPs to decrease the risk of thromboembolism and to support lactation.

NECON 10/11 **(ethinyl estradiol + norethindrone)** ▶L ♀X ▶– $$

ADULT – Contraception: 1 tab PO daily.

PEDS – Not approved in children.

FORMS – Trade only: Tabs 35 mcg ethinyl estradiol/0.5 mg norethindrone (10), 35 mcg ethinyl estradiol/1 mg norethindrone (11).

NOTES – Same as Ortho-Novum 10/11.

OB/GYN: Contraceptives—Oral Triphasic

NOTE: Not recommended in women older than 35 yo who smoke. Increased risk of thromboembolism, CVA, MI, hepatic neoplasia, and gallbladder disease. Nausea, breast tenderness, and breakthrough bleeding are common transient side effects. Nighttime dosing may minimize nausea. Effectiveness is reduced by hepatic enzyme–inducing drugs such as certain anticonvulsants and barbiturates, rifampin, rifabutin, griseofulvin, and protease inhibitors. Additionally, products that contain St. John's wort may decrease efficacy. Vomiting or diarrhea may also increase the risk of contraceptive failure. An additional form of birth control may be advisable. Advise patients to take at the same time every day. See prescribing information for instructions on missing doses. Most available in 21- and 28-day packs. Although not approved by the FDA, combined OCPs are used for dysfunctional uterine bleeding, emergency contraception, dysmenorrhea, pelvic pain, and hirsutism (with spironolactone): 1 tab PO daily. Wait 6 weeks postpartum to initiate combination OCPs to decrease the risk of thromboembolism and to support lactation.

ARANELLE **(ethinyl estradiol + norethindrone)** ▶L ♀X ▶– $$

ADULT – Contraception: 1 tab PO daily.

PEDS – Not approved in children.

FORMS – Trade only: Tabs 35 mcg ethinyl estradiol/0.5, 1, 0.5 mg norethindrone.

NOTES – Same as Tri-Norinyl.

CYCLESSA **(ethinyl estradiol + desogestrel, *Caziant*)** ▶L ♀X ▶– $$

ADULT – Contraception: 1 tab PO daily.

PEDS – Not approved in children.

FORMS – Generic/Trade: Tabs 25 mcg ethinyl estradiol/0.100 (7), 0.125 (7), 0.150 mg desogestrel (7).

NOTES – Same as Cesia, Velivet.

ENPRESSE **(ethinyl estradiol + levonorgestrel, ♣ *Triquilar*)** ▶L ♀X ▶– $$

ADULT – Contraception: 1 tab PO daily.

PEDS – Not approved in children.

UNAPPROVED ADULT – Emergency contraception: See table.

FORMS – Trade only: Tabs 30, 40, 30 mcg ethinyl estradiol/0.05, 0.075, 0.125 mg levonorgestrel.

NOTES – Same as Trivora 28.

ESTROSTEP FE **(ethinyl estradiol + norethindrone + ferrous fumarate)** ▶L ♀X ▶– $$$

ADULT – Contraception: 1 tab PO daily.

PEDS – Not approved in children.

FORMS – Generic/Trade: Tabs 20, 30, 35 mcg ethinyl estradiol/1 mg norethindrone + "placebo" tabs with 75 mg ferrous fumarate. Packs of 28 only.

NOTES – All 28 tabs must be taken. Same as Tilia Fe and Tri-Legest Fe.

ORAL CONTRACEPTIVES* ▶L CX	Estrogen (mcg)	Progestin (mg)
Monophasic		
Necon 1/50, Norinyl 1+50	50 mestranol	1 norethindrone
Ovcon-50	50 ethinyl estradiol	
Demulen 1/50, Zovia 1/50E		1 ethynodiol
Ogestrel		0.5 norgestrel
Necon 1/35, Norinyl 1+35, Nortrel 1/35, Ortho-Novum 1/35	35 ethinyl estradiol	1 norethindrone
Brevicon, Modicon, Necon 0.5/35,Nortrel 0.5/35		0.5 norethindrone
Balziva, Femcon Fe, Ovcon-35, Zenchent, Zeosa		0.4 norethindrone
Previfem		0.18 norgestimate
MonoNessa, Ortho-Cyclen, Sprintec-28		0.25 norgestimate
Demulen 1/35, Kelnor 1/35, Zovia 1/35E		1 ethynodiol
Junel 1.5/30, Junel 1.5/30 Fe, Loestrin 211.5/30, Loestrin Fe 1.5/30, Microgestin Fe 1.5/30	30 ethinyl estradiol	1.5 norethindrone
Cryselle, Lo/Ovral, Low-Ogestrel		0.3 norgestrel
Apri, Desogen, Ortho-Cept, Reclipsen		0.15 desogestrel
Levora, Nordette, Portia, Solia		0.15 levonorgestrel
Ocella, Safyral, Yasmin, Zarah		3 drospirenone
Generess Fe	25 ethinyl estradiol	0.8 norethindrone
Junel 1/20, Junel Fe 1/20, Loestrin 211/20, Loestrin Fe 1/20, Loestrin 24 Fe, Microgestin Fe 1/20	20 ethinyl estradiol	1 norethindrone
Aviane, Lessina, Lutera, Sronyx		0.1 levonorgestrel
Amethyst[†]*, Lybrel*[†]		0.09 levonorgestrel
Gianvi, Yaz		3 drospirenone
Beyaz		2 drospirenone
Azurette, Kariva, Mircette	20/10 ethinyl estradiol	0.15 desogestrel
Progestin only		
Camila, Errin, Jolivette, Micronor, Nor-Q.D., Nora-BE	none	0.35 norethindrone
Biphasic (estrogen and progestin contents vary)		
Necon 10/11	35 ethinyl estradiol	0.5/1 norethindrone
Triphasic (estrogen and progestin contents vary)		
Caziant, Cesia, Cyclessa, Velivet	25 ethinyl estradiol	0.100/0.125/0.150 desogestrel
Ortho-Novum 7/7/7, Necon 7/7/7, Nortrel 7/7/7	35 ethinyl estradiol	0.5/0.75/1 norethindrone
Aranelle, Leena, Tri-Norinyl		0.5/1/0.5 norethindrone
Enpresse, Trivora-28	30/40/30 ethinyl estradiol	0.5/0.75/0.125 levonorgestrel
Ortho Tri-Cyclen, Trinessa, Tri-Previfem, Tri-Sprintec	35 ethinyl estradiol	0.18/0.215/0.25 norgestimate
Ortho Tri-Cyclen Lo	25 ethinyl estradiol	
Estrostep Fe, Tilia Fe, Tri-Legest, Tri-Legest Fe	20/30/35 ethinyl estradiol	1 norethindrone
Quadphasic		
Natazia	3 mg/2 mg estradiol valerate	2/3/0 dienogest
Extended Cycle[††]		
Jolessa, Quasense, Seasonale	30 ethinyl estradiol	0.15 levonorgestrel
Amethia, Seasonique	30/10 ethinyl estradiol	0.15 levonorgestrel
LoSeasonique	20 ethinyl estradiol	0.1 levonorgestrel

*All: Not recommended in smokers. Increases risk of thromboembolism, CVA, MI, hepatic neoplasia, and gallbladder disease. Nausea, breast tenderness, and breakthrough bleeding are common transient side effects. Effectiveness reduced by hepatic enzyme-inducing drugs such as certain anticonvulsants and barbiturates, rifampin, rifabutin, griseofulvin, and protease inhibitors. Coadministration with St. John's wort may decrease efficacy. Vomiting or diarrhea may also increase the risk of contraceptive failure. Consider an additional form of birth control in above circumstances. See product insert for instructions on missing doses. Most available in 21-and 28-day packs.

Progestin only: Must be taken at the same time every day. Because much of the literature regarding OC adverse effects pertains mainly to estrogen/progestin combinations, the extent to which progestin-only contraceptives cause these effects is unclear. No significant interaction has been found with broad-spectrum antibiotics. The effect of St. John's wort is unclear. No placebo days, start new pack immediately after finishing current one. Available in 28-day packs. Readers may find the following website useful: www.managingcontraception.com.

[†] Approved for continuous use without a "pill-free" period.

[††] 84 active pills and 7 placebo pills.

LEENA **(ethinyl estradiol + norethindrone)** ▶L ♀X ▶– $$
ADULT – Contraception: 1 tab PO daily.
PEDS – Not approved in children.
FORMS – Trade only: Tabs 35 mcg ethinyl estradiol/0.5, 1, 0.5 mg norethindrone.
NOTES – Same as Tri-Norinyl.

NECON 7/7/7 **(ethinyl estradiol + norethindrone)** ▶L ♀X ▶– $$
ADULT – Contraception: 1 tab PO daily.
PEDS – Not approved in children.
FORMS – Trade only: Tabs 35 mcg ethinyl estradiol/0.5, 0.75, 1 mg norethindrone.
NOTES – Same as Ortho-Novum 7/7/7.

NORTREL 7/7/7 **(ethinyl estradiol + norethindrone)** ▶L ♀X ▶– $$
ADULT – Contraception: 1 tab PO daily.
PEDS – Not approved in children.
FORMS – Trade only: Tabs 35 mcg ethinyl estradiol/0.5, 0.75, 1 mg norethindrone.
NOTES – Same as Ortho-Novum 7/7/7.

ORTHO TRI-CYCLEN **(ethinyl estradiol + norgestimate, ✤ *Tri-Cyclen*)** ▶L ♀X ▶– $$
ADULT – Contraception, adult acne: 1 tab PO daily.
PEDS – Not approved in children.
FORMS – Generic/Trade: Tabs 35 mcg ethinyl estradiol/0.18, 0.215, 0.25 mg norgestimate.
NOTES – Same as Trinessa, Tri-Previfem, and Tri-Sprintec.

ORTHO TRI-CYCLEN LO **(ethinyl estradiol + norgestimate)** ▶L ♀X ▶– $$$
ADULT – Contraception: 1 tab PO daily.
PEDS – Not approved in children.
FORMS – Trade only: Tabs 25 mcg ethinyl estradiol/0.18, 0.215, 0.25 mg norgestimate.

ORTHO-NOVUM 7/7/7 **(ethinyl estradiol + norethindrone)** ▶L ♀X ▶– $$
ADULT – Contraception: 1 tab PO daily.
PEDS – Not approved in children.
FORMS – Trade only: Tabs 35 mcg ethinyl estradiol/0.5, 0.75, 1 mg norethindrone.
NOTES – Same as Necon 7/7/7 and Nortrel 7/7/7.

TRI-LEGEST **(ethinyl estradiol + norethindrone)** ▶L ♀X ▶– $$$
ADULT – Contraception: 1 tab PO daily.
PEDS – Not approved in children.
FORMS – Trade only: Tabs 20, 30, 35 mcg ethinyl estradiol/1 mg norethindrone.

TRI-LEGEST FE **(ethinyl estradiol + norethindrone + ferrous fumarate)** ▶L ♀X ▶– $$$
ADULT – Contraception: 1 tab PO daily.
PEDS – Not approved in children.
FORMS – Trade only: Tabs 20, 30, 35 mcg ethinyl estradiol/1 mg norethindrone + "placebo" tabs with 75 mg ferrous fumarate.
NOTES – Same as Estrostep Fe and Tilia Fe. All 28 tabs must be taken.

TRIVORA-28 **(ethinyl estradiol + levonorgestrel)** ▶L ♀X ▶– $$
ADULT – Contraception: 1 tab PO daily.
PEDS – Not approved in children.
UNAPPROVED ADULT – Emergency contraception: See table.
FORMS – Trade only: Tabs 30, 40, 30 mcg ethinyl estradiol/0.05, 0.075, 0.125 mg levonorgestrel.
NOTES – Same as Enpresse.

TRI-NORINYL **(ethinyl estradiol + norethindrone, ✤ *Synphasic*)** ▶L ♀X ▶– $$
ADULT – Contraception: 1 tab PO daily.
PEDS – Not approved in children.
FORMS – Trade only: Tabs 35 mcg ethinyl estradiol/0.5, 1, 0.5 mg norethindrone.
NOTES – Same as Aranelle and Leena.

TRI-PREVIFEM **(ethinyl estradiol + norgestimate)** ▶L ♀X ▶– $$
ADULT – Contraception, adult acne: 1 tab PO daily.
PEDS – Not approved in children.
FORMS – Trade only: Tabs 35 mcg ethinyl estradiol/0.18, 0.215, 0.25 mg norgestimate.
NOTES – Same as Ortho Tri-Cyclen, Trinessa, and Tri-Sprintec.

TRI-SPRINTEC **(ethinyl estradiol + norgestimate)** ▶L ♀X ▶– $$
ADULT – Contraception, adult acne: 1 tab PO daily.
PEDS – Not approved in children.
FORMS – Trade only: Tabs 35 mcg ethinyl estradiol/0.18, 0.215, 0.25 mg norgestimate.
NOTES – Same as Ortho Tri-Cyclen, Trinessa, and Tri-Previfem.

TRINESSA **(ethinyl estradiol + norgestimate)** ▶L ♀X ▶– $$
ADULT – Contraception, adult acne: 1 tab PO daily.
PEDS – Not approved in children.
FORMS – Trade only: Tabs 35 mcg ethinyl estradiol/0.18, 0.215, 0.25 mg norgestimate.
NOTES – Same as Ortho Tri-Cyclen, Tri-Previfem, and Tri-Sprintec.

VELIVET **(ethinyl estradiol + desogestrel)** ▶L ♀X ▶– $$
ADULT – Contraception: 1 tab PO daily.
PEDS – Not approved in children.
FORMS – Generic/Trade: Tabs 25 mcg ethinyl estradiol/0.100, 0.125, 0.150 mg desogestrel.
NOTES – Same as Caziant, Cesia, and Cyclessa.

OB/GYN: Contraceptives—Quad-Phasic

NATAZIA **(estradiol valerate + estradiol valerate/dienogest)** ▶L – stomach ♀X ◗–
ADULT – Contraception: 1 PO daily, start on day 1 of menstrual cycle. Heavy menstrual bleeding.
PEDS – Not approved in children.
FORMS – Trade only: Tabs 3 mg estradiol valerate (2 tabs), 2 mg estradiol valerate/2 mg dienogest (5 tabs), 2 mg estradiol valerate/3 mg dienogest (17 tabs), 1 mg estradiol valerate (2 tabs), inert (2 tabs).
NOTES – Not evaluated in BMI greater than 30.

OB/GYN: Contraceptives—Other

ETONOGESTREL (***Implanon, Nexplanon***) ▶L ♀X ◗+ $$$$$
WARNING – Increased risk of thromboembolism and CVA. Effectiveness may be reduced by hepatic enzyme-inducing drugs such as certain anticonvulsants, barbiturates, griseofulvin, rifampin. Additionally, products that contain St. John's wort may decrease efficacy; an additional form of birth control may be advisable.
ADULT – Contraception: 1 subdermal implant q 3 years.
PEDS – Not approved in children.
FORMS – Trade only: Single rod implant, 68 mg etonogestrel. Nexplanon also contains 15 mg barium sulfate.
NOTES – Not studied in women greater than 130% of ideal body wt; may be less effective if overweight. Implant should be palpable immediately after insertion.

LEVONORGESTREL (***Next Choice***) ▶L ♀X ◗– $$
ADULT – Emergency contraception: 1 tab PO ASAP but within 72 h of intercourse. 2nd tab 12 h later.
PEDS – Not approved in children.
UNAPPROVED ADULT – 2 tabs (1.5 mg) PO ASAP but within 72 h of intercourse (lesser efficacy at up to 120 h).
FORMS – OTC Trade only: Kit contains 2 tabs 0.75 mg.
NOTES – OTC if at least 17 yo; Rx if younger. Nausea uncommon; however, if vomiting occurs within 1 h, initial dose must be given again. Consider adding an antiemetic. Patients should be instructed to then contact their healthcare providers. Can be used at any time during the menstrual cycle.

LEVONORGESTREL 1S (***Plan B One-Step***) ▶L ♀X ◗– $$
ADULT – Emergency contraception: 1 tab PO ASAP but within 72 h of intercourse.
PEDS – Not approved in children.
FORMS – OTC Trade only: Tabs 1.5 mg.
NOTES – OTC if at least 17 yo; Rx if younger. Nausea uncommon; however, if vomiting occurs within 1 h, initial dose must be given again. Consider adding an antiemetic. Patients should be instructed to then contact their healthcare providers. Can be used at any time during the menstrual cycle. Lesser efficacy at up to 120 h.

NUVARING **(ethinyl estradiol vaginal ring + etonogestrel)** ▶L ♀X ◗– $$$
ADULT – Contraception: 1 ring intravaginally for 3 weeks each month.
PEDS – Not approved in children.
FORMS – Trade only: Flexible intravaginal ring, 15 mcg ethinyl estradiol/0.120 mg etonogestrel/day in 1, 3 rings/box.
NOTES – Insert on day 5 of cycle or within 7 days of the last oral contraceptive pill. The ring must remain in place continuously for 3 weeks, including during intercourse. Remove for 1 week, then insert a new ring. May be used continuously for 4 weeks and replaced immediately to skip a withdrawal week. Store at room temperature (59° to 86°F) for up to 4 months. In case of accidental removal, reinsert ASAP after rinsing with cool to lukewarm water. If removal is for longer than 3 h, use backup method until ring in place for at least 7 days.

ORTHO EVRA **(norelgestromin + ethinyl estradiol transdermal,** ✤***Evra***) ▶L ♀X ◗– $$$
WARNING – Average estrogen concentration 60% higher than common oral contraceptives (ie, 35 mcg ethinyl estradiol), which may further increase the risk of thromboembolism.
ADULT – Contraception: 1 patch q week for 3 weeks, then 1 week patch-free.
PEDS – Not approved in children.
FORMS – Trade only: Transdermal patch: 150 mcg norelgestromin/20 mcg ethinyl estradiol/day in 1, 3 patches/box.
NOTES – May be less effective in women 90 kg or greater (198 lbs). Apply new patch on the same day each week. Do not exceed 7 days between patches. Rotate application sites, avoid the waistline. Do not use earlier than 4 weeks postpartum if not breastfeeding.

EMERGENCY CONTRACEPTION

Emergency contraception within 72 h of unprotected sex.

Progestin-only methods (causes less nausea and may be more effective. Available OTC for age 17 yo or older): Plan B One-Step (levonorgestrel 1.5 mg tab): Take one pill. Next Choice (levonorgestrel 0.75 mg): Take one tab ASAP and 2nd dose 12 h later.

Progestin and estrogen method: Dose is defined as 2 pills of Ogestrel, 4 pills of Cryselle, Enpresse*, Jolessa, Levora, Lo/Ovral, Low Ogestrel, Nordette, Portia, Quasense, Seasonale, Seasonique, Solia, or Trivora*, or 5 pills of Aviane, Lessina, LoSeasonique, Lutera, or Sronyx: Take first dose ASAP and 2nd dose 12 h later. If vomiting occurs within 1 h of taking dose, consider repeating that dose with an antiemetic 1 h prior.

Emergency contraception within 120 h of unprotected sex. Ella (ulipristal 50mg): Take 1 pill. More info at: www.not-2-late.com.

*Use 0.125 mg levonorgestrel/30 mcg ethinyl estradiol tabs.

ULIPRISTAL ACETATE (*Ella*) ▶L ♀X ▶?

ADULT – Emergency contraception: 1 tab PO ASAP within 5 days of intercourse.

PEDS – Safety and efficacy are expected to be the same for postpubertal adolescents younger than 18 yo as for adults.

FORMS – Trade only: Tabs 30 mg.

NOTES – If vomiting occurs within 3 h of administration, consider repeating the dose. Can be used at any time during menstrual cycle.

OB/GYN: Estrogens

NOTE: See also Hormone Combinations. Unopposed estrogens increase the risk of endometrial cancer in postmenopausal women. Malignancy should be ruled out in cases of persistent or recurrent abnormal vaginal bleeding. In women with an intact uterus, a progestin should be administered daily throughout the month or for the last 10 to 12 days of the month. Do not use during pregnancy. May increase the risk of DVT/PE, gallbladder disease. Interactions with oral anticoagulants, certain anticonvulsants, rifampin, barbiturates, corticosteroids, and St. John's wort. Estrogens should not be used in the prevention of cardiovascular disease. In the Women's Health Initiative, the use of conjugated estrogens (Premarin) caused an increase in the risk of CVA and PE. Additionally, the combination with medroxyprogesterone increased the risk of breast cancer and MI. Women older than 65 yo with 4 years of therapy had an increased risk of dementia. Estrogens should be prescribed at the lowest effective doses and for the shortest duration. Patients should be counseled regarding the risks/benefits of HRT.

BIEST **(estradiol + estriol)** ▶L ♀X ▶- $$$

WARNING – For topical dosages: Patient should take precautions to ensure that children and pets do not make contact with skin where topical estrogen has been applied.

UNAPPROVED ADULT – Hormone replacement therapy: Once or twice daily dosing.

FORMS – Must be compounded by a pharmacist. Most common estriol/estradiol ratios 80%/20% or 50%/50%. May be formulated as cream, gel, troche, or capsule.

NOTES – Compounded bioidentical hormones are not FDA approved. These products should be considered to have the same safety issues raised by the Women's Health Initiative as those associated with hormone therapy agents that are FDA approved.

ESTERIFIED ESTROGENS (*Menest*) ▶L ♀X ▶– $$

ADULT – Moderate to severe menopausal vasomotor symptoms: 1.25 mg PO daily. Atrophic vaginitis: 0.3 to 1.25 mg PO daily. Female hypogonadism: 2.5 to 7.5 mg PO daily in divided doses for 20 days followed by a 10-day rest period. Repeat until bleeding occurs. Bilateral oophorectomy and ovarian failure: 1.25 mg PO daily. Prevention of postmenopausal osteoporosis: 0.3 to 1.25 mg PO daily.

PEDS – Not approved in children.

FORMS – Trade only: Tabs 0.3, 0.625, 1.25, 2.5 mg.

NOTES – Typical hormone replacement regimen consists of a daily estrogen dose with a progestin added either daily or for the last 10 to 12 days of the cycle.

ESTRADIOL (*Estrace, Gynodiol*) ▶L ♀X ▶– $

ADULT – Moderate to severe menopausal vasomotor symptoms and atrophic vaginitis, female hypogonadism, bilateral oophorectomy and ovarian failure: 1 to 2 mg PO daily. Prevention of postmenopausal osteoporosis: 0.5 mg PO daily.

PEDS – Not approved in children.

(cont.)

ESTRADIOL (*cont.*)

FORMS – Generic/Trade: Tabs, micronized 0.5, 1, 2 mg, scored. Trade only: 1.5 mg (Gynodiol).

NOTES – Typical hormone replacement regimen consists of a daily estrogen dose with a progestin added either daily or for the last 10 to 12 days of the cycle.

ESTRADIOL ACETATE (*Femtrace*) ▶L ♀X ▶– $$

ADULT – Moderate to severe menopausal vasomotor symptoms: 0.45 to 1.8 mg PO daily.

PEDS – Not approved in children.

FORMS – Trade only: Tabs, 0.45, 0.9, 1.8 mg.

NOTES – Typical hormone replacement regimen consists of a daily estrogen dose with a progestin added either daily or for the last 10 to 12 days of the cycle.

ESTRADIOL ACETATE VAGINAL RING (*Femring*) ▶L ♀X ▶– $$$

WARNING – A few cases of toxic shock syndrome have been reported. Bowel obstruction.

ADULT – Menopausal vasomotor symptoms or vaginal atrophy: Insert ring into the vagina and replace after 90 days.

PEDS – Not approved in children.

FORMS – Trade only: 0.05 mg/day and 0.1 mg/day.

NOTES – Should the ring fall out or be removed during the 90-day period, rinse in lukewarm water and re-insert. Ring adhesion to vaginal wall has been reported, making removal difficult.

ESTRADIOL CYPIONATE (*Depo-Estradiol*) ▶L ♀X ▶– $

ADULT – Moderate to severe menopausal vasomotor symptoms: 1 to 5 mg IM q 3 to 4 weeks. Female hypogonadism: 1.5 to 2 mg IM q month.

PEDS – Not approved in children.

ESTRADIOL GEL (*Divigel, Estrogel, Elestrin*) ▶L ♀X ▶– $$$

WARNING – Patient should take precautions to ensure that children and pets do not make contact with skin where topical estradiol has been applied.

ADULT – Moderate to severe menopausal vasomotor symptoms and atrophic vaginitis: Thinly apply contents of 1 complete pump depression to one entire arm, from wrist to shoulder (Estrogel) or upper arm (Elestrin) or contents of 1 foil packet to left or right upper thigh on alternating days. Allow to dry completely before dressing. Wash both hands thoroughly after application.

PEDS – Not approved in children.

FORMS – Trade only: Gel 0.06% in nonaerosol, metered-dose pump with #64 or #32 1.25 g doses (Estrogel), #100 0.87 g doses (Elestrin). Gel 0.1% in single-dose foil packets of 0.25, 0.5, 1.0 g, carton of 30 (Divigel).

NOTES – Depress the pump 2 times to prime. Concomitant sunscreen may increase absorption. Typical hormone replacement regimen consists of a daily estrogen dose with a progestin added either daily or for the last 10 to 12 days of the cycle.

ESTRADIOL TOPICAL EMULSION (*Estrasorb*) ▶L ♀X ▶– $$

WARNING – Patient should take precautions to ensure that children and pets do not make contact with skin where topical estradiol has been applied.

ADULT – Moderate to severe menopausal vasomotor symptoms: Apply entire contents of 1 pouch each to left and right legs (spread over thighs and calves) q am. Rub for 3 min until entirely absorbed. Allow to dry completely before dressing. Wash both hands thoroughly after application. Daily dose is two 1.74 g pouches.

PEDS – Not approved in children.

FORMS – Trade only: Topical emulsion, 56 pouches/carton.

NOTES – Typical hormone replacement regimen consists of a daily estrogen dose with a progestin added either daily or for the last 10 to 12 days of the cycle. Concomitant sunscreen may increase absorption.

ESTRADIOL TRANSDERMAL PATCH (*Alora, Climara, Esclim, Estraderm, FemPatch, Menostar, Vivelle, Vivelle Dot, ✦Estradot, Oesclim*) ▶L ♀X ▶– $$

ADULT – Moderate to severe menopausal vasomotor symptoms and atrophic vaginitis, female hypogonadism, bilateral oophorectomy, and ovarian failure: Initiate with 0.025 to 0.05 mg/day patch once or twice per week, depending on the product (see FORMS). Prevention of postmenopausal osteoporosis: 0.025 to 0.1 mg/day patch.

PEDS – Not approved in children.

FORMS – Generic/Trade: Transdermal patches doses in mg/day: Climara (once a week) 0.025, 0.0375, 0.05, 0.06, 0.075, 0.1. Trade only: FemPatch (once a week) 0.025. Esclim (twice per week) 0.025, 0.0375, 0.05, 0.075, 0.1. Vivelle, Vivelle Dot (twice per week) 0.025, 0.0375, 0.05, 0.075, 0.1. Estraderm (twice per week) 0.05, 0.1. Alora (twice per week) 0.025, 0.05, 0.075, 0.1.

NOTES – Rotate application sites, avoid the waistline. Transdermal may be preferable for women with high triglycerides and chronic liver disease.

ESTRADIOL TRANSDERMAL SPRAY (*Evamist*) ▶L ♀X ▶– $$$

WARNING – Patient should take precautions to ensure that children and pets do not make contact with skin where topical estradiol has been applied.

ADULT – Moderate to severe menopausal vasomotor symptoms: Initial: 1 spray daily to adjacent nonoverlapping inner surface of the forearm. Allow to dry for 2 min and do not wash for 30 min. Adjust up to 3 sprays daily based on clinical response.

PEDS – Not approved in children.

FORMS – Trade only: Spray: 1.53 mg estradiol per 90 mcL spray, 56 sprays per metered-dose pump.

NOTES – Depress the pump 3 times with the cover on to prime each new applicator. Hold upright and vertical for spraying; rest the plastic cone against the skin. Typical hormone replacement regimen consists of a daily estrogen dose with a progestin added either daily or for the last 10 to 12 days of the cycle.

ESTRADIOL VAGINAL RING (*Estring*) ▶L ♀X ▶– $$$

WARNING – Do not use during pregnancy. Toxic shock syndrome has been reported.

ADULT – Vaginal atrophy and lower urinary tract atrophy: Insert ring into upper third of the vaginal vault and replace after 90 days.

PEDS – Not approved in children.

FORMS – Trade only: 2 mg ring single pack.

NOTES – Should the ring fall out or be removed during the 90-day period, rinse in lukewarm water, and re-insert. Reports of ring adhesion to the vaginal wall, making ring removal difficult. Minimal systemic absorption, probable lower risk of adverse effects than systemic estrogens.

ESTRADIOL VAGINAL TAB (*Vagifem*) ▶L ♀X ▶– $$$

WARNING – Do not use during pregnancy.

ADULT – Menopausal atrophic vaginitis: Begin with 1 tab vaginally daily for 2 weeks, maintenance 1 tab vaginally twice per week.

PEDS – Not approved in children.

FORMS – Trade only: Vaginal tab: 10 mcg or 25 mcg in disposable single-use applicators, 8, 18/pack.

ESTRADIOL VALERATE (*Delestrogen*) ▶L ♀X ▶– $$

ADULT – Moderate to severe menopausal vasomotor symptoms and atrophic vaginitis, female hypogonadism, bilateral oophorectomy, and ovarian failure: 10 to 20 mg IM q 4 weeks.

PEDS – Not approved in children.

ESTROGEN VAGINAL CREAM (*Premarin, Estrace*) ▶L ♀X ▶? $$$$

ADULT – Atrophic vaginitis: Premarin: 0.5 to 2 g intravaginally daily for 1 to 2 weeks, then reduce to 0.5 g twice weekly maintenance. Estrace: 1 to 4 g intravaginally daily for 1 to 2 weeks. Gradually reduce to a maintenance dose of 1 g 1 to 3 times per week.

PEDS – Not approved in children.

FORMS – Trade only: Premarin: 0.625 mg conjugated estrogens/g in 42.5 g with or without calibrated applicator. Estrace: 0.1 mg estradiol/g in 42.5 g with calibrated applicator. Generic only: Cream 0.625 mg synthetic conjugated estrogens/g in 30 g with calibrated applicator.

NOTES – Possibility of absorption through the vaginal mucosa. Uterine bleeding might be provoked by excessive use in menopausal women. Breast tenderness and vaginal discharge due to mucus hypersecretion may result from excessive estrogenic stimulation. Endometrial withdrawal bleeding may occur if use is discontinued.

ESTROGENS CONJUGATED (*Premarin, C.E.S., Congest*) ▶L ♀X ▶– $$$

ADULT – Moderate to severe menopausal vasomotor symptoms, atrophic vaginitis, and urethritis: 0.3 to 1.25 mg PO daily. Female hypogonadism: 0.3 to 0.625 mg PO daily for 3 weeks with 1 week off q month. Bilateral oophorectomy and ovarian failure: 1.25 mg PO daily for 3 weeks with 1 week off q month. Prevention of postmenopausal osteoporosis: 0.625 mg PO daily. Abnormal uterine bleeding: 25 mg IV/IM. Repeat in 6 to 12 h if needed.

PEDS – Not approved in children.

UNAPPROVED ADULT – Prevention of postmenopausal osteoporosis: 0.3 mg PO daily. Normalizing bleeding time in patients with AV malformations or underlying renal impairment: 30 to 70 mg IV/PO daily until bleeding time normalized.

FORMS – Trade only: Tabs 0.3, 0.45, 0.625, 0.9, 1.25 mg.

ESTROGENS SYNTHETIC CONJUGATED A (*Cenestin*) ▶L ♀X ▶– $$$

ADULT – Moderate to severe menopausal vasomotor symptoms: 0.3 to 1.25 mg PO daily.

PEDS – Not approved in children.

FORMS – Trade only: Tabs 0.3, 0.45, 0.625, 0.9, 1.25 mg.

NOTES – The difference between synthetic conjugated estrogens A and B is the additional component of delta-8,9-dehydroestrone sulfate in the B preparation. The clinical significance of this is unknown.

***ESTROGENS SYNTHETIC CONJUGATED* B** (*Enjuvia*) ▶L ♀X ▶– $$

ADULT – Moderate to severe menopausal vasomotor symptoms: 0.3 to 1.25 mg PO daily.

PEDS – Not approved in children.

FORMS – Trade only: Tabs 0.3, 0.45, 0.625, 0.9, 1.25 mg.

NOTES – Typical hormone replacement regimen consists of a daily estrogen dose with a progestin either daily or for the last 10 to 12 days of the cycle. The difference between synthetic conjugated estrogens A and B is the additional component of delta-8,9-dehydroestrone sulfate in the B preparation. The clinical significance of this is unknown.

ESTROPIPATE (*Ogen, Ortho-Est*) ▶L ♀X ▶– $

ADULT – Moderate to severe menopausal vasomotor symptoms, vulvar and vaginal atrophy: 0.75 to 6 mg PO daily. Female hypogonadism, bilateral oophorectomy, or ovarian failure: 1.5 to 9 mg PO daily. Prevention of osteoporosis: 0.75 mg PO daily.

PEDS – Not approved in children.

FORMS – Generic/Trade: Tabs 0.75, 1.5, 3, 6 mg of estropipate.

NOTES – 6 mg estropipate is 5 mg sodium estrone sulfate.

***TRIEST* (estradiol + estriol + estrone)** ▶L ♀X ▶– $$$

WARNING – For topical dosages: Patient should take precautions to ensure that children and pets do not make contact with skin where topical hormone has been applied.

UNAPPROVED ADULT – Hormone replacement therapy: Once or twice daily dosing.

FORMS – Must be compounded by a pharmacist. May be formulated as capsule, cream, gel, troche, or vaginal suppository.

NOTES – Compounded bioidentical hormones are not FDA approved. These products should be considered to have the same safety issues as those associated with hormone therapy agents that are FDA approved.

OB/GYN: GnRH Agents

NOTE: Anaphylaxis has occurred with synthetic GnRH agents.

CETRORELIX ACETATE (*Cetrotide*) ▶Plasma ♀X ▶– $$$$$

ADULT – Infertility: Multiple-dose regimen: 0.25 mg SC daily during the early to mid follicular phase. Continue treatment daily until the days of hCG administration. Single-dose regimen: 3 mg SC for 1 dose usually on stimulation day 7.

PEDS – Not approved in children.

FORMS – Trade only: Injection 0.25 mg and 3 mg vials.

NOTES – Best sites for SC self-injection are on the abdomen around the navel. Storage in original carton: 0.25 mg refrigerated (36–46°F); 3 mg room temperature (77°F). Contraindicated with severe renal impairment.

GANIRELIX (*Follistim-Antagon Kit*, ✤ *Orgalutran*) ▶Plasma ♀X ▶? $$$$$

ADULT – Infertility: 250 mcg SC daily during the early to mid follicular phase. Continue treatment daily until the days of hCG administration.

PEDS – Not approved in children.

FORMS – Trade only: Injection 250 mcg/0.5 mL in prefilled, disposable syringes with 3 vials follitropin beta.

NOTES – Best sites for SC self-injection are on the abdomen around the navel or upper thigh. Store at room temperature (77°F) for up to 3 months. Protect from light. Packaging contains natural rubber latex which may cause allergic reactions.

NAFARELIN (*Synarel*) ▶L ♀X ▶– $$$$$

ADULT – Endometriosis: 200 mcg spray into 1 nostril q am and the other nostril q pm. May be increased to one 200 mcg spray into each nostril two times per day. Duration of treatment: 6 months.

PEDS – Central precocious puberty: 2 sprays into each nostril two times per day for a total of 1600 mcg/day. May be increased to 1800 mcg/day. Allow 30 sec to elapse between sprays.

FORMS – Trade only: Nasal soln 2 mg/mL in 8 mL bottle (200 mcg per spray) approximately 80 sprays/bottle.

NOTES – Ovarian cysts have occurred in the first 2 months of therapy. Symptoms of hypoestrogenism may occur. Elevations of phosphorus and eosinophil counts, and decreases in serum calcium and WBC counts have been documented. Consider norethindrone as "add back" therapy to decrease bone loss (see norethindrone).

OB/GYN: Hormone Combinations

NOTE: See also Estrogens. Unopposed estrogens increase the risk of endometrial cancer in postmenopausal women. Malignancy should be ruled out in cases of persistent or recurrent abnormal vaginal bleeding. Do not use during pregnancy. May increase the risk of DVT/PE, gallbladder disease. Interactions with oral anticoagulants, phenytoin, rifampin, barbiturates, corticosteroids, and St. John's wort. For preparations containing testosterone derivatives, observe women for signs of virilization, and lipid abnormalities. In the Women's Health Initiative, the combination of conjugated estrogens and medroxyprogesterone (PremPro) caused an increase in the risk of breast cancer, MI, CVA, and DVT/PE and did not improve overall quality of life. Women older than 65 yo with 4 years of therapy had an increased risk of dementia. Estrogen/progestin combinations should be prescribed at the lowest effective doses and for the shortest durations. Patients should be counseled regarding the risks/benefits of hormone replacement.

ACTIVELLA **(estradiol + norethindrone)** ▶L ♀X ▶– $$$
ADULT – Moderate to severe menopausal vasomotor symptoms, vulvar and vaginal atrophy, prevention of postmenopausal osteoporosis: 1 tab PO daily.
PEDS – Not approved in children.
FORMS – Trade only: Tabs 1/0.5 mg and 0.5/0.1 mg estradiol/norethindrone acetate in calendar dial pack dispenser.

ANGELIQ **(estradiol + drospirenone)** ▶L ♀X ▶– $$$
ADULT – Moderate to severe menopausal vasomotor symptoms, vulvar and vaginal atrophy: 1 tab PO daily.
PEDS – Not approved in children.
FORMS – Trade only: Tabs 1 mg estradiol/0.5 mg drospirenone.
NOTES – May cause hyperkalemia in high-risk patients due to antimineralocorticoid activity of drospirenone. Monitor potassium in patients on ACE inhibitors, ARBs, potassium-sparing diuretics, heparin, aldosterone antagonists, and NSAIDs. Should not be used if renal insufficiency, hepatic dysfunction, or adrenal insufficiency.

CLIMARA PRO **(estradiol + levonorgestrel)** ▶L ♀X ▶– $$$
ADULT – Moderate to severe menopausal vasomotor symptoms, prevention of postmenopausal osteoporosis: 1 patch weekly.
PEDS – Not approved in children.
FORMS – Trade only: Transdermal 0.045/0.015 estradiol/levonorgestrel in mg/day, 4 patches/box.
NOTES – Rotate application sites; avoid the waistline.

COMBIPATCH **(estradiol + norethindrone, ♣ *Estalis*)** ▶L ♀X ▶– $$$
ADULT – Moderate to severe menopausal vasomotor symptoms, vulvar and vaginal atrophy, female hypogonadism, bilateral oophorectomy, ovarian failure, prevention of postmenopausal osteoporosis: 1 patch twice per week.
PEDS – Not approved in children.
FORMS – Trade only: Transdermal patch 0.05 estradiol/0.14 norethindrone and 0.05 estradiol/0.25 norethindrone in mg/day, 8 patches/box.
NOTES – Rotate application sites, avoid the waistline.

EEMT **(esterified estrogens + methyltestosterone)** ▶L ♀X ▶– $$$$
ADULT – Moderate to severe menopausal vasomotor symptoms: 1 tab PO daily.
PEDS – Not approved in children.
UNAPPROVED ADULT – Menopause-associated decrease in libido: 1 tab PO daily.
FORMS – Generic only: Tabs 1.25 mg esterified estrogens/2.5 mg methyltestosterone.
NOTES – Monitor LFTs and lipids.

EEMT H.S. **(esterified estrogens + methyltestosterone)** ▶L ♀X ▶– $$$
ADULT – Moderate to severe menopausal vasomotor symptoms: 1 tab PO daily.
PEDS – Not approved in children.
UNAPPROVED ADULT – Menopause-associated decrease in libido: 1 tab PO daily.
FORMS – Generic only: Tabs 0.625 mg esterified estrogens/1.25 mg methyltestosterone.
NOTES – HS indicates half-strength. Monitor LFTs and lipids.

FEMHRT **(ethinyl estradiol + norethindrone)** ▶L ♀X ▶– $$$
WARNING – Multiple strengths; see FORMS and write specific product on Rx.
ADULT – Moderate to severe menopausal vasomotor symptoms, prevention of postmenopausal osteoporosis: 1 tab PO daily.
PEDS – Not approved in children.
FORMS – Trade only: Tabs 5/1, 2.5/0.5 mcg ethinyl estradiol/mg norethindrone, 28/blister card.

PREFEST **(estradiol + norgestimate)** ▶L ♀X ▶– $$$
ADULT – Moderate to severe menopausal vasomotor symptoms, vulvar atrophy, atrophic vaginitis, prevention of postmenopausal

(cont.)

DRUGS GENERALLY ACCEPTED AS SAFE IN PREGNANCY (selected)

Analgesics	acetaminophen, codeine*, meperidine*, methadone*, oxycodone*
Antimicrobials	azithromycin, cephalosporins, clotrimazole, erythromycins (not estolate), metronidazole, penicillins, permethrin, nitrofurantoin***, nystatin
Antivirals	acyclovir, famciclovir, valacyclovir
CV	hydralazine*, labetalol, methyldopa, nifedipine
Derm	benzoyl peroxide, clindamycin, erythromycin
Endo	insulin, levothyroxine, liothyronine
ENT	chlorpheniramine, diphenhydramine, dextromethorphan, guaifenesin, nasal steroids, nasal cromolyn
GI	antacids*, bisacodyl, cimetidine, docusate, doxylamine, famotidine, lactulose, loperamide, meclizine, metoclopramide, nizatidine, ondansetron, psyllium, ranitidine, simethicone, trimethobenzamide
Heme	Heparin, low molecular wt heparins
Psych	bupropion, buspirone, desipramine, doxepin
Pulmonary	beclomethasone, budesonide, cromolyn, montelukast, nedocromil, prednisone**, short-acting inhaled beta-2 agonists, theophylline

*Except if used long-term or in high dose at term.
**Except 1st trimester.
***Contraindicated at term and during labor and delivery.

PREFEST (*cont.*)

osteoporosis: 1 pink tab PO daily for 3 days followed by 1 white tab PO daily for 3 days, sequentially throughout the month.
PEDS – Not approved in children.
FORMS – Trade only: Tabs in 30-day blister packs 1 mg estradiol (15 pink), 1 mg estradiol/0.09 mg norgestimate (15 white).

PREMPHASE (estrogens conjugated + medroxyprogesterone) ▶L ♀X ▶– $$$
ADULT – Moderate to severe menopausal vasomotor symptoms, vulvar/vaginal atrophy, prevention of postmenopausal osteoporosis: 0.625 mg conjugated estrogens PO daily on days 1 to 14 and 0.625 mg conjugated estrogens/5 mg medroxyprogesterone PO daily on days 15 to 28.
PEDS – Not approved in children.
FORMS – Trade only: Tabs in 28 days EZ-Dial dispensers: 0.625 mg conjugated estrogens (14 tabs), 0.625 mg/5 mg conjugated estrogens/medroxyprogesterone (14 tabs).

PREMPRO (estrogens conjugated + medroxyprogesterone, ✦ ***Premplus***) ▶L ♀X ▶– $$$
WARNING – Multiple strengths; see FORMS and write specific product on Rx.
ADULT – Moderate to severe menopausal vasomotor symptoms, vulvar/vaginal atrophy, prevention of postmenopausal osteoporosis: 1 tab PO daily.
PEDS – Not approved in children.
FORMS – Trade only: Tabs in 28-day EZ-Dial dispensers: 0.625 mg/5 mg, 0.625 mg/2.5 mg, 0.45 mg/1.5 mg (Prempro low dose), or 0.3 mg/1.5 mg conjugated estrogens/medroxyprogesterone.

OB/GYN: Labor Induction / Cervical Ripening

NOTE: Fetal wellbeing should be documented prior to use.

DINOPROSTONE (***PGE2, Prepidil, Cervidil, Prostin E2***) ▶Lung ♀C ▶? $$$$$
ADULT – Cervical ripening: Gel: 1 syringe via catheter placed into cervical canal below the internal os. May be repeated q 6 h to a max of 3 doses. Vaginal insert: Place in posterior fornix. Evacuation of uterine contents after fetal death up to 28 weeks or termination of pregnancy 12 to 20th gestational week: 20 mg intravaginal suppository; repeat at 3- to 5-h intervals until abortion occurs. Do not use for more than 2 days.

(cont.)

DINOPROSTONE (*cont.*)

PEDS – Not approved in children.
FORMS – Trade only: Gel (Prepidil) 0.5 mg/3 g syringe. Vaginal insert (Cervidil) 10 mg. Vaginal supps (Prostin E2) 20 mg.
NOTES – Patient should remain supine for 15 to 30 min after gel and 2 h after vaginal insert. For hospital use only. Monitor for uterine hyperstimulation and abnormal fetal heart rate. Caution with asthma or glaucoma. Contraindicated in prior C-section or major uterine surgery due to potential for uterine rupture.

MISOPROSTOL-OB (*PGE1, Cytotec*) ▶LK ♀X ◗– $$

WARNING – Contraindicated in desired early or preterm pregnancy due to its abortifacient property. Pregnant women should avoid contact/exposure to the tabs. Uterine rupture reported with use for labor induction and medical abortion.
UNAPPROVED ADULT – Cervical ripening and labor induction: 25 mcg intravaginally q 3 to 6 h (or 50 mcg q 6 h). First trimester pregnancy failure: 800 mcg intravaginally, repeat on day 3 if expulsion incomplete. Medical abortion less than 63 days gestation: With mifepristone, see mifepristone; with methotrexate: 800 mcg intravaginally 5 to 7 days after 50 mg/m^2 PO or IM methotrexate. Preop cervical ripening: 400 mcg intravaginally 3 to 4 h before mechanical cervical dilation. Postpartum hemorrhage: 800 mcg PR for 1 dose. Oral dosing has been used but is controversial. Treatment of duodenal ulcers: 100 mcg PO four time per day.
FORMS – Generic/Trade: Oral tabs 100, 200 mcg.
NOTES – Contraindicated with prior C-section. Oral tabs can be inserted into the vagina for labor induction/cervical ripening. Monitor for uterine hyperstimulation and abnormal fetal heart rate. Risk factors for uterine rupture: Prior uterine surgery and 5 or more previous pregnancies.

OXYTOCIN (*Pitocin*) ▶LK ♀? ◗– $

WARNING – Not approved for elective labor induction, although widely used.
ADULT – Induction/stimulation of labor: 10 units in 1000 mL NS, 1 to 2 milliunits/min IV as a continuous infusion (6 to 12 mL/h). Increase in increments of 1 to 2 milliunits/min q 30 min until a contraction pattern is established, up to a max of 20 milliunits/min. Postpartum bleeding: 10 units IM after delivery of the placenta. 10 to 40 units in 1000 mL NS IV infusion, infuse 20 to 40 milliunits/min.
PEDS – Not approved in children.
UNAPPROVED ADULT – Augmentation of labor: 0.5 to 2 milliunits/min IV as a continuous infusion, increase by 1 to 2 milliunits/min q 30 min until adequate pattern of labor to a max of 40 milliunits/min.
NOTES – Use a pump to accurately control the infusion while patient is under continuous observation. Continuous fetal monitoring is required. Concurrent sympathomimetics may result in postpartum HTN. Anaphylaxis and severe water intoxication have occurred. Caution in patients undergoing a trial of labor after C-section.

OB/GYN: Ovulation Stimulants

NOTE: Potentially serious adverse effects include DVT/PE, ovarian hyperstimulation syndrome, adnexal torsion, ovarian enlargement and cysts, and febrile reactions.

CHORIOGONADOTROPIN ALFA (*hCG, Ovidrel*) ▶L ♀X ◗? $$$

ADULT – Specialized dosing for ovulation induction.
PEDS – Not approved in children.
FORMS – Trade only: Powder for injection or prefilled syringe 250 mcg.
NOTES – Best site for SC self-injection is on the abdomen below the navel. Beware of multiple gestation pregnancy and multiple adverse effects. Store in original package and protect from light. Use immediately after reconstitution.

CHORIONIC GONADOTROPIN (*hCG, Pregnyl, Novarel*) ▶L ♀X ◗? $$$

ADULT – Specialized dosing for ovulation induction.
PEDS – Not approved in children.
NOTES – Beware of multiple gestation pregnancy and multiple adverse effects. For IM use only.

CLOMIPHENE (*Clomid, Serophene*) ▶L ♀D ◗? $$$$$

ADULT – Specialized dosing for infertility.
PEDS – Not approved in children.
FORMS – Generic/Trade: Tabs 50 mg, scored.
NOTES – Beware of multiple pregnancy and multiple adverse effects.

FOLLITROPIN ALFA (*FSH, Gonal-F, Gonal-F RFF Pen*) ▶L ♀X ▶? $$$$$

ADULT – Specialized dosing for infertility.

PEDS – Not approved in children.

FORMS – Trade only: Powder for injection, 75 international units FSH activity, multidose vial 450, 1050 international units FSH activity. Prefilled, multiple-dose pen, 300 international units, 450 international units, 900 international units FSH activity with single-use disposable needles.

NOTES – Best site for SC self-injection is on the abdomen below the navel. Beware of multiple gestation pregnancy and multiple adverse effects. Store in original package and protect from light. Use immediately after reconstitution. Pen may be stored at room temperature for up to 1 month or expiration, whichever is first.

FOLLITROPIN BETA (*FSH, Follistim AQ, ✤Puregon*) ▶L ♀X ▶? $$$$$

ADULT – Specialized dosing for infertility.

PEDS – Not approved in children.

FORMS – Trade only: Cartridge, for use with the Follistim Pen, 150, 300, 600, 900 international units. Aqueous soln 75, 150 international units FSH activity.

NOTES – Best site for SC self-injection is on the abdomen below the navel. Beware of multiple gestation pregnancy and multiple adverse effects. Store in original package and protect from light. Use powder for injection immediately after reconstitution. Cartridge may be stored for up to 28 days. Store aqueous soln in refrigerator.

GONADOTROPINS (menotropins, *FSH and LH, Menopur, Pergonal, Repronex, ✤Propasi HP*) ▶L ♀X ▶? $$$$$

ADULT – Specialized dosing for infertility.

PEDS – Not approved in children.

FORMS – Trade only: Powder for injection, 75 international units FSH/LH activity.

NOTES – Best site for SC self-injection is on the abdomen below the navel. Beware of multiple gestation pregnancy and numerous adverse effects. Use immediately after reconstitution.

LUTROPIN ALFA (*Luveris*) ▶L ♀X ▶– $$$$$

ADULT – Specialized dosing for infertility.

PEDS – Not approved in children.

FORMS – Trade only: Powder for injection, 75 international units LH activity.

NOTES – For use with follitropin alfa. Best site for SC self-injection is on the abdomen below the navel. Protect from light. Use immediately after reconstitution.

UROFOLLITROPIN (*Bravelle, FSH, Fertinex*) ▶L ♀X ▶? $$$$$

ADULT – Specialized dosing for infertility and polycystic ovary syndrome.

PEDS – Not approved in children.

FORMS – Trade only: Powder for injection, 75 international units FSH activity.

NOTES – Best site for SC self-injection is on the abdomen below the navel. Beware of multiple gestation pregnancy and numerous adverse effects. Use immediately after reconstitution.

OB/GYN: Progestins

NOTE: Do not use in pregnancy. DVT, PE, cerebrovascular disorders, and retinal thrombosis may occur. Effectiveness may be reduced by hepatic enzyme–inducing drugs such as certain anticonvulsants and barbiturates, rifampin, rifabutin, griseofulvin, and protease inhibitors. The effects of St. John's wort–containing products on progestin-only pills is currently unknown. In the Women's Health Initiative, the combination of conjugated estrogens and medroxyprogesterone (PremPro) caused a statistically significant increase in the risk of breast cancer, MI, CVA, and DVT/PE. Additionally, women older than 65 yo with 4 years of therapy had an increased risk of dementia. Estrogen/progestin combinations should be prescribed at the lowest effective doses and for the shortest durations. Patients should be counseled regarding the risks/benefits of hormone replacement.

HYDROXYPROGESTERONE CAPROATE (*Makena*) ▶L + glucuronidation ♀B ▶? $$$$$

WARNING – For singleton pregnancy in women who have history of spontaneous preterm birth. Not intended in mutiple gestations or other risk factors for preterm birth.

ADULT – To reduce risk of preterm birth: 250 mg IM once weekly. Begin between gestational age 16 weeks, 0 days and 20 weeks, 6 days. Continue through birth or week 37, whichever occurs first.

PEDS – Not approved in children

FORMS – Trade only. 5 mL MDV (250 mg/mL) hydroxyprogesterone caproate in castor oil soln.

NOTES – Unique ruling from FDA that compounding pharmacists can continue to make customized hydroxyprogesterone caproate injection.

MEDROXYPROGESTERONE (*Provera*) ▶L ♀X ▶+ $

ADULT – Secondary amenorrhea: 5 to 10 mg PO daily for 5 to 10 days. Abnormal uterine bleeding: 5 to 10 mg PO daily for 5 to 10 days beginning on the 16th or 21st day of the cycle (after estrogen priming). Withdrawal bleeding usually occurs 3 to 7 days after therapy ends.

PEDS – Not approved in children.

UNAPPROVED ADULT – Add to estrogen replacement therapy to prevent endometrial hyperplasia: 10 mg PO daily for 10 to 12 days each month, or 2.5 to 5 mg PO daily. Endometrial hyperplasia: 10 to 30 mg PO daily (long-term); 40 to 100 mg PO daily (short-term) or 500 mg IM twice per week.

FORMS – Generic/Trade: Tabs 2.5, 5, 10 mg, scored.

NOTES – Breakthrough bleeding/spotting may occur. Amenorrhea usually after 6 months of continuous dosing.

MEDROXYPROGESTERONE—INJECTABLE (*Depo-Provera, depo-subQ provera 104*) ▶L ♀X ▶+ $

WARNING – Risk of significant bone loss (possibly reversible) increases with duration of use. Long-term use (more than 2 years) only recommended if other methods of birth control are inadequate or symptoms of endometriosis return after discontinuation. It is unknown if use by younger women will reduce peak bone mass.

ADULT – Contraception/endometriosis: 150 mg IM in deltoid or gluteus maximus or 104 mg SC in anterior thigh or abdomen q 13 weeks. Also used for adjunctive therapy in endometrial and renal carcinoma.

PEDS – Not approved in children.

UNAPPROVED ADULT – Dysfunctional uterine bleeding: 150 mg IM in deltoid or gluteus maximus q 13 weeks.

NOTES – Breakthrough bleeding/spotting may occur. Amenorrhea usually after 6 months. Wt gain is common. To be sure that the patient is not pregnant give this injection only during the first 5 days after the onset of a normal menstrual period or after a negative pregnancy test. May be given immediately post-pregnancy termination or postpartum, including breastfeeding women. May be given as often as 11 weeks apart. If the time between injections is greater than 14 weeks, exclude pregnancy before administering. Return to fertility can be variably delayed after last injection, with the median time to pregnancy being 10 months. Bone loss may occur with prolonged administration. Evaluate bone mineral density if considering retreatment for endometriosis.

MEGESTROL (*Megace, Megace ES*) ▶L ♀D ▶? $$$$$

ADULT – AIDS anorexia: 800 mg (20 mL) susp PO daily or 625 mg (5 mL) ES daily. Palliative treatment for advanced breast carcinoma: 40 mg (tabs) PO four times per day. Endometrial carcinoma: 40 to 320 mg/day (tabs) in divided doses.

PEDS – Not approved in children.

UNAPPROVED ADULT – Endometrial hyperplasia: 40 to 160 mg PO daily for 3 to 4 months. Cancer-associated anorexia/cachexia: 80 to 160 mg PO four times per day.

FORMS – Generic/Trade: Tabs 20, 40 mg. Susp 40 mg/mL in 240 mL. Trade only: Megace ES susp 125 mg/mL (150 mL).

NOTES – In HIV-infected women, breakthrough bleeding/spotting may occur.

NORETHINDRONE (*Aygestin, Micronor, Nor-Q.D., Camila, Errin, Jolivette, Nora-BE*) ▶L ♀D/X ▶See notes $

ADULT – Contraception: 0.35 mg PO daily. Amenorrhea, abnormal uterine bleeding: 2.5 to 10 mg PO daily for 5 to 10 days during the second half of the menstrual cycle. Endometriosis: 5 mg PO daily for 2 weeks. Increase by 2.5 mg q 2 weeks to 15 mg/day.

PEDS – Not approved in children.

UNAPPROVED ADULT – "Add back" therapy with GnRH agonists (eg, leuprolide) to decrease bone loss: 5 mg PO daily.

FORMS – Generic/Trade: Tabs scored 5 mg. Trade only: 0.35 mg tabs.

NOTES – Contraceptive doses felt compatible with breast feeding, but not higher doses.

PROGESTERONE GEL (*Crinone, Prochieve*) ▶Plasma ♀– ▶? $$$

ADULT – Secondary amenorrhea: 45 mg (4%) intravaginally every other day up to 6 doses. If no response, use 90 mg (8%) intravaginally every other day up to 6 doses. Specialized dosing for infertility.

PEDS – Not approved in children.

FORMS – Trade only: 4%, 8% single-use, prefilled applicators.

NOTES – An increase in dose from the 4% gel can only be accomplished using the 8% gel; doubling the volume of 4% does not increase absorption.

PROGESTERONE IN OIL ▶L ♀X ▶? $$

WARNING – Contraindicated in peanut allergy since some products contain peanut oil.

ADULT – Amenorrhea, uterine bleeding: 5 to 10 mg IM daily for 6 to 8 days.

PEDS – Not approved in children.

NOTES – Discontinue with thrombotic disorders, sudden or partial loss of vision, proptosis, diplopia, or migraine.

PROGESTERONE MICRONIZED (*Prometrium*) ▶L ♀B ▶+ $$

WARNING – Contraindicated in patients allergic to peanuts since caps contain peanut oil.

ADULT – Hormone therapy to prevent endometrial hyperplasia: 200 mg PO at bedtime 10 to 12 days/month. Secondary amenorrhea: 400 mg PO at bedtime for 10 days.

PEDS – Not approved in children.

UNAPPROVED ADULT – Hormone therapy to prevent endometrial hyperplasia: 100 mg at bedtime daily.

FORMS – Trade only: Caps 100, 200 mg.

NOTES – Breast tenderness, dizziness, headache, and abdominal cramping may occur.

PROGESTERONE MICRONIZED COMPOUNDED (*Progest*) ▶L ♀B? ▶? $

WARNING – For topical dosages: Patient should take precautions to ensure that children and pets do not make contact with skin where topical hormone has been applied.

UNAPPROVED ADULT – Hormone replacement therapy: Once or twice daily dosing.

FORMS – Must be compounded by a pharmacist. May be formulated as capsule, cream, gel, troche, or vaginal suppository.

NOTES – Compounded bioidentical hormones are not FDA approved. These products should be considered to have the same safety issues as those associated with hormone therapy agents that are FDA approved.

PROGESTERONE VAGINAL INSERT (*Endometrin*) ▶Plasma ♀– ▶? $$$$

ADULT – Specialized dosing for infertility.

PEDS – Not approved in children.

FORMS – Trade only: 100 mg vaginal insert.

NOTES – Do not use concomitantly with other vaginal products, such as antifungals, as this may alter absorption.

OB/GYN: Selective Estrogen Receptor Modulators

RALOXIFENE (*Evista*) ▶L ♀X ▶– $$$$

WARNING – Increases the risk of venous thromboembolism and CVA. Do not use during pregnancy.

ADULT – Postmenopausal osteoporosis prevention/treatment, breast cancer prevention: 60 mg PO daily.

PEDS – Not approved in children.

FORMS – Trade only: Tabs 60 mg.

NOTES – Contraindicated with history of venous thromboembolism. Interactions with oral anticoagulants and cholestyramine. May increase risk of DVT/PE. Discontinue use 72 h prior to and during prolonged immobilization because of DVT risk. Does not decrease (and may increase) hot flashes. Leg cramps. Triglyceride levels may increase in women with prior estrogen-associated hypertriglyceridemia (greater than 500 mg/dL).

TAMOXIFEN (*Nolvadex, Soltamox, Tamone*) ▶L ♀D ▶– $$

WARNING – Uterine malignancies, CVA, and pulmonary embolism, sometimes fatal. Visual disturbances, cataracts, hypercalcemia, increased LFTs, bone pain, fertility impairment, hot flashes, menstrual irregularities, endometrial hyperplasia and cancer, alopecia. Do not use during pregnancy.

ADULT – Breast cancer prevention in high-risk women: 20 mg PO daily for 5 years. Breast cancer: 10 to 20 mg PO two times per day for 5 years.

PEDS – Not approved in children.

UNAPPROVED ADULT – Mastalgia: 10 mg PO daily for 4 months. Anovulation: 5 to 40 mg PO two times per day for 4 days.

FORMS – Generic/Trade: Tabs 10, 20 mg. Trade only (Soltamox): Sugar-free soln 10 mg/5 mL (150 mL).

NOTES – Reliable contraception is recommended. Monitor CBCs, LFTs. Regular gynecologic and ophthalmologic examinations. Interacts with oral anticoagulants. Does not decrease hot flashes.

OB/GYN: Uterotonics

CARBOPROST (*Hemabate,* **15-methyl-prostaglandin F2 alpha**) ▶LK ♀C ▶? $$$

ADULT – Refractory postpartum uterine bleeding: 250 mcg deep IM. If necessary, may repeat at 15 to 90 min intervals up to a total dose of 2 mg (8 doses).

PEDS – Not approved in children.

NOTES – Caution with asthma. Transient fever, HTN, nausea, bronchoconstriction, and flushing. May augment oxytocics.

METHYLERGONOVINE (*Methergine*) ▶LK ♀C ▶? $$

ADULT – To increase uterine contractions and decrease postpartum bleeding: 0.2 mg IM

(cont.)

METHYLERGONOVINE (*cont.*)

after delivery of the placenta, delivery of the anterior shoulder, or during the puerperium. Repeat q 2 to 4 h prn. 0.2 mg PO three to four times per day in the puerperium for a max of 1 week.

PEDS – Not approved in children.

FORMS – Trade only: Tabs 0.2 mg.

NOTES – Contraindicated in pregnancy-induced HTN/preeclampsia. Avoid IV route due to risk of sudden HTN and CVA. If IV absolutely necessary, give slowly over no less than 1 min, monitor BP.

OB/GYN: Vaginitis Preparations

NOTE: See also STD/vaginitis table in Antimicrobials section. Many experts recommend 7 days antifungal therapy for pregnant women with *Candida vaginitis*. Many of these creams and supps are oil-based and may weaken latex condoms and diaphragms. Do not use latex products for 72 h after last dose.

BORIC ACID ▶Not absorbed ♀? ▶– $

PEDS – Not approved in children.

UNAPPROVED ADULT – Resistant vulvovaginal candidiasis: 600 mg suppository intravaginally at bedtime for 2 weeks.

FORMS – No commercial preparation; must be compounded by pharmacist. Vaginal supps 600 mg in gelatin caps.

NOTES – Reported use for azole-resistant non-albicans (*C. glabrata*) or recurrent albicans failing azole therapy. Do not use if abdominal pain, fever, or foul-smelling vaginal discharge is present. Avoid vaginal intercourse during treatment.

BUTOCONAZOLE (***Gynazole, Mycelex-3***) ▶LK ♀C ▶? $(OTC), $$$(Rx)

ADULT – Local treatment of vulvovaginal candidiasis, nonpregnant patients: Mycelex-3: 1 applicatorful (~5 g) intravaginally at bedtime for 3 days, up to 6 days, if necessary. Pregnant patients: (second and third trimesters only) 1 applicatorful (~5 g) intravaginally at bedtime for 6 days. Gynazole-1: 1 applicatorful (~5 g) intravaginally once daily.

PEDS – Not approved in children.

FORMS – OTC: Trade only (Mycelex 3): 2% vaginal cream in 5 g prefilled applicators (3s), 20 g tube with applicators. Rx: Trade only (Gynazole-1): 2% vaginal cream in 5 g prefilled applicator.

NOTES – Do not use if abdominal pain, fever, or foul-smelling vaginal discharge is present. Since small amount may be absorbed from the vagina, use during the first trimester only when essential. During pregnancy, use of a vaginal applicator may be contraindicated and manual insertion may be preferred. Vulvar/vaginal burning may occur. Avoid vaginal intercourse during treatment.

CLINDAMYCIN—VAGINAL (***Cleocin, Clindesse, ✤ Dalacin***) ▶L ♀– ▶+ $$

ADULT – Bacterial vaginosis: Cleocin: 1 applicatorful (~100 mg clindamycin phosphate in 5 g cream) intravaginally at bedtime for 7 days, or 1 suppository at bedtime for 3 days. Clindesse: 1 applicatorful cream single dose.

PEDS – Not approved in children.

FORMS – Generic/Trade: 2% vaginal cream in 40 g tube with 7 disposable applicators (Cleocin). Vag suppository (Cleocin Ovules) 100 mg (3) with applicator. 2% vaginal cream in a single-dose prefilled applicator (Clindesse).

NOTES – Clindesse may degrade latex/rubber condoms and diaphragms for 5 days after the last dose (Cleocin for up to 3 days). Not recommended during pregnancy despite B rating, as it does not prevent the adverse effects of bacterial vaginosis (eg, preterm birth, neonatal infection). Cervicitis, vaginitis, and vulvar irritation may occur. Avoid vaginal intercourse during treatment.

CLOTRIMAZOLE—VAGINAL (***Mycelex 7, Gyne-Lotrimin, ✤ Canesten, Clotrimaderm***) ▶LK ♀B ▶? $

ADULT – Local treatment of vulvovaginal candidiasis: 1 applicatorful 1% cream at bedtime for 7 days. 1 applicatorful 2% cream at bedtime for 3 days. 100 mg suppository intravaginally at bedtime for 7 days. 200 mg suppository at bedtime for 3 days. Topical cream for external symptoms two times per day for 7 days.

PEDS – Not approved in children.

FORMS – OTC Generic/Trade: 1% vaginal cream with applicator (some prefilled). 2% vaginal cream with applicator and 1% topical cream in some combination packs. OTC Trade only (Gyne-Lotrimin): Vaginal suppository 100 mg (7), 200 mg (3) with applicators.

NOTES – Do not use if abdominal pain, fever, or foul-smelling vaginal discharge is present. Since small amounts of these drugs may be absorbed from the vagina, use during the 1st trimester only when essential. During pregnancy, use of a vaginal applicator may

(cont.)

CLOTRIMAZOLE—VAGINAL (*cont.*)

be contraindicated; manual insertion of tabs may be preferred. Skin rash, lower abdominal cramps, bloating, vulvar irritation may occur. Avoid vaginal intercourse during treatment.

METRONIDAZOLE—VAGINAL (***MetroGel-Vaginal, Vandazole***) ▶LK ♀B ◗? $$

ADULT – Bacterial vaginosis: 1 applicatorful (approximately 5 g containing approximately 37.5 mg metronidazole) intravaginally at bedtime or two times per day for 5 days.

PEDS – Not approved in children.

FORMS – Generic/Trade: 0.75% gel in 70 g tube with applicator.

NOTES – Cure rate same with at bedtime and twice daily dosing. Vaginally applied metronidazole could be absorbed in sufficient amounts to produce systemic effects. Caution in patients with CNS diseases due to rare reports of seizures, neuropathy, and numbness. Do not administer to patients who have taken disulfiram within the last 2 weeks. Interaction with ethanol. Caution with warfarin. *Candida cervicitis* and *vaginitis*, and vaginal, perineal, or vulvar itching may occur. Avoid vaginal intercourse during treatment.

MICONAZOLE (***Monistat, Femizol-M, M-Zole, Micozole, Monazole***) ▶LK ♀+ ◗? $

ADULT – Local treatment of vulvovaginal candidiasis: 1 applicatorful 2% cream intravaginally at bedtime for 7 days or 4% cream at bedtime for 3 days. 100 mg suppository intravaginally at bedtime for 7 days, 400 mg at bedtime for 3 days, or 1200 mg for 1 dose. Topical cream for external symptoms two times per day for 7 days.

PEDS – Not approved in children.

FORMS – OTC Generic/Trade: 2% vaginal cream in 45 g with 1 applicator or 7 disposable applicators. Vaginal suppository 100 mg (7) OTC Trade only: 400 mg (3), 1200 mg (1) with applicator. Generic/Trade: 4% vaginal cream in 25 g tubes or 3 prefilled applicators. Some in combination packs with 2% miconazole cream for external use.

NOTES – Do not use if abdominal pain, fever, or foul-smelling vaginal discharge is present. Since small amounts of these drugs may be absorbed from the vagina, use during the 1st trimester only when essential. During pregnancy, use of a vaginal applicator may be contraindicated; manual insertion of suppositories may be preferred. Vulvovaginal burning, itching, irritation, and pelvic cramps may occur. Avoid vaginal intercourse during treatment. May increase warfarin effect.

NYSTATIN—VAGINAL (***Mycostatin, ✤ Nilstat, Nyaderm***) ▶Not metabolized ♀A ◗? $$

ADULT – Local treatment of vulvovaginal candidiasis: 100,000 units tab intravaginally at bedtime for 2 weeks.

PEDS – Not approved in children.

FORMS – Generic only: Vaginal tabs 100,000 units in 15s with applicator.

NOTES – Topical azole products more effective. Do not use if abdominal pain, fever, or foul-smelling vaginal discharge is present. During pregnancy use of a vaginal applicator may be contraindicated; manual insertion of tabs may be preferred. Avoid vaginal intercourse during treatment.

TERCONAZOLE (***Terazol***) ▶LK ♀C ◗– $$

ADULT – Local treatment of vulvovaginal candidiasis: 1 applicatorful 0.4% cream intravaginally at bedtime for 7 days. 1 applicatorful 0.8% cream intravaginally at bedtime for 3 days. 80 mg suppository intravaginally at bedtime for 3 days.

PEDS – Not approved in children.

FORMS – All forms supplied with applicators: Generic/Trade: Vaginal cream 0.4% (Terazol 7) in 45 g tube, 0.8% (Terazol 3) in 20 g tube. Vaginal suppository (Terazol 3) 80 mg (#3).

NOTES – Do not use if abdominal pain, fever, or foul-smelling vaginal discharge is present. Since small amounts of these drugs may be absorbed from the vagina, use during the 1st trimester only when essential. During pregnancy, use of a vaginal applicator may be contraindicated; manual insertion of supps may be preferred. Avoid vaginal intercourse during treatment. Vulvovaginal irritation, burning, and pruritus may occur.

TIOCONAZOLE (***Monistat 1-Day, Vagistat-1***) ▶Not absorbed ♀C ◗– $

ADULT – Local treatment of vulvovaginal candidiasis: 1 applicatorful (~ 4.6 g) intravaginally at bedtime for 1 dose.

PEDS – Not approved in children.

FORMS – OTC Trade only: Vaginal ointment: 6.5% (300 mg) in 4.6 g prefilled single-dose applicator.

NOTES – Do not use if abdominal pain, fever, or foul-smelling vaginal discharge is present. Since small amounts of these drugs may be absorbed from the vagina, use during the first trimester only when essential. During pregnancy, use of a vaginal applicator may be contraindicated. Avoid vaginal intercourse during treatment. Vulvovaginal burning and itching may occur.

OB/GYN: Other OB/GYN Agents

DANAZOL (***Danocrine***, ✤ ***Cyclomen***) ▶L ♀X ▶– $$$$$

ADULT – Endometriosis: Start 400 mg PO two times per day, then titrate downward to a dose sufficient to maintain amenorrhea for 3 to 6 months, up to 9 months. Fibrocystic breast disease: 100 to 200 mg PO two times per day for 4 to 6 months.

PEDS – Not approved in children.

UNAPPROVED ADULT – Menorrhagia: 100 to 400 mg PO daily for 3 months. Cyclical mastalgia: 100 to 200 mg PO two times per day for 4 to 6 months.

FORMS – Generic only: Caps 50, 100, 200 mg.

NOTES – Contraindications: Impaired hepatic, renal, or cardiac function. Androgenic effects may not be reversible even after the drug is discontinued. May alter voice. Hepatic dysfunction has occurred. Insulin requirements may increase in diabetics. Prolongation of PT/INR has been reported with concomitant warfarin.

MIFEPRISTONE (***Mifeprex, RU-486***) ▶L ♀X ▶? $$$$$

WARNING – Rare cases of sepsis and death have occurred. Surgical intervention may be necessary with incomplete abortions. Patients need to be given info on where such services are available and what do in case of an emergency.

ADULT – Termination of pregnancy, up to 49 days: Day 1: 600 mg PO. Day 3: 400 mcg misoprostol (unless abortion confirmed). Day 14: Confirmation of pregnancy termination.

PEDS – Not approved in children.

UNAPPROVED ADULT – Termination of pregnancy, up to 63 days: 200 mg PO followed by 800 mcg misoprostol intravaginally 24 to 72 h later.

FORMS – Trade only: Tabs 200 mg.

NOTES – Bleeding/spotting and cramping most common side effects. Prolonged heavy bleeding may be a sign of incomplete abortion. Contraindications: Ectopic pregnancy, IUD use, adrenal insufficiency and long-term steroid use, use of anticoagulants, hemorrhagic disorders and porphyrias. CYP3A4 inducers may increase metabolism and lower levels. Available through physician offices only.

PREMESIS-RX **(pyridoxine + folic acid + cyanocobalamin + calcium carbonate)** ▶L ♀A ▶+ $$

ADULT – Treatment of pregnancy-induced nausea: 1 tab PO daily.

PEDS – Unapproved in children.

FORMS – Trade only: Tabs 75 mg vitamin B6 (pyridoxine), sustained-release, 12 mcg vitamin B12 (cyanocobalamin), 1 mg folic acid, and 200 mg calcium carbonate.

NOTES – May be taken in conjunction with prenatal vitamins.

RHO IMMUNE GLOBULIN (***HyperRHO S/D, MICRhoGAM, RhoGAM, Rhophylac, WinRho SDF***) ▶L ♀C ▶? $$$$$

ADULT – Prevention of hemolytic disease of the newborn if mother Rh– and baby is or might be Rh+: 300 mcg vial IM to mother at 28 weeks gestation followed by a second dose within 72 h of delivery. Doses more than 1 vial may be needed if large fetal–maternal hemorrhage occurs during delivery (see complete prescribing information to determine dose). Following amniocentesis, miscarriage, abortion, or ectopic pregnancy at least 13 weeks gestation: 1 vial (300 mcg) IM. Less than 12 weeks gestation: 1 vial (50 mcg) microdose IM. Immune thrombocytopenic purpura (ITP), nonsplenectomized (WinRho): 250 units/kg/dose (50 mcg/kg/dose) IV for 1 dose if hemoglobin is greater than 10 g/dL or 125 to 200 units/kg/dose (25 to 40 mcg/kg/dose) IV for 1 dose if hemoglobin is less than 10 g/dL. Additional doses of 125 to 300 units/kg/dose (25 to 60 mcg/kg/dose) IV may be given as determined by patient's response.

PEDS – Immune thrombocytopenic purpura (ITP), nonsplenectomized (WinRho): 250 units/kg/dose (50 mcg/kg/dose) IV for 1 dose if hemoglobin is greater than 10 g/dL or 125 to 200 units/kg/dose (25 to 40 mcg/kg/dose) IV for 1 dose if hemoglobin is less than 10 g/dL. Additional doses of 125 to 300 units/kg/dose (25 to 60 mcg/kg/dose) IV may be given as determined by patient's response.

UNAPPROVED ADULT – Rh-incompatible transfusion: Specialized dosing.

NOTES – One 300 mcg vial prevents maternal sensitization to the Rh factor if the fetomaternal hemorrhage is less than 15 mL fetal RBCs (30 mL of whole blood). When the fetomaternal hemorrhage exceeds this (as estimated by Kleihauer-Betke testing), administer more than one 300 mcg vial.

ONCOLOGY: Alkylating agents

ALTRETAMINE (***Hexalen***) ▶L ♀D ▶– $ varies by therapy

WARNING – Peripheral neuropathy, bone marrow suppression, fertility impairment, N/V, alopecia. Instruct patients to report promptly fever, sore throat, signs of local infection, bleeding from any site, or symptoms suggestive of anemia.

ADULT – Chemotherapy doses vary by indication. Ovarian cancer.

PEDS – Not approved in children.

UNAPPROVED ADULT – Lung, breast, cervical cancer, non-Hodgkin's lymphoma.

FORMS – Trade only: Caps 50 mg.

NOTES – Reliable contraception is recommended. Monitor CBCs. Cimetidine increases toxicity. MAOIs may cause severe orthostatic hypotension.

BENDAMUSTINE (***Treanda***) ▶Plasma ♀D ▶– $ varies by therapy

WARNING – Anaphylaxis, bone marrow suppression, nephrotoxicity, Stevens-Johnson syndrome, toxic epidermal necrolysis. Instruct patients to report promptly fever, sore throat, signs of local infection, bleeding from any site, or symptoms suggestive of anemia. Take precautions to avoid extravasation, including monitoring intravenous infusion site during and after administration.

ADULT – Chemotherapy doses vary by indication. CLL, non-Hodgkin's lymphoma.

PEDS – Not approved in children.

NOTES – Reliable contraception is recommended. Monitor CBCs and renal function.

BUSULFAN (***Myleran, Busulfex***) ▶LK ♀D ▶– $ varies by therapy

WARNING – Secondary malignancies, bone marrow suppression, adrenal insufficiency, hyperuricemia, pulmonary fibrosis, seizures (must initiate prophylactic anticonvulsant therapy prior to use of busulfan), cellular dysplasia, hepatic veno-occlusive disease, fertility impairment, alopecia. Instruct patients to report promptly fever, sore throat, signs of local infection, bleeding from any site, symptoms suggestive of anemia, or yellow discoloration of the skin or eyes.

ADULT – Chemotherapy doses vary by indication. Tabs: CML. Injection: Conditioning regimen prior to allogeneic hematopoietic progenitor cell transplantation for CML. in combination with cyclophosphamide.

PEDS – Chemotherapy doses vary by indication. Tabs: CML. Safety of the injection has not been established.

UNAPPROVED ADULT – High dose in conjunction with stem cell transplant for leukemia and lymphoma.

FORMS – Trade only (Myleran) Tabs 2 mg. Busulfex injection for hospital/oncology clinic use; not intended for outpatient prescribing.

NOTES – Reliable contraception is recommended. Monitor CBCs and LFTs. Hydration and allopurinol to decrease adverse effects of uric acid. Acetaminophen and itraconazole decrease busulfan clearance. Phenytoin increases clearance.

CARMUSTINE (***BCNU, BiCNU, Gliadel***) ▶Plasma ♀D ▶– $ varies by therapy

WARNING – Secondary malignancies, bone marrow suppression, pulmonary fibrosis, nephrotoxicity, hepatotoxicity, ocular nerve fiber-layer infarcts and retinal hemorrhages, fertility impairment, alopecia. Local soft tissue toxicity/extravasation can occur if carmustine is infused too quickly. Infusions should run over at least 2 h. Wafer: Seizures, brain edema and herniation, intracranial infection. Instruct patients to report promptly fever, sore throat, signs of local infection, bleeding from any site, symptoms suggestive of anemia, or yellow discoloration of the skin or eyes.

ADULT – Chemotherapy doses vary by indication. Injection: Glioblastoma, brainstem glioma, medulloblastoma, astrocytoma, ependymoma and metastatic brain tumors, multiple myeloma with prednisone; Hodgkin's disease and non-Hodgkin's lymphomas, in combination regimens. Wafer: Glioblastoma multiforme, adjunct to surgery. High-grade malignant glioma, adjunct to surgery and radiation.

PEDS – Not approved in children.

UNAPPROVED ADULT – Mycosis fungoides, topical soln.

NOTES – Reliable contraception is recommended. Monitor CBCs, PFTs, LFTs, and renal function. May decrease phenytoin and digoxin levels. Cimetidine may increase myelosuppression. Significant absorption to PVC containers will occur. Carmustine must be dispensed in glass or non-PVC containers.

CHLORAMBUCIL (***Leukeran***) ▶L ♀D ▶– $ varies by therapy

WARNING – Secondary malignancies, bone marrow suppression, seizures, fertility impairment, alopecia. Instruct patients to report promptly fever, sore throat, signs of local infection, bleeding from any site, or symptoms suggestive of anemia.

(cont.)

CHLORAMBUCIL (*cont.*)

ADULT – Chemotherapy doses vary by indication. CLL. Lymphomas including indolent lymphoma and Hodgkin's disease.

PEDS – Not approved in children.

UNAPPROVED ADULT – Uveitis and meningoencephalitis associated with Behcet's disease. Idiopathic membranous nephropathy. Ovarian carcinoma.

FORMS – Trade only: Tabs 2 mg.

NOTES – Reliable contraception is recommended. Monitor CBCs. Avoid live vaccines.

CYCLOPHOSPHAMIDE (***Cytoxan, Neosar***) ▶L ♀D ▶– $ varies by therapy

WARNING – Secondary malignancies, leukopenia, cardiac toxicity, acute hemorrhagic cystitis, hypersensitivity, fertility impairment, alopecia. Instruct patients to report promptly fever, sore throat, signs of local infection, bleeding from any site, symptoms suggestive of anemia, or yellow discoloration of the skin or eyes.

ADULT – Chemotherapy doses vary by indication. Non-Hodgkin's lymphomas, Hodgkin's disease. Multiple myeloma. Disseminated neuroblastoma. Adenocarcinoma of the ovary. Retinoblastoma. Carcinoma of the breast. CLL. CML. AML. Mycosis fungoides.

PEDS – Chemotherapy doses vary by indication. ALL. "Minimal change" nephrotic syndrome.

UNAPPROVED ADULT – Wegener's granulomatosis, other steroid-resistant vasculitides. Severe progressive RA. Systemic lupus erythematosus. Multiple sclerosis. Polyarteritis nodosa. Lung, testicular, and bladder cancer, sarcoma.

FORMS – Generic only: Tabs 25, 50 mg. Injection for hospital/oncology clinic use; not intended for outpatient prescribing.

NOTES – Reliable contraception is recommended. Monitor CBCs, urine for red cells. Allopurinol may increase myelosuppression. Thiazides may prolong leukopenia. May reduce digoxin levels, reduce fluoroquinolone activity. May increase anticoagulant effects. Coadministration with mesna reduces hemorrhagic cystitis when used in high doses.

DACARBAZINE (***DTIC-Dome***) ▶LK ♀C ▶– $ varies by therapy

WARNING – Extravasation associated with severe necrosis. Secondary malignancies, bone marrow suppression, hepatotoxicity, anorexia, N/V, anaphylaxis, alopecia. Instruct patients to report promptly fever, sore throat, signs of local infection, bleeding from any site, symptoms suggestive of anemia, or yellow discoloration of the skin or eyes.

ADULT – Chemotherapy doses vary by indication. Metastatic melanoma. Hodgkin's disease, in combination regimens.

PEDS – Not approved in children.

UNAPPROVED ADULT – Malignant pheochromocytoma, in combination regimens. Sarcoma.

NOTES – Monitor CBCs and LFTs.

IFOSFAMIDE (***Ifex***) ▶L ♀D ▶– $ varies by therapy

WARNING – Secondary malignancies, hemorrhagic cystitis, confusion, coma, bone marrow suppression, hematuria, nephrotoxicity, alopecia. Instruct patients to report promptly fever, sore throat, signs of local infection, bleeding from any site, symptoms suggestive of anemia, or yellow discoloration of the skin or eyes.

ADULT – Chemotherapy doses vary by indication. Germ cell testicular cancer, in combination regimens.

PEDS – Not approved in children.

UNAPPROVED ADULT – Bladder cancer, cervical cancer, ovarian cancer, non-small cell and small cell lung cancers, Hodgkin's and non-Hodgkin's lymphomas, ALL, osteosarcoma, and soft tissue sarcomas.

UNAPPROVED PEDS – Ewing's sarcoma, osteosarcoma, soft tissue sarcomas, neuroblastoma.

FORMS – Powder for reconstitution: 1 g and 3 g vials. Solution for injection: 50 mg/mL 20 mL and 60 mL vials.

NOTES – Reliable contraception is recommended. Monitor CBCs, renal function, and urine for red cells. Coadministration with mesna reduces hemorrhagic cystitis. Requires extensive hydration to minimize bladder toxicity.

LOMUSTINE (***CeeNu, CCNU***) ▶L ♀D ▶– $ varies by therapy

WARNING – Secondary malignancies, bone marrow suppression, hepatotoxicity, nephrotoxicity, pulmonary fibrosis, fertility impairment, alopecia. Instruct patients to report promptly fever, sore throat, signs of local infection, bleeding from any site, symptoms suggestive of anemia, or yellow discoloration of the skin or eyes.

ADULT – Chemotherapy doses vary by indication. Brain tumors. Hodgkin's disease, in combination regimens.

PEDS – Chemotherapy doses vary by indication. Brain tumors. Hodgkin's disease, in combination regimens.

(cont.)

LOMUSTINE (*cont.*)

FORMS – Trade only: Caps 10, 40, 100 mg.

NOTES – Reliable contraception is recommended. Monitor CBCs, LFTs, PFTs, and renal function. Avoid alcohol.

MECHLORETHAMINE (***Mustargen***) ▶Plasma ♀D ▶– $ varies by therapy

WARNING – Extravasation associated with severe necrosis. Secondary malignancies, bone marrow suppression, amyloidosis, herpes zoster, anaphylaxis, fertility impairment, alopecia. Instruct patients to report promptly fever, sore throat, signs of local infection, bleeding from any site, or symptoms suggestive of anemia.

ADULT – Chemotherapy doses vary by indication. Intravenous: Hodgkin's disease (Stages III and IV). Lymphosarcoma. Chronic myelocytic or chronic lymphocytic leukemia. Polycythemia vera. Mycosis fungoides. Bronchogenic carcinoma. Intrapleurally, intraperitoneally, or intrapericardially: Metastatic carcinoma resulting in effusion.

PEDS – Not approved in children.

UNAPPROVED ADULT – Cutaneous mycosis fungoides: Topical soln or ointment.

UNAPPROVED PEDS – Hodgkin's disease (Stages III and IV), in combination regimens.

NOTES – Reliable contraception is recommended. Monitor CBCs.

MELPHALAN (***Alkeran***) ▶Plasma ♀D ▶– $ varies by therapy

WARNING – Secondary malignancies, bone marrow suppression, anaphylaxis, fertility impairment, alopecia. Instruct patients to report promptly fever, sore throat, signs of local infection, bleeding from any site, or symptoms suggestive of anemia.

ADULT – Chemotherapy doses vary by indication. Multiple myeloma and nonresectable epithelial ovarian carcinoma.

PEDS – Not approved in children.

UNAPPROVED ADULT – Non-Hodgkin's lymphoma in high doses for stem cell transplant, testicular cancer.

FORMS – Trade only: Tabs 2 mg. Injection for hospital/clinic use; not intended for outpatient prescribing.

NOTES – Reliable contraception is recommended. Monitor CBCs. Avoid live vaccines.

PROCARBAZINE (***Matulane***) ▶LK ♀D ▶– $ varies by therapy

WARNING – Secondary malignancies, bone marrow suppression, hemolysis and Heinz-Ehrlich inclusion bodies in erythrocytes, hypersensitivity, fertility impairment, alopecia. Peds: Tremors, convulsions, and coma have occurred. Instruct patients to report promptly fever, sore throat, signs of local infection, bleeding from any site, symptoms suggestive of anemia, black tarry stools, or vomiting of blood.

ADULT – Chemotherapy doses vary by indication. Hodgkin's disease (Stages III and IV), in combination regimens.

PEDS – Chemotherapy doses vary by indication. Hodgkin's disease (Stages III and IV), in combination regimens.

FORMS – Trade only: Caps 50 mg.

NOTES – Reliable contraception is recommended. Monitor CBCs. Renal/hepatic function impairment may predispose toxicity. UA, LFTs, and BUN weekly. May decrease digoxin levels. May increase effects of opioids, sympathomimetics, TCAs. Ingestion of foods with high tyramine content may result in a potentially fatal hypertensive crisis. Alcohol may cause a disulfiram-like reaction.

STREPTOZOCIN (***Zanosar***) ▶Plasma ♀C ▶– $ varies by therapy

WARNING – Extravasation associated with severe necrosis. Secondary malignancies, nephrotoxicity, N/V, hepatotoxicity, decrease in hematocrit, hypoglycemia, fertility impairment, alopecia.

ADULT – Chemotherapy doses vary by indication. Metastatic islet cell carcinoma of the pancreas.

PEDS – Not approved in children.

NOTES – Hydration important. Monitor renal function, CBCs, and LFTs.

TEMOZOLOMIDE (***Temodar***, ✤***Temodal***) ▶Plasma ♀D ▶– $ varies by therapy

WARNING – Secondary malignancies, bone marrow suppression, fertility impairment, alopecia. Instruct patients to report promptly fever, sore throat, signs of local infection, bleeding from any site, or symptoms suggestive of anemia. Cases of interstitial pneumonitis, alveolitis, and pulmonary fibrosis have been reported.

ADULT – Chemotherapy doses vary by indication. Anaplastic astrocytoma, glioblastoma multiforme.

PEDS – Not approved in children.

UNAPPROVED ADULT – Metastatic melanoma, renal cell carcinoma. Cutaneous T-cell lymphomas.

FORMS – Trade only: Caps 5, 20, 100, 140, 180, 250 mg. Temozolomide is also available as a 100 mg powder for injection.

NOTES – Reliable contraception is recommended. Monitor CBCs. Valproic acid decreases clearance.

THIOTEPA (*Thioplex*) ▶L ♀D ▶– $ varies by therapy

WARNING – Secondary malignancies, bone marrow suppression, hypersensitivity, fertility impairment, alopecia. Instruct patients to report promptly fever, sore throat, signs of local infection, bleeding from any site, symptoms suggestive of anemia, black tarry stools, or vomiting of blood.

ADULT – Chemotherapy doses vary by indication. Adenocarcinoma of the breast or ovary. Control of intracavitary malignant effusions. Superficial papillary carcinoma of the urinary bladder. Hodgkin's disease. Lymphosarcoma.

PEDS – Not approved in children.

NOTES – Reliable contraception is recommended. Monitor CBCs.

ONCOLOGY: Antibiotics

BLEOMYCIN (*Blenoxane*) ▶K ♀D ▶– $ varies by therapy

WARNING – Pulmonary fibrosis, skin toxicity, nephro/hepatotoxicity, alopecia, and severe idiosyncratic reaction consisting of hypotension, mental confusion, fever, chills, and wheezing. Because of the possibility of an anaphylactoid reaction, lymphoma patients should be treated with 2 units or less for the first 2 doses. If no acute reaction occurs, then the regular dosage schedule may be followed.

ADULT – Chemotherapy doses vary by indication. Squamous cell carcinoma of the head and neck. Carcinoma of the skin, penis, cervix, and vulva. Hodgkin's and non-Hodgkin's lymphoma. Testicular carcinoma. Malignant pleural effusion: Sclerosing agent.

PEDS – Not approved in children.

UNAPPROVED ADULT – Treatment of ovarian germ cell tumors.

NOTES – Reliable contraception is recommended. Frequent chest x-rays. May decrease digoxin and phenytoin levels. Risk of pulmonary toxicity increases with lifetime cumulative dose greater than 400 units.

DACTINOMYCIN (*Cosmegen*) ▶Not metabolized ♀C ▶– $ varies by therapy

WARNING – Extravasation associated with severe necrosis. Contraindicated with active chickenpox or herpes zoster. Erythema and vesiculation (with radiation), bone marrow suppression, alopecia. Instruct patients to report promptly fever, sore throat, signs of local infection, bleeding from any site, or symptoms suggestive of anemia.

ADULT – Chemotherapy doses vary by indication. Wilms' tumor. Rhabdomyosarcoma. Metastatic and nonmetastatic choriocarcinoma. Nonseminomatous testicular carcinoma. Ewing's sarcoma. Sarcoma botryoides. Most in combination regimens.

PEDS – Chemotherapy doses vary by indication. See adult. Contraindicated in infants younger than 6 mo.

NOTES – Monitor CBCs.

DAUNORUBICIN (*DaunoXome, Cerubidine*) ▶L ♀D ▶– $ varies by therapy

WARNING – Extravasation associated with severe necrosis. Cardiac toxicity, more frequent in children. Bone marrow suppression, infusion-related reactions. Instruct patients to report promptly fever, sore throat, signs of local infection, bleeding from any site, or symptoms suggestive of anemia.

ADULT – Chemotherapy doses vary by indication. First-line treatment of advanced HIV-associated Kaposi's sarcoma (DaunoXome). AML, in combination regimens. ALL (Cerubidine).

PEDS – Chemotherapy doses vary by indication. ALL (Cerubidine). DaunoXome not approved in children.

NOTES – Reliable contraception is recommended. Monitor CBCs, cardiac, renal and hepatic function (toxicity increased with impaired function). Transient urine discoloration (red).

DOXORUBICIN LIPOSOMAL (*Doxil, ✤ Caelyx, Myocet*) ▶L ♀D ▶– $ varies by therapy

WARNING – Extravasation associated with severe necrosis. Cardiac toxicity, more frequent in children. Bone marrow suppression, infusion-associated reactions, necrotizing colitis, mucositis, hyperuricemia, palmar-plantar erythrodysesthesia. Secondary malignancies. Instruct patients to report promptly fever, sore throat, signs of local infection, bleeding from any site, or symptoms suggestive of anemia.

ADULT – Chemotherapy doses vary by indication. Advanced HIV-associated Kaposi's sarcoma, multiple myeloma, ovarian carcinoma.

PEDS – Not approved in children.

UNAPPROVED ADULT – Breast cancer, Hodgkin's lymphoma, non-Hodgkin's lymphoma, soft tissue sarcomas.

NOTES – Heart failure with cumulative doses. Monitor ejection fraction, CBCs, LFTs, uric acid levels, and renal function (toxicity increased with impaired function). Reliable contraception is recommended. Transient urine discoloration (red).

DOXORUBICIN NON-LIPOSOMAL (*Adriamycin, Rubex*) ▶L ♀D ▶– $ varies by therapy

WARNING – Extravasation associated with severe necrosis. Cardiac toxicity, more frequent in children. Bone marrow suppression, infusion-associated reactions, necrotizing colitis, mucositis, hyperuricemia, alopecia. Secondary malignancies. Instruct patients to report promptly fever, sore throat, signs of local infection, bleeding from any site, or symptoms suggestive of anemia.

ADULT – Chemotherapy doses vary by indication. ALL. AML. Wilms' tumor. Neuroblastoma. Soft tissue and bone sarcomas. Breast carcinoma. Ovarian carcinoma. Transitional cell bladder carcinoma. Thyroid carcinoma. Hodgkin's and non-Hodgkin's lymphomas. Bronchogenic carcinoma. Gastric carcinoma.

PEDS – Chemotherapy doses vary by indication: See ADULT.

UNAPPROVED ADULT – Sarcoma, small cell lung cancer.

NOTES – Heart failure with cumulative doses. Monitor ejection fraction, CBCs, LFTs, uric acid levels, and renal function (toxicity increased with impaired function). Reliable contraception is recommended. Transient urine discoloration (red).

EPIRUBICIN (*Ellence, ✤Pharmorubicin*) ▶L ♀D ▶– $ varies by therapy

WARNING – Extravasation associated with severe necrosis. Cardiac toxicity, bone marrow suppression, secondary malignancy (AML), hyperuricemia, fertility impairment, alopecia. Instruct patients to report promptly fever, sore throat, signs of local infection, bleeding from any site, or symptoms suggestive of anemia.

ADULT – Chemotherapy doses vary by indication. Adjuvant therapy for breast cancer, axillary-node positive.

PEDS – Not approved in children.

UNAPPROVED ADULT – Neoadjuvant and metastatic breast cancer. Cervical cancer, esophageal cancer, gastric cancer, soft tissue sarcomas, uterine sarcoma.

NOTES – Reliable contraception is recommended. Monitor CBCs, cardiac, hepatic and renal function (toxicity increased with impaired function). Cimetidine increases levels. Transient urine discoloration (red).

IDARUBICIN (*Idamycin*) ▶? ♀D ▶– $ varies by therapy

WARNING – Extravasation associated with severe necrosis. Cardiac toxicity, bone marrow suppression, hyperuricemia, alopecia. Instruct patients to report promptly fever, sore throat, signs of local infection, bleeding from any site, or symptoms suggestive of anemia.

ADULT – Chemotherapy doses vary by indication. AML, in combination regimens.

PEDS – Not approved in children.

UNAPPROVED ADULT – ALL, CML.

NOTES – Reliable contraception is recommended. Monitor CBCs, LFTs, cardiac and renal function (toxicity increased with impaired function).

MITOMYCIN (*Mutamycin, Mitomycin-C*) ▶L ♀D ▶– $ varies by therapy

WARNING – Extravasation associated with severe necrosis. Bone marrow suppression, hemolytic uremic syndrome, nephrotoxicity, adult respiratory distress syndrome, alopecia. Instruct patients to report promptly fever, sore throat, signs of local infection, bleeding from any site, or symptoms suggestive of anemia.

ADULT – Chemotherapy doses vary by indication. Disseminated adenocarcinoma of stomach, pancreas, or colorectum, in combination regimens.

PEDS – Not approved in children.

UNAPPROVED ADULT – Superficial bladder cancer, intravesical route; pterygia, adjunct to surgical excision: Ophthalmic soln.

NOTES – Reliable contraception is recommended. Monitor CBCs and renal function.

MITOXANTRONE (*Novantrone*) ▶LK ♀D ▶– $ varies by therapy

WARNING – Secondary malignancies (AML), bone marrow suppression, cardiac toxicity/heart failure, hyperuricemia, increased LFTs. Instruct patients to report promptly fever, sore throat, signs of local infection, bleeding from any site, or symptoms suggestive of anemia.

ADULT – Chemotherapy doses vary by indication. AML, in combination regimens. Symptomatic patients with hormone refractory prostate cancer. Multiple sclerosis (secondary progressive, progressive relapsing, or worsening relapsing-remitting): 12 mg/m^2 of BSA IV q 3 months.

PEDS – Not approved in children.

UNAPPROVED ADULT – Breast cancer. Non-Hodgkin's lymphoma. ALL, CML, ovarian carcinoma. Sclerosing agent for malignant pleural effusions.

NOTES – Reliable contraception is recommended. Monitor CBCs and LFTs. Baseline echocardiogram and repeat echoes prior to each dose are recommended. Transient urine and sclera discoloration (blue-green).

VALRUBICIN (*Valstar,* ♣ *Valtaxin*) ▶K ♀C ◗– $ varies by therapy
WARNING – Induces complete responses in only 1 in 5 patients. Delaying cystectomy could lead to development of lethal metastatic bladder cancer. Irritable bladder symptoms, alopecia.
ADULT – Chemotherapy doses vary by indication. Bladder cancer, intravesical therapy of BCG-refractory carcinoma in situ.
PEDS – Not approved in children.
NOTES – Reliable contraception is recommended. Transient urine discoloration (red).

ONCOLOGY: Antimetabolites

AZACITIDINE (*Vidaza*) ▶K ♀D ◗– $ varies by therapy
WARNING – Contraindicated with malignant hepatic tumors. Bone marrow suppression. Fertility impairment. Instruct patients to report promptly fever, sore throat, or signs of local infection or bleeding from any site.
ADULT – Chemotherapy doses vary by indication. Myelodysplastic syndrome subtypes.
PEDS – Not approved in children.
NOTES – Reliable contraception is recommended. Men should not father children while on this drug. Monitor CBC, renal and hepatic function.

CAPECITABINE (*Xeloda*) ▶L ♀D ◗– $ varies by therapy
WARNING – Increased INR and bleeding with warfarin. Contraindicated in severe renal dysfunction (CrCl less than 30 mL/min). Severe diarrhea, fertility impairment, palmar-plantar erythrodysesthesia or chemotherapy-induced acral erythema, cardiac toxicity, hyperbilirubinemia, neutropenia, alopeci, typhlitis. Instruct patients to report promptly fever, sore throat, or signs of local infection or bleeding from any site.
ADULT – Chemotherapy doses vary by indication. Metastatic breast and colorectal cancer.
PEDS – Not approved in children.
UNAPPROVED ADULT – Gastric cancer, esophageal cancer, pancreatic cancer, hepatocellular carcinoma, ovarian cancer, metastatic renal cell cancer, neuroendocrine tumors, metastatic CNS lesions.
FORMS – Trade only: Tabs 150, 500 mg.
NOTES – Reliable contraception is recommended. Antacids containing aluminum hydroxide and magnesium hydroxide increase levels. May increase phenytoin levels. Contraindicated with known dihydropyrimidine dehydrogenase (DPD) deficiency.

CLADRIBINE (*Leustatin,* **chlorodeoxyadenosine**) ▶intracellular ♀D ◗– $ varies by therapy
WARNING – Bone marrow suppression, nephrotoxicity, neurotoxicity, fever, fertility impairment, alopecia. Instruct patients to report promptly fever, sore throat, signs of local infection, bleeding from any site, or symptoms suggestive of anemia.
ADULT – Chemotherapy doses vary by indication. Hairy cell leukemia.
PEDS – Not approved in children.
UNAPPROVED ADULT – Advanced cutaneous T-cell lymphomas. Chronic lymphocytic leukemia, non-Hodgkin's lymphomas. AML. Autoimmune hemolytic anemia. Mycosis fungoides. Sezary syndrome. Progressive multiple sclerosis.
NOTES – Reliable contraception is recommended. Monitor CBCs and renal function.

CLOFARABINE (*Clolar*) ▶K ♀D ◗– $ varies by therapy
WARNING – Myelodysplastic syndrome, bone marrow suppression, tumor lysis syndrome, hepatotoxicity. Instruct patients to report promptly fever, sore throat, or signs of local infection, bleeding from any site, or symptoms suggestive of anemia.
ADULT – Not approved in adults.
PEDS – Age 1 to 21 yo: Chemotherapy doses vary by indication. Relapsed or refractory acute lymphoblastic leukemia.
NOTES – Reliable contraception is recommended. Monitor CBCs, LFTs, and renal function.

CYTARABINE (*Cytosar-U, Tarabine, Depo-Cyt, AraC*) ▶LK ♀D ◗– $ varies by therapy
WARNING – Bone marrow suppression, hepatotoxicity, N/V/D, hyperuricemia, pancreatitis, peripheral neuropathy, "cytarabine syndrome" (fever, myalgia, bone pain, occasional chest pain, maculopapular rash, conjunctivitis, and malaise), alopecia. Neurotoxicity. Chemical arachnoiditis (N/V, headache, and fever) with Depo-Cyt. Instruct patients to report promptly fever, sore throat, or signs of local infection, bleeding from any site, symptoms suggestive of anemia, or yellow discoloration of the skin or eyes.
ADULT – Chemotherapy doses vary by indication. AML. ALL. CML. Prophylaxis and treatment of meningeal leukemia. intrathecal

(cont.)

CYTARABINE (*cont.*)

(Cytosar-U, Tarabine). Lymphomatous meningitis, intrathecal (Depo-Cyt).

PEDS – Chemotherapy doses vary by indication. AML. ALL. Chronic myelocytic leukemia. Prophylaxis and treatment of meningeal leukemia, intrathecal (Cytosar-U, Tarabine). Depo-Cyt not approved in children.

NOTES – Reliable contraception is recommended. Monitor CBCs, LFTs, and renal function. Decreases digoxin levels. Chemical arachnoiditis can be reduced by coadministration of dexamethasone. Use dexamethasone eye drops with high doses.

DECITABINE (***Dacogen***) ▸L ♀D ▸– $ varies by therapy

WARNING – Bone marrow suppression, pulmonary edema. Instruct patients to report promptly fever, sore throat, or signs of local infection, bleeding from any site, or symptoms suggestive of anemia.

ADULT – Myelodysplastic syndromes. Treatment regimen: Option 1: Administer at a dose of 15 mg/m^2 by continuous IV infusion over 3 h repeated q 8 h for 3 days. Repeat cycle q 6 weeks. Option 2: Administer at a dose of 20 mg/m^2 by continuous IV infusion over 1 h repeated daily for 5 days. Repeat cycle q 4 weeks.

PEDS – Not approved in children.

NOTES – Reliable contraception is recommended. Men should not father children during and 2 months after therapy. Monitor CBCs, baseline LFTs.

FLOXURIDINE (***FUDR***) ▸L ♀D ▸– $ varies by therapy

WARNING – Bone marrow suppression, nephrotoxicity, increased LFTs, alopecia. Instruct patients to report promptly fever, sore throat, or signs of local infection, bleeding from any site, or symptoms suggestive of anemia.

ADULT – Chemotherapy doses vary by indication. GI adenocarcinoma metastatic to the liver given by intrahepatic arterial pump.

PEDS – Not approved in children.

NOTES – Reliable contraception is recommended. Monitor CBCs, LFTs, and renal function.

FLUDARABINE (***Fludara***) ▸Serum ♀D ▸– $ varies by therapy

WARNING – Neurotoxicity (agitation, blindness, and coma), progressive multifocal leukoencephalopathy and death, bone marrow suppression, hemolytic anemia, thrombocytopenia, ITP, Evan's syndrome, acquired hemophilia, pulmonary toxicity, fertility impairment, hyperuricemia, alopecia. Instruct patients to report promptly fever, sore throat, or signs of local infection, bleeding from any site, or symptoms suggestive of anemia.

ADULT – Chemotherapy doses vary by indication. Chronic lymphocytic leukemia.

PEDS – Not approved in children.

UNAPPROVED ADULT – Non-Hodgkin's lymphoma. Mycosis fungoides. Hairy-cell leukemia. Hodgkin's disease.

NOTES – Reliable contraception is recommended. Monitor CBCs and renal function; watch for hemolysis.

FLUOROURACIL (***Adrucil, 5-FU***) ▸L ♀D ▸– $ varies by therapy

WARNING – Increased INR and bleeding with warfarin. Bone marrow suppression, angina, fertility impairment, alopecia, diarrhea, mucositis, hand and foot syndrome (palmar-plantar erythrodysesthesia). Instruct patients to report promptly fever, sore throat, signs of local infection, bleeding from any site, or symptoms suggestive of anemia.

ADULT – Chemotherapy doses vary by indication. Colon, rectum, breast, stomach, and pancreatic carcinoma. Dukes' stage C colon cancer with irinotecan or leucovorin after surgical resection.

PEDS – Not approved in children.

UNAPPROVED ADULT – Head and neck, renal cell, prostate, ovarian, esophageal, anal, and topical to skin for basal and squamous cell carcinoma.

NOTES – Reliable contraception is recommended. Monitor CBCs.

GEMCITABINE (***Gemzar***) ▸intracellular ♀D ▸– $ varies by therapy

WARNING – Bone marrow suppression, fever, rash, increased LFTs, proteinuria, hematuria, alopecia. Instruct patients to report promptly fever, sore throat, signs of local infection, bleeding from any site, or symptoms suggestive of anemia.

ADULT – Chemotherapy doses vary by indication. Adenocarcinoma of the pancreas. Non-small cell lung cancer, in combination regimens. Metastatic breast cancer, in combination regimens. Advanced ovarian cancer.

PEDS – Not approved in children.

NOTES – Reliable contraception is recommended. Monitor CBCs, LFTs, and renal function.

MERCAPTOPURINE (***6-MP, Purinethol***) ▸L ♀D ▸– $ varies by therapy

WARNING – Mercaptopurine is mutagenic in animals and humans, carcinogenic in animals, and may increase the patient's risk of neoplasia. Cases of hepatosplenic T-cell lymphoma have been reported in patients treated with

(cont.)

MERCAPTOPURINE (*cont.*)

mercaptopurine for inflammatory bowel disease. The safety and efficacy of mercaptopurine in patients with inflammatory bowel disease have not been established. Bone marrow suppression, hepatotoxicity, hyperuricemia, alopecia. Instruct patients to report promptly fever, sore throat, signs of local infection, bleeding from any site, symptoms suggestive of anemia, or yellow discoloration of the skin or eyes.

ADULT – Chemotherapy doses vary by indication. ALL. AML. CML.

PEDS – Chemotherapy doses vary by indication. ALL. AML.

UNAPPROVED ADULT – Inflammatory bowel disease: Start at 50 mg PO daily, titrate to response. Typical dose range 0.5 to 1.5 mg/kg PO daily.

UNAPPROVED PEDS – Inflammatory bowel disease: 1.5 mg/kg PO daily.

FORMS – Generic/Trade: Tabs 50 mg.

NOTES – Reliable contraception is recommended. Monitor CBCs, LFTs, and renal function. Consider folate supplementation. Allopurinol and trimethoprim-sulfamethoxazole increase toxicity.

METHOTREXATE—ONCOLOGY (***Rheumatrex, Trexall***) ▶KL – intestinal flora ♀X ▶–

WARNING – Acute renal failure, third-spacing in ascites/pleural effusions/bone marrow suppression/mucositis/hepatotoxicity/pneumonitis.

ADULT – Trophoblastic neoplasms, acute lymphocytic leukemia, meningeal leukemia, breast cancer, head and neck cancer, cutaneous T-cell lymphoma, lung cancer, non-Hodgkin's Lymphoma, osteosarcoma.

PEDS – ALL, meningeal leukemia, non-Hodgkin's lymphoma, nonmetastatic osteosarcoma.

UNAPPROVED ADULT – Bladder cancer, CNS tumors, acute promyelocytic leukemia, soft tissue sarcomas, acute graft versus host disease prophylaxis.

UNAPPROVED PEDS – Dermatomyositis, juvenile idiopathic arthritis.

FORMS – Injection, powder for reconstitution, 1 g. Injection soln 25 mg/ml. Oral tabs, 2.5 mg, 5 mg, 7.5 mg, 10 mg, 15 mg.

NELARABINE (***Arranon***) ▶LK ♀D ▶– $ varies by therapy

WARNING – Peripheral neuropathy, paralysis, demyelination, severe somnolence, convulsions. Bone marrow suppression.

ADULT – Chemotherapy doses vary by indication. ALL, T-cell lymphoblastic lymphoma.

PEDS – Chemotherapy doses vary by indication. ALL, T-cell lymphoblastic lymphoma.

NOTES – Reliable contraception is recommended. Monitor renal function.

PEMETREXED (***Alimta***) ▶K ♀D ▶– $ varies by therapy

WARNING – Bone marrow suppression, rash. Instruct patients to report promptly fever, sore throat, signs of local infection, bleeding from any site, symptoms suggestive of anemia.

ADULT – Chemotherapy doses vary by indication. Malignant pleural mesothelioma, in combination with cisplatin. Nonsquamous non-small cell lung cancer. Supplement with folic acid and vitamin B12.

PEDS – Not approved in children. No efficacy in pediatric patients has been reported. Pharmacokinetics in pediatric patients are comparable to adults.

UNAPPROVED ADULT – Metastatic bladder cancer, cervical cancer, thymic malignancies.

NOTES – Reliable contraception is recommended. Monitor CBCs and renal function. Do not use in patients with CrCl less than 45 mL/min. Avoid NSAIDs around the time of administration. Drainage of mild or moderate third space fluid collection prior to ALIMTA treatment should be considered, but is probably not necessary. The effect of severe third space fluid on pharmacokinetics is not known.

PENTOSTATIN (***Nipent***) ▶K ♀D ▶– $ varies by therapy

WARNING – Bone marrow suppression, nephrotoxicity, hepatotoxicity, CNS toxicity, pulmonary toxicity, severe rash, fertility impairment, alopecia. Instruct patients to report promptly fever, sore throat, signs of local infection, bleeding from any site, symptoms suggestive of anemia, or yellow discoloration of the skin or eyes.

ADULT – Chemotherapy doses vary by indication. Hairy cell leukemia, refractory to alpha-interferon.

PEDS – Not approved in children.

UNAPPROVED ADULT – ALL, CLL, non-Hodgkin's lymphoma, mycosis fungoides.

NOTES – Reliable contraception is recommended. Monitor CBCs and renal function.

PRALATREXATE (***Folotyn***) ▶+ intracellular ♀D ▶–

WARNING – Bone marrow suppression, mucositis, and hepatotoxicity may require dosage modification. Concomitant administration of drugs that are subject to substantial renal clearance (eg, NSAIDs, trimethoprim-sulfamethoxazole) may result in delayed clearance of pralatrexate.

ADULT – 30 mg/m^2 IV once weekly for 6 out of 7 weeks. Treatment of relapsed/refractory peripheral T-cell lymphoma (PTCL).

(cont.)

PRALATREXATE (*cont.*)

PEDS – Not approved in pediatrics.

NOTES – Folic acid and vitamin B12 supplementation needed to reduce hematologic toxicity and treatment related mucositis. Folic Acid 1 to 1.25 mg PO daily should be started within 10 days prior to starting pralatrexate, and continued for 30 days post last pralatrexate dose. Vitamin B12 1000mcg IM should be administered within 10 weeks prior to starting pralatrexate, and q 8 to 10 weeks thereafter. Vitamin B12 may be given same day as pralatrexate after the initial dose.

THIOGUANINE (*Tabloid,* ♣ *Lanvis*) ▶L ♀D ◗– $ varies by therapy

WARNING – Bone marrow suppression, hepatotoxicity, hyperuricemia, alopecia. Instruct patients to report promptly fever, sore throat, signs of local infection, bleeding from any site, symptoms suggestive of anemia, or yellow discoloration of the skin or eyes.

ADULT – Chemotherapy doses vary by indication. Acute nonlymphocytic leukemias.

PEDS – Chemotherapy doses vary by indication. Acute nonlymphocytic leukemias.

FORMS – Generic only: Tabs 40 mg, scored.

NOTES – Reliable contraception is recommended. Monitor CBCs and LFTs.

ONCOLOGY: Cytoprotective Agents

AMIFOSTINE (*Ethyol*) ▶plasma ♀C ◗– $ varies by therapy

WARNING – Hypotension, hypocalcemia, N/V, hypersensitivity.

ADULT – Doses vary by indication. Reduction of renal toxicity with cisplatin. Reduction of xerostomia and mucositis with radiation.

PEDS – Not approved in children.

NOTES – Monitor calcium and BP.

DENOSUMAB (*Xgeva*) ▶? – ♀C ◗?

ADULT – Prevention of skeletal-related events in bone metastases from solid tumors. 120 mg SC q 4 weeks. On September 16, 2011, the FDA granted approval for denosumab (Prolia) as a treatment to increase bone mass in patients at high risk for fracture receiving androgen deprivation therapy (ADT) for nonmetastatic prostate cancer or adjuvant aromatase inhibitor (AI) therapy for breast cancer. In men with nonmetastatic prostate cancer, denosumab also reduced the incidence of vertebral fracture.

PEDS – Not approved in children.

UNAPPROVED ADULT – Prevention of bone loss due to androgen deprivation therapy in nonmetastatic prostate cancer, and due to aromatase inhibitor therapy in nonmetastic breast cancer. Treatment of of bone destruction caused by rheumatoid arthritis.

FORMS – 70 mg/mL injection. 1.7 mL vials (Xgeva).

DEXRAZOXANE (*Totect, Zinecard*) ▶plasma ♀C ◗– $ varies by therapy

WARNING – Additive bone marrow suppression, secondary malignancies, fertility impairment, N/V.

ADULT – Doses vary by indication. Reduction of cardiac toxicity with doxorubicin. Treatment of anthracycline extravasation; give ASAP within 6 h of extravasation. Not approved in children.

FORMS – Monitor CBCs.

GLUCARPIDASE (*Voraxaze*) ▶L ♀C ◗?

ADULT – Toxic plasma methotrexate concentrations (more than 1 micromole/L) in patients with delayed methotrexate clearance due to impaired renal function. Given IV 50 units/kg.

PEDS – Toxic plasma methotrexate concentrations (more than 1 micromole/L) in patients with delayed methotrexate clearance due to impaired renal function.

UNAPPROVED ADULT – 2000 units delivered intrathecally as soon as possible after intrathecal methotrexate overdose.

FORMS – 1000 unit powder for injection.

MESNA (*Mesnex,* ♣ *Uromitexan*) ▶plasma ♀B ◗– $ varies by therapy

WARNING – Hypersensitivity, bad taste in the mouth.

ADULT – Doses vary by indication. Reduction of hemorrhagic cystis with ifosfamide.

PEDS – Not approved in children.

UNAPPROVED ADULT – Doses vary by indication. Reduction of hemorrhagic cystis with high-dose cyclophosphamide.

UNAPPROVED PEDS – Doses vary by indication.

FORMS – Trade only: Tabs 400 mg, scored. Also available as a 100 mg/mL injection.

NOTES – False-positive test urine ketones.

PALIFERMIN (*Kepivance*) ▶plasma ♀C ◗? $ varies by therapy

ADULT – Doses vary by indication. Decreases incidence, duration, and severity of severe oral mucositis in patients receiving therapy for hematologic malignancies.

PEDS – Not approved in children.

ONCOLOGY: Hormones

ABIRATERONE ACETATE (***Zytiga***) ▶L – ♀X ▶–
WARNING – Significant increases in hepatic enzymes have been reported; may require dose reduction.
ADULT – Treatment of metastatic, castration-resistant prostate cancer in combination with prednisone after previous treatment with docetaxel. 1000 mg PO daily in combination with Prednisone 5 mg twice daily.
PEDS – Not for use in pediatrics.
FORMS – 250 mg tabs.
NOTES – Increased mineralocorticoid levels due to CYP17 inhibition. Avoid concurrent use with CYP3A4 inhibitors and inducers, as well as CYP2D6 substrates.

ANASTROZOLE (***Arimidex***) ▶L ♀X ▶– $ varies by therapy
WARNING – Patients with estrogen receptor-negative disease and patients who do not respond to tamoxifen therapy rarely respond to anastrozole. Fertility impairment, vaginal bleeding, hot flashes, alopecia, decrease in bone mineral density. Increase in cardiovascular ischemia in women with preexisting ischemic heart disease.
ADULT – Chemotherapy doses vary by indication. Locally advanced or metastatic breast cancer. Adjuvant early breast cancer.
PEDS – Not approved in children.
FORMS – Generic/Trade: Tabs 1 mg.
NOTES – Reliable contraception is recommended. Monitor CBCs. Contraindicated in premenopausal women.

BICALUTAMIDE (***Casodex***, ✤ ***Apo-Bicalutamide***) ▶L ♀X $ varies by therapy
WARNING – Hypersensitivity, hepatotoxicity, interstitial lung disease, gynecomastia/breast pain, fertility impairment, hot flashes, diarrhea, alopecia. Increased risk for cardiovascular disease and diabetes.
ADULT – Prostate cancer: 50 mg PO daily in combination with a LHRH analog (eg, goserelin or leuprolide). Not indicated in women.
PEDS – Not approved in children.
UNAPPROVED ADULT – Monotherapy for locally advanced prostate cancer at a dose of 150 mg PO daily.
FORMS – Generic/Trade: Tabs 50 mg.
NOTES – Monitor PSA levels, CBC, ECG, serum testosterone, luteinizing hormone, and LFTs. Monitor glucose closely in diabetics. Displaces warfarin, possibly increasing anticoagulant effects. Gynecomastia and breast pain occur. Avoid concomitant use with tolvaptan.

CYPROTERONE ▶L ♀X ▶– $ varies by therapy
ADULT – Prostate cancer.
PEDS – Not approved in children.
FORMS – Generic/Trade: Tabs 50 mg.
NOTES – Dose-related hepatotoxicity has occurred, monitor LFTs at initiation and during treatment. Monitor adrenocortical function periodically. May impair carbohydrate metabolism; monitor blood glucose, especially in diabetics.

DEGARELIX ▶LK ♀X ▶– $ varies by therapy
WARNING – QT prolongation.
ADULT – Advanced prostate cancer: Initial dose: 240 mg SC; maintenance: 80 mg SC q 28 days.
PEDS – Not approved in children.
NOTES – Monitor LFTs and PSA. May prolong QT interval. May decrease bone mineral density.

ESTRAMUSTINE (***Emcyt***) ▶L ♀X ▶– $ varies by therapy
WARNING – Thrombosis, including MI, glucose intolerance, HTN, fluid retention, increased LFTs, alopecia.
ADULT – Chemotherapy doses vary by indication. Hormone refractory prostate cancer.
PEDS – Not approved in children.
FORMS – Trade only: Caps 140 mg.
NOTES – Reliable contraception is recommended. Monitor LFTs, glucose, and BP. Milk, milk products, and calcium-rich foods or drugs may impair absorption.

EXEMESTANE (***Aromasin***) ▶L ♀D ▶– $ varies by therapy
WARNING – Lymphocytopenia, alopecia.
ADULT – Chemotherapy doses vary by indication. Breast cancer.
PEDS – Not approved in children.
UNAPPROVED ADULT – Chemotherapy doses vary by indication. Prevention of prostate cancer.
FORMS – Trade only: Tabs 25 mg.
NOTES – Contraindicated in premenopausal women. Reliable contraception is recommended. Monitor CBCs.

FLUTAMIDE (***Eulexin***, ✤ ***Euflex***) ▶L ♀D ▶– $ varies by therapy
WARNING – Hepatic failure, methemoglobinemia, hemolytic anemia, breast neoplasms, gynecomastia, fertility impairment, photosensitivity, alopecia.
ADULT – Prostate cancer: 250 mg PO q 8 h in combination with an LHRH analog (eg, goserelin or leuprolide). Not indicated in women.
PEDS – Not approved in children.

(cont.)

FLUTAMIDE (*cont.*)

UNAPPROVED ADULT – Hirsutism in women.

FORMS – Generic only: Caps 125 mg.

NOTES – Monitor LFTs, PSA, methemoglobin levels. Transient urine discoloration (amber or yellow-green). Avoid exposure to sunlight/use sunscreen. Increased INR with warfarin. Gynecomastia and breast pain occur.

FULVESTRANT (***Faslodex***) ▶L ♀D ▶– $ varies by therapy

WARNING – Contraindicated in pregnancy. Hypersensitivity, N/V/D, constipation, abdominal pain, hot flashes. Use with caution in patients with bleeding disorders. Hepatic impairment may require dose adjustment.

ADULT – Chemotherapy doses vary by indication. Breast cancer.

PEDS – Not approved in children.

NOTES – Reliable contraception is recommended. FDA approved only in hormone receptor–positive metastatic breast cancer in postmenopausal women with disease progression following antiestrogen therapy.

GOSERELIN (***Zoladex***) ▶LK ♀D/X ▶– $ varies by therapy

WARNING – Transient increases in sex hormones, increases in lipids, hypercalcemia, decreases in bone mineral density, vaginal bleeding, fertility impairment, hot flashes, decreased libido, alopecia.

ADULT – Prostate cancer: 3.6 mg implant SC into upper abdominal wall q 28 days, or 10.8 mg implant SC q 12 weeks. Endometriosis: 3.6 mg implant SC q 28 days or 10.8 mg implant q 12 weeks for 6 months. Specialized dosing for breast cancer.

PEDS – Not approved in children.

UNAPPROVED ADULT – Adjuvant prostate cancer. Palliative treatment of breast cancer. 3.6 mg implant SC q 28 days indefinitely. Endometrial thinning prior to ablation for dysfunctional uterine bleeding: 3.6 mg SC 4 weeks prior to surgery or 3.6 mg SC q 4 weeks for 2 doses with surgery 2 to 4 weeks after last dose.

FORMS – Trade only: Implants 3.6, 10.8 mg.

NOTES – Transient increases in testosterone and estrogen occur. Hypercalcemia may occur in patients with bone metastases. Vaginal bleeding may occur during the first 2 months of treatment and should stop spontaneously. Reliable contraception is recommended. Consider norethindrone as "add back" therapy to decrease bone loss (see norethindrone).

HISTRELIN (***Vantas, Supprelin LA***) ▶Not metabolized ♀X ▶– $ varies by therapy

WARNING – Worsening of symptoms, especially during the 1st weeks of therapy: Increase in bone pain, difficulty urinating. Decreases in bone mineral density. Increased risk of cardiovascular disease and diabetes in men with prostate cancer.

ADULT – Palliative treatment of advanced prostate cancer: Insert 1 implant SC in the upper arm surgically q 12 months. May repeat if appropriate after 12 months.

PEDS – Central precocious puberty (Supprelin LA), in age older than 2 yo: Insert 1 implant SC in the inner upper arm surgically. May repeat if appropriate after 12 months.

FORMS – Trade only: 50 mg implant.

NOTES – Causes transient increase of testosterone level during the first weeks of treatment which may create or exacerbate symptoms. Patients with metastatic vertebral lesions and/or urinary tract obstruction should be closely observed during the 1st few weeks of therapy. Avoid wetting arm for 24 h after implant insertion and from heavy lifting or strenuous exertion of the involved arm for 7 days after insertion. Measure testosterone levels and PSA periodically. May decrease bone density. Monitor LH, FSH, estradiol or testosterone, height, and bone age in children with central precocious puberty at 1 month post implantation and q 6 months thereafter.

LETROZOLE (***Femara***) ▶LK ♀D ▶– $$$$$

WARNING – Fertility impairment, decreases in lymphocytes, increased LFTs, alopecia.

ADULT – 2.5 mg PO daily. Adjuvant treatment of postmenopausal, hormone receptor positive, early breast cancer. Extended adjuvant treatment of early breast cancer after 5 years of tamoxifen therapy. Advanced breast cancer with disease progression after antiestrogen therapy, hormone receptor positive or hormone receptor unknown, locally advanced or metastatic breast cancer.

PEDS – Not approved in children.

UNAPPROVED ADULT – Ovarian (epithelial) cancer. Endometrial cancer.

FORMS – Trade only: Tabs 2.5 mg.

NOTES – Reliable contraception is recommended. Monitor CBCs, LFTs, and lipids.

LEUPROLIDE (***Eligard, Lupron Depot, Lupron Depot-Ped***) ▶L ♀X ▶– $ varies by therapy

WARNING – Possible increase of diabetes and cardiovascular disease in men receiving leuprolide for prostate cancer. Worsening of symptoms: Increase in bone pain, difficulty urinating. Decreases in bone mineral density. Anaphylaxis, alopecia.

ADULT – Advanced prostate cancer: Lupron: 1 mg SC daily. Eligard: 7.5 mg SC q month, 22.5 mg SC q 3 months, 30 mg SC q 4 months,

(cont.)

LEUPROLIDE (*cont.*)

or 45 mg SC q 6 months. Lupron depot: 7.5 mg IM q month, 22.5 mg IM q 3 months or 30 mg IM q 4 months. Viadur: 65 mg SC implant q 12 months. Endometriosis or uterine leiomyomata (fibroids): 3.75 mg IM q month or 11.25 mg IM q 3 months for total therapy of 6 months (endometriosis) or 3 months (fibroids). Administer concurrent iron for fibroid-associated anemia.

PEDS – Central precocious puberty: Injection: 50 mcg/kg/day SC. Increase by 10 mcg/kg/day until total down regulation. Depot-Ped: 0.3 mg/kg q 4 weeks IM (minimum dose 7.5 mg). Increase by 3.75 mg q 4 weeks until adequate down regulation.

UNAPPROVED ADULT – Treatment of breast cancer, infertility, menses cessation in patients receiving high-dose chemotherapy, prostatic hyperplasia.

NOTES – For prostate cancer, monitor testosterone, prostatic acid phosphatase, and PSA levels. Transient increases in testosterone and estrogen occur. For endometriosis, a fractional dose of the 3-month Depot preparation is not equivalent to the same dose of the monthly formulation. Rotate the injection site periodically. Consider norethindrone as "add back" therapy to decrease bone loss (see norethindrone).

NILUTAMIDE (***Nilandron***) ▶L ♀C ▶– $ varies by therapy

WARNING – Interstitial pneumonitis, hepatitis, aplastic anemia (isolated cases), delay in adaptation to the dark, hot flashes, alcohol intolerance, alopecia.

ADULT – Prostate cancer: 300 mg PO daily for 30 days, then 150 mg PO daily. Begin therapy on same day as surgical castration.

PEDS – Not approved in children.

FORMS – Trade only: Tabs 150 mg.

NOTES – Monitor CBCs, LFTs, and chest X-rays. Caution patients who experience delayed adaptation to the dark about driving at night or through tunnels; suggest wearing tinted glasses. May increase phenytoin and theophylline levels. Avoid alcohol.

TOREMIFENE (***Fareston***) ▶L ♀D ▶– $ varies by therapy

WARNING – QT prolongation that is dose and concentration dependent. Use is contraindicated in the presence of uncorrected hypokalemia or hypomagnesemia. Hypercalcemia and tumor flare, endometrial hyperplasia, thromboembolism, hot flashes, nausea, increased LFTs, vaginal bleeding, fertility impairment, rare myelosuppression, alopecia.

ADULT – Chemotherapy doses vary by indication. Breast cancer.

PEDS – Not approved in children.

UNAPPROVED ADULT – Treatment of soft tissue sarcoma.

FORMS – Trade only: Tabs 60 mg.

NOTES – Avoid concurrent use with strong CYP3A4 inhibitors and QTc-prolonging agents. Reliable contraception is recommended. Monitor CBCs, calcium levels, and LFTs. May increase effects of anticoagulants.

TRIPTORELIN (***Trelstar Depot***) ▶LK ♀X ▶– $ varies by therapy

WARNING – Transient increases in sex hormones, bone pain, neuropathy, hematuria, urethral/bladder outlet obstruction, spinal cord compression, anaphylaxis, hot flashes, impotence, alopecia.

ADULT – Chemotherapy doses vary by indication. Prostate cancer.

PEDS – Not approved in children.

TRIPTORELIN (***Trelstar***) ▶tissues – ? ♀X ▶–

WARNING – Anaphylactic shock, hypersensitivity, and angioedema have been reported. Tumor Flare: Transient increase in serum testosterone levels can occur within the first few weeks of treatment. This may worsen prostate cancer and result in spinal cord compression and urinary tract obstruction.

ADULT – Palliative treatment of advanced prostate cancer. Administered as a single intramuscular injection: 3.75 mg q 4 weeks. 11.25 mg q 12 weeks. 22.5 mg q 24 weeks.

PEDS – Not indicated in pediatrics.

FORMS – Injectable suspension: 3.75 mg, 11.25 mg, 22.5 mg.

NOTES – $—varies by therapy.

ONCOLOGY: Immunomodulators

ALDESLEUKIN (***Proleukin*, interleukin-2**) ▶K ♀C ▶– $ varies by therapy

WARNING – Capillary leak syndrome, resulting in hypotension and reduced organ perfusion. Exacerbation of autoimmune diseases and symptoms of CNS metastases, impaired neutrophil function, hepato/nephrotoxicity, mental status changes, decreased thyroid function, anemia, thrombocytopenia, fertility impairment, alopecia.

ADULT – Chemotherapy doses vary by indication. Renal-cell carcinoma. Metastatic melanoma.

(cont.)

ALDESLEUKIN (*cont.*)

PEDS – Not approved in children.

UNAPPROVED ADULT – Kaposi's sarcoma. Colorectal cancer. Non-Hodgkin's lymphoma. Acute myeloid leukemia (AML).

NOTES – Monitor CBCs, electrolytes, LFTs, renal function, and chest X-rays. Baseline PFTs. Avoid iodinated contrast media. Antihypertensives potentiate hypotension.

BCG (***Bacillus of Calmette & Guerin, Pacis, TheraCys, Tice BCG,*** ✤ ***Oncotice, Immucyst***) ▶Not metabolized ♀C ▶? $ varies by therapy

WARNING – Hypersensitivity, hematuria, urinary frequency, dysuria, bacterial UTI, flu-like syndrome, alopecia.

ADULT – Chemotherapy doses vary by indication. Carcinoma in situ of the urinary bladder, intravesical.

PEDS – Not approved in children.

NOTES – Bone marrow depressants, immunosuppressants, and antimicrobial therapy may impair response. Increase fluid intake after treatments.

DENILEUKIN (***Ontak***) ▶Plasma ♀C ▶– $ varies by therapy

WARNING – Hypersensitivity, vascular leak syndrome (hypotension, edema, hypoalbuminemia), visual loss, thrombosis, rash, diarrhea, alopecia.

ADULT – Chemotherapy doses vary by indication. Cutaneous T-cell lymphoma.

PEDS – Not approved in children.

UNAPPROVED ADULT – Mycosis fungoides, Sezary syndrome. Second-line treatment for peripheral T-cell lymphoma.

NOTES – Monitor CBCs, LFTs, and renal function. Visual loss is usually persistent.

EVEROLIMUS (***Afinitor***) ▶L ♀D ▶– $ varies by therapy

WARNING – Noninfectious pneumonitis, hyperglycemia, bone marrow suppression. Avoid live vaccines.

ADULT – Chemotherapy doses vary by indication. Advanced renal cell carcinoma. Progressive neuroendocrine tumors of pancreatic origin (PNET) in patients with unresectable, locally advanced, or metastatic disease. Subependymal giant cell astrocytoma (SEGA) associated with tuberous sclerosis. Advanced breast cancer in postmenopausal women. Renal angiomyolipoma associated with tuberous sclerosis comples (TSC), who do not require immediate surgery.

PEDS – Not approved in children.

UNAPPROVED ADULT – Treatment of relapsed or refractory Waldenstrom's macroglobulinemia (WM).

NOTES – Reliable contraception is recommended. Drugs that induce the CYP3A4 system such as phenytoin, phenobarbital, rifampin may decrease concentrations. Inhibitors such as clarithromycin, itraconazole, ketoconazole, and ritonavir may increase concentrations. Avoid live vaccines. Monitor CBC, hepatic and renal function, glucose, and lipid profile. Increased risk of proteinuria when used in combination with cyclosporine.

INTERFERON ALFA-2A (***Roferon-A***) ▶Plasma ♀C ▶– $ varies by therapy

WARNING – GI hemorrhage, CNS reactions, leukopenia, increased LFTs, anemia, neutralizing antibodies, depression/suicidal behavior, alopecia.

ADULT – Discontinued by manufacturer February 2008. Chemotherapy doses vary by indication. Hairy cell leukemia. AIDS-related Kaposi's sarcoma. CML.

PEDS – Not approved in children.

UNAPPROVED ADULT – Superficial bladder tumors. Carcinoid tumor. Cutaneous T-cell lymphoma. Essential thrombocythemia. Non-Hodgkin's lymphoma.

NOTES – Discontinued by manufacturer February 2008, only included here for completeness. Reliable contraception is recommended. Monitor CBCs and LFTs. Hydration important. Decreases clearance of theophylline.

LENALIDOMIDE (***Revlimid***) ▶K ♀X ▶– $ varies by therapy

WARNING – Potential for human birth defects, potential for an increased risk of developing secondary malignancies, bone marrow suppression, DVT, and PE. Instruct patients to report promptly fever, sore throat, signs of local infection, bleeding from any site, or symptoms suggestive of anemia.

ADULT – Chemotherapy doses vary by indication. Myelodysplastic syndromes in patients with deletion 5q and transfusion-dependent anemia (with or without cytogenetic abnormalities). Multiple myeloma in combination with dexamethasone in patients who have received at least one prior therapy.

PEDS – Not approved in children.

FORMS – Trade only: Caps 5, 10, 15, 25 mg.

NOTES – Analog of thalidomide; can cause birth defects or fetal death. Lenalidomide, a thalidomide analogue, caused limb abnormalities in a developmental monkey study similar to birth defects caused by thalidomide in humans. If lenalidomide is used during pregnancy, it may cause birth defects or death to a developing baby. Pregnancy must be excluded before start of treatment. Prevent pregnancy during treatment by the use of two reliable methods of contraception. Available only through a restricted distribution program.

(cont.)

LENALIDOMIDE (*cont.*)

Reliable contraception is mandated; males must use a latex condom. Monitor CBCs. Do not break, chew, or open the caps. Adjust dose for CrCl less than 60 mL/min.

PEGINTERFERON ALFA-2B (*Sylatron*) ▶K – ♀C ▶?

WARNING – May cause or aggravate severe depression. Suicide or suicidal ideation.

ADULT – Sylatron brand indicated for adjuvant treatment of melanoma. 6 mcg/kg/week SC for 8 doses, followed by 3 mg/kg/week up to 5 years.

PEDS – No approved oncology indication in pediatrics.

FORMS – Powder for injection.

SIPULEUCEL-T (*Provenge*) ▶? –

WARNING – Acute infusion reactions may occur within 1 day of infusion. Cerebrovascular events, including hemorrhagic and ischemic strokes, were observed in clinical trials.

ADULT – Treatment of metastatic hormone-refractory prostate cancer in patients who are symptomatic or minimally symptomatic. Administer a total of 3 doses at 2-week intervals.

PEDS – Not approved in children.

FORMS – Infusion, premixed in preservative-free LR. Greater than 50 million autologous CD54+ cells activated with PAP-GM-CSF (250 mL).

NOTES – No pregnancy or lactation data. Not indicated for use in women. Premedication with oral acetaminophen and diphenhydramine is recommended to minimize infusion reactions.

TEMSIROLIMUS (*Torisel*) ▶L ♀C ▶– $ varies by therapy

WARNING – Hypersensitivity, interstitial lung disease, bowel perforation, renal failure, hyperglycemia, bone marrow suppression. Avoid live vaccines.

ADULT – Chemotherapy doses vary by indication. Advanced renal cell carcinoma.

PEDS – Not approved in children.

UNAPPROVED ADULT – Relapsed or refractory mantle cell lymphoma.

NOTES – Reliable contraception is recommended. Drugs that induce the CYP3A4 system such as phenytoin, phenobarbital, rifampin may decrease concentrations. Inhibitors such as clarithromycin, itraconazole, ketoconazole, and ritonavir may increase concentrations. Avoid live vaccines. Monitor CBC, hepatic and renal function, glucose and lipid profile. Premedicate with an H1 antagonist 30 min prior to infusion to prevent infusion reactions, edema, pain, rash, mucositis, myelosuppression, weakness, hepatic and renal impairment, infection.

THALIDOMIDE (*Thalomid*) ▶Plasma ♀X ▶? $$$$$

WARNING – Pregnancy category X. Has caused severe, life-threatening human birth defects. Available only through special restricted distribution program. Prescribers and pharmacists must be registered in this program in order to prescribe or dispense. During therapy with thalidomide, patients with a history of seizures or with other risk factors for the development of seizures should be monitored closely for clinical changes that could precipitate acute seizure activity.

ADULT – Chemotherapy doses vary by indication. Multiple myeloma with dexamethasone. Erythema nodosum leprosum: 100 to 400 mg PO at bedtime. Use low end of dose range for initial episodes and if wt less than 50 kg.

PEDS – Not approved in children.

UNAPPROVED ADULT – Graft-vs-host reactions after bone marrow transplant, Crohn's disease, Waldenstrom's macroglobinemia. Langerhans cell histiocytosis, AIDs–related aphthous stomatitis.

UNAPPROVED PEDS – Clinical trials show beneficial effects when combined with dexamethasone in multiple myeloma.

FORMS – Trade only: Caps 50, 100, 150, 200 mg.

ONCOLOGY: Miscellaneous

ARSENIC TRIOXIDE (*Trisenox*) ▶L ♀D ▶– $ varies by therapy

WARNING – APL differentiation syndrome: Fever, dyspnea, wt gain, pulmonary infiltrates and pleural/pericardial effusions, occasionally with impaired myocardial contractility and episodic hypotension, with or without leukocytosis. QT prolongation, AV block, torsades de pointes, N/V/D, hyperglycemia, alopecia.

ADULT – Chemotherapy doses vary by indication. Acute promyelocytic leukemia, refractory.

PEDS – Not approved in children younger than 5 yo. Chemotherapy doses vary by indication. Acute promyelocytic leukemia, refractory.

UNAPPROVED ADULT – Chemotherapy doses vary by indication. Chronic myeloid leukemia. ALL.

NOTES – Reliable contraception is recommended. Monitor ECG, electrolytes, renal function, CBCs, and PT.

ASPARAGINASE (*Elspar*, ♣ *Kidrolase*) ▶? ♀C ◗– $ varies by therapy

WARNING – Contraindicated with previous/current pancreatitis. Anaphylaxis, bone marrow suppression, bleeding, hyperglycemia, pancreatitis, hepato/nephrotoxicity, alopecia. Instruct patients to report promptly fever, sore throat, signs of local infection, bleeding from any site, or symptoms suggestive of anemia.

ADULT – Chemotherapy doses vary by indication. ALL, in combination regimens.

PEDS – Chemotherapy doses vary by indication. ALL, in combination regimens.

NOTES – Toxicity greater in children. Monitor CBCs, LFTs, renal function, PT, glucose, and amylase. May interfere with interpretation of thyroid function tests.

ASPARAGINASE ERWINIA CHRYSANTHEMI (*Erwinaze*, ♣ *Erwinase*) ▶? – ♀C ◗?

ADULT – A component of a multi-agent chemotherapeutic regimen for the treatment of patients with acute lymphoblastic leukemia (ALL) who have developed hypersensitivity to *E. coli*–derived asparaginase.

PEDS – Approved in adults and children with ALL.

FORMS – Powder for injection.

BEXAROTENE (*Targretin*) ▶L ♀X ◗– $ varies by therapy

WARNING – Gel: Rash, pruritus, contact dermatitis. Caps: Lipid abnormalities, increased LFTs, pancreatitis, hypothyroidism, leukopenia, cataracts, photosensitivity, alopecia.

ADULT – Chemotherapy doses vary by indication. Cutaneous T-cell lymphoma.

PEDS – Not approved in children.

FORMS – Trade only: 1% gel (60 g). Caps 75 mg.

NOTES – Gel: Do not use with DEET (insect repellant) or occlusive dressings. Caps: Monitor lipids, LFTs, thyroid function tests, CBCs. Multiple drug interactions; consult product insert for info. Reliable contraception is recommended.

BORTEZOMIB (*Velcade*) ▶L ♀D ◗– $ varies by therapy

WARNING – Peripheral neuropathy, orthostatic hypotension, heart failure, pneumonia, acute respiratory distress syndrome, thrombocytopenia, neutropenia, N/V/D. Instruct patients to report promptly acute onset of dyspnea, cough and low-grade fever, and bleeding from any site. Acute liver failure has been reported rarely. Use with caution in patients with hepatic dysfunction.

ADULT – Chemotherapy doses vary by indication. Multiple myeloma, mantle cell lymphoma. In the United States may given IV or SC.

PEDS – Not approved in children.

UNAPPROVED ADULT – Waldenstrom's macroglobulinemia, peripheral T-cell lymphoma, cutaneous T-cell lymphoma, systemic light chain amyloidosis.

FORMS – Single use 3.5 mg vials.

NOTES – Reliable contraception is recommended. Monitor CBCs.

LEUCOVORIN (*Wellcovorin*, **folinic acid**) ▶gut ♀C ◗? $ varies by therapy

WARNING – Allergic sensitization.

ADULT – Doses vary by indication. Reduction of toxicity due to folic acid antagonists (ie, methotrexate). Colorectal cancer with 5-FU. Megaloblastic anemias.

PEDS – Not approved in children.

FORMS – Generic only: Tabs 5, 10, 15, 25 mg. Injection for hospital/oncology clinic use; not intended for outpatient prescribing.

NOTES – Monitor methotrexate concentrations and CBCs.

LEVOLEUCOVORIN (*Fusilev*) ▶gut ♀C ◗? $ varies by therapy

WARNING – Allergic sensitization.

ADULT – Doses vary by indication. Reduction of toxicity due to high-dose methotrexate for osteosarcoma. Indicated for use in combination chemotherapy with 5-fluorouracil in the palliative treatment of patients with advanced metastatic colorectal cancer. Antidote for impaired methotrexate elimination and for inadvertent overdosage of folic acid antagonists.

PEDS – Not approved in children.

FORMS – 50 mg powder for injection.

NOTES – Monitor methotrexate concentrations and CBCs.

MITOTANE (*Lysodren*) ▶L ♀C ◗– $ varies by therapy

WARNING – Adrenal insufficiency, depression. Instruct patients to report promptly if N/V, loss of appetite, diarrhea, mental depression, skin rash or darkening of the skin occurs. N/V/D, alopecia.

ADULT – Chemotherapy doses vary by indication. Adrenal cortical carcinoma, inoperable.

PEDS – Not approved in children.

FORMS – Trade only: Tabs 500 mg.

NOTES – Hold after shock or trauma; give systemic steroids. Behavioral and neurological assessments at regular intervals when continuous treatment more than 2 years. May decrease steroid and warfarin effects. Reliable contraception is recommended.

PEGASPARGASE (*Oncaspar*) ▶? ♀C ▶– $ varies by therapy

WARNING – Contraindicated with previous/current pancreatitis. Hypersensitivity, including anaphylaxis. Bone marrow suppression, bleeding, hyperuricemia, hyperglycemia, hepato/nephrotoxicity, CNS toxicity, N/V/D, alopecia.

ADULT – Chemotherapy doses vary by indication. ALL, in combination regimens.

PEDS – Chemotherapy doses vary by indication. ALL, in combination regimens.

NOTES – Monitor CBCs, LFTs, renal function, amylase, glucose, and PT. Bleeding potentiated with warfarin, heparin, dipyridamole, aspiri, or NSAIDs.

PORFIMER (*Photofrin*) ▶? ♀C ▶– $ varies by therapy

WARNING – Photosensitivity, ocular sensitivity, chest pain, respiratory distress, constipation.

ADULT – Chemotherapy doses vary by indication. Esophageal cancer. Endobronchial non-small cell lung cancer. High-grade dysplasia in Barrett's esophagus. (All with laser therapy.)

PEDS – Not approved in children.

NOTES – Avoid concurrent photosensitizing drugs.

RASBURICASE (*Elitek*, ✤ *Fasturtec*) ▶L ♀C ▶– $$$$$

WARNING – May cause hypersensitivity reactions including anaphylaxis, hemolysis (G6PD-deficient patients), methemoglobinemia, interference with uric acid measurements.

ADULT – Uric acid elevation prevention with leukemia, lymphoma, and solid tumor malignancies receiving anticancer therapy: 0.2 mg/kg IV over 30 min daily for up to 5 days.

PEDS – Uric acid elevation prevention in children (1 mo to 17 yo) with leukemia, lymphoma, and solid tumor malignancies receiving anticancer therapy: 0.2 mg/kg IV over 30 min daily for up to 5 days.

NOTES – Safety and efficacy have been established only for one 5-day treatment course. Hydrate IV if at risk for tumor lysis syndrome. Screen for G6PD deficiency in high-risk patients.

ROMIDEPSIN (*Istodax*) ▶L – ♀D ▶–

WARNING – QTc prolongation/ECG changes have been observed. High potential for drug interactions. Pancytopenias.

ADULT – 14 mg/m^2 IV days 1, 8, and 15 of a 28-day cycle. Treatment of cutaneous T-cell lymphoma in patients who have received at least one prior systemic therapy. Refractory peripheral T-cell lymphoma.

PEDS – Not approved in children.

FORMS – 10 mg powder for reconstitution.

TRETINOIN—ONCOLOGY (*Vesanoid*) ▶L ♀D ▶– $ varies by therapy

WARNING – Retinoic acid-APL (RA-APL) syndrome: Fever, dyspnea, wt gain, pulmonary edema, pulmonary infiltrates and pleural/pericardial effusions, occasionally with impaired myocardial contractility and episodic hypotension, with or without leukocytosis. Reversible hypercholesterolemia/hypertriglyceridemia, increased LFTs, alopecia. Contraindicated in paraben-sensitive patients.

ADULT – Chemotherapy doses vary by indication. Acute promyelocytic leukemia.

PEDS – Not approved in children.

UNAPPROVED PEDS – Acute promyelocytic leukemia. Limited data.

FORMS – Generic/Trade: Caps 10 mg.

NOTES – Reliable contraception is recommended. Monitor CBCs, coagulants, LFTs, triglycerides, and cholesterol levels. Ketoconazole increases levels.

VISMODEGIB (*Erivedge*) ▶oxidation – glucuronidation ♀D ▶–

WARNING – Vismodegib has been approved with a boxed warning stating that use of this drug can result in embryo-fetal death or severe birth defects. Pregnancy status must be verified prior to initiation of treatment, and both male and female patients need to be advised of these risks. Women need to be advised of the need for contraception and men of the potential risk for vismodegib exposure through semen.

ADULT – 150 mg orally once daily for basal cell carcinoma (BCC) that has metastasized or relapsed after treatment with surgery, or for patients who are not candidates for surgery or radiation.

PEDS – Not approved in children.

FORMS – 150 mg caps.

VORINOSTAT (*Zolinza*) ▶L ♀D ▶– $$$$$

WARNING – PE/DVT, anemia, thrombocytopenia, QT prolongation.

ADULT – Chemotherapy doses vary by indication. Cutaneous T-cell lymphoma.

PEDS – Not approved in children.

FORMS – Trade only: Caps 100 mg.

NOTES – Reliable contraception is recommended. Monitor CBCs, electrolytes, renal function, EKG.

ONCOLOGY: Mitotic Inhibitors

CABAZITAXEL (*Jevtana*) ▶L – ♀D ▶–

WARNING – Neutropenia, febrile neutropenia: Neutropenic deaths have been reported. Severe hypersensitivity reactions can occur. Mortality related to diarrhea has been reported. Renal failure, including cases with fatal outcomes, has been reported. Patients older than 65 yo were more likely to experience fatal outcomes not related to disease. Should not be given to patients with hepatic impairment.

ADULT – Indicated in combination with prednisone for treatment of patients with hormone-refractory metastatic prostate cancer previously treated with a docetaxel-containing treatment regimen. 25 mg/m² administered IV q 3 weeks in combination with oral prednisone 10 mg administered daily throughout treatment.

PEDS – Not indicated in pediatrics.

FORMS – Single use vial 60 mg/1.5 mL, supplied with diluent (5.7 mL).

NOTES – Premedication regimen required 30 minutes before each dose: Antihistamine, corticosteroid (dexamethasone 8 mg or equivalent steroid), and H2 antagonist.

DOCETAXEL (*Taxotere*) ▶L ♀D ▶– $ varies by therapy

WARNING – Severe hypersensitivity with anaphylaxis, bone marrow suppression, fluid retention, neutropenia, rash, erythema of the extremities, nail hypo- or hyperpigmentation, hepatotoxicity, treatment-related mortality, paresthesia/dysesthesia, asthenia, fertility impairment, alopecia. Instruct patients to report promptly fever, sore throat, or signs of local infection.

ADULT – Chemotherapy doses vary by indication. Breast cancer. Non-small cell lung cancer. Hormone-refractory, metastatic prostate cancer. Advanced gastric adenocarcinoma with cisplatin and fluorouracil. Squamous cell carcinoma of the head and neck.

PEDS – Not approved in children.

UNAPPROVED ADULT – Gastric cancer. Melanoma. Non-Hodgkin's lymphoma. Ovarian cancer. Pancreatic cancer. Prostate cancer. Small-cell lung cancer. Soft-tissue sarcoma. Urothelial cancer. Adjuvant and neoadjuvant breast cancer.

NOTES – Reliable contraception is recommended. Monitor CBCs and LFTs. CYP3A4 inhibitors or substrates may lead to significant increases in blood concentrations.

ERIBULIN (*Halaven*) ▶feces – ♀D ▶–

WARNING – Dose reduction may be required in patients with hepatic impairment or renal impairment.

ADULT – Metastatic breast cancer in patients who have previously received at least two chemotherapeutic regimens for the treatment of metastatic disease. Prior therapy should have included an anthracycline and a taxane in either the adjuvant or metastatic setting.

PEDS – Not approved in children.

FORMS – IV only.

NOTES – Dose is 1.4 mg/m² on days 1 and 8 q 21 days.

IXABEPILONE (*Ixempra*) ▶L ♀D ▶– $ varies by therapy

WARNING – Contraindicated in patients with AST or ALT greater than 2.5 ULN or bilirubin more than 1 times ULN upper limit of normal or higher. Contraindicated in patients with hypersensitivity reactions to products containing Cremophor EL (polyoxyethylated castor oil). Neutropenia. Instruct patients to report promptly fever, sore throat, signs of local infection, or anemia. Peripheral neuropathy (sensory and motor) occurs commonly. Dose reductions, delays, or discontinuations may be necessary. Usually occurs during the first 3 cycles of treatment.

ADULT – Chemotherapy doses vary by indication. Metastatic or locally advanced breast cancer.

PEDS – Not approved in children.

FORMS – 15 mg and 45 mg powder for injection.

NOTES – CYP450 inhibitors such as ketoconazole may increase concentration; inducers such as rifampin, phenytoin, or carbamazepine may reduce levels Patients should receive an H1 and H2 blocker 1 hour prior to ixabepilone infusion to minimize hypersensitivity reactions. If patients experience such a reaction, they should also receive a corticosteroid prior to the next dose.

PACLITAXEL (*Taxol, Abraxane, Onxol*) ▶L ♀D ▶– $ varies by therapy

WARNING – Anaphylaxis, bone marrow suppression, cardiac conduction abnormalities, peripheral neuropathy, fertility impairment, alopecia. Contraindicated in patients with hypersensitivity reactions to products containing Cremophor EL (polyoxyethylated castor oil). Instruct patients to report promptly fever, sore throat, signs of local infection or anemia.

(cont.)

PACLITAXEL (*cont.*)

ADULT – Chemotherapy doses vary by indication. Ovarian cancer. Metastatic breast cancer. Non-small cell lung cancer, in combination regimens. AIDS-related Kaposi's sarcoma.

PEDS – Not approved in children.

UNAPPROVED ADULT – Advanced head and neck cancer. Small-cell lung cancer. Adenocarcinoma of the upper GI tract. Gastric, esophageal, and colon adenocarcinoma. Hormone-refractory prostate cancer. Non-Hodgkin's lymphoma. Transitional cell carcinoma of the urothelium. Adenocarcinoma or unknown primary, adjuvant, and neoadjuvant breast cancer, uterine cancer. Pancreatic cancer. Polycystic kidney disease.

NOTES – Abraxane is a form of paclitaxel bound to albumin. Reliable contraception is recommended. Monitor CBCs. Ketoconazole, felodipine, diazepam, and estradiol may increase paclitaxel.

VINBLASTINE (*Velban, VLB*) ▶L ♀D ▶– $ varies by therapy

WARNING – Extravasation associated with severe necrosis. Leukopenia, fertility impairment, bronchospasm, alopecia. Instruct patients to report promptly fever, sore throat, or signs of local infection.

ADULT – Chemotherapy doses vary by indication. Hodgkin's disease. Non-Hodgkin's lymphoma. Histiocytic lymphoma. Mycosis fungoides. Advanced testicular carcinoma. Kaposi's sarcoma. Letterer-Siwe disease (histiocytosis X). Choriocarcinoma. Breast cancer.

PEDS – Not approved in children.

UNAPPROVED ADULT – Non-small cell lung cancer, renal cancer, CML.

NOTES – Reliable contraception is recommended. May decrease phenytoin levels. Erythromycin/drugs that inhibit CYP450 enzymes may increase toxicity.

VINCRISTINE (*Oncovin, Vincasar, VCR*) ▶L ♀D ▶– $ varies by therapy

WARNING – Extravasation associated with severe necrosis. CNS toxicity, hypersensitivity, bone marrow suppression, hyperuricemia, bronchospasm, fertility impairment, alopecia. Instruct patients to report promptly fever, sore throat, signs of local infection, or anemia.

ADULT – Chemotherapy doses vary by indication. ALL. Hodgkin's disease. Non-Hodgkin's lymphomas. Rhabdomyosarcoma. Neuroblastoma. Wilms' tumor. All in combination regimens.

PEDS – Chemotherapy doses vary by indication. Acute leukemia. Sarcoma, multiple myeloma.

UNAPPROVED ADULT – Idiopathic thrombocytopenic purpura. Kaposi's sarcoma. Breast cancer. Bladder cancer.

NOTES – Reliable contraception is recommended. Monitor CBCs. May decrease phenytoin and digoxin levels.

VINORELBINE (*Navelbine*) ▶L ♀D ▶– $ varies by therapy

WARNING – Extravasation associated with severe necrosis. Granulocytopenia, pulmonary toxicity, bronchospasm, peripheral neuropathy, increased LFTs, alopecia. Instruct patients to report promptly fever, sore throat, or signs of local infection.

ADULT – Chemotherapy doses vary by indication. Non-small cell lung cancer, alone or in combination regimens.

PEDS – Not approved in children.

UNAPPROVED ADULT – Breast cancer. Cervical carcinoma. Desmoid tumors. Kaposi's sarcoma. Ovarian, Hodgkin's disease, head and neck cancer.

NOTES – Reliable contraception is recommended. Monitor CBCs. Drugs that inhibit CYP450 enzymes may increase toxicity.

ONCOLOGY: Monoclonal Antibodies

ALEMTUZUMAB (*Campath,* ♣*MabCampath*) ▶? ♀C ▶– $ varies by therapy

WARNING – Idiopathic thrombocytopenic purpura, bone marrow suppression, hemolytic anemia, hypersensitivity, and immunosuppression.

ADULT – Chemotherapy doses vary by indication. B-cell chronic lymphocytic leukemia.

PEDS – Not approved in children.

NOTES – Monitor CBC.

BEVACIZUMAB (*Avastin*) ▶? ♀C ▶– $ varies by therapy

WARNING – CVA, MI, TIA, angina, GI perforation, wound dehiscence, serious hemorrhage, HTN, heart failure, nephrotic syndrome, reversible posterior leukoencephalopathy syndrome (brain capillary leak syndrome), nasal septum perforation. Tracheoesophageal fistula has been reported. Microangiopathic hemolytic anemia (MAHA) in patients on concomitant sunitinib malate. Females of reproductive potential should be informed of increased reproductive failure. Increased risk of venous thromboembolic (VTE) and bleeding events in patients receiving anticoagulation therapy after first VTE event while receiving bevacizumab.

(cont.)

BEVACIZUMAB (*cont.*)

ADULT – Chemotherapy doses vary by indication. Metastatic colorectal carcinoma; unresectable, locally advanced, recurrent, or metastatic nonsquamous, non-small cell lung cancer; glioblastoma; metastatic renal cell cancer.

PEDS – Not approved in children.

UNAPPROVED ADULT – Metastatic breast cancer, recurrent ovarian cancer, recurrent cervical cancer, soft tissue sarcomas, age-related macular degeneration.

NOTES – Monitor BP and UA for protein. Do not use in combination with sunitinib.

BRENTUXIMAB VEDOTIN (***Adcetris***) ▶oxidation – feces ♀D ▶–

WARNING – Peripheral motor neuropathy, infusion reactions, including anaphylaxis, (premedication is required), progressive multifocal leukoencephalopathy. Use of brentuximab is contraindicated with bleomycin due to increased risk for pulmonary toxicity.

ADULT – Treatment of Hodgkin's lymphoma after failure of at least 2 prior chemotherapy regimens (in patient ineligible for transplant) or after stem cell transplant failure. Systemic anaplastic large cell lymphoma (sALCL) after failure of at least one prior chemotherapy regimen.

PEDS – Not approved in children.

FORMS – 50 mg powder for injection.

CETUXIMAB (***Erbitux***) ▶? ♀C ▶– $ varies by therapy

WARNING – Anaphylaxis, cardiopulmonary arrest/sudden death, pulmonary toxicity, rash, sepsis, renal failure, pulmonary embolus, hypomagnesemia.

ADULT – Chemotherapy doses vary by indication. Metastatic colorectal carcinoma, head and neck squamous cell carcinoma. In combination with platinum-based therapy plus 5-florouracil (5-FU) for the first-line treatment of patients with recurrent locoregional disease and/or metastatic squamous cell carcinoma of the head and neck (SCCHN). Use in combination with FOLFIRI (irinotecan, 5-fluorouracil, leucovorin) for first-line treatment of patients with K-ras mutation-negative (wild-type), EGFR-expressing metastatic colorectal cancer (mCRC).

PEDS – Not approved in children. Safety and effectiveness in children not established. No new safety signals identified in pediatric patients after pharmacokinetic evaluation.

UNAPPROVED ADULT – EGFR-expressing advanced non-small cell lung cancer.

NOTES – Monitor renal function and electrolytes including magnesium. Caution with known CAD, heart failure, or arrhythmias. Premedication with an H1 antagonist and a 1-h observation period after infusion is recommended due to potential for anaphylaxis. Use is not recommended in patients with codon 12 or 13 KRAS mutations.

IBRITUMOMAB (***Zevalin***) ▶L ♀D ▶– $ varies by therapy

WARNING – Contraindicated in patients with allergy to murine proteins. Hypersensitivity. Serious infusion reactions, some fatal, may occur within 24 h of rituximab infusion. Prolonged and severe cytopenias occur in most patients. Severe cutaneous and mucocutaneous reactions, some fatal, reported with Zevalin therapeutic regimen. Do not exceed 32 mCi (1184 MBq) of Y-90 Zevalin.

ADULT – Chemotherapy doses vary by indication. Non-Hodgkin's lymphoma.

PEDS – Not approved in children.

NOTES – Reliable contraception is recommended. Monitor CBCs.

IPILIMUMAB (***Yervoy***) ▶endogenous – ♀C ▶–

WARNING – Severe and fatal immune-mediated adverse reactions due to T-cell activation and proliferation. Interacts with Vitamin K antagonists and cardiac glycosides.

ADULT – Unresectable or metastatic melanoma. 3 mg/kg q 3 weeks for 4 doses.

PEDS – Not approved in children.

FORMS – IV.

NOTES – Scheduled doses will need to be withheld for moderate immune-mediated reactions and symptomatic endocrine disorders. Permanently discontinue drug if cannot complete treatment course within 16 weeks of initial dose.

OFATUMUMAB (***Arzerra***) ▶immune system – ♀C ▶?

WARNING – May cause cause serious infusion reactions. Premedicate with acetaminophen, an antihistamine, and a corticosteroid. May cause prolonged cytopenias. Progressive multifocal leukoencephalopathy (PML) can occur. Hepatitis B reactivation may occur. Intestinal obstruction may occur.

ADULT – 300 mg IV initial dose (dose 1), followed 1 week later by 2000 mg IV weekly for 7 doses (doses 2 through 8), followed 4 weeks later by 2000 mg IV q 4 weeks for 4 doses (doses 9 through 12). Treatment of patients with chronic lymphocytic leukemia (CLL) refractory to fludarabine and alemtuzumab.

PEDS – Not approved in children.

(cont.)

OFATUMUMAB (*cont.*)

NOTES – Premedicate 30 min to 2 h prior to ofatumumab infusion with acetaminopen, antihistamine, and corticosteroid. See product labeling for dose reduction guidelines of corticosteroids.

PANITUMUMAB (***Vectibix***) ▶Not metabolized ♀C ◗– $ varies by therapy

WARNING – Skin exfoliation, severe dermatologic reactions complicated by sepsis and death. Anaphylaxis.

ADULT – Chemotherapy doses vary by indication. Metastatic colorectal carcinoma.

PEDS – Not approved in children.

NOTES – Reliable contraception is recommended. Monitor potassium and magnesium.

PERTUZUMAB (***Perjeta***) ▶? – ♀D ◗–

WARNING – BOXED WARNING regarding embryo-fetal toxicity and birth defects.

ADULT – Use in combination with trastuzumab and docetaxel for the treatment of patients with HER2-positive metastatic breast cancer who have not received prior anti-HER2 therapy or chemotherapy for metastatic disease. Initial dose, 840 mg IV, followed by 420 mg q 3 weeks thereafter.

PEDS – Not approved in children.

FORMS – 420 mg/14 mL single-use vial.

RITUXIMAB (***Rituxan***) ▶Not metabolized ♀C ◗– $ varies by therapy

WARNING – Contraindicated if allergy to murine proteins. Fatal infusion reactions, tumor lysis syndrome, severe mucocutaneous reactions, cardiac arrhythmias, nephrotoxicity, bowel obstruction/perforation, hypersensitivity, neutropenia, thrombocytopenia, anemia, serious viral infections with death. Hepatitis B virus (HBV) reactivation with fulminant hepatitis, hepatic failure, and death can occur in patients treated with Rituxan. The median time to the diagnosis of hepatitis among patients with hematologic malignancies was approximately 4 months after the initiation of Rituxan and approximately 1 month after the last dose. Screen patients at high risk of HBV infection before initiation of Rituxan. Closely monitor carriers of hepatitis B for clinical and laboratory signs of active HBV infection for several months following Rituxan therapy. Discontinue Rituxan and any concomitant chemotherapy in patients who develop viral hepatitis, and institute appropriate treatment, including antiviral therapy. Insufficient data exist regarding the safety of resuming Rituxan in patients who develop hepatitis subsequent to HBV reactivation. Cases of fatal progressive multifocal leukoencephalopathy have been reported.

ADULT – RA: 1000 mg IV infusion weekly for 2 doses in combination with methotrexate and methylprednisolone 100 mg IV pretreatment. Chemotherapy doses vary by indication. Non-Hodgkin's lymphoma. Rheumatoid arthritis with methotrexate. Treatment of patients previously treated for CD20-positive chronic lymphocytic leukemia (CLL) in combination with fludarabine and cyclophosphamide (FC). Wegener's granulomatosis (with glucocorticoids), Microscopic polyangiitis (with glucocorticoids).

PEDS – Not approved in children.

UNAPPROVED ADULT – Immune thrombocytopenic purpura (ITP), thrombotic thrombocytopenic purpura (TTP), multiple sclerosis, Hodgkin's lymphoma, treatment of systemic autoimmune diseases other than RA, treatment of steroid-refractory chronic graft-vs-host disease.

UNAPPROVED PEDS – Autoimmune hemolytic anemia in children.

NOTES – Monitor CBCs.

TOSITUMOMAB (***Bexxar***) ▶Not metabolized ♀X ◗– $ varies by therapy

WARNING – Contraindicated in patients with allergy to murine proteins. Hypersensitivity, anaphylaxis, infusion reactions, neutropenia, thrombocytopenia, anemia. Hypothyroidism.

ADULT – Chemotherapy doses vary by indication. Follicular, non-Hodgkin's lymphoma unresponsive to rituximab.

PEDS – Not approved in children.

NOTES – This product is a combination of tositumomab + iodine-131 tositumomab. Reliable contraception is recommended. Monitor CBC, TSH.

TRASTUZUMAB (***Herceptin***) ▶Not metabolized ♀B ◗– $ varies by therapy

WARNING – Hypersensitivity, including fatal anaphylaxis, fatal infusion-related reactions, pulmonary events including ARDS and death, ventricular dysfunction and heart failure. Anemia, leukopenia, diarrhea, alopecia.

ADULT – Chemotherapy doses vary by indication. Breast cancer with tumors overexpressing the HER2/neu protein. HER2-overexpressing metastatic gastric or gastroesophageal junction adenocarcinoma with cisplatin and a fluoropyrimidine.

PEDS – Not approved in children.

NOTES – Monitor with ECG, echocardiogram, or MUGA scan. CBCs.

ONCOLOGY: Platinum-Containing Agents

CARBOPLATIN (*Paraplatin*) ▶K ♀D ▶– $ varies by therapy

WARNING – Secondary malignancies, bone marrow suppression, increased in patients with renal insufficiency; emesis, anaphylaxis, nephrotoxicity, peripheral neuropathy, increased LFTs, alopecia. Instruct patients to report promptly fever, sore throat, signs of local infection, bleeding from any site, symptoms suggestive of anemia, or yellow discoloration of the skin or eyes.

ADULT – Chemotherapy doses vary by indication. Ovarian carcinoma.

PEDS – Not approved in children.

UNAPPROVED ADULT – Small-cell lung cancer, in combination regimens. Squamous cell carcinoma of the head and neck. Advanced endometrial cancer. Acute leukemia. Seminoma of testicular cancer. Non-small cell lung cancer. Adenocarcinoma of unknown primary. Cervical cancer. Bladder carcinoma. Breast cancer. Hodgkin's Lymphoma. Mesiothelioma. Melanoma. Neuroendocrine tumors. Non-Hodgkin's Lymphoma. Prostate cancer. Sarcomas. Small cell lung cancer.

NOTES – Reliable contraception is recommended. Monitor CBCs, LFTs, and renal function. May decrease phenytoin levels.

CISPLATIN (*Platinol-AQ*) ▶K ♀D ▶– $ varies by therapy

WARNING – Secondary malignancies, nephrotoxicity, bone marrow suppression, N/V, very highly emetogenic, ototoxicity, anaphylaxis, hepatotoxicity, vascular toxicity, hyperuricemia, electrolyte disturbances, optic neuritis, papilledema and cerebral blindness, neuropathies, muscle cramps, alopecia. Amifostine can be used to reduce renal toxicity in patients with advanced ovarian cancer. Instruct patients to report promptly fever, sore throat, signs of local infection, bleeding from any site, symptoms suggestive of anemia, or yellow discoloration of the skin or eyes. An increased risk of cisplatin-induced ototoxicity in children has been associated with variants in the thiopurine S-methyltransferase (TPMT) gene.

ADULT – Chemotherapy doses vary by indication. Metastatic testicular and ovarian tumors, bladder cancer.

PEDS – Not approved in children.

UNAPPROVED ADULT – Esophageal cancer, gastric cancer, non-small cell lung cancer and small cell lung cancer, head and neck cancer, endometrial cancer, cervical cancer, neoadjuvant bladder sparing chemotherapy, sarcoma.

NOTES – Reliable contraception is recommended. Monitor CBCs, LFTs, renal function, and electrolytes. Audiometry. Aminoglycosides potentiate renal toxicity. Decreases phenytoin levels. Patients older than 65 yo may be more susceptible to nephrotoxicity, bone marrow suppression, and peripheral neuropathy. Verify any dose of cisplatin exceeding 100 mg/m^2 per course of therapy.

OXALIPLATIN (*ELOXATIN*) ▶LK ♀D ▶– $ varies by therapy

WARNING – Anaphylactic reactions to ELOXATIN have been reported, and may occur within minutes of ELOXATIN administration. Epinephrine, corticosteroids, and antihistamines have been employed to alleviate symptoms. Neuropathy, pulmonary fibrosis, bone marrow suppression, transient vision loss, N/V/D, fertility impairment. Instruct patients to report promptly fever, sore throat, signs of local infection, bleeding from any site, or symptoms suggestive of anemia.

ADULT – Chemotherapy doses vary by indication. Colorectal cancer with 5-FU + leucovorin.

PEDS – Not approved in children.

UNAPPROVED ADULT – Esophageal cancer, gastric cancer, non-Hodgkin's lymphoma, ovarian cancer, testicular cancer, hepatobiliary cancer, pancreatic cancer.

NOTES – Reliable contraception is recommended. Monitor CBCs and renal function.

ONCOLOGY: Radiopharmaceuticals

SAMARIUM 153 (*Quadramet*) ▶Not metabolized ♀C ▶– $ varies by therapy

WARNING – Bone marrow suppression, flare reactions. Instruct patients to report promptly fever, sore throat, signs of local infection, or anemia.

ADULT – Chemotherapy doses vary by indication. Osteoblastic metastatic bone lesions, relief of pain.

PEDS – Not approved in children.

UNAPPROVED ADULT – Ankylosing spondylitis. Paget's disease. RA.

(cont.)

SAMARIUM 153 (*cont.*)

NOTES – Reliable contraception is recommended. Monitor CBCs. Radioactivity in excreted urine for 12 h after dose.

STRONTIUM-89 (***Metastron***) ▶K ♀D ▶– $ varies by therapy

WARNING – Bone marrow suppression, flare reactions, flushing sensation. Instruct patients to report promptly fever, sore throat, signs of local infection, or anemia.

ADULT – Chemotherapy doses vary by indication. Painful skeletal metastases, relief of bone pain.

PEDS – Not approved in children.

NOTES – Reliable contraception is recommended. Monitor CBCs. Radioactivity in excreted urine for 12 h after dose.

ONCOLOGY: Topoisomerase Inhibitors

ETOPOSIDE (***VP-16, Etopophos, Toposar, VePesid***) ▶K ♀D ▶– $ varies by therapy

WARNING – Bone marrow suppression, anaphylaxis, hypotension, CNS depression, alopecia. Instruct patients to report promptly fever, sore throat, or signs of local infection.

ADULT – Chemotherapy doses vary by indication. Testicular cancer. Small cell lung cancer, in combination regimens.

PEDS – Not approved in children.

UNAPPROVED ADULT – AML. Hodgkin's disease. Non-Hodgkin's lymphomas. Kaposi's sarcoma. Neuroblastoma. Choriocarcinoma. Rhabdomyosarcoma. Hepatocellular carcinoma. Epithelial ovarian, non-small and small cell lung, testicular, gastric, endometrial, and breast cancers. ALL. Soft tissue sarcoma.

FORMS – Generic/Trade: Caps 50 mg. Injection for hospital/clinic use; not intended for outpatient prescribing.

NOTES – Reliable contraception is recommended. Monitor CBCs, LFTs, and renal function. May increase INR with warfarin.

IRINOTECAN (***Camptosar***) ▶L ♀D ▶– $ varies by therapy

WARNING – Diarrhea and dehydration (may be life-threatening), bone marrow suppression (worse with radiation), orthostatic hypotension, colitis, hypersensitivity, pancreatitis. Instruct patients to report promptly diarrhea, fever, sore throat, signs of local infection, bleeding from any site, or symptoms suggestive of anemia.

ADULT – Chemotherapy doses vary by indication. Metastatic carcinoma of the colon or rectum, in combination regimens.

PEDS – Not approved in children.

UNAPPROVED ADULT – Non-small cell lung cancer and small cell lung cancer, ovarian and cervical cancer.

NOTES – Enzyme-inducing drugs such as phenytoin, phenobarbital, carbamazepine, rifampin, and St. John's wort decrease concentrations and possibly effectiveness. Ketoconazole is contraindicated during therapy. Atazanavir increases concentrations. Reliable contraception is recommended. Monitor CBCs. May want to withhold diuretics during active N/V. Avoid laxatives. Loperamide/fluids/electrolytes for diarrhea. Consider atropine for cholinergic symptoms during the infusion. Patients who are homozygous for the UGT1A1*28 allele are at increased risk for neutropenia. Dosage reductions may be necessary.

TENIPOSIDE (***Vumon, VM-26***) ▶K ♀D ▶– $ varies by therapy

WARNING – Bone marrow suppression, anaphylaxis, hypotension, CNS depression, alopecia. Instruct patients to report promptly fever, sore throat, or signs of local infection.

ADULT – Not approved in adult patients.

PEDS – Chemotherapy doses vary by indication. ALL, refractory, in combination regimens.

NOTES – Reliable contraception is recommended. Monitor CBCs, LFTs, and renal function.

TOPOTECAN (***Hycamtin***) ▶Plasma ♀D ▶– $ varies by therapy

WARNING – Bone marrow suppression (primary neutropenia), severe bleeding, interstitial lung disease. Instruct patients to report promptly fever, sore throat, signs of local infection, bleeding from any site, or symptoms suggestive of anemia.

ADULT – Chemotherapy doses vary by indication. Ovarian and cervical cancer. Small-cell lung cancer, relapsed.

PEDS – Not approved in children.

FORMS – Trade only: Caps 0.25, 1 mg. 4 mg powder for injection.

NOTES – Reliable contraception is recommended. Monitor CBCs.

ONCOLOGY: Tyrosine Kinase Inhibitors

AXITINIB (*INLYTA*) ▶L – ♀D ▶–

WARNING – Hypertension including hypertensive crisis has been observed. Blood pressure should be well controlled prior to initiating INLYTA. Monitor for hypertension and treat as needed. Arterial and venous thrombotic events have been observed and can be fatal. Hemorrhagic events have been observed and can be fatal.

ADULT – Treatment of patients with advanced renal cell carcinoma (RCC) after failure of one prior systemic therapy. The starting dose of INLYTA is 5 mg twice daily without regard to food.

PEDS – Not approved in children.

FORMS – 1 mg and 5 mg tablets.

CRIZOTINIB (*Xalkori*) ▶L – ♀D ▶–

WARNING – Severe, fatal pneumonitis, elevations in liver enzymes, QT prolongation.

ADULT – Locally advanced or metastatic non-small cell lung cancer in patients who express an abnormal ALK (anaplastic lymphoma kinase) gene.

PEDS – Not approved in children.

FORMS – 200mg and 250mg oral capsules

DASATINIB (*Sprycel*) ▶L ♀D ▶– $ varies by therapy

WARNING – Bone marrow suppression, hemorrhage, prolonged QT interval, pleural effusion, congestive heart failure, and myocardial infarction and left ventricular dysfunction. Dasatinib may increase the risk of a rare but serious condition in which there is abnormally high blood pressure in the arteries of the lungs (pulmonary arterial hypertension [PAH]). Symptoms of PAH may include shortness of breath, fatigue, and swelling of the body (eg, the ankles and legs). In reported cases, patients developed PAH after starting dasatinib, including after more than 1 year of treatment.

ADULT – Chemotherapy doses vary by indication. CML. ALL.

PEDS – Not approved in children.

UNAPPROVED ADULT – Post allogeneic stem cell transplant treatment of CML.

FORMS – Trade only: Tabs 20, 50, 70, 100 mg.

NOTES – Reliable contraception is recommended. Monitor LFTs, CBCs, and wt. Monitor for signs and symptoms of fluid retention. Increased by ketoconazole, erythromycin, itraconazole, clarithromycin, ritonavir, atazanavir, indinavir, nelfinavir, saquinavir, and telithromycin. Decreased by rifampin, phenytoin, carbamazepine, phenobarbital, and dexamethasone. Increases simvastatin. Antacids should be taken at least 2 h pre- or post-dose. Avoid H2 blockers and PPIs.

ERLOTINIB (*Tarceva*) ▶L ♀D ▶– $ varies by therapy

WARNING – Interstitial lung disease, acute renal failure, hepatic failure, GI perforations, exfoliative skin disorders, MI, CVA, microangiopathic hemolytic anemia, corneal perforation. Elevated INR and potential bleeding. Patients taking warfarin or other coumarin-derivative anticoagulants should be monitored regularly for changes in prothrombin time or INR.

ADULT – Chemotherapy doses vary by indication. Non-small cell lung cancer, pancreatic cancer. Monotherapy for the maintenance treatment of patients with locally advanced or metastatic non-small cell lung cancer whose disease has not progressed after four cycles of platinum-based first-line chemotherapy.

PEDS – Not approved in children.

FORMS – Trade only: Tabs 25, 100, 150 mg.

NOTES – Reliable contraception is recommended. Hepato-renal syndrome has been reported; monitor LFTs and SCr. CYP3A4 inhibitors such as ketoconazole increase concentrations. CYP3A4 inducers such as rifampin decrease concentrations. Increases INR in patients on warfarin. Monitor LFTs. Avoid concomitant use of erlotinib with H2 blockers and PPIs.

GEFITINIB (*Iressa*) ▶L ♀D ▶– $ varies by therapy

WARNING – Pulmonary toxicity, corneal erosion, N/V. Instruct patients to report promptly acute onset of dyspnea, cough, and low-grade fever.

ADULT – Chemotherapy doses vary by indication. Non-small cell lung cancer.

PEDS – Not approved in children.

FORMS – Trade only: Tabs 250 mg.

NOTES – Reliable contraception is recommended. Monitor LFTs. Potent inducers of CYP3A4 (eg, rifampin, phenytoin) decrease concentration; use 500 mg. May increase warfarin effect; monitor INR. Potent inhibitors of CYP3A4 (eg, ketoconazole, itraconazole) increase toxicity. Ranitidine increases concentrations.

IMATINIB (*Gleevec*) ▶L ♀D ▶– $ varies by therapy

WARNING – Cases of fatal tumor lysis syndrome have been reported. Use caution in patients with high tumor burden, or high tumor proliferative rate. Bone marrow suppression, increased LFTs, hemorrhage, erythema multiforme, Stevens-Johnson syndrome, N/V, pulmonary edema, CHF, muscle cramps. May cause growth retardation in children. Use caution when driving a car or operating machinery.

ADULT – Chemotherapy doses vary by indication. CML. GI stromal tumors (GISTs), Ph+ ALL, agressive systemic mastocytosis, dermatofibrosarcoma protuberans, hypereosinophillic syndrome, myelodysplastic/myeloproliferative disease associated with platelet-derived growth factor recptor mutations.

PEDS – Chemotherapy doses vary by indication. CML.

UNAPPROVED ADULT – Treatment of desmoid tumors, post stem cell transplant follow-up treatment in CML.

FORMS – Trade only: Tabs 100, 400 mg.

NOTES – Reliable contraception is recommended. Monitor LFTs, CBCs, and wt. Monitor for signs and symptoms of fluid retention. Increased by ketoconazole, erythromycin, itraconazole, clarithromycin. Decreased by phenytoin, carbamazepine, rifampin, phenobarbital, St. John's wort. Increases acetaminophen levels and warfarin effects. Monitor INR. Reduce dose with renal insufficiency.

LAPATINIB (*Tykerb*) ▶L ♀D ▶– $ varies by therapy

WARNING – Hepatotoxicity has been reported with lapatinib. May be severe or fatal. Decreased LVEF, QT prolongation, hepatotoxicity, interstitial lung disease, pneumonitis, severe diarrhea.

ADULT – Chemotherapy doses vary by indication. Treatment of HER2-overexpressing advanced or metastatic breast cancer in combination with capecitabine, in patients who have received prior therapy including an anthracycline, a taxane, and trastuzumab. Also indicated in combination with letrozole for the treatment of postmenopausal women with hormone receptor–positive metastatic breast cancer that overexpresses the HER2 receptor for whom hormonal therapy is indicated.

PEDS – Not approved in children.

FORMS – Trade only: Tabs 250 mg.

NOTES – Monitor LFTs, CBCs, and wt. Monitor for signs and symptoms of fluid retention. Increased by ketoconazole, erythromycin, itraconazole, clarithromycin. Decreased by phenytoin, carbamazepine, rifampin, phenobarbital, St. John's wort. Increases acetaminophen levels and warfarin effects. Monitor INR. Reduce dose with renal insufficiency. Reliable contraception is recommended. Modify dose for cardiac and other toxicities, severe hepatic impairment, and CYP3A4 drug interactions.

NILOTINIB (*Tasigna*) ▶L ♀D ▶– $ varies by therapy

WARNING – Prolonged QT interval and sudden death, bone marrow suppression, intracranial hemorrhage, pneumonia, elevated lipase. Progressive peripheral arterial occlusive disease. Must be administered on an empty stomach. Food increases bioavailability which may then cause prolonged QTc.

ADULT – Chemotherapy doses vary by indication. Treatment of newly diagnosed adult patients with Philadelphia chromosome–positive chronic myeloid leukemia (Ph+ CML in chronic phase). Treatment of chronic phase (CP) and accelerated phase (AP) Ph+ CML in adult patients resistant to or intolerant to prior therapy that included imatinib.

PEDS – Not approved in children.

FORMS – Trade only: Caps 200 mg.

NOTES – Contraindicated with hypokalemia, hypomagnesemia, or long QT syndrome. Reliable contraception is recommended. Monitor EKG, LFTs, CBCs, and lipase. Serum levels of nilotinib increased by potent CYP450 inhibitors such as ketoconazole and decreased by CYP450 inducers such as rifampin. Avoid food at least 2 h pre-dose or 1 h post-dose. Food effects: Food increases blood levels of nilotinib.

PAZOPANIB (*Votrient*) ▶L + ♀D ▶– $$$$$

WARNING – Severe and fatal hepatotoxicty have occurred. Observe LFTs prior to and during treatment. Prolonged QT intervals and torsades de pointes have been observed. Fatal hemorrhagic events have occurred. Arterial thrombotic events have occurred and can be fatal.

ADULT – 800 mg orally once daily without food. Treatment of advanced renal cell carcinoma. Treatment of advanced soft tissue sarcoma in patients who have received prior chemotherapy.

PEDS – Not indicated in pediatrics.

FORMS – Trade only: Tabs 200 mg.

SORAFENIB (*Nexavar*) ▶L ♀D ▶– $ varies by therapy

WARNING – Increased risk of bleeding, cardiac ischemia/infarction, GI perforation. Sorafenib in combination with carboplatin and paclitaxel is contraindicated in patients with

(cont.)

SORAFENIB (*cont.*)

squamous cell lung cancer. Co-administration of oral neomycin causes a decrease in sorafenib exposure

ADULT – Chemotherapy doses vary by indication. Advanced renal cell carcinoma. Unresectable hepatocellular carcinoma.

PEDS – Not approved in children.

UNAPPROVED ADULT – Advanced thyroid cancer, recurrent or metastatic angiosarcoma, imatinib-resistant GIST.

FORMS – Trade only: Tabs 200 mg.

NOTES – Take 1 h before or 2 h after meals for best absorption. Monitor BP. Monitor INR with warfarin. Reliable contraception is recommended. Hepatic impairment may reduce concentrations. Increases docetaxel and doxorubicin.

SUNITINIB (*Sutent*) ▶L ♀D ▶– $ varies by therapy

WARNING – Hepatotoxicity has been observed in clinical trials and post-marketing experience. This hepatotoxicity may be severe, and deaths have been reported. Prolonged QT intervals and torsades de pointes has been observed. Hemorrhagic events including tumor-related hemorrhage have occurred. Decrease in LVEF with possible clinical CHF, adrenal toxicity, serious and fatal GI complications, bone marrow suppression, bleeding, HTN, yellow skin discoloration, depigmentation of hair or skin, thyroid dysfunction. Cases of tumor lysis syndrome, some fatal, have been observed in clinical trials and have been reported in post-marketing experience, primarily in patients with RCC or GIST treated with sunitinib.

ADULT – Chemotherapy doses vary by indication. GI stromal tumors (GIST), advanced renal cell carcinoma. Treatment of progressive, well differentiated pancreatic neuroendocrine tumors (pNET) in patients with unresectable, locally advanced, or metastatic disease.

PEDS – Not approved in children.

UNAPPROVED ADULT – Treatment of advanced thyroid cancer, treatment of pancreatic neuroendocrine tumors, treatment of non-GIST soft tissue sarcomas.

FORMS – Trade only: Caps 12.5, 25, 50 mg.

NOTES – Reliable contraception is recommended. CYP3A4 inhibitors such as ketoconazole increase concentrations. CYP3A4 inducers such as rifampin and St. John's wort can decrease concentrations. Increases INR in patients on warfarin. Monitor CBC.

RUXOLITINIB (*Jakafi*) ▶L – ♀C ▶–

ADULT – Treatment of intermediate or high-risk myelofibrosis. Doses based on platelet count.

PEDS – Not approved in children.

FORMS – 5 mg, 10 mg, 15 mg, 20 mg, 25 mg tabs.

VANDETANIB (*Caprelsa*) ▶K – ♀? ▶–

WARNING – QT prolongation, torsades de pointes and sudden death.

ADULT – Unresectable locally advanced or metastatic medullary thyroid carcinoma.

PEDS – Not approved in peds.

FORMS – 100 mg and 300 mg oral capsules.

VEMURAFENIB (*Zelboraf*) ▶? – ♀D ▶–

WARNING – Cutaneous squamous cell carcinomas were detected in 24% of patients receiving vemurafenib in clinical trials. Hypersensitivity reactions, uveitis, severe dermatologic reactions, QT prolongation, and liver enzyme abnormalities.

ADULT – Unresectable or metastatic melanoma in patients with the BRAFV600E mutation. Dose is 960 mg orally twice daily.

PEDS – Not approved in pediatric patients children.

FORMS – 240 mg oral tabs.

OPHTHALMOLOGY: Antiallergy—Decongestants & Combinations

NOTE: Overuse can cause rebound dilation of blood vessels. Do not administer while wearing soft contact lenses. Wait 10 min after use before inserting contact lenses. On average, each mL of eye drop soln contains approximately 20 gtts. Reserve ointment formulations for bedtime use due to severe vision blurring. Most eye medications can be administered 1 gtt at a time despite common manufacturer recommendations of 1 to 2 gtts concurrently. Even a single gtt is typically more than the eye can hold, and thus a second gtt is wasteful and increases the possibility of systemic toxicity. If 2 gtts of the medication are desired, separate single gtts by at least 5 min.

NAPHAZOLINE (*Albalon, All Clear, AK-Con, Naphcon, Clear Eyes*) ▶? ♀C ▶? $

ADULT – Ocular vasoconstrictor/decongestant: 1 to 2 gtts four times per day for up to 3 days.

PEDS – Not approved for age younger than 6 yo. Give 1 to 2 gtts four times per day for up to 3 days for age 6 yo or older.

FORMS – OTC Generic/Trade: Soln 0.012, 0.025% (15, 30 mL). Rx Generic/Trade: 0.1% (15 mL).

NOTES – Avoid in patients with cardiovascular disease, HTN, narrow-angle glaucoma.

NAPHCON-A (naphazoline + pheniramine, Visine-A) ▶L ♀C ▶? $
ADULT – Ocular decongestant: 1 gtt four times per day prn for up to 3 days.
PEDS – Not approved for age younger than 6 yo. Use adult dose for age 6 yo or older.
FORMS – OTC Trade only: Soln 0.025% + 0.3% (15 mL).
NOTES – Avoid in patients with cardiovascular disease, HTN, narrow-angle glaucoma, age younger than 6 yo.

VASOCON-A (naphazoline + antazoline) ▶L ♀C ▶? $
ADULT – Ocular decongestant: 1 gtt four times per day prn for up to 3 days.
PEDS – Not approved for children younger than 6 yo. Use adult dose for age 6 yo or older.
FORMS – OTC Trade only: Soln 0.05% + 0.5% (15 mL).
NOTES – Avoid in patients with cardiovascular disease, HTN, narrow-angle glaucoma.

OPHTHALMOLOGY: Antiallergy—Dual Antihistamine & Mast Cell Stabilizer

NOTE: Wait at least 10 to 15 min after use before inserting contact lenses. On average, each mL of eye drop soln contains approximately 20 gtts. Reserve ointment formulations for bedtime use due to severe vision blurring. Most eye medications can be administered 1 gtt at a time despite common manufacturer recommendations of 1 to 2 gtts concurrently. Even a single gtt is typically more than the eye can hold and thus a second gtt is both wasteful and increases the possibility of systemic toxicity. If 2 gtts of the medication are desired, separate single gtts by at least 5 min.

AZELASTINE—OPHTHALMIC (***Optivar***) ▶L ♀C ▶? $$$
ADULT – Allergic conjunctivitis: 1 gtt two times per day.
PEDS – Not approved for age younger than 3 yo. Use adult dose for age 3 yo or older.
FORMS – Trade/generic: Soln 0.05% (6 mL).

EPINASTINE (***Elestat***) ▶K ♀C ▶? $$$$
ADULT – Allergic conjunctivitis: 1 gtt two times per day.
PEDS – Not approved for age younger than 2 yo. Use adult dose for age 2 yo or older.
FORMS – Trade only: Soln 0.05% (5 mL).

KETOTIFEN—OPHTHALMIC (***Alaway, Zaditor***) ▶Minimal absorption ♀C ▶? $
ADULT – Allergic conjunctivitis: 1 gtt in each eye q 8 to 12 h.
PEDS – Allergic conjunctivitis: 1 gtt in each eye q 8 to 12 h age older than 3 yo.
FORMS – OTC Generic/Trade: Soln 0.025% (5 mL, 10 mL).

OLOPATADINE (***Pataday, Patanol***) ▶K ♀C ▶? $$$$
ADULT – Allergic conjunctivitis: 1 gtt of 0.1% soln in each eye two times per day (Patanol) or 1 gtt of 0.2% soln in each eye daily (Pataday).
PEDS – Not approved for age younger than 3 yo. Use adult dose for age 3 yo or older.
FORMS – Trade only: Soln 0.1% (5 mL, Patanol), 0.2% (2.5 mL, Pataday).
NOTES – Do not administer while wearing soft contact lenses. Allow 6 to 8 h between doses.

OPHTHALMOLOGY: Antiallergy—Pure Antihistamines

NOTE: Antihistamines may aggravate dry eye symptoms. Wait 10 min after use before inserting contact lenses. On average, each mL of eye drop soln contains approximately 20 gtts. Reserve ointment formulations for bedtime use due to severe vision blurring. Most eye medications can be administered 1 gtt at a time despite common manufacturer recommendations of 1 to 2 gtts concurrently. Even a single gtt is typically more than the eye can hold and thus a second gtt is both wasteful and increases the possibility of systemic toxicity. If 2 gtts of the medication are desired, separate single gtts by at least 5 min.

ALCAFTADINE (***Lastacaft***) ▶not absorbed – ♀B ▶? $$$
ADULT – Allergic conjunctivitis: 1gtt in each eye daily.
PEDS – 2 years or older: Allergic conjunctivitis: 1gtt in each eye daily.
FORMS – Soln 0.25%, 3 mL.

BEPOTASTINE (***Bepreve***) ▶L (but minimal absorption) – ♀C ▶? $$$
ADULT – Allergic conjunctivitis: 1 gtt two times per day.
PEDS – Not studied in children younger than 2 yo.
FORMS – Trade only: Soln 1.5% (2.5, 5, 10 mL)

(cont.)

BEPOTASTINE (*cont.*)
NOTES – Remove contact lenses prior to instillation.

EMEDASTINE (*Emadine*) ▸L ♀B ▸? $$$
ADULT – Allergic conjunctivitis: 1 gtt daily to four times per day.
PEDS – Not approved for age younger than 3 yo. Use adult dose for age 3 yo or older.
FORMS – Trade only: Soln 0.05% (5 mL).

LEVOCABASTINE—OPHTHALMIC (*Livostin*) ▸Minimal absorption ♀C ▸? $$$
ADULT – Allergic conjunctivitis: 1 gtt two to four times per day for 2 weeks.
PEDS – Not approved for age younger than 12 yo. Use adult dose for age 12 yo or older.
FORMS – Trade only: Susp 0.05% (5, 10 mL).
NOTES – Wait 10 min after use before inserting contact lenses.

OPHTHALMOLOGY: Antiallergy—Pure Mast Cell Stabilizers

NOTE: Works best as preventative agent; use continually during at risk season. Wait 10 min after use before inserting contact lenses. On average, each mL of eye drop soln contains approximately 20 gtts. Reserve ointment formulations for bedtime use due to severe vision blurring. Most eye medications can be administered 1 gtt at a time despite common manufacturer recommendations of 1 to 2 gtts concurrently. Even a single gtt is typically more than the eye can hold and thus a second gtt is both wasteful and increases the possibility of systemic toxicity. If 2 gtts of the medication are desired, separate single gtts by at least 5 min.

CROMOLYN—OPHTHALMIC (*Crolom, Opticrom*) ▸LK ♀B ▸? $$
ADULT – Allergic conjunctivitis: 1 to 2 gtts 4 to 6 times per day.
PEDS – Not approved for age younger than 4 yo. Use adult dose for age 4 yo or older.
FORMS – Generic/Trade: Soln 4% (10 mL).
NOTES – Response may take up to 6 weeks.

LODOXAMIDE (*Alomide*) ▸K ♀B ▸? $$$
ADULT – Allergic conjunctivitis: 1 to 2 gtts in each eye four times per day for up to 3 months.
PEDS – Not approved for age younger than 2 yo. Use adult dose for age 2 yo or older.
FORMS – Trade only: Soln 0.1% (10 mL).
NOTES – Do not administer while wearing soft contact lenses.

NEDOCROMIL—OPHTHALMIC (*Alocril*) ▸L ♀B ▸? $$$
ADULT – Allergic conjunctivitis: 1 to 2 gtts in each eye two times per day.
PEDS – Allergic conjunctivitis: 1 to 2 gtts in each eye two times per day. Not approved for age younger than 3 yo.
FORMS – Trade only: Soln 2% (5 mL).
NOTES – Soln normally appears slightly yellow.

PEMIROLAST (*Alamast*) ▸? ♀C ▸? $$$
ADULT – Allergic conjunctivitis: 1 to 2 gtts in each eye four times per day.
PEDS – Not approved for age younger than 3 yo. Use adult dose for 3 yo or older.
FORMS – Trade only: Soln 0.1% (10 mL).
NOTES – Decreased itching may be seen within a few days, but full effect may require up to 4 weeks.

OPHTHALMOLOGY: Antibacterials—Aminoglycosides

NOTE: On average, each mL of eye drop soln contains approximately 20 gtts. Reserve ointment formulations for bedtime use due to severe vision blurring. Most eye medications can be administered 1 gtt at a time despite common manufacturer recommendations of 1 to 2 gtts concurrently. Even a single gtt is typically more than the eye can hold and thus a second gtt is both wasteful and increases the possibility of systemic toxicity. If 2 gtts of the medication are desired, separate single gtts by at least 5 min.

GENTAMICIN—OPHTHALMIC (*Garamycin, Genoptic, Gentak,* ✦ *Diogent*) ▸K ♀C ▸? $
ADULT – Ocular infections: 1 to 2 gtts q 2 to 4 h or ½ inch ribbon of ointment two to three times per day.
PEDS – Not approved in children.
UNAPPROVED ADULT – Up to 2 gtts q 1 h have been used for severe infections.
UNAPPROVED PEDS – Ocular infections: 1 to 2 gtts q 4 h or ½ inch ribbon of ointment two to three times per day.
FORMS – Generic/Trade: Soln 0.3% (5, 15 mL) Ointment 0.3% (3.5 g tube).
NOTES – For severe infections, use up to 2 gtts q 1 h.

TOBRAMYCIN—OPHTHALMIC (*Tobrex*) ▶K ♀B ▶– $

ADULT – Ocular infections, mild to moderate: 1 to 2 gtts q 4 h or ½ inch ribbon of ointment two to three times per day. Ocular infections, severe: 2 gtts q 1 h, then taper to q 4 h or ½ inch ribbon of ointment q 3 to 4 h, then taper to two to three times per day.

PEDS – Use adult dose for age 2 mo or older.

UNAPPROVED PEDS – Ocular infections, mild to moderate: 1 to 2 gtts q 4 h or ½ inch ribbon of ointment two to three times per day. Ocular infections, severe: 2 gtts q 1 h, then taper to q 4 h or ½ inch ribbon of ointment q 3 to 4 h, then taper to two to three times per day.

FORMS – Generic/Trade: Soln 0.3% (5 mL). Trade only: Ointment 0.3% (3.5 g tube).

OPHTHALMOLOGY: Antibacterials—Fluoroquinolones

NOTE: Avoid the overuse of fluoroquinolones for conjunctivitis. Ocular administration has not been shown to cause arthropathy. On average, each mL of eye drop soln contains approximately 20 gtts. Reserve ointment formulations for bedtime use due to severe vision blurring. Most eye medications can be administered 1 gtt at a time despite common manufacturer recommendations of 1 to 2 gtts concurrently. Even a single gtt is typically more than the eye can hold and thus a second gtt is both wasteful and increases the possibility of systemic toxicity. If 2 gtts of the medication are desired, separate single gtts by at least 5 min.

BESIFLOXACIN (*Besivance*) ▶LK ♀C ▶? $$$

ADULT – 1 gtt three times per day for 7 days.

PEDS – Not approved for age younger than 1 yo. Use adult dose for age 1 yo or older.

FORMS – Trade: Soln 0.6% (5 mL).

NOTES – Do not wear contacts during use.

CIPROFLOXACIN—OPHTHALMIC (*Ciloxan*) ▶LK ♀C ▶? $$

ADULT – Corneal ulcers/keratitis: 2 gtts q 15 min for 6 h, then 2 gtts q 30 min for 1 day; then 2 gtts q 1 h for 1 day, and 2 gtts q 4 h for 3 to 14 days. Bacterial conjunctivitis: 1 to 2 gtts q 2 h while awake for 2 days, then 1 to 2 gtts q 4 h while awake for 5 days; or ½ inch ribbon ointment three times per day for 2 days, then ½ inch ribbon two times per day for 5 days.

PEDS – Bacterial conjunctivitis: Use adult dose for age 1 yo or older (soln) and age 2 yo or older (ointment). Not approved below these ages.

FORMS – Generic/Trade: Soln 0.3% (2.5, 5, 10 mL). Trade only: Ointment 0.3% (3.5 g tube).

NOTES – May cause white precipitate of active drug at site of epithelial defect that may be confused with a worsening infection. Resolves within 2 weeks and does not necessitate discontinuation.

GATIFLOXACIN—OPHTHALMIC (*Zymaxid*, ♣ *Zymar*) ▶K ♀C ▶? $$$

ADULT – Bacterial conjunctivitis: 1 to 2 gtts q 2 h while awake (up to 8 times per day on days 1 and 2), then 1 to 2 gtts 4 times per day on days 3 thru 7.

PEDS – Not approved for age younger than 1 yo. Use adult dose for age 1 yo or older.

FORMS – Trade only: Soln 0.3% (5 mL).

LEVOFLOXACIN—OPHTHALMIC (*Iquix*, *Quixin*) ▶KL ♀C ▶? $$$

ADULT – Bacterial conjunctivitis, Quixin: 1 to 2 gtts q 2 h while awake (up to 8 times per day) on days 1 and 2, then 1 to 2 gtts q 4 h (up to 4 times per day) on days 3 to 7. Corneal ulcers, Iquix: 1 to 2 gtts q 30 min to 2 h while awake and q 4 to 6 h overnight on days 1 to 3, then 1 to 2 gtts q 1 to 4 h while awake on day 4 to completion of therapy.

PEDS – Bacterial conjunctivitis, Quixin: 1 to 2 gtts q 2 h while awake (up to 8 times per day) on days 1 and 2, then 1 to 2 gtts q 4 h (up to 4 times/day) on days 3 to 7 for age older than 1 yo only. Corneal ulcers, Iquix: 1 to 2 gtts q 30 min to 2 h while awake and q 4 to 6 h overnight on days 1 to 3, then 1 to 2 gtts q 1 to 4 h while awake on day 4 to completion of therapy for age older than 6 yo only.

FORMS – Trade only: Soln 0.5% (Quixin, 5 mL), 1.5% (Iquix, 5 mL).

MOXIFLOXACIN—OPHTHALMIC (*Vigamox*, *Moxeza*) ▶LK ♀C ▶? $$$

ADULT – Bacterial conjunctivitis: 1 gtt in each affected eye three times per day for 7 days (Vigamox) or 1 gtt in each affected eye two times per day for 7 days (Moxeza).

PEDS – Use adult dose for age 1 yo or older.

FORMS – Trade only: Soln 0.5% (3 mL, Vigamox and Moxeza).

OFLOXACIN—OPHTHALMIC (*Ocuflox*) ▶LK ♀C ▶? $$

ADULT – Corneal ulcers/keratitis: 1 to 2 gtts q 30 min while awake and 1 to 2 gtts 4 to 6 h after retiring for 2 days, then 1 to 2 gtts q 1 h

(cont.)

OFLOXACIN—OPHTHALMIC (*cont.*)

while awake for 5 days, then 1 to 2 gtts four times per day for 3 days. Bacterial conjunctivitis: 1 to 2 gtts q 2 to 4 h for 2 days, then 1 to 2 gtts four times per day for 5 days.

PEDS – Bacterial conjunctivitis: Use adult dose for age 1 yo or older, not approved age younger than 1 yo.

FORMS – Generic/Trade: Soln 0.3% (5, 10 mL).

OPHTHALMOLOGY: Antibacterials—Other

NOTE: On average, each mL of eye drop soln contains approximately 20 gtts. Reserve ointment formulations for bedtime use due to severe vision blurring. Most eye medications can be administered 1 gtt at a time despite common manufacturer recommendations of 1 to 2 gtts concurrently. Even a single gtt is typically more than the eye can hold and thus a second gtt is both wasteful and increases the possibility of systemic toxicity. If 2 gtts of the medication are desired, separate single gtts by at least 5 min.

AZITHROMYCIN—OPHTHALMIC (*Azasite*) ▶L ♀B ▶? $$$

ADULT – Ocular infections: 1 gtt two times per day for 2 days, then 1 gtt daily for 5 more days.

PEDS – Ocular infections: 1 gtt two times per day for 2 days, then 1 gtt daily for 5 more days for age 1 yo or older.

FORMS – Trade only: Soln 1% (2.5 mL).

BACITRACIN—OPHTHALMIC (*AK Tracin*) ▶Minimal absorption ♀C ▶? $

ADULT – Ocular infections: Apply ¼ to ½ inch ribbon of ointment q 3 to 4 h or two to four times per day for 7 to 10 days.

PEDS – Not approved in children.

UNAPPROVED PEDS – Ocular infections: Apply ½ inch ribbon of ointment q 3 to 4 h or two to four times per day for 7 to 10 days.

FORMS – Generic/Trade: Ointment 500 units/g (3.5 g tube).

ERYTHROMYCIN—OPHTHALMIC (*Ilotycin, AK-Mycin*) ▶L ♀B ▶+ $

ADULT – Ocular infections, corneal ulceration: ½ inch ribbon of ointment q 3 to 4 h or 2 to 6 times per day. For chlamydial infections: two times per day for 2 months or two times per day for the first 5 days of each month for 6 months.

PEDS – Ophthalmia neonatorum prophylaxis: ½ inch ribbon to both eyes within 1 h of birth.

FORMS – Generic only: Ointment 0.5% (1, 3.5 g tube).

♣ **FUSIDIC ACID—OPHTHALMIC** ▶L ♀? ▶? $

ADULT – Canada only. Eye infections: 1 gtt in both eyes q 12 h for 7 days.

PEDS – Canada only. Eye infections: 1 gtt in both eyes q 12 h for 7 days for age 2 yo or older.

FORMS – Canada trade only: gtts 1%. Multidose tubes of 3, 5 g. Single-dose preservative-free tubes of 0.2 g in a box of 12.

NEOSPORIN OINTMENT—OPHTHALMIC **(neomycin + bacitracin + polymyxin)** ▶K ♀C ▶? $

ADULT – Ocular infections: ½ inch ribbon of ointment q 3 to 4 h for 7 to 10 days or ½ inch ribbon two to three times per day for mild to moderate infection.

PEDS – Not approved in children.

UNAPPROVED PEDS – ½ inch ribbon of ointment q 3 to 4 h for 7 to 10 days.

FORMS – Generic only: Ointment. (3.5 g tube).

NOTES – Contact dermatitis can occur after prolonged use.

NEOSPORIN SOLUTION—OPHTHALMIC **(neomycin + polymyxin + gramicidin)** ▶KL ♀C ▶? $$

ADULT – Ocular infections: 1 to 2 gtts q 4 to 6 h for 7 to 10 days.

PEDS – Not approved in children.

UNAPPROVED PEDS – 1 to 2 gtts q 4 to 6 h for 7 to 10 days.

FORMS – Generic/Trade: Soln (10 mL).

NOTES – Contact dermatitis can occur after prolonged use.

POLYSPORIN—OPHTHALMIC **(polymyxin + bacitracin)** ▶K ♀C ▶? $$

ADULT – Ocular infections: ½ inch ribbon of ointment q 3 to 4 h for 7 to 10 days or ½ inch ribbon two to three times per day for mild to moderate infection.

PEDS – Not approved in children.

UNAPPROVED PEDS – Ocular infections: ½ inch ribbon of ointment q 3 to 4 h for 7 to 10 days.

FORMS – Generic only: Ointment (3.5 g tube).

POLYTRIM—OPHTHALMIC **(polymyxin + trimethoprim)** ▶KL ♀C ▶? $

ADULT – Ocular infections: 1 to 2 gtts q 4 to 6 h (up to 6 gtts per day) for 7 to 10 days.

PEDS – Not approved for age younger than 2 mo. Use adult dose for age 2 mo or older.

FORMS – Generic/Trade: Soln (10 mL).

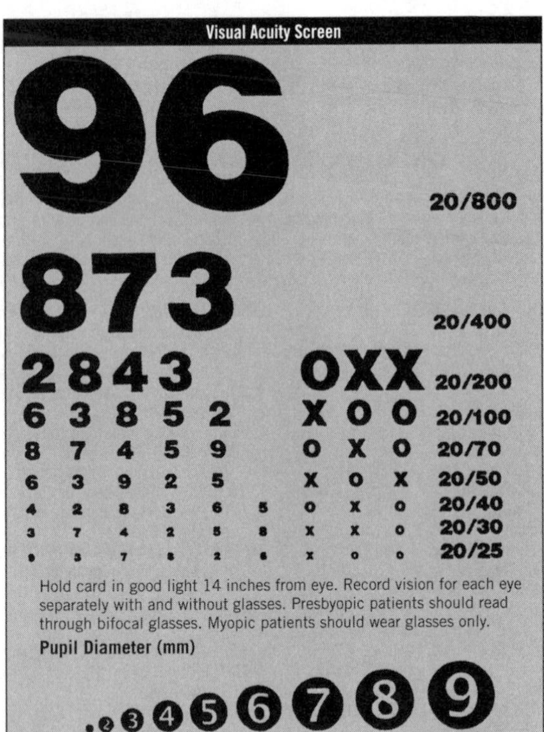

SULFACETAMIDE—OPHTHALMIC (*Bleph-10, Sulf-10*) ▶K ♀C ▶– $

ADULT – Ocular infections, corneal ulceration: 1 to 2 gtts q 2 to 3 h initially, then taper by decreasing frequency as condition allows over 7 to 10 days or ½ inch ribbon of ointment q 3 to 4 h initially, then taper 7 to 10 days. Trachoma: 2 gtts q 2 h with systemic antibiotic such as doxycycline or azithromycin.

PEDS – Not approved age younger than 2 mo. Use adult dose for age 2 mo or older.

FORMS – Generic/Trade: Soln 10% (15 mL), Ointment 10% (3.5 g tube). Generic only: Soln 30% (15 mL).

NOTES – Ointment may be used as an adjunct to soln.

OPHTHALMOLOGY: Antiviral Agents

GANCICLOVIR (*Zirgan*) ▶Minimal absorption ♀C ▶? $$$$

ADULT – Herpetic keratitis: 1 gtt five times per day (approximately q 3 h) until ulcer heals, then 1 gtt three times per day for 7 days.

PEDS – Not approved in children younger than 2 yo. Use adult dosing for age 2 yo and older.

FORMS – Trade only: Gel 0.15% (5g).

NOTES – Do not wear contact lenses.

TRIFLURIDINE (*Viroptic*) ▶Minimal absorption ♀C ▶– $$$

ADULT – Herpetic keratitis: 1 gtt q 2 h to max 9 gtts per day. After re-epithelialization, decrease dose to 1 gtt q 4 to 6 h while awake for 7 to 14 days. Max of 21 days of treatment.

PEDS – Not approved age younger than 6 yo. Use adult dose for age 6 yo or older.

FORMS – Generic/Trade Soln 1% (7.5 mL).

NOTES – Avoid continuous use more than 21 days; may cause keratitis and conjunctival scarring. Urge frequent use of topical lubricants (ie, tear substitutes) to minimize surface damage.

OPHTHALMOLOGY: Corticosteroid & Antibacterial Combinations

NOTE: Recommend that only ophthalmologists or optometrists prescribe due to infection, cataract, corneal/scleral perforation, and glaucoma risk from prolonged use. Monitor intraocular pressure. Gradually taper when discontinuing. Shake suspensions well before using. On average, each mL of eye drop soln contains approximately 20 gtts. Reserve ointment formulations for bedtime use due to severe vision blurring. Most eye medications can be administered 1 gtt at a time despite common manufacturer recommendations of 1 to 2 gtts concurrently. Even a single gtt is typically more than the eye can hold and thus a second gtt is both wasteful and increases the possibility of systemic toxicity. If 2 gtts of the medication are desired, separate single gtts by at least 5 min.

BLEPHAMIDE **(prednisolone—ophthalmic + sulfacetamide)** ▶KL ♀C ▶? $

ADULT – Steroid-responsive inflammatory condition with bacterial infection or risk of bacterial infection: Start 1 to 2 gtts q 1 h during the day and q 2 h during the night, then 1 gtt q 4 h and at bedtime; or ½ inch ribbon to lower conjunctival sac 3 to 4 times/day and 1 to 2 times at night.

PEDS – Not approved in children younger than 6 yo.

FORMS – Generic/Trade: Soln/Susp (5, 10 mL), Trade only: Ointment (3.5 g tube).

CORTISPORIN—OPHTHALMIC **(neomycin + polymyxin + hydrocortisone—ophthalmic)** ▶LK ♀C ▶? $

ADULT – Steroid-responsive inflammatory condition with bacterial infection or risk of bacterial infection: 1 to 2 gtts or ½ inch ribbon of ointment q 3 to 4 h or more frequently prn.

PEDS – Not approved in children.

UNAPPROVED PEDS – 1 to 2 gtts or ½ inch ribbon of ointment q 3 to 4 h.

FORMS – Generic only: Susp (7.5 mL), Ointment (3.5 g tube).

MAXITROL **(dexamethasone—ophthalmic + neomycin + polymyxin)** ▶KL ♀C ▶? $

ADULT – Steroid-responsive inflammatory condition with bacterial infection or risk of bacterial infection: Ointment: Place a small amount (about ½ inch) in the affected eye 3 to 4 times per day or apply at bedtime as an adjunct with gtts. Susp: Instill 1 to 2 gtts into affected eye(s) 4 to 6 times daily; in severe disease, gtts may be used hourly and tapered to discontinuation.

PEDS – Not approved in children.

FORMS – Generic/Trade: Susp (5 mL), Ointment (3.5 g tube).

PRED G **(prednisolone—ophthalmic + gentamicin)** ▶KL ♀C ▶? $$

ADULT – Steroid-responsive inflammatory condition with bacterial infection or risk of bacterial infection: Start 1 to 2 gtts q 1 h during the days and q 2 h during the night, then 1 gtt 2 to 4 times daily or ½ inch ribbon of ointment 1 to 3 times per day.

PEDS – Not approved in children.

FORMS – Trade only: Susp (2, 5, 10 mL), Ointment (3.5 g tube).

TOBRADEX **(tobramycin + dexamethasone—ophthalmic)** ▶L ♀C ▶? $$$

ADULT – Steroid-responsive inflammatory condition with bacterial infection or risk of bacterial infection: 1 to 2 gtts q 2 h for 1 to 2 days, then 1 to 2 gtts q 4 to 6 h; or ½ inch ribbon of ointment three to four times per day.

PEDS – 1 to 2 gtts q 2 h for 1 to 2 days, then 1 to 2 gtts q 4 to 6 h; or ½ inch ribbon of ointment three to four times per day for age 2 yo or older.

FORMS – Trade only (tobramycin 0.3%/dexamethasone 0.1%): Susp (2.5, 5, 10 mL) Trade/generic: (tobramycin 0.3%/dexamethasone 0.1%): Ointment (3.5 g tube).

TOBRADEX ST **(tobramycin + dexamethasone—ophthalmic)** ▶L ♀C ▶? $$$

ADULT – Steroid-responsive inflammatory condition with bacterial infection or risk of bacterial infection: 1 gtt q 2 h for 1 to 2 days, then 1 gtt q 4 to 6 h.

PEDS – 2 yo or older: 1 gtt q 2 h for 1 to 2 days, then 1 gtt q 4 to 6 h.

FORMS – Trade only: Tobramycin 0.3%/dexamethasone 0.05%: Susp (2.5, 5, 10 mL).

VASOCIDIN **(prednisolone—ophthalmic + sulfacetamide)** ▶KL ♀C ▶? $
ADULT – Steroid-responsive inflammatory condition with bacterial infection or risk of bacterial infection: Start 1 to 2 gtts q 1 h during the day and q 2 h during the night, then 1 gtt q 4 to 8 h.
PEDS – Not approved in children.
FORMS – Generic only: Soln (5, 10 mL).

ZYLET **(loteprednol + tobramycin)** ▶LK ♀C ▶? $$$
ADULT – 1 to 2 gtts q 1 to 2 h for 1 to 2 days then 1 to 2 gtts q 4 to 6 h.
PEDS – Not approved in children.
FORMS – Trade only: Susp 0.5% loteprednol + 0.3% tobramycin (2.5, 5, 10 mL).

OPHTHALMOLOGY: Corticosteroids

NOTE: Recommend that only ophthalmologists or optometrists prescribe due to infection, cataract, corneal/scleral perforation, and glaucoma risk. Monitor intraocular pressure. Gradually taper when discontinuing. Shake susp well before using. On average, each mL of eye drop soln contains approximately 20 gtts. Reserve ointment formulations for bedtime use due to severe vision blurring. Most eye medications can be administered 1 gtt at a time despite common manufacturer recommendations of 1 to 2 gtts concurrently. Even a single gtt is typically more than the eye can hold and thus a second gtt is both wasteful and increases the possibility of systemic toxicity. If 2 gtts of the medication are desired, separate single gtts by at least 5 min.

DIFLUPREDNATE (***Durezol***) ▶Not absorbed ♀C ▶? $$$$
ADULT – 1 gtt into affected eye four times per day, beginning 24 h after surgery for 2 weeks, then 1 gtt into affected eye two times per day for 1 week, then taper based on response.
PEDS – Not approved in children.
FORMS – Trade only: Ophthalmic emulsion 0.05% (2.5, 5 mL).
NOTES – If used for more than 10 days, monitor intraocular pressure.

FLUOCINOLONE—OPHTHALMIC (***Retisert***) ▶Not absorbed ♀C ▶? $$$$$
PEDS – Not approved in children younger than 12 yo.
FORMS – Implantable tablet 0.59 mg only available from manufacturer.
NOTES – Releases 0.6 mcg/day decreasing over about 1 month, then 0.3 to 0.4 mcg/day over about 30 months. Within 34 weeks 60% require medication to control intraocular pressure and within 2 years nearly all phakic eyes develop cataracts.

FLUOROMETHOLONE (***FML, FML Forte, Flarex***) ▶L ♀C ▶? $$
ADULT – 1 to 2 gtts q 1 to 2 h or ½ inch ribbon of ointment q 4 h for 1 to 2 days, then 1 to 2 gtts two to four times per day or ½ inch of ointment one to three times per day.
PEDS – Not approved age younger than 2 yo. Use adult dose for age 2 yo or older.
FORMS – Trade only: Susp 0.1% (5, 10, 15 mL), 0.25% (2, 5, 10, 15 mL), Ointment 0.1% (3.5 g tube).
NOTES – Fluorometholone acetate (Flarex) is more potent than fluorometholone (FML, FML Forte). Use caution in glaucoma.

LOTEPREDNOL (***Alrex, Lotemax***) ▶L ♀C ▶? $$$
ADULT – 1 to 2 gtts four times per day, may increase to 1 gtt q 1 h during first weeks of therapy prn. Postop inflammation: 1 to 2 gtts four times per day or ½ inch four times daily beginning 24 h after surgery.
PEDS – Not approved in children.
FORMS – Trade only: Susp 0.2% (Alrex 5, 10 mL), 0.5% (Lotemax 2.5, 5, 10, 15 mL). Oint 3.5 g.

PREDNISOLONE—OPHTHALMIC (***Pred Forte, Pred Mild, Inflamase Forte, Econopred Plus, ♣ AK Tate, Diopred***) ▶L ♀C ▶? $$
ADULT – Soln: 1 to 2 gtts (up to q 1 h during day and q 2 h at night), when response observed, then 1 gtt q 4 h, then 1 gtt three to four times per day. Susp: 1 to 2 gtts two to four times per day.
PEDS – Not approved in children.
FORMS – Generic/Trade: Soln, Susp 1% (5, 10, 15 mL). Trade only (Pred Mild): Susp 0.12% (5, 10 mL), Susp (Pred Forte) 1% (1 mL).
NOTES – Prednisolone acetate (Pred Mild, Pred Forte) is more potent than prednisolone sodium phosphate (AK-Pred, Inflamase Forte).

RIMEXOLONE (***Vexol***) ▶L ♀C ▶? $$
ADULT – Postop inflammation: 1 to 2 gtts four times per day for 2 weeks. Uveitis: 1 to 2 gtts q 1 h while awake for 1 week, then 1 gtt q 2 h while awake for 1 week, then taper.
PEDS – Not approved in children.
FORMS – Trade only: Susp 1% (5, 10 mL).
NOTES – Prolonged use associated with corneal/scleral perforation and cataracts.

TRIAMCINOLONE—VITREOUS (*Triesence*) ▶L ♀D ▶? ?
ADULT – Administered intravitreally.
PEDS – Not approved in children.
NOTES – Do not use in patients with systemic fungal infections.

OPHTHALMOLOGY: Glaucoma Agents—Beta-Blockers

NOTE: May be absorbed and cause side effects and drug interactions associated with systemic beta-blocker therapy. Use caution in cardiac conditions and asthma. Advise patients to apply gentle pressure over nasolacrimal duct for 5 min after instillation to minimize systemic absorption. On average, each mL of eye drop soln contains approximately 20 gtts. Reserve ointment formulations for bedtime use due to severe vision blurring. Most eye medications can be administered 1 gtt at a time despite common manufacturer recommendations of 1 to 2 gtts concurrently. Even a single gtt is typically more than the eye can hold and thus a second gtt is both wasteful and increases the possibility of systemic toxicity. If 2 gtts of the medication are desired, separate single gtts by at least 5 min.

BETAXOLOL—OPHTHALMIC (*Betoptic, Betoptic S*) ▶LK ♀C ▶? $$
ADULT – Chronic open-angle glaucoma or ocular HTN: 1 to 2 gtts two times per day.
PEDS – Chronic open-angle glaucoma or ocular HTN: 1 to 2 gtts two times per day.
FORMS – Trade only: Susp 0.25% (10, 15 mL). Generic only: Soln 0.5% (5, 10, 15 mL).
NOTES – Selective beta-1-blocking agent. Shake susp before use.

CARTEOLOL—OPHTHALMIC (*Ocupress*) ▶KL ♀C ▶? $
ADULT – Chronic open-angle glaucoma or ocular HTN: 1 gtt two times per day.
PEDS – Not approved in children.
FORMS – Generic only: Soln 1% (5, 10, 15 mL).
NOTES – Nonselective beta-blocker but has intrinsic sympathomimetic activity.

LEVOBUNOLOL (*Betagan*) ▶? ♀C ▶– $$
ADULT – Chronic open-angle glaucoma or ocular HTN: 1 to 2 gtts (0.5%) one to two times per day or 1 to 2 gtts (0.25%) two times per day.
PEDS – Not approved in children.
FORMS – Generic/Trade: Soln 0.25% (5, 10 mL), 0.5% (5, 10, 15 mL).
NOTES – Nonselective beta-blocker.

METIPRANOLOL (*Optipranolol*) ▶? ♀C ▶? $
ADULT – Chronic open-angle glaucoma or ocular HTN: 1 gtt two times per day.
PEDS – Not approved in children.
FORMS – Generic/Trade: Soln 0.3% (5, 10 mL).
NOTES – Nonselective beta-blocker.

TIMOLOL—OPHTHALMIC (*Betimol, Timoptic, Timoptic XE, Istalol, Timoptic Ocudose*) ▶LK ♀C ▶+ $$
ADULT – Chronic open-angle glaucoma or ocular HTN: 1 gtt (0.25 or 0.5%) two times per day or 1 gtt of gel-forming soln (0.25 or 0.5% Timoptic XE) daily or 1 gtt (0.5% Istalol soln) daily.
PEDS – Chronic open-angle glaucoma or ocular HTN: 1 gtt (0.25 or 0.5%) of gel-forming soln daily.
FORMS – Generic/Trade: Soln 0.25, 0.5% (5, 10, 15 mL), Preservative-free soln (Timoptic Ocudose) 0.25% (0.2 mL), Gel-forming soln (Timoptic XE) 0.25, 0.5% (5 mL).
NOTES – Administer other eye meds at least 10 min before Timoptic XE. Greatest effect if Timoptic XE is administered in the morning. Nonselective beta-blocker.

OPHTHALMOLOGY: Glaucoma Agents—Carbonic Anhydrase Inhibitors

NOTE: Sulfonamide derivatives; verify absence of sulfa allergy before prescribing. On average, each mL of eye drop soln contains approximately 20 gtts. Reserve ointment formulations for bedtime use due to severe vision blurring. Most eye medications can be administered 1 gtt at a time despite common manufacturer recommendations of 1 to 2 gtts concurrently. Even a single gtt is typically more than the eye can hold and thus a second gtt is both wasteful and increases the possibility of systemic toxicity. If 2 gtts of the medication ARE desired, separate single gtts by at least 5 min.

BRINZOLAMIDE (*Azopt*) ▶LK ♀C ▶? $$$
ADULT – Chronic open-angle glaucoma or ocular HTN: 1 gtt three times per day.
PEDS – Not approved in children.
FORMS – Trade only: Susp 1% (10, 15 mL).
NOTES – Do not administer while wearing soft contact lenses. Wait 10 min after use before inserting contact lenses.

DORZOLAMIDE (*Trusopt*) ▶KL ♀C ▶– $$$
ADULT – Chronic open-angle glaucoma or ocular HTN: 1 gtt three times per day.
PEDS – Chronic open-angle glaucoma or ocular HTN: 1 gtt three times per day.
FORMS – Generic/Trade: Soln 2% (10 mL).
NOTES – Do not administer while wearing soft contact lenses. Keep bottle tightly capped to avoid crystal formation. Wait 10 min after use before inserting contact lenses.

METHAZOLAMIDE ▶LK ♀C ▶? $$
ADULT – Glaucoma: 100 to 200 mg PO initially, then 100 mg PO q 12 h until desired response. Maintenance dose: 25 to 50 mg PO (up to three times per day).
PEDS – Not approved in children.
FORMS – Generic only: Tabs 25, 50 mg.
NOTES – Mostly metabolized in the liver thus less chance of renal calculi than with acetazolamide.

OPHTHALMOLOGY: Glaucoma Agents—Combinations and Other

NOTE: On average, each mL of eye drop soln contains approximately 20 gtts. Reserve ointment formulations for bedtime use due to severe vision blurring. Most eye medications can be administered 1 gtt at a time despite common manufacturer recommendations of 1 to 2 gtts concurrently. Even a single gtt is typically more than the eye can hold and thus a second gtt is both wasteful and increases the possibility of systemic toxicity. If 2 gtts of the medication are desired, separate single gtts by at least 5 min.

COMBIGAN **(brimonidine + timolol)** ▶LK ♀C ▶– $$$
ADULT – Chronic open-angle glaucoma or ocular HTN: 1 gtt q 12 h.
PEDS – Not approved in age younger than 2 yo. Use adult dosing in 2 yo or older.
FORMS – Trade only: Soln brimonidine 0.2% + timolol 0.5% (5, 10 mL).
NOTES – Do not administer while wearing soft contact lenses. Wait 10 min after use before inserting contact lenses. Contraindicated with MAOIs. See beta-blocker warnings.

COSOPT **(dorzolamide + timolol)** ▶LK ♀D ▶– $$$
ADULT – Chronic open-angle glaucoma or ocular HTN: 1 gtt two times per day.
PEDS – Not approved in children younger than 2 yo. In children older than 2 yo, use adult dose.
FORMS – Generic/Trade: Soln dorzolamide 2% + timolol 0.5% (5, 10 mL).
NOTES – Do not administer while wearing soft contact lenses. Wait 10 min after use before inserting contact lenses. Not recommended if severe renal or hepatic dysfunction. Use caution in sulfa allergy. See beta-blocker warnings.

OPHTHALMOLOGY: Glaucoma Agents—Miotics

NOTE: Observe for cholinergic systemic effects (eg, salivation, lacrimation, urination, diarrhea, GI upset, excessive sweating). On average, each mL of eye drop soln contains approximately 20 gtts. Reserve ointment formulations for bedtime use due to severe vision blurring. Most eye medications can be administered 1 gtt at a time despite common manufacturer recommendations of 1 to 2 gtts concurrently. Even a single gtt is typically more than the eye can hold and thus a second gtt is both wasteful and increases the possibility of systemic toxicity. If 2 gtts of the medication are desired, separate single gtts by at least 5 min.

ACETYLCHOLINE (*Miochol-E*) ▶Acetylcholinesterases ♀? ▶? $$
ADULT – Intraoperative miosis or pressure lowering: 0.5 mL to 2 mL injected intraocularly.
PEDS – Not approved in children.

CARBACHOL (*Isopto Carbachol, Miostat*) ▶? ♀C ▶? $$
ADULT – Glaucoma: 1 gtt three times per day. Intraoperative miosis or pressure lowering: 0.5 mL injected intraocularly.
PEDS – Not approved in children.
FORMS – Trade only: Soln (Isopto Carbachol) 1.5, 3% (15 mL). Intraocular soln (Miostat) 0.01%.

ECHOTHIOPHATE IODIDE (*Phospholine Iodide*) ▶? ♀C ▶? $$$
ADULT – Glaucoma: 1 gtt two times per day.
PEDS – Accommodative esotropia: 1 gtt daily (0.06%) or 1 gtt every other day (0.125%).
FORMS – Trade only: Soln 0.125% (5 mL).
NOTES – Use lowest effective dose strength. Use extreme caution if asthma, spastic GI diseases, GI ulcers, bradycardia, hypotension, recent MI, epilepsy, Parkinson's disease, history of retinal detachment. Stop 3 weeks before general anesthesia as may cause prolonged succinylcholine paralysis. Discontinue if cardiac effects noted.

PILOCARPINE—OPHTHALMIC (*Pilopine HS, Isopto Carpine*) ▶Plasma ♀C ▶? $

ADULT – Reduction of intraocular pressure with open-angle glaucoma, acute angle-closure glaucoma, prevention of postoperative elevated intraocular pressure associated with laser surgery, induction of miosis: 1 gtt up to four times per day or ½ inch ribbon (4% gel) at bedtime.

PEDS – Glaucoma: 1 gtt up to four times per day.

FORMS – Generic/Trade: Soln 0.5% (15 mL), 1% (2 mL, 15 mL), 2% (2 mL, 15 mL), 4% (2 mL, 15 mL), 6% (15 mL). Trade only (Pilopine HS): Gel 4% (4 g tube).

NOTES – Do not administer while wearing soft contact lenses. Wait at least 15 min after use before inserting contact lenses. Causes miosis. May cause blurred vision and difficulty with night vision.

OPHTHALMOLOGY: Glaucoma Agents—Prostaglandin Analogs

NOTE: Do not administer while wearing soft contact lenses. Wait 10 min after use before inserting contact lenses. May aggravate intraocular inflammation. On average, each mL of eye drop soln contains approximately 20 gtts. Reserve ointment formulations for bedtime use due to severe vision blurring. Most eye medications can be administered 1 gtt at a time despite common manufacturer recommendations of 1 to 2 gtts concurrently. Even a single gtt is typically more than the eye can hold and thus a second gtt is both wasteful and increases the possibility of systemic toxicity. If 2 gtts of the medication are desired, separate single gtts by at least 5 min.

BIMATOPROST (*Lumigan, Latisse*) ▶LK ♀C ▶? $$$

ADULT – Chronic open-angle glaucoma or ocular HTN: 1 gtt to affected eyes at bedtime. Hypotrichosis of the eyelashes (Latisse): Apply at bedtime to the skin of the upper eyelid margin at the base of the eyelashes.

PEDS – Not approved in children.

FORMS – Trade only: Soln 0.01%, 0.03% (Lumigan, 2.5, 5, 7.5 mL), (Latisse, 3 mL with 60 sterile, disposable applicators).

NOTES – Concurrent administration of bimatoprost for hypotrichosis and intraocular pressure–lowering prostaglandin analogs in ocular hypertensive patients may decrease the intraocular pressure–lowering effect. Monitor closely for changes in intraocular pressure.

LATANOPROST (*Xalatan*) ▶LK ♀C ▶? $$$

ADULT – Chronic open-angle glaucoma or ocular HTN: 1 gtt at bedtime.

PEDS – Not approved in children.

FORMS – Trade only: Soln 0.005% (2.5 mL).

TAFLUPROST (*Zioptan*) ▶L – ♀C ▶? $$$

ADULT – Chronic open-angle glaucome or ocular HTN: 1 gtt in each affect eye q pm.

PEDS – Not approved in children.

FORMS – Trade: Soln 0.0015%

NOTES – Can cause pigmentation of iris, periorbital tissue, and eyelashes.

TRAVOPROST (*Travatan, Travatan Z*) ▶L ♀C ▶? $$$

ADULT – Chronic open-angle glaucoma or ocular HTN: 1 gtt at bedtime.

PEDS – Not approved in children.

FORMS – Trade only: Soln (Travatan), benzalkonium chloride-free (Travatan Z) 0.004% (2.5, 5 mL).

NOTES – Wait 10 min after use before inserting contact lenses. Avoid if prior or current intraocular inflammation.

OPHTHALMOLOGY: Glaucoma Agents—Sympathomimetics

NOTE: Do not administer while wearing soft contact lenses. Wait 10 min after use before inserting contact lenses. On average, each mL of eye drop soln contains approximately 20 gtts. Reserve ointment formulations for bedtime use due to severe vision blurring. Most eye medications can be administered 1 gtt at a time despite common manufacturer recommendations of 1 to 2 gtts concurrently. Even a single gtt is typically more than the eye can hold and thus a second gtt is both wasteful and increases the possibility of systemic toxicity. If 2 gtts of the medication are desired, separate single gtts by at least 5 min.

APRACLONIDINE (*Iopidine*) ▶KL ♀C ▶? $$$$

ADULT – Perioperative intraocular pressure elevation: 1 gtt (1%) 1 h prior to surgery, then 1 gtt immediately after surgery.

PEDS – Not approved in children.

FORMS – Generic/Trade: Soln 0.5% (5, 10 mL). Trade only: Soln 1% (0.1 mL).

NOTES – Rapid tachyphylaxis may occur. Do not use long term.

BRIMONIDINE (*Alphagan P*, ♣ *Alphagan*) ▶L ♀B ◗? $$

ADULT – Chronic open-angle glaucoma or ocular HTN: 1 gtt three times per day.

PEDS – Glaucoma: 1 gtt three times per day for age older than 2 yo.

FORMS – Trade only: Soln 0.1% (5, 10, 15 mL). Generic/Trade: Soln 0.15% (5, 10, 15 mL). Generic only: Soln 0.2% (5, 10, 15 mL).

NOTES – Contraindicated in patients receiving MAOIs. Twice daily dosing may have similar efficacy.

DIPIVEFRIN (*Propine*) ▶Eye/plasma/L ♀B ◗? $

ADULT – Chronic open-angle glaucoma or ocular HTN: 1 gtt two times per day.

PEDS – Glaucoma: 1 gtt two times per day.

FORMS – Generic/Trade: Soln 0.1% (5, 10, 15 mL).

OPHTHALMOLOGY: Macular Degeneration

PEGAPTANIB (*Macugen*) ▶Minimal absorption ♀B ◗? $$$$$

ADULT – "Wet" macular degeneration: 0.3 mg intravitreal injection q 6 weeks.

PEDS – Not approved in children.

RANIBIZUMAB (*Lucentis*) ▶Intravitreal ♀C ◗? $$$$$

ADULT – Treatment of neovascular (wet) macular degeneration: 0.5 mg intravitreal injection q 28 days. If monthly injections not feasible, can administer q 3 months, but this regimen is less effective. Macular edema following retinal vein occlusion: 0.5 mg intravitreal injection q 28 days.

PEDS – Not approved in children.

NOTES – Increased CVA risk noted with higher doses (0.5 mg) and with prior CVA.

VERTEPORFIN (*Visudyne*) ▶L/plasma ♀C ◗? $$$$$

ADULT – Treatment of exudative age-related macular degeneration: 6 mg/m² IV over 10 min; laser light therapy 15 min after start of infusion.

PEDS – Not approved in children.

NOTES – Severe risk of photosensitivity for 5 days; must avoid exposure to sunlight.

OPHTHALMOLOGY: Mydriatics & Cycloplegics

NOTE: Use caution in infants. On average, each mL of eye drop soln contains approximately 20 gtts. Reserve ointment formulations for bedtime use due to severe vision blurring. Most eye medications can be administered 1 gtt at a time despite common manufacturer recommendations of 1 to 2 gtts concurrently. Even a single gtt is typically more than the eye can hold and thus a second gtt is both wasteful and increases the possibility of systemic toxicity. If 2 gtts of the medication are desired separate single gtts by at least 5 min.

ATROPINE—OPHTHALMIC (*Isopto Atropine, Atropine Care*) ▶L ♀C ◗+ $

ADULT – Uveitis: 1 to 2 gtts of 0.5% or 1% soln daily to four times per day, or ⅛ to ¼ inch ribbon (1% ointment) daily (up to three times per day). Refraction: 1 to 2 gtts of 1% soln 1 h before procedure or ⅛ to ¼ inch ribbon one to three times per day.

PEDS – Uveitis: 1 to 2 gtts of 0.5% soln one to three times per day) or ⅛ to ¼ inch ribbon one to three times per day. Refraction: 1 to 2 gtts (0.5%) two times per day for 1 to 3 days before procedure or ⅛ inch ribbon (1% ointment) for 1 to 3 days before procedure.

UNAPPROVED PEDS – Amblyopia: 1 gtt in good eye daily.

FORMS – Generic/Trade: Soln 1% (2, 5, 15 mL). Generic only: Ointment 1% (3.5 g tube).

NOTES – Cycloplegia may last up to 5 to 10 days and mydriasis may last up to 7 to 14 days. Each drop of a 1% soln contains 0.5 mg atropine. Treat atropine overdose with physostigmine 0.25 mg every 15 min until symptoms resolve.

CYCLOPENTOLATE (*AK-Pentolate, Cyclogyl, Pentolair*) ▶? ♀C ◗? $

ADULT – Refraction: 1 to 2 gtts (1% or 2%), repeat in 5 to 10 min prn. Give 45 min before procedure.

PEDS – May cause CNS disturbances in children. Refraction: 1 to 2 gtts (0.5%, 1%, or 2%), repeat in 5 to 10 min prn. Give 45 min before procedure.

FORMS – Generic/Trade: Soln 1% (2, 15 mL). Trade only (Cyclogyl): 0.5% (15 mL), 1% (5 mL), 2% (2, 5, 15 mL).

NOTES – Cycloplegia may last 6 to 24 h; mydriasis may last 1 day.

HOMATROPINE (*Isopto Homatropine*) ▶? ♀C ◗? $

ADULT – Refraction: 1 to 2 gtts (2%) or 1 gtt (5%) in eye(s) immediately before procedure,

(cont.)

HOMATROPINE (*cont.*)

repeat q 5 to 10 min prn. Max 3 doses. Uveitis: 1 to 2 gtts (2 to 5%) two to three times per day or as often as q 3 to 4 h.

PEDS – Refraction: 1 gtt (2%) in eye(s) immediately before procedure, repeat q 10 min prn. Uveitis: 1 gtt (2%) two to three times per day.

FORMS – Trade only: Soln 2% (5 mL), 5% (15 mL). Generic/Trade: Soln 5% (5 mL).

NOTES – Cycloplegia and mydriasis last 1 to 3 days.

PHENYLEPHRINE—OPHTHALMIC (***AK-Dilate, Altafrin, Mydfrin, Refresh***) ▶Plasma, L ♀C ▶? $

ADULT – Ophthalmologic exams: 1 to 2 gtts (2.5%, 10%) before procedure. Ocular surgery: 1 to 2 gtts (2.5%, 10%) before surgery. Red eyes: 1 or 2 gtts (0.12%) in affected eyes up to four times daily.

PEDS – Not routinely used in children.

UNAPPROVED PEDS – Ophthalmologic exams: 1 gtt (2.5%) before procedure. Ocular surgery: 1 gtt (2.5%) before surgery.

FORMS – Rx Generic/Trade: Soln 2.5% (2, 3, 5, 15 mL), 10% (5 mL). OTC Trade only (Altafrin and Refresh): Soln 0.12% (15 mL).

NOTES – Overuse can cause rebound dilation of blood vessels. No cycloplegia; mydriasis may last up to 5 h. Systemic absorption, especially with 10% soln, may be associated with sympathetic stimulation (eg, increased BP).

TROPICAMIDE (***Mydriacyl, Tropicacyl***) ▶? ♀C ▶? $

ADULT – Dilated eye exam: 1 to 2 gtts (0.5%) in eye(s) 15 to 20 min before exam, repeat q 30 min prn.

PEDS – Not approved in children.

FORMS – Generic/Trade: Soln 0.5% (15 mL), 1% (3, 15 mL). Generic only: Soln 1% (2 mL).

NOTES – Mydriasis may last 6 h and has weak cycloplegic effects.

OPHTHALMOLOGY: Non-Steroidal Anti-Inflammatories

NOTE: On average, each mL of eye drop soln contains approximately 20 gtts. Reserve ointment formulations for bedtime use due to severe vision blurring. Most eye medications can be administered 1 gtt at a time despite common manufacturer recommendations of 1 to 2 gtts concurrently. Even a single gtt is typically more than the eye can hold and thus a second gtt is both wasteful and increases the possibility of systemic toxicity. If 2 gtts of the medication are desired separate single gtts by at least 5 min.

BROMFENAC—OPHTHALMIC (***Bromday***) ▶Minimal absorption ♀C, D (3rd trimester) ▶? $$$$$

ADULT – Postop inflammation and pain following cataract surgery: 1 gtt in each affected eye once daily beginning 1 day prior to surgery and continuing for 14 days after surgery.

PEDS – Not approved in children.

FORMS – Trade only: Soln 0.09% (1.7 mL, 2.5 mL).

NOTES – Not for use with soft contact lenses. Contains sodium sulfite and may cause allergic reactions.

DICLOFENAC—OPHTHALMIC (***Voltaren, ✤ Voltaren Ophtha***) ▶L ♀C ▶? $$$

ADULT – Postop inflammation following cataract surgery: 1 gtt four times per day for 1 to 2 weeks. Ocular photophobia and pain associated with corneal refractive surgery: 1 to 2 gtt to operative eye(s) 1 h prior to surgery and 1 to 2 gtt within 15 min after surgery, then 1 gtt four times per day prn for no more than 3 days.

PEDS – Not approved in children.

FORMS – Generic/Trade: Soln 0.1% (2.5, 5 mL).

NOTES – Contraindicated for use with soft contact lenses.

FLURBIPROFEN—OPHTHALMIC (***Ocufen***) ▶L ♀C ▶? $

ADULT – Inhibition of intraoperative miosis: 1 gtt q 30 min beginning 2 h prior to surgery (total of 4 gtts).

PEDS – Not approved in children.

UNAPPROVED ADULT – Treatment of cystoid macular edema, inflammation after glaucoma or cataract laser surgery, uveitis syndromes.

FORMS – Generic/Trade: Soln 0.03% (2.5 mL).

KETOROLAC—OPHTHALMIC (***Acular, Acular LS***) ▶L ♀C ▶? $$$$

ADULT – Allergic conjunctivitis: 1 gtt (0.5%) four times per day. Postop inflammation following cataract surgery: 1 gtt (0.5%) four times per day beginning 24 h after surgery for 1 to 2 weeks. Postop corneal refractive surgery: 1 gtt (0.4%) prn for up to 4 days.

PEDS – Not approved age younger than 3 yo. Use adult dose for age 3 yo or older.

FORMS – Generic/Trade: Soln (Acular LS) 0.4% (5 mL). Trade only: Acular 0.5% (3, 5, 10 mL), preservative-free Acular 0.45% unit dose (0.4 mL).

NOTES – Do not administer while wearing soft contact lenses. Wait 10 min after use before inserting contact lenses. Avoid use in late pregnancy.

NEPAFENAC (***Nevanac***) ▶Minimal absorption ♀C, D in third trimester ▶? $$$
ADULT – Postop inflammation following cataract surgery: 1 gtt three times per day beginning 24 h before cataract surgery and continued for 2 weeks after surgery.
PEDS – Not approved in children.
FORMS – Trade only: Susp 0.1% (3 mL).
NOTES – Not for use with contact lenses. Caution if previous allergy to aspirin or other NSAIDs.

OPHTHALMOLOGY: Other Ophthalmologic Agents

ARTIFICIAL TEARS (***Tears Naturale, Hypotears, Refresh Tears, GenTeal, Systane***) ▶Minimal absorption ♀A ▶+ $
ADULT – Ophthalmic lubricant: 1 to 2 gtts prn.
PEDS – Ophthalmic lubricant: 1 to 2 gtts prn.
FORMS – OTC Generic/Trade: Soln (15, 30 mL, among others).

CYCLOSPORINE—OPHTHALMIC (***Restasis***) ▶Minimal absorption ♀C ▶? $$$$
ADULT – Keratoconjunctivitis sicca (chronic dry eye disease): 1 gtt in each eye q 12 h.
PEDS – Not approved in children.
FORMS – Trade only: Emulsion 0.05% (0.4 mL single-use vials).
NOTES – Wait 10 min after use before inserting contact lenses. May take 1 month to note clinical improvement.

FLUORESCEIN (***Fluor-I-Strip, Fluor-I-Strip AT, Ful-Glo***) ▶Minimal absorption ♀? ▶? $
ADULT – Following ocular anesthetic: Apply enough stain to bulbar conjunctiva to assess integrity of cornea.
PEDS – Following ocular anesthetic: Apply enough stain to bulbar conjunctiva to assess integrity of cornea.
FORMS – Trade only (Fluor-I-Strip AT): Fluorescein 1 mg in sterile ophthalmic strip. (Fluor-I-Strip): Fluorescein 9 mg in sterile ophthalmic strip.
NOTES – Do not use with soft contact lenses

HYDROXYPROPYL CELLULOSE (***Lacrisert***) ▶Minimal absorption ♀+ ▶+ $$$
ADULT – Moderate to severe dry eyes: 1 insert in each eye daily. Some patients may require twice daily use.
PEDS – Not approved in children.
FORMS – Trade only: Ocular insert 5 mg.
NOTES – Do not use with soft contact lenses.

LIDOCAINE—OPHTHALMIC (***Akten***) ▶L ♀B ▶? ?
ADULT – Do not prescribe for unsupervised use. Corneal toxicity may occur with repeated use. Local anesthetic: 2 gtts before procedure, repeat prn.
PEDS – Not approved in children.
FORMS – Generic only: Gel 3.5% (5 mL).

PETROLATUM (***Lacrilube, Dry Eyes, Refresh PM, ♣ Duolube***) ▶Minimal absorption ♀A ▶+ $
ADULT – Ophthalmic lubricant: Apply ¼ to ½ inch ointment to inside of lower lid prn.
PEDS – Ophthalmic lubricant: Apply ¼ to ½ inch ointment to inside of lower lid prn.
FORMS – OTC Trade only: Ointment (3.5, 7 g) tube.

PROPARACAINE (***Ophthaine, Ophthetic, ♣ Alcaine***) ▶L ♀C ▶? $
ADULT – Do not prescribe for unsupervised use. Corneal toxicity may occur with repeated use. Local anesthetic: 1 to 2 gtts before procedure. Repeat q 5 to 10 min for 1 to 3 doses (suture or foreign body removal) or for 5 to 7 doses (ocular surgery).
PEDS – Not approved in children.
FORMS – Generic/Trade: Soln 0.5% (15 mL).

TETRACAINE—OPHTHALMIC (***Pontocaine***) ▶Plasma ♀C ▶? $
ADULT – Do not prescribe for unsupervised use. Corneal toxicity may occur with repeated use. Local anesthetic: 1 to 2 gtts before procedure.
PEDS – Not approved in children.
FORMS – Generic only: Soln 0.5% (15 mL), unit-dose vials (0.7, 2 mL).

TRYPAN BLUE (***Vision Blue, Membrane Blue***) ▶Not absorbed ♀C ▶? $$
ADULT – Aid during ophthalmic surgery by staining anterior cap: Inject into anterior chamber of eye.
PEDS – Not approved in children.
FORMS – Trade only: 0.06% (Vision Blue) Ophthalmic soln (0.5 mL), 0.15% (Membrane Blue) Ophthalmic soln (0.5 mL).

PSYCHIATRY: Antidepressants—Heterocyclic Compounds

NOTE: Gradually taper when discontinuing cyclic antidepressants to avoid withdrawal symptoms. Seizures, orthostatic hypotension, arrhythmias, and anticholinergic side effects may occur. Do not use with MAOIs. Antidepressants increase the risk of suicidal thinking and behavior in children, adolescents, and young adults; carefully weigh the risks and benefits before starting and monitor patients closely. Use of serotonergic drugs in late third trimester of pregnancy can lead to prolonged hospitalizations, need for respiratory support, and tube feeding.

AMITRIPTYLINE (*Elavil*) ▶L ♀D ▶– $$
ADULT – Depression: Start 25 to 100 mg PO at bedtime; gradually increase to usual effective dose of 50 to 300 mg/day.
PEDS – Depression, adolescents: Use adult dosing. Not approved in children younger than 12 yo.
UNAPPROVED ADULT – Migraine prophylaxis and/or chronic pain: 10 to 100 mg/day. Fibromyalgia: 25 to 50 mg/day.
UNAPPROVED PEDS – Depression, age younger than 12 yo: Start 1 mg/kg/day PO divided three times per day for 3 days, then increase to 1.5 mg/kg/day. Max 5 mg/kg/day.
FORMS – Generic: Tabs 10, 25, 50, 75, 100, 150 mg. Elavil brand name no longer available; has been retained in this entry for name recognition purposes only.
NOTES – Tricyclic, tertiary amine; primarily inhibits serotonin reuptake. Demethylated to nortriptyline, which primarily inhibits norepinephrine reuptake. Usual therapeutic range is 150 to 300 ng/mL (amitriptyline + nortriptyline).

AMOXAPINE ▶L ♀C ▶– $$$
ADULT – Rarely used; other drugs preferred. Depression: Start 25 to 50 mg PO two to three times per day; increase by 50 to 100 mg two to three times per day after 1 week. Usual effective dose is 150 to 400 mg/day. Max 600 mg/day.
PEDS – Not approved in children younger than 16 yo.
FORMS – Generic only: Tabs 25, 50, 100, 150 mg.
NOTES – Tetracyclic; primarily inhibits norepinephrine reuptake. Dose 300 mg/day or less may be given once daily at bed time.

CLOMIPRAMINE (*Anafranil*) ▶L ♀C ▶+ $$$
ADULT – OCD: Start 25 mg PO at bedtime; gradually increase over 2 weeks to usual effective dose of 150 to 250 mg/day. Max 250 mg/day.
PEDS – OCD, age 10 yo or older: Start 25 mg PO at bedtime, then increase gradually over 2 weeks to 3 mg/kg/day or 100 mg/day, max 200 mg/day. Not approved for age younger than 10 yo.
UNAPPROVED ADULT – Depression: 100 to 250 mg/day. Panic disorder: 12.5 to 150 mg/day. Chronic pain: 100 to 250 mg/day.
FORMS – Generic/Trade: Caps 25, 50, 75 mg.
NOTES – Tricyclic, tertiary amine; primarily inhibits serotonin reuptake.

DESIPRAMINE (*Norpramin*) ▶L ♀C ▶+ $$
ADULT – Depression: Start 25 to 100 mg PO given once daily or in divided doses. Gradually increase to usual effective dose of 100 to 200 mg/day, max 300 mg/day.
PEDS – Depression, adolescents: 25 to 100 mg/day. Not approved in children.
FORMS – Generic/Trade: Tabs 10, 25, 50, 75, 100, 150 mg.
NOTES – Tricyclic, secondary amine; primarily inhibits norepinephrine reuptake. Usual therapeutic range is 125 to 300 ng/mL. May cause fewer anticholinergic side effects than tertiary amines. Use lower doses in adolescents or elderly.

DOXEPIN (*Sinequan, Silenor*) ▶L ♀C ▶– $$
ADULT – Depression and/or anxiety: Start 75 mg PO at bedtime. Gradually increase to usual effective dose of 75 to 150 mg/day, max 300 mg/day. Insomnia (Silenor): 6 mg PO 30 min before bedtime, 3 mg in age 65 yo or older.
PEDS – Adolescents: Use adult dosing. Not approved in children younger than 12 yo.
UNAPPROVED ADULT – Chronic pain: 50 to 300 mg/day. Pruritus: Start 10 to 25 mg at bedtime. Usual effective dose is 10 to 100 mg/day.
FORMS – Generic/Trade: Caps 10, 25, 50, 75, 100, 150 mg. Oral concentrate 10 mg/mL.
NOTES – Tricyclic, tertiary amine; primarily inhibits norepinephrine reuptake. Do not mix oral concentrate with carbonated beverages. Some patients with mild symptoms may respond to 25 to 50 mg/day.

IMIPRAMINE (*Tofranil, Tofranil PM*) ▶L ♀D ▶– $$$
ADULT – Depression: Start 75 to 100 mg PO at bedtime or in divided doses; gradually increase to max 300 mg/day.
PEDS – Enuresis age 6 yo or older: 10 to 25 mg/day PO given 1 h before bedtime, then increase in increments of 10 to 25 mg at 1- to 2-week intervals not to exceed 50 mg/day in 6 to 12 yo or 75 mg/day in children age older than 12 yo. Do not exceed 2.5 mg/kg/day.
UNAPPROVED ADULT – Panic disorder: Start 10 mg PO at bedtime, titrate to usual effective dose of 50 to 300 mg/day. Enuresis: 25 to 75 mg PO at bedtime.
UNAPPROVED PEDS – Depression, children: Start 1.5 mg/kg/day PO divided three times per day; increase by 1 to 1.5 mg/kg/day q 3 to 4 days to max 5 mg/kg/day.
FORMS – Generic/Trade: Tabs 10, 25, 50 mg. Caps 75, 100, 125, 150 mg (as pamoate salt).
NOTES – Tricyclic, tertiary amine; inhibits serotonin and norepinephrine reuptake. Demethylated to desipramine, which primarily inhibits norepinephrine reuptake.

MAPROTILINE (*Ludiomil*) ▶KL ♀B ▶? $$$

ADULT – Rarely used; other drugs preferred. Depression: Start 25 mg PO daily, then gradually increase by 25 mg q 2 weeks to max 225 mg/day. Usual effective dose is 150 to 225 mg/day. Max 200 mg/day for chronic use.

PEDS – Not approved in children.

FORMS – Generic only: Tabs 25, 50, 75 mg.

NOTES – Tetracyclic—primarily inhibits norepinephrine reuptake.

NORTRIPTYLINE (*Aventyl, Pamelor*) ▶L ♀D ▶+ $$$

ADULT – Depression: Start 25 mg PO given once daily or divided two to four times per day. Gradually increase to usual effective dose of 75 to 100 mg/day, max 150 mg/day.

PEDS – Not approved in children.

UNAPPROVED ADULT – Panic disorder: Start 25 mg PO at bedtime, titrate to usual effective dose of 50 to 150 mg/day. Smoking cessation: Start 25 mg PO daily 14 days prior to quit date. Titrate to 75 mg/day as tolerated. Continue for 6 weeks or more after quit date. Chronic pain: Start 10 to 25 mg PO q am or at bedtime. Max 150 mg/day.

UNAPPROVED PEDS – Depression, age 6 to 12 yo: 1 to 3 mg/kg/day PO divided three to four times per day or 10 to 20 mg/day PO divided three to four times per day.

FORMS – Generic/Trade: Caps 10, 25, 50, 75 mg. Oral soln 10 mg/5 mL.

NOTES – Tricyclic, secondary amine; primarily inhibits norepinephrine reuptake. Usual therapeutic range is 50 to 150 ng/mL. May cause fewer anticholinergic side effects than tertiary amines. May be used in combination with nicotine replacement for smoking cessation.

PROTRIPTYLINE (*Vivactil*) ▶L ♀C ▶+ $$$$

ADULT – Depression: 15 to 40 mg/day PO divided three to four times per day. Maximum dose is 60 mg/day.

PEDS – Not approved in children.

FORMS – Trade only: Tabs 5, 10 mg.

NOTES – Tricyclic, secondary amine; primarily inhibits norepinephrine reuptake. May cause fewer anticholinergic side effects than tertiary amines. Dose increases should be made in the morning.

TRIMIPRAMINE (*Surmontil*) ▶L ♀C ▶? $$$$

ADULT – Depression: Start 25 mg PO at bedtime; gradually increase to 75 to 150 mg/day. Max 300 mg/day.

PEDS – Not approved in children.

FORMS – Trade only: Caps 25, 50, 100 mg.

NOTES – Tricyclic, tertiary amine—primarily inhibits norepinephrine reuptake.

VILAZODONE (*Viibryd*) ▶L – ♀C ▶?

ADULT – Major depressive disorder: Start 10 mg PO once daily for 7 days. Then increase to 20 mg/day for another 7 days; then increase to target dose of 40 mg/day.

PEDS – Not approved for use in children.

FORMS – Trade only: Tabs 10, 20, 40 mg.

NOTES – Give this medication with food. Bioavailability is reduced up to 50% if taken on empty stomach.

PSYCHIATRY: Antidepressants—Monoamine Oxidase Inhibitors (MAOIs)

NOTE: May interfere with sleep; avoid at bedtime dosing. Must be on tyramine-free diet throughout treatment, and for 2 weeks after discontinuation. Numerous drug interactions; risk of hypertensive crisis and serotonin syndrome with many medications, including OTC. Allow at least 2 weeks wash-out when converting from an MAOI to an SSRI (6 weeks after fluoxetine), TCA, or other antidepressant. Contraindicated with carbamazepine or oxcarbazepine. Antidepressants increase the risk of suicidal thinking and behavior in children, adolescents, and young adults; carefully weigh the risks and benefits before starting and monitor patients closely.

ISOCARBOXAZID (*Marplan*) ▶L ♀C ▶? $$$

ADULT – Depression: Start 10 mg PO two times per day; increase by 10 mg q 2 to 4 days. Usual effective dose is 20 to 40 mg/day. Max 60 mg/day divided two to four times per day.

PEDS – Not approved in children younger than 16 yo.

FORMS – Trade only: Tabs 10 mg.

NOTES – Requires MAOI diet.

♣ **MOCLOBEMIDE** ▶L ♀C ▶– $$

ADULT – Canada only. Depression: Start 300 mg/day PO divided two times per day after meals. May increase after 1 week to max 600 mg/day.

PEDS – Not approved in children.

FORMS – Generic/Trade: Tabs 150, 300 mg. Generic only: Tabs 100 mg.

NOTES – No dietary restrictions. Do not use with TCAs; use caution with conventional MAOIs, other antidepressants, epinephrine, thioridazine, sympathomimetics, dextromethorphan, meperidine, and other opiates. Reduce dose in severe hepatic dysfunction.

PHENELZINE (*Nardil*) ▶L ♀C ▶? $$$

ADULT – Depression: Start 15 mg PO three times per day. Usual effective dose is 60 to 90 mg/day in divided doses.

PEDS – Not approved in children younger than 16 yo.

FORMS – Trade only: Tabs 15 mg.

NOTES – Requires MAOI diet. May increase insulin sensitivity. Contraindicated with meperidine.

SELEGILINE—TRANSDERMAL (*Emsam*) ▶L ♀C ▶? $$$$$

ADULT – Depression: Start 6 mg/24 h patch q 24 h. Adjust dose in 2-week intervals or more to max 12 mg/24 h.

PEDS – Not approved in children.

FORMS – Trade only: Transdermal patch 6 mg/day, 9 mg/24 h, 12 mg/24 h.

NOTES – MAOI diet is required for doses 9 mg/day or higher. Intense urges (eg, gambling and sexual) have been reported. Consider discontinuing the medication or reducing the dose if these occur.

TRANYLCYPROMINE (*Parnate*) ▶L ♀C ▶– $$

ADULT – Depression: Start 10 mg PO q am; increase by 10 mg/day at 1- to 3-week intervals to usual effective dose of 10 to 40 mg/day divided two times per day. Max 60 mg/day.

PEDS – Not approved in children younger than 16 yo.

FORMS – Generic/Trade: Tabs 10 mg.

NOTES – Requires MAOI diet.

PSYCHIATRY: Antidepressants—Selective Serotonin Reuptake Inhibitors (SSRIs)

NOTE: Gradually taper when discontinuing SSRIs to avoid withdrawal symptoms. Observe patients for worsening depression or the emergence of suicidality, anxiety, agitation, panic attacks, insomnia, irritability, hostility, impulsivity, akathisia, mania, or hypomania, particularly early in therapy or after increases in dose. Antidepressants increase the risk of suicidal thinking and behavior in children, adolescents, and young adults; carefully weigh the risks and benefits before starting treatment and then monitor patients closely. Use of SSRIs during the third trimester of pregnancy has been associated with neonatal complications including respiratory (including persistent pulmonary HTN), GI, and feeding problems, as well as seizures and withdrawal symptoms. Balance these risks against those of withdrawal and depression for the mother. Paroxetine should be avoided throughout pregnancy. Do not use sibutramine with SSRIs. Increased risk of abnormal bleeding; use caution when combined with NSAIDs or aspirin. SSRIs have been associated with serotonin syndrome and neuroleptic malignant syndrome. Use cautiously and observe closely for serotonin syndrome if SSRI is used with a triptan or other serotonergic drugs. SSRIs and SNRIs have been associated with hyponatremia, which is often associated with SIADH. The elderly and those taking diuretics may be at increased risk.

CITALOPRAM (*Celexa*) ▶LK ♀C but – in third trimester ▶– $$$

ADULT – Depression: Start 20 mg PO daily. May increase after 1 or more weeks to max 40 mg PO daily or 20 mg daily if older than 60 yo.

PEDS – Not approved in children.

FORMS – Generic/Trade: Tabs 10, 20, 40 mg. Oral soln 10 mg/5 mL. Generic only: Oral disintegrating tab 10, 20, 40 mg.

NOTES – Do not use with MAOIs or tryptophan.

ESCITALOPRAM (*Lexapro*, ✤ *Cipralex*) ▶LK ♀C but - in 3rd trimester ▶– $$$

ADULT – Depression, generalized anxiety disorder: Start 10 mg PO daily; may increase to max 20 mg PO daily after 1st week.

PEDS – Depression, age 12 yo and older: Start 10 mg PO daily. May increase to max 20 mg/day.

UNAPPROVED ADULT – Social anxiety disorder: 5 to 20 mg PO daily.

FORMS – Generic/Trade: Tabs 5, 10, 20 mg. Trade only: Oral soln 1 mg/mL.

NOTES – Do not use with MAOIs. Doses greater than 20 mg daily have not been shown to be superior to 10 mg daily. Escitalopram is the active isomer of citalopram.

FLUOXETINE (*Prozac, Prozac Weekly, Sarafem*) ▶L ♀C but – in 3rd trimester ▶– $$$

ADULT – Depression, OCD: Start 20 mg PO q am; may increase after several weeks to usual effective dose of 20 to 40 mg/day, max 80 mg/day. Depression, maintenance therapy: 20 to 40 mg/day (standard-release) or 90 mg PO once weekly (Prozac Weekly) starting 7 days after last standard-release dose. Bulimia: 60 mg PO q am; may need to titrate up to this dose slowly over several days. Panic disorder: Start 10 mg PO q am; titrate to 20 mg/day after 1 week, max 60 mg/day. Premenstrual dysphoric disorder (Sarafem): 20 mg PO daily given continuously throughout the menstrual cycle (continuous dosing) or 20 mg PO daily for 14 days prior to menses (intermittent dosing); max 80 mg daily. Doses greater than

(cont.)

FLUOXETINE (*cont.*)

20 mg/day can be divided two times per day (in morning and at noon). Bipolar depression, olanzapine plus fluoxetine: Start 5 mg olanzapine plus 20 mg fluoxetine daily in the evening. Increase to usual range of 5 to 12.5 mg olanzapine plus 20 to 50 mg fluoxetine as tolerated. Treatment-resistant depression, olanzapine plus fluoxetine: Start 5 mg olanzapine plus 20 mg fluoxetine daily in the evening. Increase to usual range of 5 to 20 mg olanzapine plus 20 to 50 mg fluoxetine as tolerated.

PEDS – Depression, age 7 to 17 yo: 10 to 20 mg PO q am (10 mg for smaller children), max 20 mg/day. OCD: Start 10 mg PO q am, max 60 mg/day (30 mg/day for smaller children).

UNAPPROVED ADULT – Hot flashes: 20 mg PO daily. Posttraumatic stress disorder: 20 to 80 mg PO daily. Social anxiety disorder: 10 to 60 mg PO daily.

FORMS – Generic/Trade: Tabs 10 mg. Caps 10, 20, 40 mg. Oral soln 20 mg/5 mL. Caps (Sarafem) 10, 20 mg. Trade only: Tabs (Sarafem) 10, 15, 20 mg. Caps delayed-release (Prozac Weekly) 90 mg. Generic only: Tabs 20, 40 mg.

NOTES – Half-life of parent is 1 to 3 days and for active metabolite norfluoxetine is 6 to 14 days. Do not use with thioridazine, MAOIs, cisapride, or tryptophan; use caution with lithium, phenytoin, TCAs, and warfarin. Pregnancy exposure has been associated with premature delivery, low birth wt, and lower Apgar scores. Decrease dose with liver disease. Increases risk of mania with bipolar disorder.

FLUVOXAMINE (*Luvox, Luvox CR*) ▶L ♀C but – in third trimester ▶– $$$$

ADULT – OCD: Start 50 mg PO at bedtime, then increase by 50 mg/day q 4 to 7 days to usual effective dose of 100 to 300 mg/day divided two times per day. Max 300 mg/day.

PEDS – OCD (children age 8 yo or older): Start 25 mg PO at bedtime; increase by 25 mg/day q 4 to 7 days to usual effective dose of 50 to 200 mg/day divided two times per day. Max 200 mg/day (8 to 11 yo) or 300 mg/day (older than 11 yo). Therapeutic effect may be seen with lower doses in girls.

FORMS – Generic/Trade: Tabs 25, 50, 100 mg. Trade only: Caps extended-release 100, 150 mg.

NOTES – Do not use with thioridazine, pimozide, alosetron, cisapride, tizanidine, tryptophan, or MAOIs; use caution with benzodiazepines, theophylline, TCAs, and warfarin. Luvox brand not currently on US market.

PAROXETINE (*Paxil, Paxil CR, Pexeva*) ▶LK ♀D ▶? $$$

ADULT – Depression: Start 20 mg PO q am; increase by 10 mg/day at intervals of 1 week or more to usual effective dose of 20 to 50 mg/day, max 50 mg/day. Depression, controlled-release tabs: Start 25 mg PO q am; may increase by 12.5 mg/day at intervals of 1 week or more to usual effective dose of 25 to 62.5 mg/day; max 62.5 mg/day. OCD: Start 20 mg PO q am; increase by 10 mg/day at intervals of 1 week or more to usual recommended dose of 40 mg/day; max 60 mg/day. Panic disorder: Start 10 mg PO q am; increase by 10 mg/day at intervals of 1 week or more to target dose of 40 mg/day; max 60 mg/day. Panic disorder, controlled-release tabs: Start 12.5 mg/day; increase by 12.5 mg/day at intervals of 1 week or more to usual effective dose of 12.5 to 75 mg/day; max 75 mg/day. Social anxiety disorder: Start 20 mg PO q am (which is the usual effective dose); max 60 mg/day. Social anxiety disorder, controlled-release tabs: Start 12.5 mg PO q am; may increase at intervals of 1 week or more to max 37.5 mg/day. Generalized anxiety disorder: Start 20 mg PO q am (which is the usual effective dose); max 50 mg/day. Posttraumatic stress disorder: Start 20 mg PO q am; usual effective dose is 20 to 40 mg/day; max 50 mg/day. Premenstrual dysphoric disorder (PMDD), continuous dosing: Start 12.5 mg PO q am (controlled-release tabs); may increase dose after 1 week to max 25 mg q am. PMDD, intermittent dosing (given for 2 weeks prior to menses): Start 12.5 mg PO q am (controlled-release tabs), max 25 mg/day.

PEDS – Not recommended for use in children or adolescents due to increased risk of suicidality.

UNAPPROVED ADULT – Hot flashes related to menopause or breast cancer: 20 mg PO daily (tabs), or 12.5 to 25 mg PO daily (controlled-release tabs).

FORMS – Generic/Trade: Tabs 10, 20, 30, 40 mg. Oral susp 10 mg/5 mL. Controlled-release tabs 12.5, 25 mg. Trade only: (Paxil CR) 37.5 mg.

NOTES – Start at 10 mg/day and do not exceed 40 mg/day in elderly or debilitated patients or those with renal or hepatic impairment. Paroxetine is an inhibitor of CYP2D6, and is contraindicated with thioridazine, pimozide, MAOIs, linezolid,and tryptophan; use caution with barbiturates, cimetidine, phenytoin, theophylline, TCAs, risperidone, atomoxetine, and warfarin. Taper gradually after long-term use; reduce by 10 mg/day q week to 20 mg/day;

(cont.)

PAROXETINE (*cont.*)

continue for 1 week at this dose, and then stop. If withdrawal symptoms develop, then restart at prior dose and taper more slowly. Pexeva is paroxetine mesylate and is a generic equivalent for paroxetine HCl. Some data suggest paroxetine may reduce the efficacy of tamoxifen. Avoid the combination if possible.

SERTRALINE (*Zoloft*) ▶LK ♀C but – in third trimester ▶+ $$$

ADULT – Depression, OCD: Start 50 mg PO daily; may increase after 1 week. Usual effective dose is 50 to 200 mg/day, max 200 mg/day. Panic disorder, posttraumatic stress disorder, social anxiety disorder: Start 25 mg PO daily; may increase after 1 week to 50 mg PO daily. Usual effective dose is 50 to 200 mg/day; max 200 mg/day. PMDD, continuous dosing: Start 50 mg PO daily; max 150 mg/day. PMDD, intermittent dosing (given for 14 days prior to menses): Start 50 mg PO daily for 3 days, then increase to max 100 mg/day.

PEDS – OCD, age 6 to 12 yo: Start 25 mg PO daily, max 200 mg/day. OCD, age 13 yo or older: Use adult dosing.

UNAPPROVED PEDS – Major depressive disorder: Start 25 mg PO daily; usual effective dose is 50 to 200 mg/day.

FORMS – Generic/Trade: Tabs 25, 50, 100 mg. Oral concentrate 20 mg/mL (60 mL).

NOTES – Do not use with cisapride, tryptophan, or MAOIs; use caution with cimetidine, warfarin, pimozide, or TCAs. Must dilute oral concentrate before administration. Administration during pregnancy has been associated with premature delivery, low birth wt, and lower Apgar scores.

PSYCHIATRY: Antidepressants—Serotonin-Norepinephrine Reuptake Inhibitors (SNRIs)

NOTE: Monitor for the emergence of anxiety, agitation, panic attacks, insomnia, irritability, hostility, impulsivity, akathisia, mania, or hypomania, and for worsening depression or the emergence of suicidality, particularly early in therapy or after increases in dose. Antidepressants increase the risk of suicidal thinking and behavior in children, adolescents, and young adults; carefully weigh the risks and benefits before starting treatment, and then monitor closely. SSRIs and SNRIs have been associated with hyponatremia, which is often associated with SIADH. The elderly and those taking diuretics may be at increased risk. Do not use with MAOIs. SNRIs have been associated with serotonin syndrome and neuroleptic malignant syndrome when used alone and especially in combination with other serotonergic drugs.

DESVENLAFAXINE (*Pristiq*) ▶LK ♀C ▶? $$$$

ADULT – Depression: 50 mg PO daily. Max 400 mg/day.

PEDS – Not approved for use in children.

FORMS – Trade only: Tabs extended-release 50, 100 mg.

NOTES – There is no evidence that doses greater than 50 mg/day offer additional benefit. Reduce dose to 50 mg PO every other day in severe renal impairment (CrCl less than 30 mL/min). Caution in cardiovascular, cerebrovascular, or lipid disorders. Gradually taper when discontinuing therapy to avoid withdrawal symptoms after prolonged use. Exposure to SSRIs or SNRIs during the 3rd trimester of pregnancy has been associated with neonatal complications including respiratory, GI, and feeding problems, as well as seizures and withdrawal symptoms. Balance these risks against those of withdrawal and depression for the mother.

DULOXETINE (*Cymbalta*) ▶L ♀C ▶? $$$$

ADULT – Depression: 20 mg PO two times per day; max 60 mg/day given once daily or divided two times per day. Generalized anxiety disorder: Start 30 to 60 mg PO daily, max 120 mg/day. Diabetic peripheral neuropathic pain: 60 mg PO daily, max 60 mg/day. Fibromyalgia: Start 30 to 60 mg PO daily, max 60 mg/day.

PEDS – Not approved in children.

FORMS – Trade only: Caps 20, 30, 60 mg.

NOTES – Avoid in renal insufficiency (CrCl less than 30 mL/min), hepatic insufficiency, or substantial alcohol use. Do not use with thioridazine, MAOIs, or potent inhibitors of CYP1A2; use caution with inhibitors of CYP2D6. Small BP increases have been observed. Exposure during the 3rd trimester of pregnancy has been associated with neonatal complications including respiratory, GI, and feeding problems, as well as seizures and withdrawal symptoms; balance these risks against those of withdrawal and depression for the mother.

VENLAFAXINE (*Effexor, Effexor XR*) ▶LK ♀C but – in 3rd trimester ▶? $$$$

ADULT – Depression: Start 37.5 to 75 mg PO daily (Effexor XR) or 75 mg/day divided two to three times per day (Effexor). Increase in 75-mg increments q 4 days to usual effective dose of 150 to 225 mg/day, max 225 mg/day (Effexor XR) or 375 mg/day (Effexor).

(cont.)

VENLAFAXINE (*cont.*)

Generalized anxiety disorder: Start 37.5 to 75 mg PO daily (Effexor XR); increase in 75-mg increments q 4 days to max 225 mg/day. Social anxiety disorder: 75 mg PO daily (Effexor XR). Panic disorder: Start 37.5 mg PO daily (Effexor XR), may titrate by 75 mg/day at weekly intervals to max 225 mg/day.

PEDS – Not approved in children. May increase the risk of suicidality in children and teenagers.

UNAPPROVED ADULT – Hot flashes (primarily in cancer patients): 37.5 to 75 mg/day of the extended-release form.

FORMS – Generic/Trade: Caps extended-release 37.5, 75, 150 mg. Tabs 25, 37.5, 50, 75, 100 mg. Generic only: Tabs extended-release 37.5, 75, 150, 225 mg.

NOTES – Noncyclic, serotonin-norepinephrine reuptake inhibitor (SNRI). Decrease dose in renal or hepatic impairment. Monitor for increases in BP. Do not give with MAOIs; use caution with cimetidine and haloperidol. Use caution and monitor for serotonin syndrome if used with triptans. Gradually taper when discontinuing therapy to avoid withdrawal symptoms after prolonged use. Hostility, suicidal ideation, and self-harm have been reported when used in children. Exposure during the 3rd trimester of pregnancy has been associated with neonatal complications including respiratory, GI, and feeding problems, as well as seizures and withdrawal symptoms. Balance these risks against those of withdrawal and depression for the mother. Mydriasis and increased intraocular pressure can occur; use caution in glaucoma.

PSYCHIATRY: Antidepressants—Other

NOTE: Monitor for the emergence of anxiety, agitation, panic attacks, insomnia, irritability, hostility, impulsivity, akathisia, mania, or hypomania, and for worsening depression or the emergence of suicidality, particularly early in therapy or after increases in dose. Antidepressants increase the risk of suicidal thinking and behavior in children, adolescents, and young adults; carefully weigh the risks and benefits before starting treatment, and then monitor closely.

BUPROPION (***Wellbutrin, Wellbutrin SR, Wellbutrin XL, Aplenzin, Zyban, Buproban***) ▶LK ♀C ▶– $$$$

ADULT – Depression: Start 100 mg PO two times per day (immediate-release tabs); can increase to 100 mg three times per day after 4 to 7 days. Usual effective dose is 300 to 450 mg/day, max 150 mg/dose and 450 mg/day. Depression, sustained-release tabs (Wellbutrin SR): Start 150 mg PO q am; may increase to 150 mg two times per day after 4 to 7 days, max 400 mg/day. Give the last dose no later than 5 pm. Depression, extended-release tabs (Wellbutrin XL): Start 150 mg PO q am; may increase to 300 mg q am after 4 days, max 450 mg q am. Depression, extended-release (Aplenzin): Start 174 mg PO q am; increase to target dose of 348 mg/day after 4 days or more. May increase to max dose of 522 mg/day after 4 weeks or more. Seasonal affective disorder, extended-release tabs (Wellbutrin XL): Start 150 mg PO q am in autumn; may increase after 1 week to target dose of 300 mg q am, max 300 mg/day. In the spring, decrease to 150 mg/day for 2 weeks and then discontinue. Smoking cessation (Zyban, Buproban): Start 150 mg PO q am for 3 days, then increase to 150 mg PO two times per day for 7 to 12 weeks. Allow 8 h between doses, with the last dose given no later than 5 pm. Max 150 mg PO two times per day. Target quit date should be after at least 1 week of therapy. Stop if there is no progress toward abstinence by the 7th week. Write "dispense behavioral modification kit" on first script.

PEDS – Not approved in children.

UNAPPROVED ADULT – ADHD: 150 to 450 mg/day PO.

UNAPPROVED PEDS – ADHD: 1.4 to 5.7 mg/kg/day PO.

FORMS – Generic/Trade (for depression, bupropion HCl): Tabs 75, 100 mg. Sustained-release tabs 100, 150, 200 mg. Extended-release tabs 150, 300 mg (Wellbutrin XL). Generic/Trade (Smoking cessation): Sustained-release tabs 150 mg (Zyban, Buproban). Trade only: Extended-release (Aplenzin, bupropion hydrobromide) tabs 174, 348, 522 mg.

NOTES – Weak inhibitor of dopamine reuptake. Do not use with MAOIs. Seizures occur in 0.4% of patients taking 300 to 450 mg/day. Contraindicated in seizure disorders, eating disorders, or with abrupt alcohol or sedative withdrawal. Wellbutrin SR, Zyban, and Buproban are all the same formulation. Equivalent doses: 174 HBr = 150 mg HCl, 348 mg HBr = 300 mg HCl, 522 mg HBr = 450

(cont.)

BUPROPION (*cont.*)

mg HCl. Consider dose reductions for hepatic and renal impairment. Has been associated with false-positive urine test results for amphetamines when using immunoassay procedures.

MIRTAZAPINE (***Remeron, Remeron SolTab***) ▶LK ♀C ▶? $$

ADULT – Depression: Start 15 mg PO at bedtime, increase after 1 to 2 weeks to usual effective dose of 15 to 45 mg/day.

PEDS – Not approved in children.

FORMS – Generic/Trade: Tabs 15, 30, 45 mg. Tabs orally disintegrating (SolTab) 15, 30, 45 mg. Generic only: Tabs 7.5 mg.

NOTES – 0.1% risk of agranulocytosis. May cause drowsiness, increased appetite, and wt gain. Do not use with MAOIs.

NEFAZODONE ▶L ♀C ▶? $$$

WARNING – Rare reports of life-threatening liver failure. Discontinue if signs or symptoms of liver dysfunction develop. Brand name product withdrawn from the market in the United States and Canada.

ADULT – Depression: Start 100 mg PO two times per day. Increase by 100 to 200 mg/day at 1-week intervals or longer to usual effective dose of 150 to 300 mg PO two times per day, max 600 mg/day. Start 50 mg PO two times per day in elderly or debilitated patients.

PEDS – Not approved in children.

FORMS – Generic only: Tabs 50, 100, 150, 200, 250 mg.

NOTES – Do not use with cisapride, MAOIs, pimozide, or triazolam; use caution with alprazolam. Many other drug interactions.

TRAZODONE (***Desyrel, Oleptro***) ▶L ♀C ▶– $

ADULT – Depression: Start 50 to 150 mg/day PO in divided doses, increase by 50 mg/day q 3 to 4 days. Usual effective dose is 400 to 600 mg/day. Extended release: Start 150 mg PO at bedtime. May increase by 75 mg/day q 3 days to max 375 mg/day.

PEDS – Not approved in children.

UNAPPROVED ADULT – Insomnia: 50 to 100 mg PO at bedtime, max 150 mg/day.

UNAPPROVED PEDS – Depression, 6 to 18 yo: Start 1.5 to 2 mg/kg/day PO divided two to three times per day; may increase q 3 to 4 days to max 6 mg/kg/day.

FORMS – Trade only: Extended release tabs (Oleptro) 150, 300 mg. Generic only: Tabs 50, 100, 150, 300 mg.

NOTES – May cause priapism. Rarely used as monotherapy for depression; most often used as a sleep aid and adjunct to another antidepressant. Use caution with CYP3A4 inhibitors or inducers.

♣**TRYPTOPHAN** ▶K ♀? ▶? $$

ADULT – Canada only. Adjunct to antidepressant treatment for affective disorders: 8 to 12 g/day in 3 to 4 divided doses.

PEDS – Not indicated.

FORMS – Trade only: L-tryptophan tabs 250, 500, 750, 1000 mg.

NOTES – Caution in diabetics; may worsen glycemic control.

PSYCHIATRY: Antimanic (Bipolar) Agents

LAMOTRIGINE (***Lamictal, Lamictal CD, Lamictal ODT, Lamictal XR***) ▶LK ♀C (see notes) ▶– $$$$

WARNING – Potentially life-threatening rashes (eg, Stevens-Johnson syndrome, toxic epidermal necrolysis) have been reported in 0.3% of adults and 0.8% of children, usually within 2 to 8 weeks of initiation; discontinue at first sign of rash. Drug interaction with valproate; see adjusted dosing guidelines. Recent data suggest an increased risk of suicidal ideation or behaviors with antiepileptic drugs. Monitor closely for signs of depression, anxiety, hostility, and hypomania/mania. Symptoms may develop within 1 week of initiation and risk continues through at least 24 weeks.

ADULT – Bipolar disorder (maintenance): Start 25 mg PO daily, 50 mg PO daily if on carbamazepine or other enzyme-inducing drugs, or 25 mg PO every other day if on valproate. Increase for weeks 3 to 4 to 50 mg/day, 50 mg twice per day if on enzyme-inducing drugs, or 25 mg/day if on valproate, then adjust over weeks 5 to 7 to target doses of 200 mg/day, 400 mg/day divided twice per day if on enzyme-inducing drugs, or 100 mg/day if on valproate. See Neurology section for epilepsy dosing.

PEDS – Not approved in children.

FORMS – Generic/Trade: Chewable dispersible tabs (Lamictal CD) 5, 25 mg. Tabs 25, 100, 150, 200 mg. Trade only: Orally disintegrating tabs (ODT) 25, 50, 100, 200 mg. Extended-release tabs (XR) 25, 50, 100, 200 mg.

NOTES – Drug interactions with valproate and enzyme-inducing antiepileptic drugs (ie, carbamazepine, phenobarbital, phenytoin, primidone); may need to adjust dose. May

(cont.)

LAMOTRIGINE (*cont.*)

increase carbamazepine toxicity. Preliminary evidence suggests that exposure during the 1st trimester of pregnancy is associated with a risk for cleft palate and/or cleft lip. Please report all fetal exposure to the Lamotrigine Pregnancy Registry (800-336-2176) and the North American Antiepileptic Drug Pregnancy Registry (888-233-2334).

LITHIUM (***Eskalith, Eskalith CR, Lithobid,*** ✤ ***Lithane***) ▶K ♀D ▶– $

WARNING – Lithium toxicity can occur at therapeutic levels.

ADULT – Acute mania: Start 300 to 600 mg PO two to three times per day; usual effective dose is 900 to 1800 mg/day. Bipolar maintenance: usually 900 to 1200 mg/day titrated to therapeutic trough level of 0.6 to 1.2 mEq/L.

PEDS – Age 12 yo or older: Use adult dosing.

UNAPPROVED PEDS – Mania (age younger than 12 yo): Start 15 to 60 mg/kg/day PO divided three to four times per day. Adjust weekly to achieve therapeutic levels.

FORMS – Generic/Trade: Caps 300, Extended-release tabs 300, 450 mg. Generic only: Caps 150, 600 mg, Tabs 300 mg, Syrup 300 mg/5 mL.

NOTES – Steady-state levels occur in 5 days (later in elderly or renally impaired patients). Usual therapeutic trough levels are 1.0 to 1.5 mEq/L (acute mania) or 0.6 to 1.2 mEq/L (maintenance). 300 mg = 8 mEq or mmol. A dose increase of 300 mg/day will increase the level by approx 0.2 mEq/L. Monitor renal and thyroid function, avoid dehydration or salt restriction, and watch closely for polydipsia or polyuria. Diuretics, ACE inhibitors, angiotensin receptor blockers, and NSAIDs may increase lithium levels (aspirin and sulindac OK). Dose-related side effects (eg, tremor, GI upset) may improve by dividing doses three to four times per day or using extended-release tabs. Monitor renal function and electrolytes.

TOPIRAMATE (***Topamax***) ▶K ♀D ▶? $$$$$

WARNING – Recent data suggest an increased risk of suicidal ideation or behaviors with antiepileptic drugs. Monitor closely for signs of depression, anxiety, hostility, and hypomania/mania. Symptoms may develop within 1 week of initiation and risk continues through at least 24 weeks.

ADULT – See Neurology section.

PEDS – Not approved for psychiatric use in children; see Neurology section.

UNAPPROVED ADULT – Bipolar disorder: Start 25 to 50 mg/day PO; titrate prn to max 400 mg/day divided two times per day. Alcohol dependence: Start 25 mg/day PO; titrate weekly to max 150 mg two times per day.

FORMS – Trade: Tabs 25, 50, 100, 200 mg. Sprinkle Caps 15, 25 mg.

NOTES – Give ½ usual adult dose to patients with renal impairment (CrCl less than 70 mL/min). Cognitive symptoms, confusion, renal stones, glaucoma, and wt loss may occur. Risk of oligohidrosis and hyperthermia, particularly in children; use caution in warm ambient temperatures and/or with vigorous physical activity. Hyperchloremic, nonanion gap metabolic acidosis may occur; monitor serum bicarbonate and reduce dose or taper off if this occurs. Report fetal exposure to North American Antiepileptic Drug Pregnancy Registry (888-233-2334).

VALPROIC ACID—PSYCH (***Depakote, Depakote ER, Stavzor,*** **divalproex,** ✤ ***Epival***) ▶L ♀D ▶+ $$$$

WARNING – Fatal hepatic failure has occurred, especially in children younger than 2 yo with multiple anticonvulsants and comorbidities. Monitor LFTs frequently during first 6 months. Life-threatening pancreatitis has been reported after initial or prolonged use. Evaluate for abdominal pain, N/V, and/or anorexia and discontinue if pancreatitis occurs. May be more teratogenic than other anticonvulsants (eg, carbamazepine, lamotrigine, and phenytoin). Hepatic failure and clotting disorders have also occurred when used during pregnancy. Recent data suggest an increased risk of suicidal ideation or behaviors with antiepileptic drugs. Monitor closely for signs of depression, anxiety, hostility, and hypomania/mania. Symptoms may develop within 1 week of initiation and risk continues through at least 24 weeks.

ADULT – Mania: Start 250 mg PO three times per day (Depakote or Stavzor) or 25 mg/kg once daily (Depakote ER); titrate to therapeutic level. Max 60 mg/kg/day.

PEDS – Not approved for mania in children.

UNAPPROVED PEDS – Bipolar disorder, manic or mixed phase (age older than 2 yo): Start 125 to 250 mg PO two times per day or 15 mg/kg/day in divided doses. Titrate to therapeutic trough level of 45 to 125 mcg/mL, max 60 mg/kg/day.

FORMS – Generic only: Syrup (Valproic acid) 250 mg/5 mL. Generic/Trade: Delayed-release tabs (Depakote) 125, 250, 500 mg. Extended-release tabs (Depakote ER) 250, 500 mg. Delayed-release sprinkle caps (Depakote)

(cont.)

VALPROIC ACID—PSYCH (*cont.*)

125 mg. Trade only (Stavzor): Delayed-release caps 125, 250, 500 mg.

NOTES – Contraindicated in urea cycle disorders or hepatic dysfunction. Reduce dose in the elderly. Recommended therapeutic trough level is 50 to 125 mcg/mL for Depakote and 85 to 125 mcg/mL for Depakote ER, though higher levels have been used. Many drug interactions. Hyperammonemia, GI irritation, or thrombocytopenia may occur. Depakote ER is approximately 10% less bioavailable than Depakote. Depakote releases divalproex sodium over 8 to 12 h (one to four times per day dosing) and Depakote ER releases divalproex sodium over 18 to 24 h (daily dosing).

PSYCHIATRY: Antipsychotics—First Generation (Typical)

NOTE: Antipsychotic potency is determined by affinity for D2 receptors. Extrapyramidal side effects (EPS) including tardive dyskinesia and dystonia may occur with antipsychotics. Use cautiously in patients with Parkinson's disease. High-potency agents are more likely to cause EPS and hyperprolactinemia. Can be given at bedtime, but may be divided initially to decrease side effects and daytime sedation. Antipsychotics have been associated with an increased risk of venous thromboembolism, especially early in therapy. Assess for other risk factors and monitor carefully. Off-label use for dementia-related psychosis in the elderly has been associated with increased mortality.

CHLORPROMAZINE (*Thorazine*) ▶LK ♀C ▶– $$$

ADULT – Psychotic disorders: 10 to 50 mg PO two to three times per day or 25 to 50 mg IM, can repeat in 1 h. Severe cases may require 400 mg IM q 4 to 6 h up to maximum of 2000 mg/day IM. Hiccups: 25 to 50 mg PO/IM three to four times per day. Persistent hiccups may require 25 to 50 mg in 0.5 to 1 liter NS by slow IV infusion.

PEDS – Severe behavioral problems/psychotic disorders age 6 mo to 12 yo: 0.5 mg/kg PO q 4 to 6 h prn or 1 mg/kg PR q 6 to 8 h prn or 0.5 mg/kg IM q 6 to 8 h prn.

FORMS – Generic only: Tabs 10, 25, 50, 100, 200 mg. Generic/Trade: Oral concentrate 30 mg/mL, 100 mg/mL. Trade only: Syrup 10 mg/5 mL, Supps 25, 100 mg.

NOTES – Monitor for hypotension with IM or IV use.

FLUPENTHIXOL (**flupentixol**, ✤ ***Fluanxol, Fluanxol Depot***) ▶? ♀? ▶– $$

ADULT – Canada only. Schizophrenia/psychosis: Tabs initial dose: 3 mg PO daily in divided doses, maintenance 3 to 12 mg daily in divided doses. IM initial dose 5 to 20 mg IM q 2 to 4 weeks, maintenance 20 to 40 mg q 2 to 4 weeks. Higher doses may be necessary in some patients.

PEDS – Not approved in children.

FORMS – Trade only: Tabs 0.5, 3 mg.

NOTES – Relatively nonsedating antipsychotic.

FLUPHENAZINE (***Prolixin***, ✤ ***Modecate***) ▶LK ♀C ▶? $$$

ADULT – Psychotic disorders: Start 0.5 to 10 mg/day PO divided q 6 to 8 h. Usual effective dose 1 to 20 mg/day. Max dose is 40 mg/day PO or 1.25 to 10 mg/day IM divided q 6 to 8 h. Max dose is 10 mg/day IM. May use long-acting formulations (enanthate/decanoate) when patients are stabilized on a fixed daily dose. Approximate conversion ratio: 12.5 to 25 mg IM/SC (depot) q 3 weeks is equivalent to 10 to 20 mg/day PO.

PEDS – Not approved in children.

FORMS – Generic/Trade: Tabs 1, 2.5, 5, 10 mg. Elixir 2.5 mg/5 mL. Oral concentrate 5 mg/mL.

NOTES – Do not mix oral concentrate with coffee, tea, cola, or apple juice.

HALOPERIDOL (***Haldol***) ▶LK ♀C ▶– $$

ADULT – Psychotic disorders, Tourette syndrome: 0.5 to 5 mg PO two to three times per day. Usual effective dose is 6 to 20 mg/day, maximum dose is 100 mg/day or 2 to 5 mg IM q 1 to 8 h prn. May use long-acting (depot) formulation when patients are stabilized on a fixed daily dose. Approximate conversion ratio: 100 to 200 mg IM (depot) q 4 weeks is equivalent to 10 mg/day PO haloperidol.

PEDS – Psychotic disorders, age 3 to 12 yo: 0.05 to 0.15 mg/kg/day PO divided two to three times per day. Tourette syndrome or nonpsychotic behavior disorders, age 3 to 12 yo: 0.05 to 0.075 mg/kg/day PO divided two to three times per day. Increase dose by 0.5 mg q week to max dose of 6 mg/day. Not approved for IM administration in children.

UNAPPROVED ADULT – Acute psychosis and combative behavior: 5 to 10 mg IV/IM, repeat prn in 10 to 30 min. IV route associated with QT prolongation, torsades de pointes, and sudden death; use ECG monitoring.

UNAPPROVED PEDS – Psychosis age 6 to 12 yo: 1 to 3 mg/dose IM (as lactate) q 4 to 8 h, max 0.15 mg/kg/day.

(cont.)

HALOPERIDOL (*cont.*)

FORMS – Generic only: Tabs 0.5, 1, 2, 5, 10, 20 mg. Oral concentrate 2 mg/mL.

NOTES – Therapeutic range is 2 to 15 ng/mL.

LOXAPINE (***Loxitane***, ✤ ***Loxapac***) ▶LK ♀C ▶– $$$$

ADULT – Psychotic disorders: Start 10 mg PO two times per day, usual effective dose is 60 to 100 mg/day divided two to four times per day. Max dose is 250 mg/day.

PEDS – Not approved in children.

FORMS – Generic/Trade: Caps 5, 10, 25, 50 mg.

✤ **METHOTRIMEPRAZINE** ▶L ♀? ▶? $

ADULT – Canada only. Anxiety/analgesia: 6 to 25 mg PO per day given three times per day. Sedation: 10 to 25 mg bedtime. Psychoses, intense pain: Start 50 to 75 mg PO per day given in 2 to 3 doses, max 1000 mg/day. Postop pain: 20 to 40 mg PO or 10 to 25 mg IM q 8 h. Anesthesia premedication: 10 to 25 mg IM or 20 to 40 mg PO q 8 h with last dose of 25 to 50 mg IM 1 h before surgery. Limit therapy to less than 30 days.

PEDS – Canada only. 0.25 mg/kg/day given in 2 to 3 doses, max 40 mg/day for age younger than 12 yo.

FORMS – Canada only: Generic/Trade: Tabs 2, 5, 25, 50 mg.

MOLINDONE (***Moban***) ▶LK ♀C ▶? $$$$$

ADULT – Psychotic disorders: Start 50 to 75 mg/day PO divided three to four times per day, usual effective dose is 50 to 100 mg/day. Max dose is 225 mg/day.

PEDS – Adolescents: Adult dosing. Not approved in children younger than 12 yo.

FORMS – Trade only: Tabs 5, 10, 25, 50 mg. Drug no longer manufactured and only available while current supplies last.

ANTIPSYCHOTIC RELATIVE ADVERSE EFFECTS[a]

Generation	Antipyschotic	Anticholinergic	Sedation	Hypotension	EPS	Weight Gain	Diabetes/ Hyperglycemia	Dyslipidemia
1st	chlorpromazine	+++	+++	++	++	++	?	?
1st	fluphenazine	++	+	+	++++	++	?	?
1st	haloperidol	+	+	+	++++	++	0	?
1st	loxapine	++	+	+	++	+	?	?
1st	molindone	++	++	+	++	+	?	?
1st	perphenazine	++	++	+	++	+	+/?	?
1st	pimozide	+	+	+	+++	?	?	?
1st	thioridazine	++++	+++	+++	+	+++	+/?	?
1st	thiothixene	+	++	++	+++	++	?	/
1st	trifluoperazine	++	+	+	+++	++	?	?
2nd	aripiprazole	++	+	0	0	0/+	0	0
2nd	asenapine	+	+	++	++	+	?	?
2nd	clozapine	++++	+++	+++	0	+++	+	+
2nd	iloperidone	++	+	+++	+	++	?	?
2nd	olanzapine	+++	++	+	0[b]	+++	+	+
2nd	paliperidone	+	+	++	++	++	?	?
2nd	risperidone	+	++	+	+[b]	++	?	?
2nd	quetiapine	+	+++	++	0	++	?	?
2nd	ziprasidone	+	+	0	0	0/+	0	0

[a]Risk of specific adverse effects is graded from 0 (absent) to ++++ (high). ? = Limited or inconsistent comparative data.

[b]Extrapyramidal symptoms (EPS) are dose-related and are more likely for risperidone greater than 6 to 8 mg/day, olanzapine greater than 20 mg/day. Akathisia risk remains unclear and may not be reflected in these ratings. There are limited comparative data for aripiprazole iloperidone, paliperidone, and asenapine relative to other second-generation antipsychotics.

References: Goodman & Gilman 11e p461-500, *Applied Therapeutics* 8e p78, APA schizophrenia practice guideline, *Psychiatry Q* 2002; 73:297, *Diabetes Care* 2004;27:596, *Pharmacotherapy. A Pathophysiologic Approach*, 8. pg 1158, 2011.

PERPHENAZINE ▶LK ♀C ▶? $$$
ADULT – Psychotic disorders: Start 4 to 8 mg PO three times per day or 8 to 16 mg PO two to four times per day (hospitalized patients), max PO dose is 64 mg/day. Can give 5 to 10 mg IM q 6 h, max IM dose is 30 mg/day.
PEDS – Not approved in children.
FORMS – Generic only: Tabs 2, 4, 8, 16 mg. Oral concentrate 16 mg/5 mL.
NOTES – Do not mix oral concentrate with coffee, tea, cola, or apple juice.

PIMOZIDE (***Orap***) ▶L ♀C ▶– $$$
ADULT – Tourette syndrome: Start 1 to 2 mg/day PO in divided doses, increase q 2 days to usual effective dose of 1 to 10 mg/day. Max dose is 0.2 mg/kg/day up to 10 mg/day.
PEDS – Tourette syndrome: older than 12 yo: 0.05 mg/kg PO at bedtime, increase q 3 days to max 0.2 mg/kg/day up to 10 mg/day.
FORMS – Trade only: Tabs 1, 2 mg.
NOTES – QT prolongation may occur. Monitor ECG at baseline and periodically throughout therapy. Contraindicated with macrolide antibiotics, nefazodone, sertraline, citalopram, and escitalopram. Use caution with inhibitors of CYP3A4.

THIORIDAZINE (***Mellaril***) ▶LK ♀C ▶? $$
WARNING – Can cause QTc prolongation, torsade de pointes–type arrhythmias, and sudden death.
ADULT – Psychotic disorders: Start 50 to 100 mg PO three times per day, usual effective dose is 200 to 800 mg/day divided two to four times per day. Max dose is 800 mg/day.
PEDS – Behavioral disorders, 2 to 12 yo: 10 to 25 mg PO two to three times per day, max dose is 3 mg/kg/day.
FORMS – Generic only: Tabs 10, 15, 25, 50, 100, 150, 200 mg. Oral concentrate 30, 100 mg/mL.
NOTES – Not recommended as 1st-line therapy. Contraindicated in patients with a history of cardiac arrhythmias, congenital long QT syndrome, or those taking fluvoxamine, propranolol, pindolol, drugs that inhibit CYP2D6 (eg, fluoxetine, paroxetine), and other drugs that prolong the QTc interval. Only use for patients with schizophrenia who do not respond to other antipsychotics. Monitor baseline ECG and potassium. Pigmentary retinopathy with doses greater than 800 mg/day.

THIOTHIXENE (***Navane***) ▶LK ♀C ▶? $$$
ADULT – Psychotic disorders: Start 2 mg PO three times per day. Usual effective dose is 20 to 30 mg/day, max dose is 60 mg/day PO.
PEDS – Adolescents: Adult dosing. Not approved in children younger than 12 yo.
FORMS – Generic/Trade: Caps 1, 2, 5, 10. Oral concentrate 5 mg/mL. Trade only: Caps 20 mg.

TRIFLUOPERAZINE (***Stelazine***) ▶LK ♀C ▶– $$$
ADULT – Psychotic disorders: Start 2 to 5 mg PO two times per day. Usual effective dose is 15 to 20 mg/day; some patients may require 40 mg/day or more. Anxiety: 1 to 2 mg PO two times per day for up to 12 weeks. Max dose is 6 mg/day.
PEDS – Psychotic disorders, age 6 to 12 yo: 1 mg PO one to two times per day, gradually increase to max dose of 15 mg/day.
FORMS – Generic/Trade: Tabs 1, 2, 5, 10 mg. Trade only: Oral concentrate 10 mg/mL.
NOTES – Dilute oral concentrate just before giving.

♣**ZUCLOPENTHIXOL** (***Clopixol***) ▶L ♀? ▶? $$$$
ADULT – Canada only. Antipsychotic. Tabs: Start 10 to 50 mg PO daily, maintenance 20 to 60 mg daily. Injectable: Accuphase (acetate) 50 to 150 mg IM q 2 to 3 days, Depot (decanoate) 150 to 300 mg IM q 2 to 4 weeks.
PEDS – Not approved in children.
FORMS – Trade, Canada only: Tabs 10, 20 mg (Clopixol).

PSYCHIATRY: Antipsychotics—Second Generation (Atypical)

NOTE: Tardive dyskinesia, neuroleptic malignant syndrome, drug-induced parkinsonism, dystonia, and other extrapyramidal side effects may occur with antipsychotic medications. Atypical antipsychotics have been associated with wt gain, dyslipidemia, hyperglycemia, and diabetes mellitus; monitor closely. Off-label use for dementia-related psychosis in the elderly has been associated with increased mortality. Antipsychotics have been associated with an increased risk of venous thromboembolism, particularly early in therapy; assess for other risk factors and monitor carefully. Antipsychotics when used for schizophrenia or bipolar disorder have been associated with an increased risk of suicidal thinking and behavior. Monitor closely.

ARIPIPRAZOLE (***Abilify, Abilify Discmelt***) ▶L ♀C ▶? $$$$$
WARNING – Antipsychotics when used for schizophrenia or bipolar disorder have been

(cont.)

ARIPIPRAZOLE (*cont.*)

associated with an increased risk of suicidal thinking and behavior. Monitor closely.

ADULT – Schizophrenia: Start 10 to 15 mg PO daily. Max 30 mg daily. Bipolar disorder (acute and maintenance for manic or mixed episodes): Start 30 mg PO daily; reduce dose to 15 mg/day if higher dose poorly tolerated. 15 mg PO daily. May increase to 30 mg/day based on response and tolerability. Agitation associated with schizophrenia or bipolar disorder: 9.75 mg IM recommended. May consider 5.25 to 15 mg if indicated. May repeat after 2 h up to max 30 mg/day. Depression, adjunctive therapy: Start 2 to 5 mg PO daily. Increase by 5 mg/day at intervals of 1 week or more to max 15 mg/day.

PEDS – Schizophrenia, 13 to 17 yo: Start 2 mg PO daily. May increase to 5 mg/day after 2 days, and to target dose of 10 mg/day after 2 more days. Max 30 mg/day. Bipolar disorder (acute and maintenance for manic or mixed episodes, monotherapy or adjunctive to lithium or valproate), 10 to 17 yo: Start 2 mg PO daily. May increase to 5 mg/day after 2 days, and to target dose of 10 mg/day after 2 more days. Increase by 5 mg/day to max 30 mg/day. Irritability associated with autism: Start 2 mg PO daily. Increase by 5 mg/day prn up to max 15 mg/day.

FORMS – Trade only: Tabs 2, 5, 10, 15, 20, 30 mg. Oral soln 1 mg/mL (150 mL). Orally disintegrating tabs (Discmelt) 10, 15, 20, 30 mg.

NOTES – Low EPS and tardive dyskinesia risk. Increase dose when used with CYP3A4 inducers such as carbamazepine. Decrease usual dose by at least half when used with CYP3A4 or CYP2D6 inhibitors such as ketoconazole, fluoxetine, or paroxetine. Increase dose by ½ to 20 to 30 mg/day when used with CYP3A4 inducers such as carbamazepine. Reduce when inducer is stopped.

ASENAPINE (*Saphris*) ▶L ♀C ◗–

WARNING – Antipsychotics when used for schizophrenia or bipolar disorder have been associated with an increased risk of suicidal thinking and behavior. Monitor closely.

ADULT – Schizophrenia: Initial and maintenance, 5 mg sublingual two times per day. Max 10 mg/day. Bipolar disorder, acute manic or mixed episodes: Start 5 mg subligual two times per day (adjunctive) or 10 mg subligual two times per day (monotherapy). Max 20 mg/day.

PEDS – Not approved for use in children.

FORMS – Trade: Sublingual tabs 5, 10 mg.

NOTES – Must be used sublingually and not chewed or crushed.

CLOZAPINE (*Clozaril, FazaClo ODT*) ▶L ♀B ◗– $$$$$

WARNING – Risk of agranulocytosis is 1 to 2%, monitor WBC and ANC counts q week for 6 months, then q 2 weeks thereafter, and weekly for 4 weeks after discontinuation. Contraindicated if WBC less than 3500 or ANC less than 2000/mm^3. Discontinue if WBC less than 3000/mm^3. May decrease monitoring to q 4 weeks after 12 months if WBC greater than 3500/mm^3 and ANC greater than 2000/mm^3. See prescribing information for more details. Risk of myocarditis (particularly during the first month), seizures, orthostatic hypotension, and cardiopulmonary arrest. Antipsychotics when used for schizophrenia or bipolar disorder have been associated with an increased risk of suicidal thinking and behavior. Monitor closely.

ADULT – Severe, medically refractory schizophrenia or schizophrenia/schizoaffective disorder with suicidal behavior: Start 12.5 mg PO one or two times per day; increase by 25 to 50 mg/day to usual effective dose of 300 to 450 mg/day, max 900 mg/day. Retitrate if stopped for more than 3 to 4 days.

PEDS – Not approved in children.

FORMS – Generic/Trade: Tabs 25, 100 mg. Generic only: Tabs 12.5, 50, 200 mg. Trade only: Orally disintegrating tab (Fazaclo ODT) 12.5, 25, 100 mg (scored).

NOTES – Patients rechallenged with clozapine after an episode of leukopenia are at increased risk of agranulocytosis, and must undergo weekly monitoring for 12 months. Register all occurrences of leukopenia, discontinuation, and/or rechallenge to the Clozaril National Registry at 1-800-448-5938. Much lower risk of EPS and tardive dyskinesia than other neuroleptics. May be effective for treatment-resistant patients who have not responded to conventional agents. May cause significant wt gain, dyslipidemia, hyperglycemia, or new onset diabetes; monitor wt, fasting blood glucose, and triglycerides before initiation and at regular intervals during treatment. Excessive sedation or respiratory depression may occur when used with CNS depressants, particularly benzodiazepines. If an orally disintegrating tab is split, then discard the remaining portion.

ILOPERIDONE (*Fanapt*) ▶L ♀C ◗– ?

ADULT – Schizophrenia, acute: Start 1 mg PO two times per day. Increase to 2 mg PO two times per day on day 2, then increase total daily dose by 2 mg/dose each day to usual effective range of 6 to 12 mg PO two times per day. Max 24 mg/day.

(cont.)

ILOPERIDONE (*cont.*)

PEDS – Not approved in children.

FORMS – Trade: Tabs 1, 2, 4, 6, 8, 10, 12 mg.

NOTES – Dose must be titrated slowly to avoid orthostatic hypotension. Retitrate the dose if off the drug more than 3 days. Reduce dose by 50% if given with strong inhibitors of CYP2D6 or CYP3A4. Avoid use with other drugs that prolong the QT interval.

LURASIDONE (*Latuda*) ▶K – ♀B ▶?

ADULT – Schizophrenia: Start 40 mg PO daily. Effective dose range 40 to 120 mg/day, max 160 mg/day.

PEDS – Not approved for use in children.

FORMS – Trade only: Tabs 20, 40, 80, 120 mg.

NOTES – Max dose 40 mg/day in moderate to severe renal or hepatic insufficiency. Take with a meal of at least 350 Cal. Do not use with strong CYP3A4 inhibitors.

OLANZAPINE (*Zyprexa, Zyprexa Zydis, Zyprexa Relprevv*) ▶L ♀C ▶– $$$$$

WARNING – Antipsychotics when used for schizophrenia or bipolar disorder have been associated with an increased risk of suicidal thinking and behavior. Monitor closely.

ADULT – Agitation in acute bipolar mania or schizophrenia: Start 10 mg IM (2.5 to 5 mg in elderly or debilitated patients); may repeat after 2 h to max 30 mg/day. Schizophrenia, oral therapy: Start 5 to 10 mg PO daily. Increase weekly to usual effective dose of 10 to 15 mg/day, max 20 mg/day. Schizophrenia, extended-release injection: Dose based on prior oral dose and ranges from 150 mg to 300 mg deep IM (gluteal) q 2 weeks or 300 mg to 405 mg q 4 weeks. See prescribing information. Bipolar disorder, maintenance treatment or monotherapy for acute manic or mixed episodes: Start 10 to 15 mg PO daily. Increase by 5 mg/day at intervals after 24 h. Clinical efficacy seen at doses of 5 to 20 mg/day, max 20 mg/day. Bipolar disorder, adjunctive therapy for acute mixed or manic episodes: Start 10 mg PO daily; usual effective dose is 5 to 20 mg/day, max 20 mg/day. Bipolar depression, olanzapine plus fluoxetine: Start 5 mg olanzapine plus 20 mg fluoxetine daily in the evening. Increase to usual range of 5 to 12.5 mg olanzapine plus 20 to 50 mg fluoxetine as tolerated. Treatment-resistant depression, olanzapine plus fluoxetine: Start 5 mg olanzapine plus 20 mg fluoxetine daily in the evening. Increase to usual range of 5 to 20 mg olanzapine plus 20 to 50 mg fluoxetine as tolerated.

PEDS – Schizophrenia and bipolar manic or mixed episodes (13 to 17 yo): Start 2.5 to 5 mg PO once daily. Increase to target of 10 mg/day. Max 20 mg/day.

UNAPPROVED ADULT – Augmentation of SSRI therapy for OCD: Start 2.5 to 5 mg PO daily, max 20 mg/day. Posttraumatic stress disorder, adjunctive therapy: Start 5 mg PO daily, max 20 mg/day.

UNAPPROVED PEDS – Bipolar disorder, manic or mixed phase: Start 2.5 mg PO daily; increase by 2.5 mg/day q 3 days to max 20 mg/day.

FORMS – Generic/Trade: Tabs 2.5, 5, 7.5, 10, 15, 20 mg. Tabs orally disintegrating (Zyprexa Zydis) 5, 10, 15, 20 mg. Trade only: Long-acting injection (Zyprexa Relprevv) 210, 300, 405 mg/vial.

NOTES – Use for acute manic episodes associated with bipolar disorder. May cause significant wt gain, dyslipidemia, hyperglycemia, or new onset diabetes; monitor wt, fasting blood glucose, and triglycerides before initiation and at regular intervals during treatment. Monitor for orthostatic hypotension, particularly when given IM. IM injection can also be associated with bradycardia and hypoventilation especially if used with other drugs that have these effects. Use caution with benzodiazepines. Use of Zyprexa Relprevv requires registration in the Zyprexa Relprevv Patient Care Program 1-877-772-9390.

PALIPERIDONE (*Invega, Invega Sustenna*) ▶KL ♀C ▶– $$$$$

WARNING – Antipsychotics when used for schizophrenia or bipolar disorder have been associated with an increased risk of suicidal thinking and behavior. Monitor closely.

ADULT – Schizophrenia and schizoaffective disorder (adjunctive and monotherapy): Start 6 mg PO q am. 3 mg/day may be sufficient in some. Max 12 mg/day. Extended-release injection: Start 234 mg IM (deltoid) and then 156 mg IM 1 week later. Recommended monthly dose 117 mg IM (deltoid or gluteal) or within range of 36 to 234 mg based on response.

PEDS – Adolescents (12 to 17 yo): Start 3 mg PO once daily. Max 6 mg/day (weight less than 51 kg) or 12 mg/day (51 kg and greater). Not approved in children under 12 yo.

FORMS – Trade only: Extended-release tabs 1.5, 3, 6, 9 mg.

NOTES – Active metabolite of risperidone. For CrCl 50 to 79 mL/min start 3 mg/day with a max of 6 mg/day. For CrCl 10 to 50 mL/min start 1.5 mg/day with a max of 3 mg/day.

QUETIAPINE (***Seroquel, Seroquel XR***) ▶LK ♀C ▶– $$$$$

WARNING – Antipsychotics when used for schizophrenia or bipolar disorder have been associated with an increased risk of suicidal thinking and behavior. Monitor closely.

ADULT – Schizophrenia: Start 25 mg PO two times per day (regular tabs); increase by 25 to 50 mg two to three times per day on days 2 and 3, and then to target dose of 300 to 400 mg/day divided two to three times per day on day 4. Usual effective dose is 150 to 750 mg/day, max 800 mg/day. Schizophrenia, extended-release tabs: Start 300 mg PO daily in evening, increase by up to 300 mg/day at intervals of more than 1 day to usual effective range of 400 to 800 mg/day. Acute bipolar mania, monotherapy or adjunctive: Start 50 mg PO two times per day on day 1, then increase to no higher than 100 mg two times per day on day 2, 150 mg two times per day on day 3, and 200 mg two times per day on day 4. May increase prn to 300 mg two times per day on day 5 and 400 mg two times per day thereafter. Usual effective dose is 400 to 800 mg/day. Acute bipolar mania, monotherapy or adjunctive, extended-release: Start 300 mg PO in evening on day 1, 600 mg day 2, and 400 to 800 mg/day thereafter. Bipolar depression, regular and extended release: 50 mg, 100 mg, 200 mg, and 300 mg per day for days 1 to 4, respectively, administered at bedtime. May increase prn to 400 mg at bedtime on day 5 and 600 mg at bedtime on day 8. Bipolar maintenance: Use dose required to maintain remission of symptoms. Major depressive disorder, adjunctive to antidepressants, extended release: Start 50 mg evening of day 1, may increase to 150 mg on day 3. Max 300 mg/day.

PEDS – Schizophrenia (13 to 17 yo): Start 50 mg PO day 1, 100 mg day 2, 200 mg day 3, 300 mg day 4, and 400 mg day 5, all given two to three times per day. Recommended range 400 to 800 mg/day. Max 800 mg/day. Acute bipolar mania (10 to 17 yo): Start 50 mg PO day 1, 100 mg day 2, 200 mg day 3, 300 mg day 4, 400 mg day 5, all given two to three times per day. Recommended range 400 to 600 mg/day. Bipolar maintenance: Use dose required to maintain remission of symptoms.

UNAPPROVED ADULT – Augmentation of SSRI therapy for OCD: Start 25 mg PO two times per day, max 300 mg/day. Adjunctive for post-traumatic stress disorder: Start 25 mg daily, max 300 mg/day.

UNAPPROVED PEDS – Bipolar disorder (manic or mixed phase): Start 12.5 mg PO two times per day (children) or 25 mg PO two times per day (adolescents); max 150 mg PO three times per day.

FORMS – Trade only: Tabs 25, 50, 100, 200, 300, 400 mg. Extended-release tabs 50, 150, 200, 300, 400 mg.

NOTES – Eye exam for cataracts recommended q 6 months. Low risk of EPS and tardive dyskinesia. May cause significant wt gain, dyslipidemia, hyperglycemia, or new onset diabetes; monitor wt, fasting blood glucose, and triglycerides before initiation and at regular intervals during treatment. Use lower doses and slower titration in elderly patients or hepatic dysfunction. Extended-release tabs should be taken without food or after light meal.

RISPERIDONE (***Risperdal, Risperdal Consta***) ▶LK ♀C ▶– $$$$$

WARNING – Antipsychotics when used for schizophrenia or bipolar disorder have been associated with an increased risk of suicidal thinking and behavior. Monitor closely.

ADULT – Schizophrenia: Start 2 mg/day PO given once daily or divided two times per day; increase by 1 to 2 mg/day at intervals of 24 h or more. Start 0.5 mg/dose and titrate by no more than 0.5 mg two times per day in elderly, debilitated, hypotensive, or renally or hepatically impaired patients; increases to doses greater than 1.5 mg two times per day should occur at intervals of 1 week or more. Usual effective dose is 4 to 8 mg/day given once daily or divided two times per day; max 16 mg/day. Long-acting injection (Consta) for schizophrenia: Start 25 mg IM q 2 weeks while continuing oral dose for 3 weeks. May increase q 4 weeks to max 50 mg q 2 weeks. Bipolar mania: Start 2 to 3 mg PO daily; may adjust by 1 mg/day at 24-h intervals to max 6 mg/day.

PEDS – Autistic disorder irritability (5 to 16 yo): Start 0.25 mg (wt less than 20 kg) or 0.5 mg (wt 20 kg or greater) PO daily. May increase after 4 days to 0.5 mg/day (wt less than 20 kg) or 1.0 mg/day (wt 20 kg or greater). Maintain at least 14 days. May then increase at 14-day intervals or more by increments of 0.25 mg/day (wt less than 20 kg) or 0.5 mg/day (wt 20 kg or greater) to max 1.0 mg/day for wt less than 20 kg, max 2.5 mg/day for wt 20 to 44 kg or max 3.0 mg/day for wt greater than 45 kg. Schizophrenia (13 to 17 yo): Start 0.5 mg PO daily; increase by 0.5 to 1 mg/day at intervals of 24 h or more to target dose of 3 mg/day. Max 6 mg/day. Bipolar mania (10 to 17 yo): Start 0.5 mg PO daily; increase by 0.5 to 1

(cont.)

RISPERIDONE (*cont.*)

mg/day at intervals of 24 h or more to recommended dose of 2.5 mg/day. Max 6 mg/day.

UNAPPROVED ADULT – Augmentation of SSRI therapy for OCD: Start 1 mg/day PO, max 6 mg/day. Adjunctive therapy for posttraumatic stress disorder: Start 0.5 mg PO at bedtime, max 3 mg/day.

UNAPPROVED PEDS – Psychotic disorders, mania, aggression: 0.5 to 1.5 mg/day PO.

FORMS – Generic/Trade: Tabs 0.25, 0.5, 1, 2, 3, 4 mg. Oral soln 1 mg/mL (30 mL). Orally disintegrating tabs 0.5, 1, 2, 3, 4 mg. Generic only: Orally disintegrating tabs 0.25 mg.

NOTES – Has a greater tendency to produce extrapyramidal side effects (EPS) than other atypical antipsychotics. EPS reported in neonates following use in third trimester of pregnancy. May cause wt gain, hyperglycemia, or new onset diabetes; monitor closely. Patients with Parkinson's disease and dementia have increased sensitivity to side effects such as EPS, confusion, falls, and neuroleptic malignant syndrome. Soln is compatible with water, coffee, orange juice, and low-fat milk; is not compatible with cola or tea. Place orally disintegrating tabs on tongue and do not chew. Establish tolerability with oral form before starting long-acting injection. Alternate injections between buttocks. May also give in deltoid.

ZIPRASIDONE (***Geodon***, ***✤ Zeldox***) ▶L ♀C ▶– $$$$$

WARNING – May prolong QTc. Avoid with drugs that prolong QTc or in those with long QT syndrome or cardiac arrhythmias. Antipsychotics when used for schizophrenia or bipolar disorder have been associated with an increased risk of suicidal thinking and behavior. Monitor closely.

ADULT – Schizophrenia: Start 20 mg PO two times per day with food; may increase at greater than 2-day intervals to max 80 mg PO two times per day. Acute agitation in schizophrenia: 10 to 20 mg IM. May repeat 10 mg dose q 2 h or 20 mg dose q 4 h, to max 40 mg/day. Bipolar mania: Start 40 mg PO two times per day with food; may increase to 60 to 80 mg two times per day on day 2. Usual effective dose is 40 to 80 mg two times per day.

PEDS – Not approved in children.

FORMS – Trade only: Caps 20, 40, 60, 80 mg, Susp 10 mg/mL.

NOTES – Drug interactions with carbamazepine and ketoconazole.

PSYCHIATRY: Anxiolytics/Hypnotics—Barbiturates

BUTABARBITAL (***Butisol***) ▶LK ♀D ▶?©III $$$

ADULT – Rarely used; other drugs preferred. Sedative: 15 to 30 mg PO three to four times per day. Hypnotic: 50 to 100 mg PO at bedtime for up to 2 weeks.

PEDS – Preop sedation: 2 to 6 mg/kg PO before procedure, max 100 mg.

FORMS – Trade only: Tabs 30, 50 mg. Elixir 30 mg/5 mL.

MEPHOBARBITAL (***Mebaral***) ▶LK ♀D ▶?©IV $$$

ADULT – Rarely used; other drugs preferred. Sedative: 32 to 100 mg PO three to four times per day, usual dose is 50 mg PO three to four times per day.

PEDS – Sedative: 16 to 32 mg PO three to four times per day.

FORMS – Trade only: Tabs 32, 50, 100 mg.

SECOBARBITAL (***Seconal***) ▶LK ♀D ▶+©II $

ADULT – Rarely used; other drugs preferred. Hypnotic: 100 mg PO at bedtime for up to 2 weeks.

PEDS – Pre-anesthetic: 2 to 6 mg/kg PO up to 100 mg.

FORMS – Trade only: Caps 100 mg.

TUINAL **(amobarbital + secobarbital)** ▶LK ♀D ▶?©II $$

ADULT – Rarely used; other drugs preferred. Hypnotic: 1 cap PO at bedtime.

PEDS – Not approved in children.

FORMS – Trade only: Caps 100 (50 mg amobarbital + 50 mg secobarbital).

PSYCHIATRY: Anxiolytics/Hypnotics—Benzodiazepines—Long Half-Life (25–100 h)

NOTE: To avoid withdrawal, gradually taper when discontinuing after prolonged use. Use cautiously in the elderly; may accumulate and lead to side effects, psychomotor impairment. Sedative-hypnotics have been associated with severe allergic reactions and complex sleep behaviors including sleep driving. Use caution and discuss with patients.

BROMAZEPAM (***✤ Lectopam***) ▶L ♀D ▶– $

ADULT – Canada only. 6 to 18 mg/day PO in equally divided doses.

PEDS – Not approved in children.

FORMS – Generic/Trade: Tabs 1.5, 3, 6 mg.

(cont.)

BROMAZEPAM (*cont.*)

NOTES – Do not exceed 3 mg/day initially in the elderly or debilitated. Gradually taper when discontinuing after prolonged use. Half-life approximately 20 h in adults but increased in elderly. Cimetidine may prolong elimination.

CHLORDIAZEPOXIDE (***Librium***) ▶LK ♀D ▶–©IV $$

ADULT – Anxiety: 5 to 25 mg PO three to four times per day or 25 to 50 mg IM/IV three to four times per day (acute/severe anxiety). Acute alcohol withdrawal: 50 to 100 mg PO/IM/IV, repeat q 3 to 4 h prn up to 300 mg/day.

PEDS – Anxiety, age older than 6 yo: 5 to 10 mg PO two to four times per day.

FORMS – Generic/Trade: Caps 5, 10, 25 mg.

NOTES – Half-life 5 to 30 h.

CLONAZEPAM (***Klonopin, Klonopin Wafer, ♣ Rivotril, Clonapam***) ▶LK ♀D ▶–©IV $

ADULT – Panic disorder: 0.25 mg PO two times per day, increase by 0.125 to 0.25 mg q 3 days to max dose of 4 mg/day. Akinetic or myoclonic seizures: Start 0.5 mg PO three times per day. Increase by 0.5 to 1 mg q 3 days prn. Max 20 mg/day.

PEDS – Akinetic or myoclonic seizures, Lennox-Gastaut syndrome (petit mal variant), or absence seizures (10 yo or younger or 30 kg or less): 0.01 to 0.03 mg/kg/day PO divided two to three times per day. Increase by 0.25 to 0.5 mg q 3 days prn. Max 0.1 to 0.2 mg/kg/day divided three times per day.

UNAPPROVED ADULT – Neuralgias: 2 to 4 mg PO daily. Restless legs syndrome: Start 0.25 mg PO at bedtime. Max 2 mg at bedtime. REM sleep behavior disorder: 1 to 2 mg PO at bedtime.

FORMS – Generic/Trade: Tabs 0.5, 1, 2 mg. Orally disintegrating tabs (approved for panic disorder only) 0.125, 0.25, 0.5, 1, 2 mg.

NOTES – Half-life 18 to 50 h. Usual therapeutic range is 20 to 80 ng/mL. Contraindicated in hepatic failure or acute narrow-angle glaucoma.

CLORAZEPATE (***Tranxene, Tranxene SD***) ▶LK ♀D ▶–©IV $

ADULT – Anxiety: Start 7.5 to 15 mg PO at bedtime or two to three times per day, usual effective dose is 15 to 60 mg/day. Acute alcohol withdrawal: 60 to 90 mg/day on 1st day divided two to three times per day, gradually reduce dose to 7.5 to 15 mg/day over 5 days. Max dose is 90 mg/day. May transfer patients to single-dose tabs (Tranxene-SD) when dose stabilized.

PEDS – Not approved in children younger than 9 yo.

FORMS – Generic/Trade: Tabs 3.75, 7.5, 15 mg. Trade only (Tranxene SD): Tabs extended-release 11.25, 22.5 mg.

NOTES – Half-life 40 to 50 h.

DIAZEPAM (***Valium, Diastat, Diastat AcuDial, ♣ Diazemuls***) ▶LK ♀D ▶–©IV $

ADULT – Status epilepticus: 5 to 10 mg IV. Repeat q 10 to 15 min prn to max 30 mg. Epilepsy, adjunctive therapy: 2 to 10 mg PO two to four times per day. Increased seizure activity: 0.2 to 0.5 mg/kg PR (rectal gel) to max 20 mg/day. Skeletal muscle spasm, spasticity related to cerebral palsy, paraplegia, athetosis, "stiff man syndrome": 2 to 10 mg PO/PR three to four times per day. 5 to 10 mg IM/IV initially, then 5 to 10 mg q 3 to 4 h prn. Decrease dose in elderly. Anxiety: 2 to 10 mg PO two to four times per day or 2 to 20 mg IM/IV, repeat dose in 3 to 4 h prn. Alcohol withdrawal: 10 mg PO three to four times per day for 24 h then 5 mg PO three to four times per day prn.

PEDS – Skeletal muscle spasm: 0.04 to 0.2 mg/kg/dose IV/IM q 2 to 4 h. Max dose 0.6 mg/kg within 8 h. Status epilepticus, age 1 mo to 5 yo: 0.2 to 0.5 mg IV slowly q 2 to 5 min to max 5 mg. Status epilepticus, age older than 5 yo: 1 mg IV slowly q 2 to 5 min to max 10 mg. Repeat q 2 to 4 h prn. Epilepsy, adjunctive therapy, muscle spasm, and anxiety disorders, age older than 6 mo: 1 to 2.5 mg PO three to four times per day; gradually increase as tolerated and needed. Increased seizure activity (rectal gel, age older than 2 yo): 0.5 mg/kg PR (2 to 5 yo), 0.3 mg/kg PR (6 to 11 yo), or 0.2 mg/kg PR (age older than 12 yo). Max 20 mg. May repeat in 4 to 12 h prn.

UNAPPROVED ADULT – Loading dose strategy for alcohol withdrawal: 10 to 20 mg PO or 10 mg slow IV in closely monitored setting, then repeat similar or lower doses q 1 to 2 h prn until sedated. Further doses should be unnecessary due to long half-life. Restless legs syndrome: 0.5 to 4 mg PO at bedtime.

FORMS – Generic/Trade: Tabs 2, 5, 10 mg. Generic only: Oral soln 5 mg/5 mL. Oral concentrate (Intensol) 5 mg/mL. Trade only: Rectal gel (Diastat) 2.5, 5, 10, 15, 20 mg. Rectal gel (Diastat AcuDial) 10, 20 mg.

NOTES – Half-life 20 to 80 h. Respiratory and CNS depression may occur. Caution in liver disease. Abuse potential. Long half-life may increase the risk of adverse effects in the elderly. Cimetidine, oral contraceptives, disulfiram, fluoxetine, isoniazid, ketoconazole, metoprolol, propoxyphene, propranolol, and valproic acid may increase

(cont.)

DIAZEPAM (*cont.*)

diazepam concentrations. Diazepam may increase digoxin and phenytoin concentrations. Rifampin may increase the metabolism of diazepam. Avoid combination with protease inhibitors. Diastat AcuDial is for home use and allows dosing from 5 to 20 mg in 2.5-mg increments.

FLURAZEPAM (*Dalmane*) ▶LK ♀X ▶–©IV $

ADULT – Insomnia: 15 to 30 mg PO at bedtime.
PEDS – Not approved in children age younger than 15 yo.
FORMS – Generic/Trade: Caps 15, 30 mg.
NOTES – Half-life 70 to 90 h. For short-term treatment of insomnia.

PSYCHIATRY: Anxiolytics/Hypnotics—Benzodiazepines—Medium Half-Life (10 to 15 h)

NOTE: To avoid withdrawal, gradually taper when discontinuing after prolonged use. Sedative-hypnotics have been associated with severe allergic reactions and complex sleep behaviors including sleep driving. Use caution and discuss with patients.

ESTAZOLAM (*ProSom*) ▶LK ♀X ▶–©IV $$

ADULT – Insomnia: 1 to 2 mg PO at bedtime for up to 12 weeks. Reduce dose to 0.5 mg in elderly, small, or debilitated patients.
PEDS – Not approved in children.
FORMS – Generic/Trade: Tabs 1, 2 mg.
NOTES – For short-term treatment of insomnia. Avoid with ketoconazole or itraconazole; caution with less potent inhibitors of CYP3A4.

LORAZEPAM (*Ativan*) ▶LK ♀D ▶–©IV $

ADULT – Anxiety: Start 0.5 to 1 mg PO two to three times per day, usual effective dose is 2 to 6 mg/day. Max dose is 10 mg/day PO. Anxiolytic/sedation: 0.04 to 0.05 mg/kg IV/IM; usual dose 2 mg, max 4 mg. Insomnia: 2 to 4 mg PO at bedtime. Status epilepticus: 4 mg IV over 2 min. May repeat in 10 to 15 min.
PEDS – Not approved in children.
UNAPPROVED ADULT – Alcohol withdrawal: 1 to 2 mg PO/IM/IV q 2 to 4 h prn or 2 mg PO/IM/IV q 6 h for 24 h then 1 mg q 6 h for 8 doses. Chemotherapy-induced N/V: 1 to 2 mg PO/SL/IV/IM q 6 h.
UNAPPROVED PEDS – Status epilepticus: 0.05 to 0.1 mg/kg IV over 2 to 5 min. May repeat 0.05 mg/kg for 1 dose in 10 to 15 min. Do not exceed 4 mg as single dose. Anxiolytic/Sedation: 0.05 mg/kg/dose q 4 to 8 h PO/IV, max 2 mg/dose. Chemotherapy-induced N/V: 0.05 mg/kg PO/IV q 8 to 12 h prn, max 3 mg/dose; or 0.02 to 0.05 mg/kg IV q 6 h prn, max 2 mg/dose.
FORMS – Generic/Trade: Tabs 0.5, 1, 2 mg. Generic only: Oral concentrate 2 mg/mL.
NOTES – Half-life 10 to 20 h. No active metabolites. For short-term treatment of insomnia.

NITRAZEPAM (♣*Mogadan*) ▶L ♀C ▶– $

ADULT – Canada only. Insomnia: 5 to 10 mg PO at bedtime.
PEDS – Canada only. Myoclonic seizures: 0.3 to 1 mg/kg/day in 3 divided doses.
FORMS – Generic/Trade: Tabs 5, 10 mg.
NOTES – Use lower doses in elderly/debilitated patients.

TEMAZEPAM (*Restoril*) ▶LK ♀X ▶–©IV $

ADULT – Insomnia: 7.5 to 30 mg PO at bedtime for 7 to 10 days.
PEDS – Not approved in children.
FORMS – Generic/Trade: Caps 7.5, 15, 22.5, 30 mg.
NOTES – Half-life 8 to 25 h. For short-term treatment of insomnia.

PSYCHIATRY: Anxiolytics/Hypnotics—Benzodiazepines—Short Half-Life (< 12 h)

ALPRAZOLAM (*Xanax, Xanax XR, Niravam*) ▶LK ♀D ▶–©IV $

ADULT – Anxiety: Start 0.25 to 0.5 mg PO three times per day, may increase q 3 to 4 days to max 4 mg/day. Use 0.25 mg PO two times per day in elderly or debilitated patients. Panic disorder: Start 0.5 mg PO three times per day (or 0.5 to 1 mg PO daily of Xanax XR), may increase by up to 1 mg/day q 3 to 4 days to usual effective dose of 5 to 6 mg/day (3 to 6 mg/day for Xanax XR), max dose is 10 mg/day.
PEDS – Not approved in children.
FORMS – Generic/Trade: Tabs 0.25, 0.5, 1, 2 mg. Tabs extended-release 0.5, 1, 2, 3 mg. Orally disintegrating tab (Niravam) 0.25, 0.5, 1, 2 mg. Generic only: Oral concentrate (Intensol) 1 mg/mL.
NOTES – Half-life 12 h, but need to give three times per day. Divide administration time evenly during waking hours to avoid interdose symptoms. Do not give with antifungals (eg, ketoconazole, itraconazole); use caution with macrolides, propoxyphene, oral

(cont.)

ALPRAZOLAM (*cont.*)

contraceptives, TCAs, cimetidine, antidepressants, anticonvulsants, paroxetine, sertraline, and others that inhibit CYP3A4.

OXAZEPAM (*Serax*) ▶LK ♀D ▶–©IV $$$

ADULT – Anxiety: 10 to 30 mg PO three to four times per day. Acute alcohol withdrawal: 15 to 30 mg PO three to four times per day.

PEDS – Not approved in children younger than 6 yo.

UNAPPROVED ADULT – Restless legs syndrome: Start 10 mg PO at bedtime. Max 40 mg at bedtime.

FORMS – Generic/Trade: Caps 10, 15, 30 mg. Trade only: Tabs 15 mg.

NOTES – Half-life 8 h.

TRIAZOLAM (*Halcion*) ▶LK ♀X ▶–©IV $

ADULT – Hypnotic: 0.125 to 0.25 mg PO at bedtime for 7 to 10 days, max 0.5 mg/day. Start 0.125 mg/day in elderly or debilitated patients.

PEDS – Not approved in children.

UNAPPROVED ADULT – Restless legs syndrome: Start 0.125 mg PO at bedtime. Max 0.5 mg at bedtime.

FORMS – Generic/Trade: Tabs 0.125, 0.25 mg.

NOTES – Half-life 2 to 3 h. Anterograde amnesia may occur. Do not use with protease inhibitors, ketoconazole, itraconazole, or nefazodone; use caution with macrolides, cimetidine, and other CYP3A4 inhibitors.

PSYCHIATRY: Anxiolytics/Hypnotics—Other

NOTE: Sedative-hypnotics have been associated with severe allergic reactions and complex sleep behaviors including sleep driving. Use caution and discuss with patients.

BUSPIRONE (*BuSpar, Vanspar*) ▶K ♀B ▶– $$$

ADULT – Anxiety: Start 15 mg "dividose" daily (7.5 mg PO two times per day), increase by 5 mg/day q 2 to 3 days to usual effective dose of 30 mg/day, max dose is 60 mg/day.

PEDS – Not approved in children.

FORMS – Generic/Trade: Tabs 5, 10, Dividose Tabs 15, 30 mg (scored to be easily bisected or trisected). Generic only: Tabs 7.5 mg.

NOTES – Slower onset than benzodiazepines; optimum effect requires 3 to 4 weeks of therapy. Do not use with MAOIs; caution with itraconazole, cimetidine, nefazodone, erythromycin, and other CYP3A4 inhibitors.

CHLORAL HYDRATE (*Aquachloral Supprettes, Somnote*) ▶LK ♀C ▶+©IV $

ADULT – Sedative: 250 mg PO/PR three times per day after meals. Hypnotic: 500 to 1000 mg PO/PR at bedtime. Acute alcohol withdrawal: 500 to 1000 mg PO/PR q 6 h prn.

PEDS – Sedative: 25 mg/kg/day PO/PR divided three to four times per day, up to 500 mg three times per day. Hypnotic: 50 mg/kg PO/PR at bedtime, up to max 1 g. Preanesthetic: 25 to 50 mg/kg PO/PR before procedure.

UNAPPROVED PEDS – Sedative: Higher than approved doses 75 to 100 mg/kg PO/PR.

FORMS – Generic only: Syrup 500 mg/5 mL, rectal supps 500 mg. Trade only: Caps 500 mg. Rectal supps: 325, 650 mg.

NOTES – Give syrup in ½ glass of fruit juice or water.

ESZOPICLONE (*Lunesta*) ▶L ♀C ▶?©IV $$$$

ADULT – Insomnia: 2 mg PO at bedtime prn, max 3 mg. Elderly: 1 mg PO at bedtime prn, max 2 mg.

PEDS – Not approved for children.

FORMS – Trade only: Tabs 1, 2, 3 mg.

NOTES – Half-life is approximately 6 h. Take immediately before bedtime.

RAMELTEON (*Rozerem*) ▶L ♀C ▶? $$$$

ADULT – Insomnia: 8 mg PO at bedtime.

PEDS – Not approved for children.

FORMS – Trade only: Tabs 8 mg.

NOTES – Do not take with/after high-fat meal. No evidence of dependence or abuse liability. Inhibitors or CYP1A2, 3A4, and 2C9 may increase serum level and effect. Avoid with severe liver disease. May decrease testosterone and increase prolactin.

ZALEPLON (*Sonata,* ✤*Starnoc*) ▶L ♀C ▶–©IV $$$$

ADULT – Insomnia: 5 to 10 mg PO at bedtime prn, max 20 mg.

PEDS – Not approved in children.

FORMS – Generic/Trade: Caps 5, 10 mg.

NOTES – Half-life is approximately 1 h. Useful if problems with sleep initiation or morning grogginess. For short-term treatment of insomnia. Take immediately before bedtime or after going to bed and experiencing difficulty falling asleep. Use 5 mg dose in patients with mild to moderate hepatic impairment, elderly patients, and in patients taking cimetidine.

(cont.)

ZALEPLON (*cont.*)

Possible drug interactions with rifampin, phenytoin, carbamazepine, and phenobarbital. Do not use for benzodiazepine or alcohol withdrawal.

ZOLPIDEM (***Ambien, Ambien CR, Zolpimist, Edluar,*** ♣ ***Sublinox***) ▶L ♀C ◗+©IV $$$$

ADULT – Adult: Insomnia: Standard tabs: 10 mg PO at bedtime; age older than 65 yo or debilitated: 5 mg PO at bedtime. Oral spray: 10 mg PO at bedtime; age older than 65 yo or debilitated: 5 mg PO at bedtime. Controlled-release tabs: 12.5 mg PO at bedtime; age older than 65 yo or debilitated: 6.25 mg PO at bedtime.

PEDS – Not approved in children.

FORMS – Generic/Trade: Tabs 5, 10 mg. Trade only: Controlled-release tabs 6.25, 12.5 mg, oral spray 5 mg/actuation (Zolpimist), sublingual tab 5, 10 mg (Edluar).

NOTES – Half-life is 2.5 h. Ambien regular-release is for short-term treatment of insomnia characterized by problems with sleep initiation. CR is useful for problems with sleep initiation and maintenance, and has been studied for up to 24 weeks. Do not use for benzodiazepine or alcohol withdrawal. Oral spray is sprayed into the mouth over the tongue. Device must be primed with 5 pumps prior to first use or if not used for 14 days.

♣ **ZOPICLONE** (***Imovane***) ▶L ♀D ◗– $

ADULT – Canada only. Short-term treatment of insomnia: 5 to 7.5 mg PO at bedtime. In elderly or debilitated, use 3.75 mg at bedtime initially, and increase prn to 5 to 7.5 mg at bedtime. Max 7.5 mg at bedtime.

PEDS – Not approved in children.

FORMS – Generic/Trade: Tabs 5, 7.5 mg. Generic only: Tabs 3.75 mg.

NOTES – Treatment should usually not exceed 7 to 10 days without reevaluation.

PSYCHIATRY: Combination Drugs

LIMBITROL (**chlordiazepoxide + amitriptyline,** ***Limbitrol DS***) ▶LK ♀D ◗–©IV $$$

ADULT – Rarely used; other drugs preferred. Depression/anxiety: 1 tab PO three to four times per day, may increase up to 6 tabs/day.

PEDS – Not approved in children younger than 12 yo.

FORMS – Generic/Trade: Tabs 5/12.5, 10/25 mg chlordiazepoxide/amitriptyline.

SYMBYAX (**olanzapine + fluoxetine**) ▶LK ♀C ◗– $$$$$

WARNING – Observe patients started on SSRIs for worsening depression or emergence of suicidal thoughts or behaviors in children, adolescents, and young adults, especially early in therapy or after increases in dose. Monitor for emergence of anxiety, agitation, panic attacks, insomnia, irritability, hostility, impulsivity, akathisia, mania, and hypomania. Carefully weigh risks and benefits before starting and then monitor such individuals closely. The use of atypical antipsychotics to treat behavioral problems in patients with dementia has been associated with higher mortality rates. Atypical antipsychotics have been associated with wt gain, dyslipidemia, hyperglycemia, and diabetes mellitus; monitor closely.

ADULT – Bipolar type 1 with depression and treatment-resistant depression: Start 6/25 mg PO at bedtime. Max 18/75 mg/day.

PEDS – Not approved in children younger than 12 yo.

FORMS – Trade only: Caps (olanzapine/fluoxetine) 3/25, 6/25, 6/50, 12/25, 12/50 mg.

NOTES – Efficacy beyond 8 weeks not established. Monitor wt, fasting glucose, and triglycerides before initiation and periodically during treatment. Contraindicated with thioridazine; do not use with cisapride, thioridazine, tryptophan, or MAOIs; caution with lithium, phenytoin, TCAs, aspirin, NSAIDs, and warfarin. Pregnancy exposure to fluoxetine associated with premature delivery, low birth wt, and lower Apgar scores. Decrease dose with liver disease or patients predisposed to hypotension.

TRIAVIL (**perphenazine + amitriptyline**) ▶LK ♀D ◗? $$

ADULT – Rarely used; other drugs preferred. Depression/anxiety: 2 to 4 mg perphenazine plus 10 to 25 mg amitriptyline PO three to four times per day or 4 mg perphenazine plus 50 mg amitriptyline two times per day. Max total per day is 16 mg perphenazine or 200 mg of amitriptyline.

PEDS – Not approved in children.

FORMS – Generic only: Tabs (perphenazine/amitriptyline) 2/10, 2/25, 4/10, 4/25, 4/50 mg.

PSYCHIATRY: Drug Dependence Therapy

ACAMPROSATE (***Campral***) ▶K ♀C ◗? $$$$

ADULT – Maintenance of abstinence from alcohol: 666 mg (2 tabs) PO three times per day. Start after alcohol withdrawal and when patient is abstinent.

PEDS – Not approved in children.

FORMS – Trade only: Tabs delayed-release 333 mg.

NOTES – Reduce dose to 333 mg if CrCl 30 to 50 mL/min. Contraindicated if CrCl less than 30 mL/min.

DISULFIRAM (***Antabuse***) ▶L ♀C ◗? $$$

WARNING – Never give to an intoxicated patient.

ADULT – Maintenance of sobriety: 125 to 500 mg PO daily.

PEDS – Not approved in children.

FORMS – Trade only: Tabs 250, 500 mg.

NOTES – Patient must abstain from any alcohol for at least 12 h before using. Disulfiram-alcohol reaction may occur for up to 2 weeks after discontinuing disulfiram. Metronidazole and alcohol in any form (eg, cough syrups, tonics) contraindicated. Hepatotoxicity.

NALTREXONE (***ReVia, Depade, Vivitrol***) ▶LK ♀C ◗? $$$$

WARNING – Hepatotoxicity with higher than approved doses.

ADULT – Alcohol dependence: 50 mg PO daily. Extended-release injectable susp: 380 mg IM q 4 weeks or monthly. Opioid dependence following detoxification: Start 25 mg PO daily, increase to 50 mg PO daily if no signs of withdrawal. Extended-release injectable susp: 380 mg IM q 4 weeks or monthly.

PEDS – Not approved in children.

FORMS – Generic/Trade: Tabs 50 mg. Trade only (Vivitrol): Extended-release injectable susp kits 380 mg.

NOTES – Avoid if recent (past 7 to 10 days) ingestion of opioids. Conflicting evidence of efficacy for chronic, severe alcoholism. Extended-release injectable suspension (Vivitrol) should be given in the gluteal muscle and use alternate side each month.

NICOTINE GUM (***Nicorette, Nicorette DS***) ▶LK ♀C ◗– $$$$

ADULT – Smoking cessation: Gradually taper 1 piece (2 mg) q 1 to 2 h for 6 weeks, 1 piece (2 mg) q 2 to 4 h for 3 weeks, then 1 piece (2 mg) q 4 to 8 h for 3 weeks. Max 30 pieces/day of 2 mg gum or 24 pieces/day of 4 mg gum. Use 4 mg pieces (Nicorette DS) for high cigarette use (more than 24 cigarettes/day).

PEDS – Not approved in children.

FORMS – OTC/Generic/Trade: Gum 2, 4 mg.

NOTES – Chew slowly and park between cheek and gum periodically. May cause N/V, hiccups. Coffee, juices, wine, and soft drinks may reduce absorption. Avoid eating/drinking for 15 min before/during gum use. Available in original, orange, or mint flavor. Do not use beyond 6 months.

NICOTINE INHALATION SYSTEM (***Nicotrol Inhaler, ♣ Nicorette inhaler***) ▶LK ♀D ◗– $$$$$

ADULT – Smoking cessation: 6 to 16 cartridges/day for 12 weeks.

PEDS – Not approved in children.

FORMS – Trade only: Oral inhaler 10 mg/cartridge (4 mg nicotine delivered), 42 cartridges/box.

NICOTINE LOZENGE (***Commit, Nicorette***) ▶LK ♀D ◗– $$$$$

ADULT – Smoking cessation: In those who smoke within 30 min of waking use 4 mg lozenge; others use 2 mg. Take 1 to 2 lozenges q 1 to 2 h for 6 weeks, then q 2 to 4 h in weeks 7 to 9, then q 4 to 8 h in weeks 10 to 12. Length of therapy 12 weeks.

PEDS – Not approved in children.

FORMS – OTC Generic/Trade: Lozenge 2, 4 mg in 48, 72, 168 count packages.

NOTES – Allow lozenge to dissolve and do not chew. Do not eat or drink within 15 min before use. Avoid concurrent use with other sources of nicotine.

NICOTINE NASAL SPRAY (***Nicotrol NS***) ▶LK ♀D ◗– $$$$$

ADULT – Smoking cessation: 1 to 2 doses each h, each dose is 2 sprays, 1 in each nostril (1 spray contains 0.5 mg nicotine). Minimum recommended: 8 doses/day, max 40 doses/day.

PEDS – Not approved in children.

FORMS – Trade only: Nasal soln 10 mg/mL (0.5 mg/inhalation); 10 mL bottles.

NICOTINE PATCHES (***Habitrol, NicoDerm CQ, Nicotrol***) ▶LK ♀D ◗– $$$$

ADULT – Smoking cessation: Start 1 patch (14 to 22 mg) daily and taper after 6 weeks. Total duration of therapy is 12 weeks.

PEDS – Not approved in children.

FORMS – OTC/Rx/Generic/Trade: Patches 11, 22 mg/24 h. 7, 14, 21 mg/24 h (Habitrol and NicoDerm). OTC/Trade: 15 mg/16 h (Nicotrol).

NOTES – Ensure patient has stopped smoking. Dispose of patches safely; can be toxic to children, pets. Remove opaque NicoDerm CQ patch prior to MRI procedures to avoid possible burns.

SUBOXONE **(buprenorphine + naloxone)** ▶L ♀C ▶– ©III $$$$$
ADULT – Treatment of opioid dependence: Maintenance: 16 mg SL daily. Can individualize to range of 4 to 24 mg SL daily.
PEDS – Not approved in children.
FORMS – Trade only: SL tabs and film 2/0.5 mg and 8/2 mg buprenorphine/naloxone.
NOTES – Suboxone preferred over Subutex for unsupervised administration. Titrate in 2- to 4-mg increments/decrements to maintain therapy compliance and prevent withdrawal. Prescribers must complete training and apply for special DEA number. See www.suboxone.com.

VARENICLINE (***Chantix***, ✤ ***Champix***) ▶K ♀C ▶? $$$$
WARNING – Has been associated with the development of suicidal ideation, changes in behavior, depressed mood, and attempted/completed suicides, both during treatment and after withdrawal. Unclear safety in serious psychiatric conditions.
ADULT – Smoking cessation: Start 0.5 mg PO daily for days 1 to 3, then 0.5 mg two times per day, days 4 to 7, then 1 mg two times per day thereafter. Take after meals with full glass of water. Start 1 week prior to cessation and continue for 12 weeks, or patient may start the drug and stop smoking between days 8 nad 35 of treatment.
PEDS – Not approved in children.
FORMS – Trade only: Tabs 0.5, 1 mg.
NOTES – For severe renal dysfunction reduce max dose to 0.5 mg two times per day. For renal failure on hemodialysis may use 0.5 mg once daily if tolerated.

PSYCHIATRY: Stimulants/ADHD/Anorexiants

NOTE: Sudden cardiac death has been reported with stimulants and atomoxetine at usual ADHD doses; carefully assess prior to treatment and avoid if cardiac conditions or structural abnormalities. Amphetamines are associated with high abuse potential and dependence with prolonged administration. Stimulants may also cause or worsen underlying psychosis or induce a manic or mixed episode in bipolar disorder. Problems with visual accommodation have also been reported with stimulants.

ADDERALL **(dextroamphetamine + amphetamine, *Adderall XR*)** ▶L ♀C ▶– ©II $$$$
ADULT – Narcolepsy, standard-release: Start 10 mg PO q am, increase by 10 mg q week, max dose is 60 mg/day divided two to three times per day at 4- to 6-h intervals. ADHD, extended-release caps (Adderall XR): 20 mg PO daily.
PEDS – ADHD, standard-release tabs: Start 2.5 mg (3 to 5 yo) or 5 mg (age 6 yo or older) PO one to two times per day, increase by 2.5 to 5 mg q week, max 40 mg/day. ADHD, extended-release caps (Adderall XR): If age 6 to 12 yo, then start 5 to 10 mg PO daily to max 30 mg/day. If 13 to 17 yo, then start 10 mg PO daily to max 20 mg/day. Not recommended age younger than 3 yo. Narcolepsy, standard-release: Age 6 to 12 yo: Start 5 mg PO daily, increase by 5 mg q week. Age older than 12 yo: Start 10 mg PO q am, increase by 10 mg q week, max dose is 60 mg/day divided two to three times per day at 4- to 6-h intervals.
FORMS – Generic/Trade: Tabs 5, 7.5, 10, 12.5, 15, 20, 30 mg. Trade only: Caps, extended-release (Adderall XR) 5, 10, 15, 20, 25, 30 mg.
NOTES – Caps may be opened and the beads sprinkled on applesauce; do not chew beads. Adderall XR should be given upon awakening. Avoid evening doses. Monitor growth and use drug holidays when appropriate. May increase pulse and BP. May exacerbate bipolar or psychotic conditions.

ARMODAFINIL (***Nuvigil***) ▶L ♀C ▶? ©IV $$$$$
ADULT – Obstructive sleep apnea, hypopnea syndrome, and narcolepsy: 150 to 250 mg PO q am. Inconsistent evidence for improved efficacy of 250 mg/day dose. Shift work sleep disorder: 150 mg PO 1 h prior to start of shift.
PEDS – Not approved in children.
FORMS – Trade only: Tabs 50, 100, 150, 200, 250 mg.
NOTES – Weak inducer for substrates of CYP3A4/5 (eg, carbamazepine, cyclosporine) which may require dose adjustments. May inhibit metabolism of substrates of CYP2C19 (eg, omeprazole, diazepam, phenytoin). May reduce efficacy of oral contraceptives; consider alternatives during treatment. Reduce dose with severe liver impairment.

ATOMOXETINE (***Strattera***) ▶K ♀C ▶? $$$$$
WARNING – Severe liver injury and failure have been reported; discontinue if jaundice or elevated LFTs. Increases risk of suicidal thinking and behavior in children and adolescents; carefully weigh risks/benefits before starting and then monitor such individuals closely for worsening depression or emergence of suicidal thoughts or behaviors

(cont.)

ATOMOXETINE (*cont.*)

especially early in therapy or after increases in dose. Monitor for emergence of anxiety, agitation, panic attacks, insomnia, irritability, hostility, impulsivity, akathisia, mania and hypomania.

ADULT – ADHD: Start 40 mg PO daily, then increase after more than 3 days to target of 80 mg/day divided one to two times per day. Max dose 100 mg/day.

PEDS – ADHD: Children/adolescents wt 70 kg or less: Start 0.5 mg/kg daily, then increase after more than 3 days to target dose of 1.2 mg/kg/day divided one to two times per day. Max dose 1.4 mg/kg or 100 mg/day, whichever is less. If wt greater than 70 kg use adult dose.

FORMS – Trade only: Caps 10, 18, 25, 40, 60, 80, 100 mg.

NOTES – If taking strong CYP2D6 inhibitors (eg, paroxetine or fluoxetine), use same starting dose but only increase if well tolerated at 4 weeks and symptoms unimproved. Caution when coadministered with oral or parenteral albuterol or other beta-2 agonists, as increases in heart rate and BP may occur. May be stopped without tapering. Monitor growth. Give "Patient Medication Guide" when dispensed. Does not appear to exacerbate tics.

BENZPHETAMINE (***Didrex***) ▶K ♀X ▶?©III $$$

WARNING – Chronic overuse/abuse can lead to marked tolerance and psychic dependence; caution with prolonged use.

ADULT – Short-term treatment of obesity: Start with 25 to 50 mg once daily in the morning and increase if needed to 1 to 3 times daily.

PEDS – Not approved for children younger than 12 yo.

FORMS – Generic/Trade: Tabs 50 mg.

NOTES – Tolerance to anorectic effect develops within week and cross-tolerance to other drugs in class common.

CAFFEINE (***NoDoz, Vivarin, Caffedrine, Stay Awake, Quick-Pep, Cafcit***) ▶L ♀B/C ▶? $

ADULT – Fatigue: 100 to 200 mg PO q 3 to 4 h prn.

PEDS – Not approved in children younger than 12 yo, except apnea of prematurity in infants between 28 and less than 33 weeks gestational age (Cafcit): Load 20 mg/kg IV over 30 min. Maintenance 5 mg/kg PO q 24 h. Monitor for necrotizing enterocolitis.

FORMS – OTC Generic/Trade: Tabs/Caps 200 mg. Oral soln caffeine citrate (Cafcit) 20 mg/mL. OTC Trade only: Tabs extended-release 200 mg. Lozenges 75 mg.

NOTES – 2 mg caffeine citrate = 1 mg caffeine base.

COCAINE ▶L ♀? ▶?©II Varies

ADULT – Drug of abuse.

PEDS – Drug of abuse.

DEXMETHYLPHENIDATE (***Focalin, Focalin XR***) ▶LK ♀C ▶?©II $$$

ADULT – ADHD, not already on stimulants: Start 10 mg PO q am (extended-release) or 2.5 mg PO two times per day (immediate-release). Max 20 mg/day for immediate release and 40 mg/day for extended release. If taking racemic methylphenidate use conversion of 2.5 mg for each 5 mg of methylphenidate.

PEDS – ADHD and age 6 yo or older and not already on stimulants: Start 5 mg PO q am (extended-release) or 2.5 mg PO two times per day (immediate-release), max 20 mg/day (immediate-release) or 30 mg/day (extended-release). If already on racemic methylphenidate, use conversion of 2.5 mg for each 5 mg of methylphenidate.

FORMS – Generic/Trade: Tabs, immediate-release 2.5, 5, 10 mg. Trade only: Extended-release caps (Focalin XR) 5, 10, 15, 20, 30 mg.

NOTES – Avoid evening doses. Monitor growth and use drug holidays when appropriate. May increase pulse and BP. 2.5 mg is equivalent to 5 mg racemic methylphenidate. Focalin XR caps may be opened and sprinkled on applesauce, but beads must not be chewed. May exacerbate bipolar or psychotic conditions. Avoid in patients allergic to methylphenidate.

DEXTROAMPHETAMINE (***Dexedrine, Dextrostat***) ▶L ♀C ▶–©II $$$$

ADULT – Narcolepsy: Start 10 mg PO q am, increase by 10 mg/day q week, max 60 mg/day divided daily (sustained-release) or two to three times per day at 4- to 6-h intervals.

PEDS – Narcolepsy: Age 6 to 12 yo: Start 5 mg PO q am, increase by 5 mg/day q week. Age older than 12 yo: Start 10 mg PO q am, increase by 10 mg/day q week, max 60 mg/day divided daily (sustained-release) or two to three times per day at 4- to 6-h intervals. ADHD: Age 3 to 5 yo: Start 2.5 mg PO daily, increase by 2.5 mg q week. Age 6 yo or older: Start 5 mg PO one to two times per day, increase by 5 mg q week, usual max 40 mg/day divided one to three times per day at 4- to 6-h intervals. Not recommended for patients younger than 3 yo. Extended-release caps not recommended for age younger than 6 yo.

FORMS – Generic/Trade: Caps extended-release 5, 10, 15 mg. Generic only: Tabs 5, 10 mg. Oral soln 5 mg/5 mL.

NOTES – Avoid evening doses. Monitor growth and use drug holidays when appropriate. May exacerbate bipolar or psychotic conditions.

BODY MASS INDEX* (Heights are in feet and inches; weights are in pounds)

BMI	Class	4' 10"	5' 0"	5' 4"	5' 8"	6' 0"	6' 4"
<19	Underweight	<91	<97	<110	<125	<140	<156
19–24	Healthy weight	91–119	97–127	110–144	125–163	140–183	156–204
25–29	Overweight	120–143	128–152	145–173	164–196	184–220	205–245
30–40	Obese	144–191	153–204	174–233	197–262	221–293	246–328
>40	Very Obese	>191	>204	>233	>262	>293	>328

*BMI = kg/m^2 = (wt in pounds)(703)/(height in inches)^2. Anorectants appropriate if BMI ≥30 (with comoribidities ≥27); surgery an option if BMI >40 (with comorbidities 35–40). www.nhlbi.nih.gov

DIETHYLPROPION (*Tenuate, Tenuate Dospan*) ▶K ♀B ◗?©IV $

WARNING – Chronic overuse/abuse can lead to marked tolerance and psychic dependence; caution with prolonged use.

ADULT – Short-term treatment of obesity: 25 mg PO three times per day 1 h before meals and mid evening if needed or 75 mg sustained-release daily at midmorning.

PEDS – Not approved for children younger than 12 yo.

FORMS – Generic/Trade: Tabs 25 mg, Tabs, extended-release 75 mg.

NOTES – Tolerance to anorectic effect develops within week and cross-tolerance to other drugs in class common.

GUANFACINE (*Intuniv*) ▶LK – ♀B ◗?

ADULT – ADHD: Start 1 mg PO q AM. Increase by 1 mg/week to max 4 mg/day.

PEDS – ADHD (6 yo and older): Start 1 mg PO q AM. Increase by 1 mg/week to max 4 mg/day.

FORMS – Trade only: Tabs 1, 2, 3, 4 mg.

NOTES – Taper when discontinuing. Use cautiously with strong CYP3A4 inhibitors.

LISDEXAMFETAMINE (*Vyvanse*) ▶L ♀C ◗–©II $$$$

ADULT – ADHD: Start 30 mg PO q am. May increase weekly by 10 to 20 mg/day to max 70 mg/day.

PEDS – ADHD: children and adolescents ages 6 yo and older: Start 30 mg PO q am. May increase weekly by 10 to 20 mg/day to max 70 mg/day.

FORMS – Trade: Caps 20, 30, 40, 50, 60, 70 mg.

NOTES – May open cap and place contents in water for administration. Avoid evening doses. Monitor growth and use drug holidays when appropriate.

METHAMPHETAMINE (*Desoxyn*) ▶L ♀C ◗–©II $$$$

ADULT – Obesity: 5 mg PO prior to meals. Short-term use only.

PEDS – ADHD (at least 6 yo): Start 5 mg PO one to two times per day. May increase by 5 mg/dose at weekly intervals to usual effective dose of 20 to 25 mg/day. Obesity (older than 12 yo): use adult dosing.

FORMS – Generic/Trade: Tabs 5 mg.

NOTES – Should not be used for more than a few weeks for obesity.

METHYLENEDIOXYMETHAMPHETAMINE (*MDMA, Ecstacy*) ▶L ♀– ◗–©I Varies

ADULT – Drug of abuse.

PEDS – Drug of abuse.

NOTES – Commonly used at "rave" parties.

METHYLPHENIDATE (*Ritalin, Ritalin LA, Ritalin SR, Methylin, Methylin ER, Metadate ER, Metadate CD, Concerta, Daytrana,* ✤ *Biphentin*) ▶LK ♀C ◗?©II $$

ADULT – Narcolepsy: 10 mg PO two to three times per day before meals. Usual effective dose is 20 to 30 mg/day, max 60 mg/day. Use sustained-release tabs when the 8 h dosage corresponds to the titrated 8 h dosage of the conventional tabs. ADHD (Concerta): Start 18 to 36 mg PO q am, usual dose range 18 to 72 mg/day.

PEDS – ADHD age 6 yo or older: Start 5 mg PO two times per day before breakfast and lunch, increase gradually by 5 to 10 mg/day at weekly intervals to max 60 mg/day. Sustained and extended-release: Start 20 mg PO daily, max 60 mg daily. Concerta (extended-release) start 18 mg PO q am; titrate in 9- to 18-mg increments at weekly intervals to max 54 mg/day (age 6 to 12 yo) or 72 mg/day (13 to 17 yo). Consult product labeling for dose conversion from other methylphenidate regimens. Discontinue after 1 month if no improvement observed. Transdermal patch age 6 to 17 yo: Start 10 mg/9 h, may increase at weekly intervals to max dose of 30 mg/9 h. Apply 2 h prior to desired onset and remove 9 h later. Effect may last up to 12 h after application. Must alternate sites daily.

FORMS – Trade only: Tabs 5, 10, 20 mg (Ritalin, Methylin, Metadate). Tabs extended-release 10, 20 mg (Methylin ER, Metadate ER). Tabs extended-release 18, 27, 36, 54

(cont.)

METHYLPHENIDATE (*cont.*)

mg (Concerta). Caps extended-release 10, 20, 30, 40, 50, 60 mg (Metadate CD) May be sprinkled on food. Tabs sustained-release 20 mg (Ritalin SR). Caps extended-release 10, 20, 30, 40 mg (Ritalin LA). Tabs chewable 2.5, 5, 10 mg (Methylin). Oral soln 5 mg/5 mL, 10 mg/5 mL (Methylin). Transdermal patch (Daytrana) 10 mg/9 h, 15 mg/9 h, 20 mg/9 h, 30 mg/9 h. Generic only: Tabs 5, 10, 20 mg, tabs extended-release 10, 20 mg, tabs sustained-release 20 mg.

NOTES – Avoid evening doses. Avoid use with severe anxiety, tension, or agitation. Monitor growth and use drug holidays when appropriate. May increase pulse and BP. Ritalin LA may be opened and sprinkled on applesauce. Apply transdermal patch to hip below beltline to avoid rubbing it off. May exacerbate bipolar, psychotic, or seizure conditions.

MODAFINIL (***Provigil,*** ***♣Alertec***) ▶L ♀C ▶?©IV $$$$$

WARNING – Associated with serious, life-threatening rashes in adults and children; discontinue immediately if unexplained rash.

ADULT – Narcolepsy and sleep apnea/hypopnea: 200 mg PO q am. Shift work sleep disorder: 200 mg PO 1 h before shift.

PEDS – Not approved in children younger than 16 yo.

FORMS – Trade only: Tabs 100, 200 mg.

NOTES – May increase levels of diazepam, phenytoin, TCAs, warfarin, or propranolol; may decrease levels of cyclosporine, oral contraceptives, or theophylline. Reduce dose in severe liver impairment.

PHENDIMATRIZINE (***Bontril, Bontril Slow Release***) ▶K ♀C ▶?©III $$

WARNING – Chronic overuse/abuse can lead to marked tolerance and psychic dependence; caution with prolonged use.

ADULT – Short-term treatment of obesity: Start 35 mg 2 to 3 times daily 1 h before meals. Sustained-release 105 mg once in the morning before breakfast.

PEDS – Not approved in children younger than 12 yo.

FORMS – Generic/Trade: Tabs/Caps 35 mg, Caps, sustained-release 105 mg.

NOTES – Tolerance to anorectic effect develops within week and cross-tolerance to other drugs in class common.

PHENTERMINE (***Adipex-P, Ionamin, Suprenza***) ▶KL ♀C ▶–©IV $

WARNING – Chronic overuse/abuse can lead to marked tolerance and psychic dependence; caution with prolonged use.

ADULT – Obesity: 8 mg PO three times per day before meals or 1 to 2 h after meals. May give 15 to 37.5 mg PO q am or 10 to 14 h before bedtime.

PEDS – Not approved in children younger than 16 yo.

FORMS – Generic/Trade: Caps 15, 30, 37.5 mg. Tabs 37.5 mg. Trade only: Orally disintegrating tables (Suprenza) 15, 30 mg. Generic only: Caps extended-release 15, 30 mg (Ionamin)

NOTES – Indicated for short-term (8 to 12 weeks) use only. Contraindicated for use during or within 14 days of MAOIs (hypertensive crisis).

PULMONARY: Beta-Agonists—Short-Acting

NOTE: Palpitations, tachycardia, tremor, lightheadedness, nervousness, headache, and nausea may occur; these effects may be more pronounced with systemic administration. Hypokalemia can occur from the transient shift of potassium into cells, rarely leading to adverse cardiovascular effects; monitor accordingly. Potential for tolerance with continued use of short-acting beta-agonists.

ALBUTEROL (***AccuNeb, Ventolin HFA, Proventil HFA, ProAir HFA, VoSpire ER, ♣Airomir, Asmavent, salbutamol***) ▶L ♀C ▶? $$

ADULT – Acute asthma: MDI: 2 puffs q 4 to 6 h prn. Soln for inhalation: 2.5 mg nebulized three to four times per day. Dilute 0.5 mL 0.5% soln with 2.5 mL NS. Deliver over 5 to 15 min. One 3 mL unit dose (0.083%) nebulized three to four times per day. Caps for inhalation: 200 to 400 mcg inhaled q 4 to 6 h via a Rotahaler device. Prevention of exercise-induced bronchospasm: MDI: 2 puffs 10 to 30 min before exercise. Asthma: 2 to 4 mg PO three times per day to four times per day or extended-release 4 to 8 mg PO q 12 h up to 16 mg PO q 12 h.

PEDS – Acute asthma: MDI: Age 4 yo or older: 1 to 2 puffs q 4 to 6 h prn. Soln for inhalation (0.5%): 2 to 12 yo: 0.1 to 0.15 mg/kg/dose not to exceed 2.5 mg three to four times per day, diluted with NS to 3 mL. Caps for inhalation: Age 4 yo or older: 200 to 400 mcg inhaled q 4 to 6 h via a Rotahaler device. Asthma: Tabs, syrup 6 to 12 yo: 2 to 4 mg PO three to four times per

(cont.)

ALBUTEROL (*cont.*)

day, max dose 24 mg/day in divided doses or extended-release 4 mg PO q 12 h. Syrup 2 to 5 yo: 0.1 to 0.2 mg/kg/dose PO three times per day up to 4 mg three times per day. Prevention of exercise-induced bronchospasm age 4 yo or older: 2 puffs 10 to 30 min before exercise.

UNAPPROVED ADULT – COPD: MDI, soln for inhalation: Use asthma dose. Acute asthma: MDI, soln for inhalation: Dose as above q 20 min for 3 doses or until improvement. Continuous nebulization: 10 to 15 mg/h until improvement. Emergency hyperkalemia: 10 to 20 mg via MDI or soln for inhalation.

UNAPPROVED PEDS – Acute asthma: Soln for inhalation: 0.15 mg/kg (minimum dose is 2.5 mg) q 20 min for 3 doses then 0.15 to 0.3 mg/kg up to 10 mg q 1 to 4 h prn, or 0.5 mg/kg/h continuous nebulization. MDI: 4 to 8 puffs q 20 min for 3 doses then q 1 to 4 h prn. Soln for inhalation (0.5%): Age younger than 2 yo: 0.05 to 0.15 mg/kg/dose q 4 to 6 h. Syrup age younger than 2 yo: 0.3 mg/kg/24 h PO divided three times per day, max dose 12 mg/24 h. Prevention of exercise-induced bronchospasm: MDI: Age 4 yo or older: 2 puffs 10 to 30 min before exercise.

FORMS – Trade only: MDI 90 mcg/actuation, 200 metered doses/canister. "HFA" inhalers use hydrofluoroalkane propellant instead of CFCs but are otherwise equivalent. Generic/Trade: Soln for inhalation 0.021% (AccuNeb), 0.042% (AccuNeb), and 0.083% in 3 mL vials, 0.5% (5 mg/mL) in 20 mL with dropper. Tabs extended-release 4, 8 mg (VoSpire ER). Generic only: Syrup 2 mg/5 mL. Tabs immediate-release 2, 4 mg.

NOTES – Do not crush or chew extended-release tabs. Use with caution in patients on MAOIs or cyclic antidepressants; may increase cardiovascular side effects.

LEVALBUTEROL (***Xopenex, Xopenex HFA***) ▶L ♀C ▶? $$$

ADULT – Acute asthma: MDI 2 puffs q 4 to 6 h prn. Soln for inhalation: 0.63 to 1.25 mg nebulized q 6 to 8 h.

PEDS – Acute asthma: MDI age 4 yo or older: 2 puffs q 4 to 6 h prn. Soln for inhalation age 12 yo or older: Use adult dose. For age 6 to 11 yo: 0.31 mg nebulized three times per day.

FORMS – Generic/Trade: Soln for inhalation 0.31, 0.63, 1.25 mg in 3 mL and 1.25 mg in 0.5 mL unit-dose vials. Trade only: HFA MDI 45 mcg/actuation, 15 g 200/canister. "HFA" inhalers use hydrofluoroalkane propellant.

NOTES – R-isomer of albuterol. Dyspepsia may occur. Use with caution in patients on MAOIs or cyclic antidepressants; may increase cardiovascular side effects.

PIRBUTEROL (***Maxair Autohaler***) ▶L ♀C ▶? $$$$

ADULT – Acute asthma: MDI: 1 to 2 puffs q 4 to 6 h. Max dose 12 puffs/day.

PEDS – Not approved in children.

UNAPPROVED PEDS – Acute asthma age 12 yo or older: Use adult dose.

FORMS – Trade only: MDI 200 mcg/actuation, 14 g 400/canister.

NOTES – Breath-actuated autohaler.

TERBUTALINE (***Brethine, ✦ Bricanyl Turbuhaler***) ▶L ♀B ▶– $$

ADULT – Asthma: 2.5 to 5 mg PO q 6 h while awake. Max dose 15 mg/24 h. Acute asthma: 0.25 mg SC into lateral deltoid area; may repeat once within 15 to 30 min. Max dose 0.5 mg/4 h.

PEDS – Not approved in children.

UNAPPROVED ADULT – Preterm labor: 0.25 mg SC q 30 min up to 1 mg in 4 h. Infusion: 2.5 to 10 mcg/min IV, gradually increased to effective max doses of 17.5 to 30 mcg/min.

UNAPPROVED PEDS – Asthma: 0.05 mg/kg/dose PO three times per day, increase to max of 0.15 mg/kg/dose three times per day, max 5 mg/day for age 12 yo or younger, use adult dose for age older than 12 yo up to max 7.5 mg/ 24 h. Acute asthma: 0.01 mg/kg SC q 20 min for 3 doses then q 2 to 6 h prn.

FORMS – Generic/Trade: Tabs 2.5, 5 mg (Brethine scored). Generic: 1 mg/1 mL injectable. Canada only (Bricanyl): DPI 0.5 mg/actuation, 200 per DPI.

PULMONARY: Beta-Agonists—Long-Acting

NOTE: Long-acting beta-agonists may increase the risk of asthma-related death. Use only as a second agent if inadequate control with an optimal dose of inhaled corticosteroids. Do not use for rescue therapy. Palpitations, tachycardia, tremor, lightheadedness, nervousness, headache, and nausea may occur. Decreases in serum potassium can occur, rarely leading to adverse cardiovascular effects; monitor accordingly.

ARFORMOTEROL (*Brovana*) ▶L ♀C ▶? $$$$$
ADULT – COPD: 15 mcg nebulized two times per day.
PEDS – Not approved in children.
FORMS – Trade only: Soln for inhalation 15 mcg in 2 mL vial.
NOTES – Not for acute COPD exacerbations.

FORMOTEROL (*Foradil, Perforomist,* ✤ *Oxeze Turbuhaler*) ▶L ♀C ▶? $$$
ADULT – Chronic asthma, COPD: 1 puff two times per day. Prevention of exercise-induced bronchospasm: 1 puff 15 min prior to exercise. COPD: 20 mcg nebulized q 12 h.
PEDS – Chronic asthma, age 5 yo or older: 1 puff two times per day. Prevention of exercise-induced bronchospasm age 12 yo or older: Use adult dose.
FORMS – Trade only: DPI 12 mcg, 12, 60 blisters/pack (Foradil). Soln for inhalation: 20 mcg in 2 mL vial (Perforomist). Canada only (Oxeze): DPI 6, 12 mcg 60 blisters/pack. Should be used only with Aerolizer device.
NOTES – For asthma, must use in combination with inhaled steroid. Do not use additional doses for exercise if on maintenance.

INDACATEROL (*Arcapta*) ▶L – ♀C ▶?
ADULT – COPD: DPI: 75 mcg inhaled once daily.
PEDS – Not approved for children.
FORMS – Trade only: DPI: 75 mcg caps for inhalation, 30 blisters. To be used only with Nehoaler device.

SALMETEROL (*Serevent Diskus*) ▶L ♀C ▶? $$$$
ADULT – Chronic asthma/COPD: 1 puff two times per day. Prevention of exercise-induced bronchospasm: 1 puff 30 min before exercise.
PEDS – Chronic asthma age 4 yo or older: 1 puff two times per day. Prevention of exercise-induced bronchospasm: 1 puff 30 min before exercise.
FORMS – Trade only: DPI (Serevent Diskus): 50 mcg, 60 blisters.
NOTES – For asthma, must use in combination with inhaled steroid. Do not use additional doses for exercise if on maintenance. Concomitant ketoconazole increases levels and prolongs QT interval. Do not use with strong CYP3A4 inhibitors such as ritonavir, itraconazole, clarithromycin, nefazodone, etc.

PULMONARY: Combinations

ADVAIR **(fluticasone—inhaled + salmeterol,** ***Advair HFA*****)** ▶L ♀C ▶? $$$$$
WARNING – Long-acting beta-agonists may increase the risk of asthma-related death; use as an adjunct only if inadequate control with an optimal dose of inhaled corticosteroids. Avoid in significantly worsening or acute asthma. Do not use for rescue therapy. Do not stop abruptly.
ADULT – Chronic asthma: DPI: 1 puff two times per day (all strengths). MDI: 2 puffs two times per day (all strengths). COPD maintenance: DPI: 1 puff two times per day (250/50 only).
PEDS – Chronic asthma: DPI: 1 puff two times per day (100/50 only) for age 4 to 11 yo. Use adult dose for 12 yo or older.
UNAPPROVED ADULT – COPD: 500/50, 1 puff two times per day.
FORMS – Trade only: DPI: 100/50, 250/50, 500/50 mcg fluticasone/salmeterol per actuation; 60 doses/DPI. Trade only (Advair HFA): MDI 45/21, 115/21, 230/21 mcg fluticasone/salmeterol per actuation; 120 doses/canister.
NOTES – See individual components for additional information. Ritonavir and other CYP3A4 inhibitors such as ketoconazole significantly increase both salmeterol and fluticasone concentrations, resulting in prolongation of QT interval (salmeterol) and systemic effects, including adrenal suppression (fluticasone). Very rare anaphylactic reaction in patients with severe milk protein allergy. Increased risk of pneumonia in COPD.

COMBIVENT, COMBIVENT RESPIMAT **(albuterol + ipratropium)** ▶L ♀C ▶? $$$$
ADULT – COPD: MDI: 2 puffs four times per day. Max dose 12 puffs/24 h. Respimat: 1 puff four times per day. Max dose 6 inhalations/24 h.
PEDS – Not approved in children.
FORMS – Trade only: MDI: 90 mcg albuterol/18 mcg ipratropium per actuation, 200/canister. Respimat: 100 mcg albuterol/20 mcg ipratropium per inhalation, 120/canister.
NOTES – MDI contraindicated with soy or peanut allergy. Refer to components.

DULERA **(mometasone—inhaled + formoterol,** ✤ ***Zenhale*****)** ▶L – ♀C ▶? $$$$$
WARNING – Long-acting beta-agonists may increase the risk of asthma-related death; use as an adjunct only if inadequate control with an optimal dose of inhaled corticosteroids. Avoid in significantly worsening or acute asthma. Do not use for rescue therapy. Do not stop abruptly.

(cont.)

***DULERA** (cont.)*

ADULT – Asthma: 2 inhalations two times per day (all strengths).

PEDS – Asthma: Use adult dose for 12 yo or older.

UNAPPROVED ADULT – COPD: 2 puffs two times per day (all strengths).

FORMS – Trade only: MDI 100/5, 200/5 mcg mometasone/formoterol per actuation; 120 doses/canister.

NOTES – See individual components for additional information. Ritonavir and other CYP3A4 inhibitors such as ketoconazole significantly increase mometasone concentration resulting in systemic effects including adrenal suppression. Canister comes with 124 doses; patient must prime before first use and after more than 5 days of disuse by spraying 4 doses in air away from face, shaking canister after each spray.

DUONEB **(albuterol + ipratropium, ✤ *Combivent inhalation soln*)** ▶L ♀C ▶? $$$$$

ADULT – COPD: 1 unit dose nebulized four times per day; may add 2 doses/day prn to max of 6 doses/day.

PEDS – Not approved in children.

FORMS – Generic/Trade: Unit dose: 2.5 mg albuterol/0.5 mg ipratropium per 3 mL vial, premixed; 30, 60 vials/carton.

NOTES – Refer to components; 3.0 mg albuterol is equivalent to 2.5 mg albuterol base.

✤ *DUOVENT UDV* (ipratropium + fenoterol) ▶L ♀? ▶? $$$$$

ADULT – Canada only. Bronchospasm associated with asthma/COPD: 1 vial (via nebulizer) q 6 h prn.

PEDS – Canada only. Children age 12 yo or older: 1 vial (via nebulizer) q 6 h prn.

FORMS – Canada trade only: Unit dose vial (for nebulization) 0.5 mg ipratropium, 1.25 mg fenoterol in 4 mL of saline.

PREDICTED PEAK EXPIRATORY FLOW (liters/min) *Am Rev Resp Dis* 1963; 88:644

Age (yo)	Women (height in inches)					Men (height in inches)					Child (height in inches)	
	55"	60"	65"	70"	75"	60"	65"	70"	75"	80"		
20	390	423	460	496	529	554	602	649	693	740	44"	160
30	380	413	448	483	516	532	577	622	664	710	46"	187
40	370	402	436	470	502	509	552	596	636	680	48"	214
50	360	391	424	457	488	486	527	569	607	649	50"	240
60	350	380	412	445	475	463	502	542	578	618	52"	267
70	340	369	400	432	461	440	477	515	550	587	54"	293

INHALER COLORS (Body then cap—Generics may differ)

Inhaler	Colors
Advair	purple
Advair HFA	purple/light purple
Aerobid-M	grey/green
Aerospan	purple/grey
Alupent	clear/blue
Alvesco	
80 mcg	brown/red
160 mcg	red/red
Asmanex	white/pink
Atrovent HFA	clear/green
Combivent	clear/orange
Flovent HFA	orange/peach
Foradil	grey/beige

Inhaler	Colors
Maxair Autohaler	white/white
ProAir HFA	red/white
Proventil HFA	yellow/orange
Pulmicort	white/brown
QVAR	
40 mcg	beige/grey
80 mcg	mauve/grey
Serevent Diskus	green
Spiriva	grey
Ventolin HFA	light blue/navy
Xopenex HFA	blue/red

SYMBICORT **(budesonide + formoterol)** ▶L ♀C ◗? $$$$

WARNING – Long-acting beta-agonists may increase the risk of asthma-related death; use as an adjunct only if inadequate control with an optimal dose of inhaled corticosteroids. Avoid in significantly worsening or acute asthma. Do not use for rescue therapy. Do not stop abruptly.

ADULT – Chronic asthma: 2 puffs two times per day (both strengths). COPD: 2 puffs two times per day (160/4.5).

PEDS – Chronic asthma age 12 yo or older: Use adult dose.

FORMS – Trade only: MDI: 80/4.5, 160/4.5 mcg budesonide/formoterol per actuation; 120 doses/canister.

NOTES – See individual components for additional information. Ritonavir and other CYP3A4 inhibitors such as ketoconazole significantly increase budesonide concentrations, resulting in systemic effects, including adrenal suppression.

PULMONARY: Inhaled Steroids

NOTE: See Endocrine—Corticosteroids when oral steroids necessary. Beware of adrenal suppression when changing from systemic to inhaled steroids. Inhaled steroids are not for treatment of acute asthma; higher doses may be needed for severe asthma and exacerbations. Adjust to lowest effective dose for maintenance. Use of a DPI, a spacing device, and rinsing the mouth with water after each use may decrease the incidence of thrush and dysphonia. Pharyngitis and cough may occur with all products. Use with caution in patients with active or quiescent TB; untreated systemic fungal, bacterial, viral, or parasitic infections; or in patients with ocular HSV. Inhaled steroids produce small, transient reductions in growth velocity in children. Prolonged use may lead to decreases in bone mineral density and osteoporosis, thereby increasing fracture risk.

BECLOMETHASONE—INHALED (***QVAR***) ▶L ♀C ◗? $$$

ADULT – Chronic asthma: 40 mcg: 1 to 4 puffs two times per day. 80 mcg: 1 to 2 puffs two times per day.

PEDS – Chronic asthma in 5 to 11 yo: 40 mcg 1 to 2 puffs two times per day.

UNAPPROVED ADULT – Chronic asthma: NHLBI dosing schedule (puffs/day divided two times per day): Low dose: 2 to 6 puffs of 40 mcg or 1 to 3 puffs of 80 mcg. Medium dose: 6 to 12 puffs of 40 mcg or 3 to 6 puffs of 80 mcg. High dose: More than 12 puffs of 40 mcg or more than 6 puffs 80 mcg.

UNAPPROVED PEDS – Chronic asthma (5 to 11 yo): NHLBI dosing schedule (puffs/day divided two times per day): Low dose: 2 to 4 puffs of 40 mcg or 1 to 2 puffs of 80 mcg. Medium dose: 4 to 8 puffs of 40 mcg or 2 to 4 puffs of 80 mcg. High dose: More than 8 puffs of 40 mcg or more than 4 puffs of 80 mcg.

FORMS – Trade only: HFA MDI: 40, 80 mcg/actuation, 7.3 g 100 actuations/canister.

BUDESONIDE—INHALED (***Pulmicort Respules, Pulmicort Flexhaler***) ▶L ♀B ◗? $$$$

ADULT – Chronic asthma: DPI: 1 to 2 puffs daily to two times per day up to 4 puffs two times per day.

PEDS – Chronic asthma 6 to 12 yo: DPI: 1 to 2 puffs daily to two times per day. 12 mo to 8 yo: Susp for inhalation (Respules): 0.5 mg to 1 mg daily or divided two times per day.

UNAPPROVED ADULT – Chronic asthma: NHLBI dosing schedule (puffs/day daily or divided two times per day): DPI: Low dose is in the range of 1 to 3 puffs of 180 mcg or 2 to 6 puffs of 90 mcg. Medium dose is in the range of 3 to 7 puffs of 180 mcg or 6 to 13 puffs of 90 mcg. High dose more than 7 puffs of 180 mcg or more than 13 puffs of 90 mcg.

UNAPPROVED PEDS – Chronic asthma (5 to 11 yo): NHLBI dosing schedule (puffs/day daily or divided two times per day) DPI: Low dose: 1 to 2 puffs of 180 mcg or 2 to 4 puffs of 90 mcg. Medium dose: 2 to 4 puffs of 180 mcg or 4 to 9 puffs of 90 mcg. High dose is more than 4 puffs of 180 mcg or more than 9 puffs of 90 mcg. Susp for inhalation (daily or divided two times per day): Low dose is in the range of 0.25 to 0.5 mg for age 4 yo or younger and about 0.5 mg for age 5 to 11 yo. Medium dose more than 0.5 to 1 mg for age 4 yo or younger and 1 mg for age 5 to 11 yo. High dose more than 1 mg for age 4 yo or younger and 2 mg for age 5 to 11 yo. Some doses may be outside the package labeling.

FORMS – Trade only: DPI (Flexhaler) 90, 180 mcg powder/actuation 60, 120 doses respectively/canister, Respules 1 mg/2 mL unit dose. Generic/Trade: Respules 0.25, 0.5 mg/2 mL unit dose.

NOTES – Respules should be delivered via a jet nebulizer with a mouthpiece or face mask.

(cont.)

BUDESONIDE—INHALED (*cont.*)

CYP3A4 inhibitors such as ketoconazole, erythromycin, ritonavir, etc., may significantly increase systemic concentrations, possibly causing adrenal suppression. Flexhaler contains trace amounts of milk proteins; caution with severe milk protein hypersensitivity.

CICLESONIDE—INHALED (***Alvesco***) ▶L ♀C ◗? $$$$

ADULT – Chronic asthma: MDI: 80 mcg/puff: 1 to 4 puffs two times per day. 160 mcg/puff: 1 to 2 puffs two times per day.

PEDS – Chronic asthma, age 12 yo or older: Use adult dose.

FORMS – Trade only: 80 mcg/actuation, 60 per canister. 160 mcg/actuation, 60, 120 per canister.

NOTES – CYP3A4 inhibitors such as ketoconazole may significantly increase systemic concentrations, possibly causing adrenal suppression.

FLUNISOLIDE—INHALED (***AeroBid, AeroBid-M, Aerospan***) ▶L ♀C ◗? $$$

ADULT – Chronic asthma: MDI: 2 puffs two times per day up to 4 puffs two times per day.

PEDS – Chronic asthma, age: 6 to 15 yo: MDI: 2 puffs two times per day.

UNAPPROVED ADULT – Chronic asthma: NHLBI dosing schedule (puffs/day divided two times

(cont.)

INHALED STEROIDS: ESTIMATED COMPARATIVE DAILY DOSES*

Adults and Children older than 12 yo				
Drug	**Form**	**Low Dose**	**Medium Dose**	**High Dose**
beclomethasone HFA MDI	40 mcg/puff 80 mcg/puff	2–6 puffs/day 1–3 puffs/day	6–12 puffs/day 3–6 puffs/day	>12 puffs/day >6 puffs/day
budesonide DPI	90 mcg/dose 180 mcg/dose	2–6 inhalations/day 1–3 inhalations/day	6–13 inhalations/day 3–7 inhalations/day	>13 inhalations/day >7 inhalations/day
budesonide	soln for nebs	—	—	—
flunisolide HFA MDI	80 mcg/puff	4puffs/day	5–8 puffs/day	>8 puffs/day
fluticasone HFA MDI	44 mcg/puff 110 mcg/puff 220 mcg/puff	2–6 puffs/day 1–2 puffs/day 1 puffs/day	6–10 puffs/day 2–4 puffs/day 1–2 puffs/day	>10 puffs/day >4 puffs/day >2 puffs/day
fluticasone DPI	50 mcg/dose 100 mcg/dose 250 mcg/dose	2–6 inhalations/day 1–3 inhalations/day 1 inhalation/day	6–10 inhalations/day 3–5 inhalations/day 2 inhalations/day	>10 inhalations/day >5 inhalations/day >2 inhalations/day
mometasone DPI	220 mcg/dose	1 inhalations/day	2 inhalations/day	>2 inhalations/day
CHILDREN (age 5 to 11 yo)				
Drug	**Form**	**Low Dose**	**Medium Dose**	**High Dose**
beclomethasone HFA MDI	40 mcg/puff 80 mcg/puff	2–4 puffs/day 1–2 puffs/day	4–8 puffs/day 2–4 puffs/day	>8 puffs/day >4 puffs/day
budesonide DPI	90 mcg/dose 180 mcg/dose	2–4 inhalations/day 1–2 inhalations/day	4–9 inhalations/day 2–4 inhalations/day	>9 inhalations/day >4 inhalations/day
budesonide	soln for nebs	0.5 mg 0.25–0.5 mg (0–4 yo)	1 mg >0.5–1 mg (0–4 yo)	2 mg >1 mg (0–4 yo)
flunisolide HFA MDI	80 mcg/puff	2 puffs/day	4 puffs/day	≥8 puffs/day
fluticasone HFA MDI (0–11 yo)	44 mcg/puff 110 mcg/puff 220 mcg/puff	2–4 puffs/day 1–2 puff/day n/a	4–8 puffs/day 2–3 puffs/day 1–2 puffs/day	>8 puffs/day >4 puffs/day >2 puffs/day
fluticasone DPI	50 mcg/dose 100 mcg/dose 250 mcg/dose	2–4 inhalations/day 1–2 inhalations/day n/a	4–8 inhalations/day 2–4 inhalations/day 1 inhalation/day	>8 inhalations/day >4 inhalations/day >1 inhalation/day
mometasone DPI	220 mcg/dose	n/a	n/a	n/a

*HFA = Hydrofluoroalkane (propellant). MDI = metered dose inhaler. DPI = dry powder inhaler.
Reference: http://www.nhlbi.nih.gov/guidelines/asthma/asthsumm.pdf

FLUNISOLIDE—INHALED (*cont.*)

per day): Low dose: 2 to 4 puffs. Medium dose: 4 to 8 puffs. High dose: More than 8 puffs.

UNAPPROVED PEDS – Chronic asthma (5 to 11 yo): NHLBI dosing schedule (puffs/day divided two times per day): Low dose: 2 to 3 puffs. Medium dose: 4 to 5 puffs. High dose: More than 5 puffs (8 puffs or more for 80 mcg HFA).

FORMS – Trade only: MDI: 250 mcg/actuation, 100 metered doses/canister. AeroBid-M (AeroBid + menthol flavor). Aerospan HFA MDI: 80 mcg/actuation, 60, 120 metered doses/canister.

FLUTICASONE—INHALED (*Flovent HFA, Flovent Diskus*) ▶L ♀C ▶? $$$$

ADULT – Chronic asthma: MDI: 2 puffs two times per day up to 4 puffs two times per day. Max dose 880 mcg two times per day.

PEDS – Chronic asthma: 2 puffs two times per day of 44 mcg/puff for age 4 to 11 yo, Use adult dose for age 12 yo or older.

UNAPPROVED ADULT – Chronic asthma: NHLBI dosing schedule (puffs/day divided two times per day): Low dose: 2 to 6 puffs of 44 mcg MDI. Medium dose: 2 to 4 puffs of 110 mcg MDI or 2 puffs of 220 mcg MDI. High dose: More than 4 puffs 110 mcg MDI or more than 2 puffs 220 mcg MDI.

UNAPPROVED PEDS – Chronic asthma, age 11 yo or younger: NHLBI dosing schedule (puffs/day divided two times per day): Low dose: 2 to 4 puffs of 44 mcg MDI. Medium dose: 4 to 8 puffs of 44 mcg MDI. 2 to 3 puffs of 110 mcg MDI. 1 to 2 puffs of 220 mcg MDI. High dose: 4 puffs or more 110 mcg MDI. 2 puffs or more 220 mcg MDI.

FORMS – Trade only: HFA MDI: 44, 110, 220 mcg/actuation 120/canister. DPI (Flovent Diskus): 50, 100, 250 mcg/actuation delivering 44, 88, 220 mcg respectively.

NOTES – Ritonavir and other CYP3A4 inhibitors such as ketoconazole significantly increase fluticasone concentrations, resulting in systemic effects, including adrenal suppression. Increased risk of pneumonia in COPD.

MOMETASONE—INHALED (*Asmanex Twisthaler*) ▶L ♀C ▶? $$$$

ADULT – Chronic asthma: 1 to 2 puffs q pm or 1 puff two times per day. If prior oral corticosteroid therapy: 2 puffs two times per day.

PEDS – Chronic asthma: Age 12 yo or older: Use adult dose.

UNAPPROVED ADULT – Chronic asthma: NHLBI dosing schedule (puffs/day divided two times per day): Low dose: 1 puff. Medium dose: 2 puffs. High dose: More than 2 puffs.

FORMS – Trade only: DPI: 110 mcg/actuation with #30 dosage units, 220 mcg/actuation with #30, 60, 120 dosage units.

NOTES – CYP3A4 inhibitors such as ketoconazole may significantly increase concentrations.

PULMONARY: Leukotriene Inhibitors

NOTE: Not for treatment of acute asthma. Abrupt substitution for corticosteroids may precipitate Churg-Strauss syndrome. Postmarket cases of agitation, aggression, anxiousness, dream abnormalities and hallucinations, depression, insomnia, irritability, restlessness, suicidal thinking and behavior (including suicide), and tremor have been reported.

MONTELUKAST (*Singulair*) ▶L ♀B ▶? $$$$

ADULT – Chronic asthma, allergic rhinitis: 10 mg PO daily. Administer in evening for asthma. Prevention of exercise-induced bronchoconstriction: 10 mg PO 2 h before exercise.

PEDS – Chronic asthma, allergic rhinitis: Give 5 mg PO daily for age 6 to 14 yo, give 4 mg (chew tab or oral granules) PO daily for age 2 to 5 yo. Asthma age 12 to 23 mo: 4 mg (oral granules) PO daily. Allergic rhinitis age 6 to 23 mo: 4 mg (oral granules) PO daily. Prevention of exercise-induced bronchoconstriction: Age 6 yo or older: Use adult dose.

FORMS – Generic/Trade: Tabs 10 mg. Oral granules 4 mg packet, 30/box. Chewable tabs (cherry flavored) 4, 5 mg.

NOTES – Chewable tabs contain phenylalanine. Oral granules may be placed directly into the mouth or mixed with a spoonful of breastmilk, baby formula, applesauce, carrots, rice, or ice cream. If mixed with food, must be taken within 15 min. Do not mix with other liquids. Levels decreased by phenobarbital and rifampin. Dyspepsia may occur. Do not take an additional dose for exercise-induced bronchospasm if already taking other doses chronically.

ZAFIRLUKAST (*Accolate*) ▶L ♀B ▶– $$$$

WARNING – Hepatic failure has been reported.

ADULT – Chronic asthma: 20 mg PO two times per day, 1 h before meals or 2 h after meals.

PEDS – Chronic asthma age 5 to 11 yo: 10 mg PO two times per day, 1 h before meals or 2

(cont.)

ZAFIRLUKAST (*cont.*)

h after meals. Use adult dose for age 12 yo or older.

UNAPPROVED ADULT – Allergic rhinitis: 20 mg PO two times per day, 1 h before meals or 2 h after meals.

FORMS – Trade only: Tabs 10, 20 mg.

NOTES – Potentiates warfarin and theophylline. Levels decreased by erythromycin and increased by high-dose aspirin. Nausea may occur. If liver dysfunction is suspected, discontinue drug and manage accordingly. Consider monitoring LFTs.

ZILEUTON (*Zyflo CR*) ▸L ♀C ▸? $$$$$

WARNING – Contraindicated in active liver disease.

ADULT – Chronic asthma: 1200 mg PO two times per day.

PEDS – Chronic asthma age 12 yo or older: Use adult dose.

FORMS – Trade only: Tabs extended-release 600 mg.

NOTES – Monitor LFTs for elevation. Potentiates warfarin, theophylline, and propranolol. Dyspepsia and nausea may occur.

PULMONARY: Other Pulmonary Medications

ACETYLCYSTEINE—INHALED (*Mucomyst*) ▸L ♀B ▸? $

ADULT – Mucolytic nebulization: 3 to 5 mL of the 20% soln or 6 to 10 mL of the 10% soln three to four times per day. Instillation, direct or via tracheostomy: 1 to 2 mL of a 10% to 20% soln q 1 to 4 h; via percutaneous intratracheal catheter: 1 to 2 mL of the 20% soln or 2 to 4 mL of the 10% soln q 1 to 4 h.

PEDS – Mucolytic nebulization: Use adult dosing.

FORMS – Generic/Trade: Soln for inhalation 10, 20% in 4, 10, 30 mL vials.

NOTES – Increased volume of liquefied bronchial secretions may occur; maintain an open airway. Watch for bronchospasm in asthmatics. Stomatitis, N/V, fever, and rhinorrhea may occur. A slight disagreeable odor may occur and should soon disappear. A face mask may cause stickiness on the face after nebulization; wash with water. The 20% soln may be diluted with NaCl or sterile water.

ACLIDINIUM (*Tudorza*) ▸L– ♀C ▸?

ADULT – COPD: Pressair: 400 mcg two times per day.

PEDS – Not approved in children.

FORMS – Trade only: Sealed aluminum pouches 400 mcg. To be used with "Pressair" device only. Packages of 60 with Pressair device.

NOTES – Not for acute bronchospasm. Use with caution in narrow-angle glaucoma, myasthenia gravis, BPH, or bladder-neck obstruction. Paradoxical bronchospasm may occur. Eye pain or blurred vision may occur if powder enters eyes. Avoid if severe lactose allergy.

ALPHA-1 PROTEINASE INHIBITOR (**alpha-1 antitrypsin,** ***Aralast, Prolastin, Zemaira***) ▸Plasma ♀C ▸? $

WARNING – Possible transmission of viruses and Creutzfeldt-Jakob disease.

ADULT – Congenital alpha-1 proteinase inhibitor deficiency with emphysema: 60 mg/kg IV once per week.

PEDS – Not approved in children.

NOTES – Contraindicated in selected IgA deficiencies with known antibody to IgA. Hepatitis B vaccine recommended in preparation for Prolastin use.

AMINOPHYLLINE ▸L ♀C ▸? $

ADULT – Acute asthma: Loading dose if currently not receiving theophylline: 6 mg/kg IV over 20 to 30 min. Maintenance IV infusion: Dose 0.5 to 0.7 mg/kg/h, mix 1 g in 250 mL D5W (4 mg/mL) set at rate 11 mL/h delivers 0.7 mg/kg/h for wt 70 kg patient. In patients with cor pulmonale, heart failure, liver failure, use 0.25 mg/kg/h. If currently on theophylline, each 0.6 mg/kg aminophylline will increase the serum theophylline concentration by approximately 1 mcg/mL. Maintenance: 200 mg PO two to four times per day.

PEDS – Acute asthma: Loading dose if currently not receiving theophylline: 6 mg/kg IV over 20 to 30 min. Maintenance oral route age older than 1 yo: 3 to 4 mg/kg/dose PO q 6 h. Maintenance IV route for age older than 6 mo: 0.8 to 1 mg/kg/h IV infusion.

UNAPPROVED PEDS – Neonatal apnea of prematurity: Loading dose 5 to 6 mg/kg IV/PO, maintenance: 1 to 2 mg/kg/dose q 6 to 8 h IV/PO.

FORMS – Generic only: Tabs 100, 200 mg. Oral liquid 105 mg/5 mL. Canada Trade only: Tabs controlled-release (12 h) 225, 350 mg, scored.

NOTES – Aminophylline is 79% theophylline. Administer IV infusion no faster than 25 mg/min. Multiple drug interactions (especially ketoconazole, rifampin, carbamazepine, isoniazid, phenytoin, macrolides, zafirlukast, and cimetidine). Review meds before initiating treatment. Irritability, nausea, palpitations, and tachycardia may occur. Overdose may be life-threatening.

BERACTANT (*Survanta*) ▶Lung ♀? ▶? $$$$$
PEDS – RDS (hyaline membrane disease) in premature infants: Specialized dosing.

CALFACTANT (*Infasurf*) ▶Lung ♀? ▶? $$$$$
PEDS – RDS (hyaline membrane disease) in premature infants: Specialized dosing.
FORMS – Trade only: Oral susp: 35 mg/mL in 3, 6 mL vials. Preservative-free.

CROMOLYN—INHALED (*Intal, Gastrocrom,* ✤ *Nalcrom*) ▶LK ♀B ▶? $$$
ADULT – Chronic asthma: MDI: 2 to 4 puffs four times per day. Soln for inhalation: 20 mg four times per day. Prevention of exercise-induced bronchospasm: MDI: 2 puffs 10 to 15 min prior to exercise. Soln for nebulization: 20 mg 10 to 15 min prior. Mastocytosis: 200 mg PO four times per day, 30 min before meals and at bedtime.
PEDS – Chronic asthma for age older than 5 yo using MDI: 2 puffs four times per day; for age older than 2 yo using soln for nebulization 20 mg four times per day. Prevention of exercise-induced bronchospasm for age older than 5 yo using MDI: 2 puffs 10 to 15 min prior to exercise, using soln for nebulization for age older than 2 yo: 20 mg 10 to 15 min prior. Mastocytosis: Age 2 to 12 yo: 100 mg PO four times per day 30 min before meals and at bedtime.
FORMS – Trade only: MDI 800 mcg/actuation, 112, 200/canister. Oral concentrate 100 mg/5 mL in 8 amps/foil pouch (Gastrocrom). Generic/Trade: Soln for nebs: 20 mg/2 mL.
NOTES – Not for treatment of acute asthma. Pharyngitis may occur. Directions for oral concentrate: 1) Break open and squeeze liquid contents of ampule(s) into a glass of water. 2) Stir soln. 3) Drink all of the liquid.

DORNASE ALFA (*Pulmozyme*) ▶L ♀B ▶? $$$$$
ADULT – Cystic fibrosis: 2.5 mg nebulized one to two times per day.
PEDS – Cystic fibrosis age 6 yo or older: 2.5 mg nebulized one to two times per day.
UNAPPROVED PEDS – Has been used in a small number of children as young as 3 mo with similar efficacy and side effects.
FORMS – Trade only: Soln for inhalation: 1 mg/mL in 2.5 mL vials.
NOTES – Voice alteration, pharyngitis, laryngitis, and rash may occur. Do not dilute or mix with other drugs.

DOXAPRAM (*Dopram*) ▶L ♀B ▶? $$$
ADULT – Acute hypercapnia due to COPD: 1 to 2 mg/min IV, max 3 mg/min. Maximum infusion time: 2 h.
PEDS – Not approved in children.
UNAPPROVED PEDS – Apnea of prematurity unresponsive to methylxanthines: Load 2.5 to 3 mg/kg over 15 min, then 1 mg/kg/h titrated to lowest effective dose. Max: 2.5 mg/kg/h. Contains benzyl alcohol; caution in neonates.
NOTES – Monitor arterial blood gases at baseline and q 30 min during infusion. Do not use with mechanical ventilation. Contraindicated with seizure disorder, severe HTN, CVA, head injury, CAD and severe heart failure.

EPINEPHRINE RACEMIC (*S-2,* ✤ *Vaponefrin*) ▶Plasma ♀C ▶– $
ADULT – See Cardiovascular section.
PEDS – Severe croup: Soln for inhalation: 0.05 mL/kg/dose diluted to 3 mL with NS over 15 min prn not to exceed q 1 to 2 h dosing. Max dose 0.5 mL.
FORMS – Trade only: Soln for inhalation: 2.25% epinephrine in 15, 30 mL.
NOTES – Cardiac arrhythmias and HTN may occur.

IPRATROPIUM—INHALED (*Atrovent, Atrovent HFA*) ▶Lung ♀B ▶? $$$$
ADULT – COPD: MDI (Atrovent, Atrovent HFA): 2 puffs four times per day; may use additional inhalations not to exceed 12 puffs/day. Soln for inhalation: 500 mcg nebulized three to four times per day.
PEDS – Not approved in children younger than 12 yo.
UNAPPROVED PEDS – Acute asthma: MDI (Atrovent, Atrovent HFA): 1 to 2 puffs three to four times per day for age 12 yo or younger. Soln for inhalation: Give 250 mcg/dose three to four times per day for age 12 yo or younger: Give 250 to 500 mcg/dose three to four times per day for age older than 12 yo. Acute asthma: Age 2 to 18 yo: 500 mcg nebulized with 2nd and 3rd doses of albuterol.
FORMS – Trade only: Atrovent HFA MDI: 17 mcg/actuation, 200/canister. Generic/Trade: Soln for nebulization: 0.02% (500 mcg/vial) in unit dose vials.
NOTES – Atrovent MDI is contraindicated with soy or peanut allergy; HFA not contraindicated. Caution with glaucoma, myasthenia gravis, BPH, or bladder neck obstruction. Cough, dry mouth, and blurred vision may occur.

✤ **KETOTIFEN** ▶L ♀C ▶– $$
ADULT – Not approved.
PEDS – Canada only. Chronic asthma: 6 mo to 3 yo: 0.05 mg/kg PO two times per day. Children older than 3 yo: 1 mg PO two times per day.
FORMS – Generic/Trade: Tabs 1 mg. Syrup 1 mg/5 mL.

(cont.)

♣ KETOTIFEN (*cont.*)

NOTES – Several weeks may be necessary before therapeutic effect. Full clinical effectiveness is generally reached after 10 weeks.

METHACHOLINE (***Provocholine***) ▶Plasma ♀C ▶? $$

WARNING – Life-threatening bronchoconstriction can result; have resuscitation capability available.

ADULT – Diagnosis of bronchial airway hyperreactivity in nonwheezing patients with suspected asthma: 5 breaths each of ascending serial concentrations, 0.025 mg/mL to 25 mg/mL, via nebulization. The procedure ends when there is more than 20% reduction in the FEV1 compared with baseline.

PEDS – Diagnosis of bronchial airway hyperreactivity: Use adult dose.

NOTES – Avoid with epilepsy, bradycardia, peptic ulcer disease, thyroid disease, urinary tract obstruction, or other conditions that could be adversely affected by a cholinergic agent. Hold beta-blockers. Do not inhale powder.

NEDOCROMIL—INHALED (***Tilade***) ▶L ♀B ▶? $$$

ADULT – Chronic asthma: MDI: 2 puffs four times per day. Reduce dose to two to three times per day as tolerated.

PEDS – Chronic asthma age older than 6 yo: MDI: 2 puffs four times per day.

FORMS – Trade only: MDI: 1.75 mg/actuation, 112/canister.

NOTES – Product to be discontinued when supplies run out. Not for treatment of acute asthma. Unpleasant taste and dysphonia may occur.

NITRIC OXIDE (***INOmax***) ▶Lung, K ♀C ▶? $$$$

PEDS – Respiratory failure with pulmonary HTN in infants older than 34 weeks old: Specialized dosing.

NOTES – Risk of methemoglobinemia increases with concomitant nitroprusside or nitroglycerin.

OMALIZUMAB (***Xolair***) ▶Plasma, L ♀B ▶? $$$$$

WARNING – Anaphylaxis may occur; monitor closely and be prepared to treat. Anaphylaxis most commonly occurs within 1 h of administration; 78% of cases occur within 12 h.

ADULT – Moderate to severe asthma with perennial allergy when symptoms not controlled by inhaled steroids: 150 to 375 mg SC q 2 to 4 weeks, based on pretreatment serum total IgE level and body wt.

PEDS – Moderate to severe asthma with perennial allergy: Age 12 yo or older: Use adult dose.

NOTES – Not for treatment of acute asthma. Divide doses greater than 150 mg over more than 1 injection site. Monitor for signs of anaphylaxis including bronchospasm, hypotension, syncope, urticaria, angioedema.

PORACTANT (***Curosurf***) ▶Lung ♀? ▶? $$$$$

PEDS – RDS (hyaline membrane disease) in premature infants: Specialized dosing.

ROFLUMILAST (***Daliresp***, ***♣ Daxas***) ▶L – ♀C ▶– $$$$

ADULT – Severe COPD due to chronic bronchitis: 500 mcg PO daily with or without food.

PEDS – Not approved for use in children.

FORMS – Trade: Tabs 500 mcg.

NOTES – Contraindicated in moderate to severe liver disease. Inhibitors of CYP3A4 or dual CYP3A4 and 1A2 (erythromycin, ketoconazole, cimetidine) may increase concentrations. Not recommended for use with strong CYP inducers (rifampin, carbamazepine, phenobarbital, phenytoin). Not for relief of acute bronchospasm. Main effect is decreased exacerbations.

THEOPHYLLINE (***Elixophyllin, Uniphyl, Theo-24, T-Phyl, ♣ Theo-Dur, Theolair***) ▶L ♀C ▶+ $

ADULT – Chronic asthma: 5 to 13 mg/kg/day PO in divided doses. Max dose 900 mg/day.

PEDS – Chronic asthma: Initial: Age older than 1 yo and wt less than 45 kg: 12 to 14 mg/kg/day PO divided q 4 to 6 h to max of 300 mg/24 h. Maintenance: 16 to 20 mg/kg/day PO divided q 4 to 6 h to max of 600 mg/24 h. For age older than 1 yo and wt 45 kg or more: Initial: 300 mg/24 h PO divided q 6 to 8 h. Maintenance: 400 to 600 mg/24 h PO divided q 6 to 8 h. Infants age 6 to 52 weeks: [(0.2 × age in weeks) + 5] × kg = 24 h dose in mg PO divided q 6 to 8 h.

UNAPPROVED ADULT – COPD: 10 mg/kg/day PO in divided doses.

UNAPPROVED PEDS – Apnea and bradycardia of prematurity: 3 to 6 mg/kg/day PO divided q 6 to 8 h. Maintain serum concentrations 3 to 5 mcg/mL.

FORMS – Generic/Trade: Elixir 80 mg/15 mL. Trade only: Caps: Theo-24: 100, 200, 300, 400 mg. T-Phyl: 12 h SR tabs 200 mg. Theolair: Tabs 125, 250 mg. Generic only: 12 h tabs 100, 200, 300, 450 mg, 12 h caps 125, 200, 300 mg.

NOTES – Multiple drug interactions (especially ketoconazole, rifampin, carbamazepine, isoniazid, phenytoin, macrolides, zafirlukast, and cimetidine). Review meds before initiating treatment. Overdose may be life-threatening.

TIOTROPIUM (*Spiriva*) ▶K ♀C ▶– $$$$

WARNING – QT prolongation has been reported.

ADULT – COPD: Handihaler: 18 mcg inhaled daily.

PEDS – Not approved in children.

FORMS – Trade only: Caps for oral inhalation 18 mcg. To be used with "Handihaler" device only. Packages of 5, 30, 90 caps with Handihaler device.

NOTES – Not for acute bronchospasm. Administer at the same time each day. Use with caution in narrow-angle glaucoma, myasthenia gravis, BPH, or bladder-neck obstruction. Avoid touching opened cap. Glaucoma, eye pain, or blurred vision may occur if powder enters eyes. May increase dosing interval in patients with CrCl less than 50 mL/min. Avoid if severe lactose allergy.

TOXICOLOGY: Toxicology

ACETYLCYSTEINE (*N-acetylcysteine, Mucomyst, Acetadote,* ✤ *Parvolex*) ▶L ♀B ▶? $$$$

ADULT – Acetaminophen toxicity: Mucomyst: Loading dose 140 mg/kg PO or NG, then 70 mg/kg q 4 h for 17 doses. May be mixed in water or soft drink diluted to a 5% soln. Acetadote (IV): Loading dose 150 mg/kg in 200 mL of D5W infused over 60 min; maintenance dose 50 mg/kg in 500 mL of D5W infused over 4 h followed by 100 mg/kg in 1000 mL of D5W infused over 16 h.

PEDS – Acetaminophen toxicity: Same as adult dosing.

UNAPPROVED ADULT – Prevention of contrast-induced nephropathy: 600 to 1200 mg PO two times per day for 2 doses before procedure and 2 doses after procedure.

FORMS – Generic/Trade: Soln 10%, 20%. Trade only: IV (Acetadote).

NOTES – May be diluted with water or soft drink to a 5% soln; use diluted soln within 1 h. Repeat loading dose if vomited within 1 h. Critical ingestion–treatment interval for maximal protection against severe hepatic injury is between 0 and 8 h. Efficacy diminishes after 8 h and treatment initiation between 15 and 24 h post-ingestion yields limited efficacy. However, treatment should not be withheld, since the reported time of ingestion may not be correct. Anaphylactoid reactions usually occur 30 to 60 min after initiating infusion. Stop infusion, administer antihistamine or epinephrine, restart infusion slowly. If anaphylactoid reactions return or severity increases, then stop treatment.

CHARCOAL (**activated charcoal,** *Actidose-Aqua, CharcoAid, EZ-Char,* ✤ *Charcodate*) ▶Not absorbed ♀+ ▶+ $

ADULT – Gut decontamination: 25 to 100 g (1 to 2 g/kg or 10× the amount of poison ingested) PO or NG as soon as possible. May repeat q 1 to 4 h prn at doses equivalent to 12.5 g/h. When sorbitol is coadministered, use only with the first dose if repeated doses are to be given.

PEDS – Gut decontamination: 1 g/kg for age younger than 1 yo; 15 to 30 g or 1 to 2 g/kg for age 1 to 12 yo PO or NG as soon as possible. Repeat doses in children have not been established, but half the initial dose is recommended. Repeat q 2 to 6 h prn. When sorbitol is coadministered, use only with the first dose if repeated doses are to be given.

FORMS – OTC/Generic/Trade: Powder 15, 30, 40, 120, 240 g. Soln 12.5 g/60 mL, 15 g/75 mL, 15 g/120 mL, 25 g/120 mL, 30 g/120 mL, 50 g/240 mL. Susp 15 g/120 mL, 25 g/120 mL, 30 g/150 mL, 50 g/240 mL. Granules 15 g/120 mL.

NOTES – Some products may contain sorbitol to improve taste and reduce GI transit time. Chocolate milk/powder may enhance palatability for pediatric use. Not usually effective for toxic alcohols (methanol, ethylene glycol, isopropanol), heavy metals (lead, iron, bromide), arsenic, lithium, potassium, hydrocarbons, and caustic ingestions (acids, alkalis). Mix powder with 8 oz water. Greatest effect when administered within 1 h of ingestion.

DEFERIPRONE (*Ferriprox,* ✤ *Ferriprox*) ▶glucuronidation – ♀D ▶–©V $$$$$

WARNING – Ferriprox can cause agranulocytosis and neutropenia may precede this development. Measure the ANC before starting and monitor weekly. Interrupt Ferriprox if infection develops and monitor the ANC more frequently.

ADULT – Transfusional iron overload due to thalassemia syndromes when current chelation therapy is inadequate: 25 mg/kg, orally, three times per day for a total of 75 mg/kg/day. The maximum dose is 33 mg/kg, three times per day for a total of 99 mg/kg/day.

PEDS – Not approved

FORMS – 500 mg film-coated tabs with a functional score.

NOTES – Contraindicated with preexisting agranulocytosis or neutropenia. Advise patients taking Ferriprox to report immediately any symptoms indicative of infection. Inform patients that their

(cont.)

DEFERIPRONE (*cont.*)

urine might show a reddish/brown discoloration due to the excretion of the iron-deferiprone complex.

DEFEROXAMINE (***Desferal***) ▶K ♀C ◗? $$$$$

ADULT – Chronic iron overload: 500 to 1000 mg IM daily and 2 g IV infusion (no faster than 15 mg/kg/h) with each unit of blood or 1 to 2 g SC daily (20 to 40 mg/kg/day) over 8 to 24 h via continuous infusion pump. Acute iron toxicity: IV infusion up to 15 mg/kg/h (consult poison center).

PEDS – Acute iron toxicity: IV infusion up to 15 mg/kg/h (consult poison center).

NOTES – Contraindicated in renal failure/anuria unless undergoing dialysis.

DIMERCAPROL (***BAL in oil***) ▶KL ♀C ◗? $$$$$

ADULT – Specialized dosing for arsenic, mercury, gold, and lead toxicity. Consult poison center. Mild arsenic or gold toxicity: 2.5 mg/kg IM four times per day for 2 days, then two times per day for 1 day, then daily for 10 days. Severe arsenic or gold toxicity: 3 mg/kg IM q 4 h for 2 days, then four times per day for 1 day, then two times per day for 10 days. Mercury toxicity: 5 mg/kg IM initially, then 2.5 mg/kg daily to two times per day for 10 days. Begin therapy within 1 to 2 h of toxicity. Acute lead encephalopathy: 4 mg/kg IM initially, then q 4 h in combination (separate syringe) with calcium edetate for 2 to 7 days. May reduce dose to 3 mg/kg IM for less severe toxicity. Deep IM injection needed.

PEDS – Not approved in children.

UNAPPROVED PEDS – Same as adult dosing. Consult poison center.

DUODOTE **(atropine + pralidoxime)** ▶K ♀C ◗? $

ADULT – Organophosphate insecticide/nerve agent poisoning, mild symptoms: 1 injection in thigh. Severe symptoms: 3 injections in rapid succession (may administer through clothes).

PEDS – Not approved in children.

FORMS – Each auto-injector dose delivers atropine 2.1 mg + pralidoxime 600 mg.

EDETATE (***EDTA, Endrate,*** **versenate**) ▶K ♀C ◗– $$$

WARNING – Beware of elevated intracranial pressure in lead encephalopathy.

ADULT – Consult poison center. Use calcium disodium form only for lead indications. Noncalcium form (eg, Endrate) is not interchangeable and is rarely used anymore. Lead toxicity: 1000 mg/m²/day IM (divided into equal doses q 8 to 12 h) or IV (infuse total dose over 8 to 12 h) for 5 days. Interrupt therapy for 2 to 4 days, then repeat same regimen. Two courses of therapy are usually necessary. Acute lead encephalopathy: Edetate alone or in combination with dimercaprol. Lead nephropathy: 500 mg/m²/dose q 24 h for 5 doses (if creatinine 2 to 3 mg/dL), q 48 h for 3 doses (if creatinine 3 to 4 mg/dL), or once per week (if creatinine greater than 4 mg/dL). May repeat at 1 month intervals.

PEDS – Specialized dosing for lead toxicity; same as adult dosing also using calcium form. Consult poison center.

FORMS – Calcium disodium formulation used for lead poisoning, other form without calcium (eg, Endrate) is not interchangeable and rarely used anymore.

ETHANOL **(alcohol)** ▶L ♀D ◗+ $

PEDS – Not approved in children.

UNAPPROVED ADULT – Consult poison center. Specialized dosing for methanol, ethylene glycol toxicity if fomepizole is unavailable or delayed: 1000 mg/kg (10 mL/kg) of 10% ethanol (100 mg/mL) IV over 1 to 2 h then 100 mg/kg/h (1 mL/kg/h) to keep ethanol level approximately 100 mg/dL.

FLUMAZENIL (***Romazicon***) ▶LK ♀C ◗? $$$$

WARNING – Do not administer in chronic benzodiazepine use or acute overdose with TCAs due to seizure risk.

ADULT – Benzodiazepine sedation reversal: 0.2 mg IV over 15 sec, then 0.2 mg q 1 min prn up to 1 mg total dose. Usual dose is 0.6 to 1 mg. Benzodiazepine overdose reversal: 0.2 mg IV over 30 sec, then 0.3 to 0.5 mg q 30 sec prn up to 3 mg total dose.

PEDS – Benzodiazepine sedation reversal: 0.01 mg/kg up to 0.2 mg IV over 15 sec; repeat q min to max 4 additional doses.

UNAPPROVED PEDS – Benzodiazepine overdose reversal: 0.01 mg/kg IV. Benzodiazepine sedation reversal: 0.01 mg/kg IV initially (max 0.2 mg), then 0.005 to 0.01 mg/kg (max 0.2 mg) q 1 min to max total dose 1 mg. May repeat doses in 20 min, max 3 mg in 1 h.

NOTES – Onset of action 1 to 3 min, peak effect 6 to 10 min. For IV use only, preferably through an IV infusion line into a large vein. Local irritation may occur following extravasation.

FOMEPIZOLE (***Antizol***) ▶L ♀C ◗? $$$$$

ADULT – Consult poison center. Ethylene glycol or methanol toxicity: 15 mg/kg IV (load), then 10 mg/kg IV q 12 h for 4 doses, then 15 mg/kg IV q 12 h until ethylene glycol or methanol level is below 20 mg/dL. Administer doses as slow IV infusions over 30 min. Increase frequency to q 4 h during hemodialysis.

PEDS – Not approved in children.

ANTIDOTES

Toxin	Antidote/Treatment
acetaminophen	N-acetylcysteine
TCAs	sodium bicarbonate
arsenic, mercury	dimercaprol (BAL)
benzodiazepine	flumazenil
beta-blockers	glucagon
calcium channel blockers	calcium chloride, glucagon
cyanide	cyanide antidote kit, Cyanokit (hydroxocobalamin)

Toxin	Antidote/Treatment
digoxin	dig immune Fab
ethylene glycol	fomepizole
heparin	protamine
iron	deferoxamine
lead	BAL, EDTA, succimer
methanol	fomepizole
methemoglobin	methylene blue
opioids/opiates	naloxone
organophosphates	atropine + pralidoxime
warfarin	vitamin K, FFP

HYDROXOCOBALAMIN (***Cyanokit***) ▶K ♀C ▶? $$$$$

ADULT – Cyanide poisoning: 5 g IV over 15 min; may repeat prn.

PEDS – Not approved in children.

IPECAC SYRUP ▶Gut ♀C ▶? $

ADULT – Emesis: 15 to 30 mL PO, then 3 to 4 glasses of water.

PEDS – AAP no longer recommends home ipecac for poisoning. Emesis, age younger than 1 yo: 5 to 10 mL, then ½ to 1 glass of water (controversial in children younger than 1 yo). Emesis, age 1 to 12 yo: 15 mL, then 1 to 2 glasses of water. May repeat dose (15 mL) if vomiting does not occur within 20 to 30 min.

FORMS – OTC Generic only: Syrup 30 mL.

NOTES – Many believe ipecac to be contraindicated in infants age younger than 6 mo. Do not use if any potential for altered mental status (eg, seizure, neurotoxicity), strychnine, beta-blocker, calcium channel blocker, clonidine, digitalis glycoside, corrosive, petroleum distillate ingestions, or if at risk for GI bleeding (coagulopathy).

METHYLENE BLUE (***Urolene blue***) ▶K ♀C ▶? $

ADULT – Methemoglobinemia: 1 to 2 mg/kg IV over 5 min. Dysuria: 65 to 130 mg PO three times per day after meals with liberal water.

PEDS – Not approved in children.

UNAPPROVED PEDS – Methemoglobinemia: 1 to 2 mg/kg/dose IV over 5 min; may repeat in 1 h prn.

FORMS – Trade only: Tabs 65 mg.

NOTES – Avoid in G6PD deficiency. May turn urine, stool, skin, contact lenses, and undergarments blue-green.

PENICILLAMINE (***Cuprimine, Depen***) ▶K ♀D ▶– $$$$$

WARNING – Fatal drug-related adverse events have occurred, caution if penicillin allergy.

ADULT – Consult poison center: Specialized dosing for copper toxicity. 750 mg to 1.5 g/day PO for 3 months based on 24 h urinary copper excretion, max 2 g/day. May start 250 mg/day PO in patients unable to tolerate.

PEDS – Specialized dosing for copper toxicity. Consult poison center.

FORMS – Trade only: Caps 125, 250 mg; Tabs 250 mg.

NOTES – Patients may require supplemental pyridoxine 25 to 50 mg/day PO. Promotes excretion of heavy metals in urine.

PHYSOSTIGMINE (***Antilirium***) ▶LK ♀D ▶? $

WARNING – Discontinue if excessive salivation, emesis, frequent urination, or diarrhea. Rapid administration can cause bradycardia, hypersalivation, respiratory difficulties and seizures. Atropine should be available as an antagonist.

ADULT – Life-threatening anticholinergic toxicity: 2 mg IV/IM, administer IV no faster than 1 mg/min. May repeat q 10 to 30 min for severe toxicity.

PEDS – Life-threatening anticholinergic toxicity: 0.02 mg/kg IM/IV injection, administer IV no faster than 0.5 mg/min. May repeat q 15 to 30 min until a therapeutic effect or max 2 mg dose.

UNAPPROVED ADULT – Postanesthesia reversal of neuromuscular blockade: 0.5 to 1 mg IV/IM, administer IV no faster than 1 mg/min. May repeat q 10 to 30 min prn.

FORMS – Generic/Trade: 1 mg/mL in 2 mL ampules.

PRALIDOXIME (***Protopam, 2-PAM***) ▶K ♀C ▶? $$$$

ADULT – Consult poison center: Specialized dosing for organophosphate toxicity: 1 to 2 g IV infusion over 15 to 30 min or slow IV injection over 5 min or longer (max rate 200 mg/min). May repeat dose after 1 h if muscle weakness persists.

(cont.)

PRALIDOXIME (*cont.*)

PEDS – Not approved in children.

UNAPPROVED ADULT – Consult poison center: 20 to 40 mg/kg/dose IV infusion over 15 to 30 min.

UNAPPROVED PEDS – Consult poison center. 25 mg/kg load then 10 to 20 mg/kg/h or 25 to 50 mg/kg load followed by repeat dose in 1 to 2 h then q 10 to 12 h.

NOTES – Administer within 36 h of exposure when possible. Rapid administration may worsen cholinergic symptoms. Give in conjunction with atropine. IM or SC may be used if IV access is not available.

PRUSSIAN BLUE (***Radiogardase***) ▶Fecal ♀C ▶+ $$$$$

ADULT – Internal contamination with radioactive cesium/thallium: 3 g PO three times per day.

PEDS – Internal contamination with radioactive cesium/thallium, 2 to 12 yo: 1 g PO three times per day.

FORMS – Trade only: Caps 500 mg.

SUCCIMER (***Chemet***) ▶K ♀C ▶? $$$$$

PEDS – Lead toxicity 1 yo or older: Start 10 mg/kg PO or 350 mg/m^2 q 8 h for 5 days, then reduce the frequency to q 12 h for 2 weeks. Not approved in children younger than 1 yo.

FORMS – Trade only: Caps 100 mg.

NOTES – Manufacturer recommends doses of 100 mg (wt 8 to 15 kg), 200 mg (wt 16 to 23 kg), 300 mg (wt 24 to 34 kg), 400 mg (wt 35 to 44 kg), and 500 mg (wt 45 kg or greater). Can open cap and sprinkle medicated beads over food, or give them in a spoon and follow with fruit drink. Indicated for blood lead levels greater than 45 mcg/dL. Allow at least 4 weeks between edetate disodium and succimer treatment.

UROLOGY: Benign Prostatic Hyperplasia

ALFUZOSIN (***UroXatral***, ***✤Xatral***) ▶KL ♀B ▶– $$$$

WARNING – Postural hypotension with or without symptoms may develop within a few hours after administration. Avoid in moderate or severe hepatic insufficiency. Avoid coadministration with potent CYP3A4 inhibitors.

ADULT – BPH: 10 mg PO daily after a meal.

PEDS – Not approved in children.

UNAPPROVED ADULT – Promotes spontaneous passage of ureteral calculi: 10 mg PO daily usually combined with an NSAID, antiemetic, and opioid of choice.

FORMS – Generic/Trade: Tabs extended-release 10 mg.

NOTES – Caution in congenital or acquired QT prolongation and severe renal insufficiency. Intraoperative floppy iris syndrome has been observed during cataract surgery.

DUTASTERIDE (***Avodart***) ▶L ♀X ▶– $$$$

ADULT – BPH: 0.5 mg PO daily with/without tamsulosin 0.4 mg PO daily.

PEDS – Not approved in children.

FORMS – Trade only: Caps 0.5 mg.

NOTES – 6 months of therapy may be needed to assess effectiveness. Pregnant or potentially pregnant women should not handle caps due to fetal risk from absorption. Caution in hepatic insufficiency. Dutasteride will decrease PSA by 50%; new baseline PSA should be established after 3 to 6 months to assess potentially cancer-related PSA changes. Cap should be swallowed whole and not chewed or opened to avoid oropharyngeal irritation.

FINASTERIDE (***Proscar***, ***Propecia***) ▶L ♀X ▶– $$$

ADULT – Proscar: 5 mg PO daily alone or in combination with doxazosin to reduce the risk of symptomatic progression of BPH. Propecia: Androgenetic alopecia in men: 1 mg PO daily.

PEDS – Not approved in children.

UNAPPROVED ADULT – Cancer prevention in "at-risk" men older than 55 yo: 5 mg daily. Androgenetic alopecia in postmenopausal women (no evidence of efficacy): 1 mg PO daily.

FORMS – Generic/Trade: Tabs 1 mg (Propecia), 5 mg (Proscar).

NOTES – Therapy for 6 to 12 months may be needed to assess effectiveness for BPH and at least 3 months for alopecia. Pregnant or potentially pregnant women should not handle crushed tabs because of possible absorption and fetal risk. Use with caution in hepatic insufficiency. Monitor PSA before therapy; finasteride will decrease PSA by 50% in patients with BPH, even with prostate cancer. Does not appear to alter detection of prostate cancer.

JALYN (**dutasteride + tamsulosin**) ▶LK – ♀X ▶– $$$$

ADULT – BPH: 0.5 mg dutasteride plus 0.4 mg tamsulosin daily 30 minutes after a meal.

PEDS – Not approved in children.

FORMS – Trade only: Caps 0.5 mg dutasteride plus 0.4 mg tamsulosin.

NOTES – Refer to components.

SILODOSIN (***RAPAFLO***) ▶LK – ♀B ▶– $$$$

ADULT – BPH: 8 mg daily with a meal.

PEDS – Not approved in children.

(cont.)

SILODOSIN (*cont.*)

FORMS – Trade: Caps 8 mg.

NOTES – Dizziness, headache, abnormal ejaculation. Alpha-blockers are generally considered to be first-line treatment in men with more than minimal obstructive urinary symptoms. Intraoperative floppy iris syndrome with cataract surgery reported. Avoid administration with strong inhibitors of CYP3A4 (ketoconazole, clarithromycin, itraconazole, ritonavir).

TAMSULOSIN (***Flomax***) ▶LK ♀B ▶– $$$$

ADULT – BPH: 0.4 mg PO daily 30 min after the same meal each days. If an adequate response is not seen after 2 to 4 weeks, may increase dose to 0.8 mg PO daily. If therapy is interrupted for several days, restart at the 0.4 mg dose.

PEDS – Not approved in children.

UNAPPROVED ADULT – Promotes spontaneous passage of ureteral calculi: 0.4 mg PO daily usually combined with an NSAID, antiemetic, and opioid of choice.

FORMS – Generic/Trade: Caps 0.4 mg.

NOTES – Dizziness, headache, abnormal ejaculation. Alpha-blockers are generally considered to be first-line treatment in men with more than minimal obstructive urinary symptoms. Caution in serious sulfa allergy: Rare allergic reactions reported. Intraoperative floppy iris syndrome with cataract surgery reported. Caution with strong inhibitors of CYP450 2D6 (fluoxetine) or 3A4 (ketoconazole).

UROLOGY: Bladder Agents—Anticholinergics and Combinations

B&O SUPPRETTES **(belladonna + opium)** ▶L ♀C ▶?©II $$$$

ADULT – Bladder spasm: 1 suppository PR once or twice daily, max 4 doses/day.

PEDS – Not approved in children younger than 12 yo.

FORMS – Trade only: Supps 30 mg opium (15A), 60 mg opium (16A).

NOTES – Store at room temperature. Contraindicated in narrow-angle glaucoma, obstructive conditions (eg, pyloric, duodenal, or other intestinal obstructive lesions, ileus, achalasia, and obstructive uropathies).

DARIFENACIN (***Enablex***) ▶LK ♀C ▶– $$$$

ADULT – Overactive bladder with symptoms of urinary urgency, frequency, and urge incontinence: 7.5 mg PO daily. May increase to max dose 15 mg PO daily in 2 weeks. Max dose 7.5 mg PO daily with moderate liver impairment or when coadministered with potent CYP3A4 inhibitors (ketoconazole, itraconazole, ritonavir, nelfinavir, clarithromycin, and nefazodone).

PEDS – Not approved in children.

FORMS – Trade only: Tabs extended-release 7.5, 15 mg.

NOTES – Contraindicated with uncontrolled narrow-angle glaucoma, urinary and gastric retention. Avoid use in severe hepatic impairment. May increase concentration of medications metabolized by CYP2D6.

FESOTERODINE (***Toviaz***) ▶plasma ♀C ▶– $$$$

ADULT – Overactive bladder: 4 mg PO daily. Increase to 8 mg if needed. Do not exceed 4 mg daily with renal insufficiency (CrCl less than 30 mL/min) or specific coadministered drugs (see Notes).

PEDS – Not approved in children.

FORMS – Trade only: Tabs extended-release 4, 8 mg.

NOTES – Contraindicated with urinary or gastric retention, or uncontrolled glaucoma. 4 mg daily max dose in renal dysfunction or with concomitant use of CYP3A4 inhibitors (eg, erythromycin, ketoconazole, itraconazole).

FLAVOXATE (***Urispas***) ▶K ♀B ▶? $$$$

ADULT – Bladder spasm: 100 or 200 mg PO three to four times per day. Reduce dose when improved.

PEDS – Not approved in children younger than 12 yo.

FORMS – Generic/Trade: Tabs 100 mg.

NOTES – May cause dizziness, drowsiness, blurred vision, dry mouth, N/V, urinary retention. Contraindicated in glaucoma, obstructive conditions (eg, pyloric, duodenal, or other intestinal obstructive lesions, ileus, achalasia, GI hemorrhage, and obstructive uropathies).

OXYBUTYNIN (***Ditropan, Ditropan XL, Gelnique, Oxytrol,*** ✦ ***Uromax***) ▶LK ♀B ▶? $

ADULT – Bladder instability: 2.5 to 5 mg PO two to three times per day, max 5 mg PO four times per day. Extended-release tabs: 5 to 10 mg PO daily same time each day, increase 5 mg/day q week to 30 mg/day. Oxytrol: 1 patch twice per week on abdomen, hips, or buttocks. Gelnique: Apply contents of 1 sachet once daily to abdomen, upper arms/shoulders, or thighs. Rotate application sites.

PEDS – Bladder instability older than 5 yo: 5 mg PO four times per day, max dose: 5 mg PO three times per day. Extended-release, older than 6 yo: 5 mg PO daily, max 20 mg/day. Transdermal patch not approved in children.

(cont.)

OXYBUTYNIN (*cont.*)

UNAPPROVED ADULT – Case reports of use for hyperhidrosis.

UNAPPROVED PEDS – Bladder instability for age younger than 6 yo: 0.2 mg/kg/dose PO two to four times per day.

FORMS – Generic/Trade: Tabs 5 mg. Syrup 5 mg/5 mL. Tabs extended-release 5, 10, 15 mg. Trade only: Transdermal patch (Oxytrol) 3.9 mg/day. Gelnique 3%, 10% gel, 1 g unit dose.

NOTES – May cause dizziness, drowsiness, blurred vision, dry mouth, urinary retention. Contraindicated with glaucoma, urinary retention, obstructive GU or GI disease, unstable cardiovascular status, and myasthenia gravis. Transdermal patch causes less dry mouth than oral form; avoid dose reduction by cutting. Wash hands immediately after applying Gelnique.

PROSED/DS **(methenamine + phenyl salicylate + methylene blue + benzoic acid + hyoscyamine)** ▶KL ♀C ▶? $$

ADULT – Bladder spasm: 1 tab PO four times per day with liberal fluids.

PEDS – Not approved in children.

FORMS – Trade only: Tabs (methenamine 81.6 mg/phenyl salicylate 36.2 mg/methylene blue 10.8 mg/benzoic acid 9.0 mg/hyoscyamine sulfate 0.12 mg).

NOTES – May cause dizziness, drowsiness, blurred vision, dry mouth, N/V, urinary retention. May turn urine/contact lenses blue.

SOLIFENACIN (***VESIcare***) ▶LK ♀C ▶– $$$$

ADULT – Overactive bladder with symptoms of urinary urgency, frequency, or urge incontinence: 5 mg PO daily. Max dose: 10 mg PO daily (5 mg PO daily if CrCl less than 30 mL/min, moderate hepatic impairment, or concurrent ketoconazole or other potent CYP3A4 inhibitors).

PEDS – Not approved in children.

FORMS – Trade only: Tabs 5, 10 mg.

NOTES – Contraindicated with uncontrolled narrow-angle glaucoma, urinary and gastric retention. Avoid use in severe hepatic impairment. Hallucinations have been reported.

TOLTERODINE (***Detrol, Detrol LA,*** ✤ ***Unidet***) ▶L ♀C ▶– $$$$

ADULT – Overactive bladder: 2 mg PO two times per day (Detrol) or 4 mg PO daily (Detrol LA). Decrease dose to 1 mg PO two times per day (Detrol) or 2 mg PO daily (Detrol LA) if adverse symptoms, hepatic insufficiency, or specific coadministered drugs (see NOTES).

PEDS – Not approved in children.

FORMS – Trade only: Tabs 1, 2 mg. Caps extended-release 2, 4 mg.

NOTES – Contraindicated with urinary or gastric retention, or uncontrolled glaucoma. High doses may prolong the QT interval. Decrease dose to 1 mg PO two times per day or 2 mg PO daily (Detrol LA) in severe hepatic or renal dysfunction or with concomitant use of CYP3A4 inhibitors (eg, erythromycin, ketoconazole, itraconazole).

TROSPIUM (***Sanctura, Sanctura XR,*** ✤ ***Trosec***) ▶LK ♀C ▶? $$$$

ADULT – Overactive bladder with urge incontinence: 20 mg PO two times per day; give 20 mg at bedtime if CrCl is less than 30 mL/min. If age 75 yo or older may taper down to 20 mg daily. Extended-release: 60 mg PO q am, 1 h before food; this form not recommended with CrCl less than 30 mL/min.

PEDS – Not approved in children.

FORMS – Trade only: Tabs 20 mg, Caps extended-release 60 mg.

NOTES – Contraindicated with uncontrolled narrow-angle glaucoma, urinary retention, gastroparesis. May cause heat stroke due to decreased sweating. Take on an empty stomach. Improvement in signs and symptoms may be seen in a week. Causes minimum CNS side effects.

URISED **(methenamine + phenyl salicylate + atropine + hyoscyamine + benzoic acid + methylene blue)** ▶K ♀C ▶? $

ADULT – Dysuria: 2 Tabs PO four times per day.

PEDS – Dysuria, age 6 yo or older: Reduce dose based on age and wt. Not recommended for children younger than 6 yo.

FORMS – Trade only: Tabs (methenamine 40.8 mg/phenyl salicylate 18.1 mg/atropine 0.03 mg/hyoscyamine 0.03 mg/4.5 mg benzoic acid/5.4 mg methylene blue).

NOTES – Take with food to minimize GI upset. May precipitate urate crystals in urine. Avoid use with sulfonamides. May turn urine/contact lenses blue.

UTA **(methenamine + sodium phosphate + phenyl salicylate + methylene blue + hyoscyamine)** ▶KL ♀C ▶? $

ADULT – Treatment of irritative voiding; relief of inflammation, hypermotility, and pain with lower UTI; relief of urinary tract symptoms caused by diagnostic procedures: 1 cap PO four times per day with liberal fluids.

PEDS – Not recommended for age younger than 6 yo. Dosing must be individualized by physician for age older than 6 yo.

FORMS – Trade only: Caps (methenamine 120 mg/sodium phosphate 40.8 mg/phenyl salicylate 36 mg/methylene blue 10 mg/hyoscyamine 0.12 mg).

(cont.)

UTA (cont.)

NOTES – May turn urine/feces blue to blue-green. Take 2 h apart from ketoconazole. May decrease absorption of thiazide diuretics. Antacids and antidiarrheals may decrease effectiveness of methenamine.

UTIRA-C **(methenamine + sodium phosphate + phenyl salicylate + methylene blue + hyoscyamine)** ▶KL ♀C ▶? $$

ADULT – Treatment of irritative voiding; relief of inflammation, hypermotility, and pain with lower UTI; relief of urinary tract symptoms caused by diagnostic procedures: 1 cap PO four times per day with liberal fluids.

PEDS – Not recommended for age younger than 6 yo. Dosing must be individualized by physician for age older than 6 yo.

FORMS – Trade only: Tabs (methenamine 81.6 mg/sodium phosphate 40.8 mg/phenyl salicylate 36.2 mg/methylene blue 10.8 mg/hyoscyamine 0.12 mg).

NOTES – May turn urine/feces blue to blue-green. Take 2 h apart from ketoconazole. May decrease absorption of thiazide diuretics. Antacids and antidiarrheals may decrease effectiveness of methenamine.

UROLOGY: Bladder Agents—Other

BETHANECHOL (***Urecholine, Duvoid***) ▶L ♀C ▶? $$$$

ADULT – Urinary retention: 10 to 50 mg PO three to four times per day or 2.5 to 5 mg SC three to four times per day. Take 1 h before or 2 h after meals to avoid N/V. Determine the minimum effective dose by giving 5 to 10 mg PO initially and repeat at hourly intervals until response or to max 50 mg.

PEDS – Not approved in children.

UNAPPROVED PEDS – Urinary retention, abdominal distention: 0.6 mg/kg/day PO divided q 6 to 8 h or 0.12 to 0.2 mg/kg/day SC divided q 6 to 8 h.

FORMS – Generic/Trade: Tabs 5, 10, 25, 50 mg.

NOTES – May cause drowsiness, lightheadedness, and fainting. Not for obstructive urinary retention. Avoid with cardiac disease, hyperthyroidism, parkinsonism, peptic ulcer disease, and epilepsy.

DIMETHYL SULFOXIDE (***DMSO, Rimso-50***) ▶KL ♀C ▶? $$$

ADULT – Interstitial cystitis: Instill 50 mL soln into bladder by catheter and allow to remain for 15 min; expelled by spontaneous voiding. Repeat q 2 weeks until symptomatic relief is obtained; thereafter, may increase time intervals between treatments.

PEDS – Not approved in children.

NOTES – Apply analgesic lubricant gel to urethra prior to inserting the catheter to avoid spasm. May administer oral analgesics or supps containing belladonna and opium prior to instillation to reduce spasms. May give anesthesia in patients with severe interstitial cystitis and very sensitive bladders during the first, second, and third treatment. May cause lens opacities and changes in refractive index; perform eye exams before and periodically during treatment. May cause a hypersensitivity reaction by liberating histamine. Monitor liver and renal function tests and CBC q 6 months. May be harmful in patients with urinary tract malignancy; can cause DMSO-induced vasodilation. Peripheral neuropathy may occur when used with sulindac. Garlic-like taste may occur within a few min of administration; odor on breath and skin may be present and remain for up to 72 h.

MIRABEGRON (***Myrbetriq***) ▶LK – ♀C ▶?

ADULT – Overactive bladder with symptoms of urge urinary incontinence, urgency, and urinary frequency: 25 mg PO daily. May increase to 50 mg unless severe renal impairment (CrCl less than 30 mL/min) or moderate hepatic impairment (Child-Pugh Class B). Not recommended in ESRD or Child-Pugh Class C liver disease.

PEDS – Not approved in children.

FORMS – Trade only: Extended-release tabs: 25, 50 mg.

NOTES – Do not chew, crush, or split tabs. May increase blood pressure; not recommended in patients with severe uncontrolled hypertension. Moderate CYP2D6 inhibitor; may increase concentrations of CYP2D6 substrates such as metoprolol.

PENTOSAN (***Elmiron***) ▶LK ♀B ▶? $$$$$

ADULT – Interstitial cystitis: 100 mg PO three times per day 1 h before or 2 h after a meal.

PEDS – Not approved in children.

FORMS – Trade only: Caps 100 mg.

NOTES – Pain relief usually occurs at 2 to 4 months and decreased urinary frequency takes 6 months. May increase risk of bleeding, especially with NSAID use. Use with caution in hepatic or splenic dysfunction.

PHENAZOPYRIDINE (*Pyridium, Azo-Standard, Urogesic, Prodium, Pyridiate, Urodol, Baridium, UTI Relief*) ▸K ♀B ◗? $

ADULT – Dysuria: 200 mg PO three times per day after meals for 2 days.

PEDS – Dysuria in children 6 to 12 yo: 12 mg/kg/day PO divided three times per day for 2 days.

FORMS – OTC Generic/Trade: Tabs 95, 97.2 mg. Rx Generic/Trade: Tabs 100, 200 mg.

NOTES – May turn urine/contact lenses orange. Contraindicated with hepatitis or renal insufficiency.

UROQUID-ACID NO. 2 **(methenamine + sodium phosphate)** ▸K ♀C ◗? $

ADULT – Chronic/recurrent UTIs: Initial: 2 tabs PO four times per day with full glass of water. Maintenance: 2 to 4 tabs PO daily, in divided doses with full glass of water.

PEDS – Not approved in children.

FORMS – Trade only: Tabs methenamine mandelate 500 mg/sodium acid phosphate 500 mg.

NOTES – 83 mg sodium/tab. Thiazide diuretics, carbonic anhydrase inhibitors, antacids, and urinary alkalinizing agents may decrease effectiveness. Caution with concurrent salicylates, may increase levels.

UROLOGY: Erectile Dysfunction

ALPROSTADIL (*Muse, Caverject, Caverject Impulse, Edex, Prostin VR Pediatric,* **prostaglandin E1,** ✤ *Prostin VR*) ▸L ♀– ◗– $$$$

ADULT – Erectile dysfunction: 1.25 to 2.5 mcg intracavernosal injection over 5 to 10 sec initially using a ½ in, 27 or 30 gauge needle. If no response, may give next higher dose after 1 h, max 2 doses/day. May increase by 2.5 mcg and then 5 to 10 mcg incrementally on separate occasions. Dose range is 1 to 40 mcg. Alternative: 125 to 250 mcg intraurethral pellet (Muse). Increase or decrease dose on separate occasions until erection achieved. Max intraurethral dose 2 pellets/24 h. The lowest possible dose to produce an acceptable erection should be used.

PEDS – Temporary maintenance of patent ductus arteriosus in neonates: Start 0.1 mcg/kg/min IV infusion. Reduce dose to minimal amount that maintains therapeutic response. Max dose 0.4 mcg/kg/min.

UNAPPROVED ADULT – Erectile dysfunction intracorporeal injection: Specially formulated mixtures of alprostadil, papaverine, and phentolamine. 0.10 to 0.50 mL injection.

FORMS – Trade only: Syringe system (Edex) 10, 20, 40 mcg. (Caverject) 5, 10, 20, 40 mcg. (Caverject Impulse) 10, 20 mcg. Pellet (Muse) 125, 250, 500, 1000 mcg. Intracorporeal injection of locally compounded combination agents (many variations): "Bi-mix" can be 30 mg/mL papaverine + 0.5 to 1 mg/mL phentolamine, or 30 mg/mL papaverine + 20 mcg/mL alprostadil in 10 mL vials. "Tri-mix" can be 30 mg/mL papaverine + 1 mg/mL phentolamine + 10 mcg/mL alprostadil in 5, 10, or 20 mL vials.

NOTES – Contraindicated in patients at risk for priapism, with penile fibrosis (Peyronie's disease), with penile implants, in women or children, in men for whom sexual activity is inadvisable, and for intercourse with a pregnant woman. Onset of effect is 5 to 20 min.

AVANAFIL (*Stendra*) ▸L – ♀C ◗? $$$$

ADULT – Erectile dysfunction: 100 mg PO 30 minutes prior to sexual activity. Max 1 dose/day. Use lower dose (50 mg) if taking certain coadministered drugs (see notes).

PEDS – Not approved in children.

FORMS – Trade only (Stendra): Tabs 50, 100, 200 mg.

NOTES – For patients taking strong CYP3A4 inhibitors (ketoconazole, ritonavir, atazanavir, clarithromycin, indinavir, itraconazole, nefazodone, nelfinavir, saquinavir, and telithromycin), do not use. For patients taking moderate CYP3A4 inhibitors (erythromycin, amprenavir, aprepitant, diltiazem, fluconazole, fosamprenavir, and verapamil), use 50 mg dose. For patients taking alpha-blocker, use 50 mg dose. Do not initiate alpha-blocker and avanafil at same time. Not recommended for patients within 6 months of MI, CVA, life-threatening arrhythmia, or coronary revascularization; resting BP less than 90/50 or greater than 170/100; or unstable angina, angina with sexual intercourse, or NYHA Class 2 or greater.

SILDENAFIL (*Viagra*) ▸LK ♀B ◗– $$$$

ADULT – Erectile dysfunction: 50 mg PO approximately 1 h (range 0.5–4 h) before sexual activity. Usual effective dose range: 25 to 100 mg. Max 1 dose/day. Use lower dose (25 mg) if older than 65 yo, hepatic/renal impairment, or certain coadministered drugs (see notes).

PEDS – Not approved in children.

(cont.)

SILDENAFIL (*cont.*)

UNAPPROVED ADULT – Antidepressant-associated sexual dysfunction: Same dosing as ADULT.

FORMS – Trade only (Viagra): Tabs 25, 50, 100 mg. Unscored tab but can be cut in half.

NOTES – Drug interactions with cimetidine, erythromycin, ketoconazole, itraconazole, saquinavir, ritonavir, and other CYP3A4 inhibitors; use 25 mg dose. Do not exceed 25 mg/48 h with ritonavir. Doses greater than 25 mg should not be taken less than 4 h after an alpha-blocker. Caution if CVA, MI, or other cardiovascular event within last 6 months. Do not use with itraconazole, ketoconazole, ritonavir, or pulmonary veno-occlusive disease. Coadministration with CYP3A4 inducers (ie, bosentan, barbiturates, carbamazepine, phenytoin, efavirenz, nevirapine, rifampin, rifabutin) may change levels of either medication; adjust doses as needed. Use caution with CVA, MI, or life-threatening arrhythmia in last 6 months; unstable angina; BP greater than 170/110; or retinitis pigmentosa. Contraindicated in patients taking nitrates within prior/subsequent 24 h. Caution with alpha-blockers due to potential for symptomatic hypotension. There have been a few reports of sudden vision loss due to nonarteritic ischemic optic neuropathy (NAION). Patients with prior NAION are at higher risk. Sudden hearing loss with or without tinnitus, vertigo, or dizziness has been reported. Transient global amnesia has also been reported.

TADALAFIL (*Cialis*) ▶L ♀B ▶– $$$$

WARNING – Contraindicated with nitrates. Caution with alpha-blockers due to potential for symptomatic hypotension. There have been a few reports of sudden vision loss due to nonarteritic ischemic optic neuropathy (NAION). Patients with prior NAION are at higher risk. Retinal artery occlusion has been reported. Sudden hearing loss with or without tinnitus, vertigo, or dizziness has been reported. Transient global amnesia.

ADULT – Erectile dysfunction: 2.5 to 5 mg PO daily without regard to timing of sexual activity. As needed dosing: 10 mg PO prn prior to sexual activity. Optimal timing of administration unclear, but should be at least 30 to 45 min before sexual activity. May increase to 20 mg or decrease to 5 mg. Max 1 dose/day. Start 5 mg (max 1 dose/day) if CrCl 31 to 50 mL/min. Max 5 mg/day if CrCl is less than 30 mL/min on dialysis. Max 10 mg/day if mild to moderate hepatic impairment; avoid in severe hepatic impairment. Max 10 mg once in 72 h if concurrent potent CYP3A4 inhibitors. BPH with or without erectile dysfunction: 5 mg PO daily. Caution with ritonavir, see prescribing information for specific dose adjustments.

PEDS – Not approved in children.

FORMS – Trade only (Cialis): Tabs 2.5, 5, 10, 20 mg.

NOTES – If nitrates needed give at least 48 h after the last tadalafil dose. Improves erectile function for up to 36 h. Not FDA-approved for women. Not recommended if MI in prior 90 days, angina during sexual activity, NYHA Class II or greater in prior 6 months, hypotension (less than 90/50), HTN (greater than 170/100), or CVA in prior 6 months. Rare reports of prolonged erections. Do not use with ketoconazole or itraconazole.

VARDENAFIL (*Levitra*) ▶LK ♀B ▶– $$$$

WARNING – Contraindicated with nitrates (time interval for safe administration unknown). Caution with alpha-blockers due to potential for symptomatic hypotension. There have been a few reports of sudden vision loss due to nonarteritic ischemic optic neuropathy (NAION). Patients with prior NAION are at higher risk. Sudden hearing loss with or without tinnitus, vertigo, or dizziness has been reported. Seizures and seizure recurrence have been reported.

ADULT – Erectile dysfunction: 10 mg PO 1 h before sexual activity. Usual effective dose range: 5 to 20 mg. Max 1 dose/day. Use lower dose (5 mg) if age 65 yo or older or moderate hepatic impairment (max 10 mg); 2.5 mg when coadministered with certain drugs (see notes). Not FDA-approved in women.

PEDS – Not approved in children.

FORMS – Trade only: Tabs 2.5, 5, 10, 20 mg.

NOTES – See the following parenthetical vardenafil dose adjustments when taken with ritonavir (max 2.5 mg/72 h); indinavir, saquinavir, atazanavir, clarithromycin, ketoconazole 400 mg daily, or itraconazole 400 mg daily (max 2.5 mg/24 h); ketoconazole 200 mg daily, itraconazole 200 mg daily, or erythromycin (max 5 mg/24 h). Avoid with alpha-blockers and antiarrhythmics, and in congenital QT prolongation. Caution if CVA, MI, or other cardiovascular event within last 6 months, unstable angina, severe liver impairment, end-stage renal disease, or retinitis pigmentosa.

YOHIMBINE (*Yocon, Yohimex*) ▶L ♀– ▶– $

ADULT – No approved indications.

PEDS – No approved indications.

UNAPPROVED ADULT – Erectile dysfunction: 1 tab PO three times per day. If side effects (eg, tremor, tachycardia, nervousness) occur,

(cont.)

YOHIMBINE (*cont.*)

reduce to ½ tab three times per day, followed by gradual increases to 1 tab three times per day.

FORMS – Generic/Trade: Tabs 5.4 mg.

NOTES – Prescription yohimbine and yohimbine bark extract (see Herbal section) are not interchangeable. Contraindicated with renal disease. Avoid with antidepressant use, psychiatric disorders, the elderly, women, or ulcer history. Efficacy of therapy longer than 10 weeks unclear. American Urological Association does not recommend as a standard treatment due to unproven efficacy.

UROLOGY: Nephrolithiasis

ACETOHYDROXAMIC ACID (***Lithostat***) ▶K ♀X ▶? $$$$

ADULT – Chronic UTI, adjunctive therapy: 250 mg PO three to four times per day for a total dose of 10 to 15 mg/kg/day. Max dose is 1.5 g/day. Decrease dose in patients with renal impairment to no more than 1 g/day.

PEDS – Adjunctive therapy in chronic urea-splitting UTI (eg, *Proteus*): 10 mg/kg/day PO divided two to three times per day.

FORMS – Trade only: Tabs 250 mg.

NOTES – Do not use if CrCl is less than 20 mL/min. Administer on an empty stomach.

CELLULOSE SODIUM PHOSPHATE (***Calcibind***) ▶Fecal ♀C ▶+ $$$$

WARNING – Avoid in heart failure or ascites due to high sodium content.

ADULT – Absorptive hypercalciuria Type 1 (age older than 16 yo): Initial dose with urinary calcium greater than 300 mg/day (on moderate calcium-restricted diet): 5 g with each meal. Decrease dose to 5 g with supper, 2.5 g with each remaining meal when calcium declines to less than 150 mg/day. Initial dose with urinary calcium 200 to 300 mg/day (controlled calcium-restricted diet): 5 g with supper, 2.5 g with each remaining meal. Mix with water, soft drink, or fruit juice. Ingest within 30 min of meal.

PEDS – Do not use if younger than 16 yo.

FORMS – Trade only: Bulk powder 300 mg.

NOTES – Give concomitant supplement of 1.5 g magnesium gluconate with 15 g/day. 1 g magnesium gluconate with 10 g/day. Take magnesium supplement at least 1 h before or after each dose to avoid binding. May cause hyperparathyroidism. Long-term use may cause hypomagnesemia, hyperoxaluria, hypomagnesuria, depletion of trace metals (copper, zinc, iron); monitor calcium, magnesium, trace metals, and CBC q 3 to 6 months; monitor parathyroid hormone once between the first 2 weeks and 3 months, then q 3 to 6 months thereafter. Adjust or stop treatment if PTH rises above normal. Stop when inadequate hypocalciuric response (urinary calcium of less than 30 mg/5 g of cellulose sodium phosphate) occurs while patient is on moderate calcium restriction. Avoid vitamin C supplementation since metabolized to oxalate.

CITRATE (***Polycitra-K, Urocit-K, Bicitra, Oracit, Polycitra, Polycitra-LC***) ▶K ♀C ▶? $$$

ADULT – Prevention of calcium and urate kidney stones: 1 packet in water/juice PO three to four times per day with meals. 15 to 30 mL PO soln three to four times per day with meals. Tabs 10 to 20 mEq PO three to four times per day with meals. Max 100 mEq/day.

PEDS – Urinary alkalinization: 5 to 15 mL PO four times per day with meals.

FORMS – Generic/Trade: Polycitra-K packet 3300 mg potassium citrate/ea, Polycitra-K oral soln (1100 mg potassium citrate/5 mL, 480 mL). Oracit oral soln (490 mg sodium citrate/5 mL, 15, 30, 480 mL). Bicitra oral soln (500 mg sodium citrate/5 mL, 480 mL). Urocit-K wax (potassium citrate) Tabs 5, 10 mEq. Polycitra-LC oral soln (550 mg potassium citrate/500 mg sodium citrate per 5 mL, 480 mL). Polycitra oral syrup (550 mg potassium citrate/500 mg sodium citrate per 5 mL, 480 mL.

NOTES – Contraindicated in renal insufficiency, PUD, UTI, and hyperkalemia.

TIOPRONIN (***Thiola***) ▶K ♀C ▶- $$$$$

ADULT – Prevention of kidney stone in severe homozygous cystinuria with urinary cystine greater than 500 mg/day: Start 800 mg/day PO. Average dose in clinical trials is 1000 mg/day, although some patients may require less. A conservative treatment program should be attempted prior to tiopronin: See NOTES.

PEDS – Age 9 yo or older: Start 15 mg/kg/day PO divided three times per day 1 h before or 2 h after meals. Measure urinary cystine 1 month after treatment and q 3 months thereafter. Dosage should be readjusted depending on the urinary cystine value. A conservative treatment program should be attempted prior to tiopronin: See NOTES.

FORMS – Trade only: Tabs 100 mg.

(cont.)

TIOPRONIN (*cont.*)

NOTES – A conservative treatment program should be attempted before starting tiopronin: 3 L of fluid should be provided, including 2 glasses with each meal and at bedtime. Patients should be expected to awake at night to urinate; they should drink 2 or more glasses of fluids before returning to bed. Additional fluids should be consumed if there is excessive sweating or intestinal fluid loss. A minimum urine output of 2 L/day on a consistent basis should be sought. Provide a modest amount of alkali in order to maintain urinary pH at high normal range (6.5 to 7). Avoid use in patients with history of agranulocytosis, aplastic anemia, or thrombocytopenia. Monitor blood counts, platelets, serum albumin, LFTs, 24-h urinary protein, and routine analysis at 3 to 6 months during treatment. Monitor urinary cystine analysis frequently during the 1st 6 months when optimum dose is being determined, then q 6 months thereafter. Abdominal x-ray is advised yearly. Patients who had adverse reactions with d-penicillamine are more likely to have adverse reactions to tiopronin. Close supervision with close monitoring of potential side effects is mandatory.

UROLOGY: Other

AMINOHIPPURATE (*PAH*) ▸K ♀C ▸? $

ADULT – Estimation of effective renal plasma flow and measurement of functional capacity of renal tubular secretory mechanism: Specialized infusion dosing available.

PEDS – Not approved in children.

NOTES – May precipitate heart failure. Patients receiving sulfonamides, procaine or thiazolsulfone may interfere with chemical color development essential for analysis. Concomitant use of probenecid my result in erroneously low effective renal plasma flow.

INDEX

A

E

F

G

H

K

L

M

N

Q

R

S

T

U

V

APPENDIX

ADULT EMERGENCY DRUGS (selected)

ALLERGY	diphenhydramine (*Benadryl*): 25 to 50 mg IV/IM/PO. epinephrine: 0.1 to 0.5 mg IM/SC (1:1000 solution), may repeat after 20 minutes. methylprednisolone (*Solu-Medrol*): 125 mg IV/IM.
HYPERTENSION	esmolol (*Brevibloc*): 500 mcg/kg IV over 1 minute, then titrate 50 to 200 mcg/kg/min. fenoldopam (*Corlopam.*): Start 0.1 mcg/kg/min, titrate up to 1.6 mcg/kg/min. labetalol: Start 20 mg slow IV, then 40 to 80 mg IV q10 min prn up to 300 mg total cumulative dose. nitroglycerin: Start 10 to 20 mcg/min IV infusion, then titrate prn up to 100 mcg/min. nitroprusside (*Nitropress*): Start 0.3 mcg/kg/min IV infusion, then titrate prn up to 10 mcg/kg/min.
DYSRHYTHMIAS / ARREST	adenosine (*Adenocard*): PSVT (not A-fib): 6 mg rapid IV & flush, preferably through a central line or proximal IV. If no response after 1-2 minutes, then 12 mg. A third dose of 12mg may be given prn. amiodarone: V-fib or pulseless V-tach: 300 mg IV/IO; may repeat 150 mg just once. Life-threatening ventricular arrhythmia: Load 150 mg IV over 10 min, then 1 mg/min × 6 h, then 0.5 mg/min × 18 h. atropine: 0.5 to 1 mg IV, repeat q 3-5 minutes prn to maximum of 3 mg. diltiazem (*Cardizem*): Rapid A-fib: bolus 0.25 mg/kg or 20 mg IV over 2 min. May repeat 0.35 mg/kg or 25 mg 15 min after 1st dose. Infusion 5-15 mg/h. epinephrine: 1 mg IV/IO q 3-5 minutes for cardiac arrest. [1:10,000 solution]. lidocaine (Xylocaine): Load 1 mg/kg IV, then 0.5 mg/kg q 8-10 min prn to max 3 mg/kg. Maintenance 2 g in 250 mL D5W (8 mg/mL) at 1 to 4 mg/min drip (7-30 mL/h).
PRESSORS	dobutamine: 2 to 20 mcg/kg/min. 70 kg: 5 mcg/kg/min with 1 mg/mL concentration (eg, 250 mg in 250 mL D5W) = 21 mL/h. dopamine: Pressor: Start at 5 mcg/kg/min, increase prn by 5 to 10 mcg/kg/min increments at 10 min intervals, max 50 mcg/kg/min. 70 kg: 5 mcg/kg/min with 1600 mcg/mL concentration (eg, 400 mg in 250 mL D5W) = 13 mL/h. Doses in mcg/kg/min: *2-4* = (traditional renal dose, apparently <2 ineffective) dopaminergic receptors; 5-10= (cardiac dose) dopaminergic and beta1 receptors; >10 = dopaminergic, beta1, and alpha1 receptors. norepinephrine (*Levophed*): 4 mg in 500 mL D5W (8 mcg/mL), start 8 to 12 mcg/min (1 to 1.5 mL/h), usual dose once BP is stabilized 2 to 4 mcg/min. 22.5 mL/h = 3 mcg/min. phenylephrine: 20 mg in 250 mL D5W (80 mcg/mL), start 100 to 180 mcg/min (75 to 135 mL/h), usual dose once BP is stabilized 40 to 60 mcg/min (30 to 45 mL/h).
INTUBATION	etomidate (*Amidate*): 0.3 mg/kg IV. methohexital (*Brevital*): 1 to 1.5 mg/kg IV. propofol (*Diprivan*): 2.0 to 2.5 mg/kg IV. rocuronium (*Zemuron*): 0.6 to 1.2 mg/kg IV. succinylcholine (*Anectine, Quelicin*): 0.6 to 1.1 mg/kg IV. Peds (<5 yo): 2 mg/kg IV. thiopental: 3 to 5 mg/kg IV.
SEIZURES	diazepam (*Valium*): 5 to 10 mg IV, or 0.2 to 0.5 mg/kg rectal gel up to 20 mg PR. fosphenytoin (*Cerebyx*): Load 15 to 20 mg "phenytoin equivalents" (PE)/ kg IV, no faster than 100 to 150 mg PE/min. lorazepam (Ativan): Status epilepticus: 4 mg IV over 2 min, may repeat in 10-15 min. Anxiolytic/sedation: 0.04 to 0.05 mg/kg IV/IM; usual dose 2 mg, max 4 mg. phenobarbital: Status epilepticus: 15 to 20 mg/kg IV load; may give additional 5 mg/kg doses q 15-30 mins to max total dose of 30 mg/kg. phenytoin (*Dilantin*): 15 to 20 mg/kg up to 1000mg IV no faster than 50 mg/min.

CARDIAC DYSRHYTHMIA PROTOCOLS (for adults and adolescents)

Chest compressions ~100/min. Ventilations 8-10/min if intubated; otherwise 30:2 compression/ventilation ratio. Drugs that can be administered down ET tube (use 2–2.5 × usual dose): epinephrine, atropine, lidocaine, naloxone, vasopressin*.

V-Fib, Pulseless V-Tach

Airway, oxygen, CPR until defibrillator ready
Defibrillate 360 J (old monophasic), 120–200 J (biphasic), or with AED
Resume CPR × 2 min (5 cycles)
Repeat defibrillation if no response
Vasopressor during CPR:

- Epinephrine 1 mg IV/IO q 3–5 minutes, or
- Vasopressin* 40 units IV to replace 1st or 2nd dose of epinephrine

Rhythm/pulse check every ~2 minutes
Consider antiarrhythmic during CPR:

- Amiodarone 300 mg IV/IO; may repeat 150 mg just once
- Lidocaine 1.0–1.5 mg/kg IV/IO, then repeat 0.5–0.75 mg/kg to max 3 doses or 3 mg/kg
- Magnesium sulfate 1–2 g IV/IO if suspect torsades de pointes

Asystole or Pulseless Electrical Activity (PEA)

Airway, oxygen, CPR
Vasopressor (when IV/IO access):

- Epinephrine 1 mg IV/IO q 3–5 min, or
- Vasopressin* 40 units IV/IO of replace 1st or 2nd dose to epinephrine

Consider atropine 1 mg IV/IO for asystole or slow PEA. Repeat q 3–5 min up to 3 doses.
Rhythm/pulse check every ~2 minutes
Consider 6 H's: hypovolemia, hypoxia, H+acidosis, hyper/ hypokalemia, hypoglycemia, hypothermia
Consider 5 T's: Toxins, tamponade-cardiac, tension pneumothorax, thrombosis (coronary or pulmonary), trauma

Bradycardia, <60 bpm and Inadequate Perfusion

Airway, oxygen, IV
Prepare for transcutaneous pacing; don't delay if advanced heart block
Consider atropine 0.5 mg IV; may repeat q 3–5 min to max 3 mg
Consider epinephrine (2–10 mcg/min) or dopamine(2–10mcg/kg/min)
Prepare for transvenous pacing

Tachycardia with Pulses

Airway, oxygen, IV
If unstable and heart rate >150 bpm, then synchronized cardioversion
If stable narrow-QRS (<120 ms):

- Regular: Attempt vagal maneuvers, If no success, adenosine 6 mg IV, then 12 mg prn (may repeat x 1)
- Irregular: Control rate with diltiazem or beta blocker (caution in CHF or severe obstructive disease).

If stable wide-QRS (>120 ms):

- Regular and suspect V-tach: Amiodarone 150 mg IV over 10 min; repeat prn to max 2.2 g/24 h. Prepare for elective synchronized cardioversion.
- Regular and suspect SVT with aberrancy: adenosine as per narrow-QRS above.
- Irregular and A-fib: Control rate with diltiazem or beta blocker (caution in CHF/ severe obstructive pulmonary disease).
- Irregular and A-fib with pre-excitation (WPW): Avoid AV nodal blocking agents; consider amiodarone 150 mg IV over 10 min,
- Irregular and torsades de pointes: magnesium 1–2 g IV load over 5–60 min, then infusion.

bpm=beats per minute; CPR=cardiopulmonary resuscitation; ET=endotracheal; IO=intraosseous; J=Joules; ms=milliseconds; WPW=Wolff-Parkinson-White. Sources: *Circulation* 2005; 112, suppl IV; **NEJM* 2008;359:21–30 (demonstrated no benefit over epinephrine and worse long-term neurological outcomes).

ANTIVIRAL DRUGS FOR INFLUENZA	Treatment* (Duration of 5 days)	Prevention (Duration of 7 to 10 days post-exposure)†
OSELTAMIVIR *(Tamiflu)*		
Adults and adolescents age 13 years and older		
	75 mg PO bid	75 mg PO once daily
Children, 1 year of age and older‡		
Body weight ≤15 kg	30 mg PO bid	30 mg PO once daily
Body weight >15 to 23 kg	45 mg PO bid	45 mg PO once daily
Body weight >23 to 40 kg	60 mg PO bid	60 mg PO once daily
Body weight >40 kg	75 mg PO bid	75 mg PO once daily
Infants, newborn to 11 months of age‡,¶		
Age 3 to 11 months old	3 mg/kg/dose PO bid	3 mg/kg/dose PO once daily
Age younger than 3 months old§	3 mg/kg/dose PO bid	Not for routine prophylaxis in infants <3 mo
ZANAMIVIR *(Relenza)***		
Adults and children (age 7 years and older for treatment, age 5 years and older for prophylaxis)		
	10 mg (two 5-mg inhalations) bid	10 mg (two 5-mg inhalations) once daily

Adapted from http://www.cdc.gov/mmwr/pdf/rr/rr6001.pdf

*Start treatment as soon as possible; benefit is greatest when started within 2 days of symptom onset. Consider longer treatment for patients who remain severely ill after 5 days of treatment.

†Duration is 10 days after household exposure, and 7 days after most recent known exposure in other situations. For long-term care facilities and hospitals, prophylaxis should last a minimum of 14 days and up to 7 days after the most recent known case was identified.

‡In July 2011, the concentration of Tamiflu suspension was changed from 12 mg/mL to 6 mg/mL. Tamiflu prescribing information contains instructions for pharmacists to compound a 6 mg/mL suspension when Tamiflu suspension is not available. The new Tamiflu suspension is provided with a 10 mL oral dispenser measured in mL rather than mg. Capsules can be opened and mixed with sweetened fluids to mask bitter taste. Make sure units of measure on dosing instructions match dosing device provided.

¶Oseltamavir is not FDA-approved for use in infants less than 1 year old. An Emergency Use Authorization for use in infants expired in June 2010.

§This dose is not intended for premature infants. Immature renal function may lead to slow clearance and high concentrations of oseltamivir in this age group.

**Zanamivir should not be used by patients with underlying pulmonary disease. Do not attempt to use *Relenza* in a nebulizer or ventilator; lactose in the formulation may cause the device to malfunction.

bid=two times per day.

NOTES